DSM-5™
Guidebook

The Essential Companion to the
Diagnostic and Statistical
Manual of Mental Disorders,
Fifth Edition

DSM-5™
Guidebook

The Essential Companion to the
Diagnostic and Statistical
Manual of Mental Disorders,
Fifth Edition

Donald W. Black, M.D.
Jon E. Grant, M.D., M.P.H., J.D.

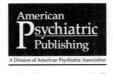

American Psychiatric Publishing
A Division of American Psychiatric Association

Washington, DC
London, England

Note: The authors have worked to ensure that all information in this book is accurate at the time of publication and consistent with general psychiatric and medical standards, and that information concerning drug dosages, schedules, and routes of administration is accurate at the time of publication and consistent with standards set by the U.S. Food and Drug Administration and the general medical community. As medical research and practice continue to advance, however, therapeutic standards may change. Moreover, specific situations may require a specific therapeutic response not included in this book. For these reasons and because human and mechanical errors sometimes occur, we recommend that readers follow the advice of physicians directly involved in their care or the care of a member of their family.

Books published by American Psychiatric Publishing (APP) represent the findings, conclusions, and views of the individual authors and do not necessarily represent the policies and opinions of APP or the American Psychiatric Association.

DSM-5™ diagnostic criteria reprinted from American Psychiatric Association: *Diagnostic and Statistical Manual of Mental Disorders,* 5th Edition. Arlington. VA, American Psychiatric Association, 2013. Copyright 2013, American Psychiatric Association. Used with permission.

If you would like to buy between 25 and 99 copies of this or any other American Psychiatric Publishing title, you are eligible for a 20% discount; please contact Customer Service at appi@psych.org or 800-368-5777. If you wish to buy 100 or more copies of the same title, please e-mail us at bulksales@psych.org for a price quote.

Copyright © 2014 American Psychiatric Association
ALL RIGHTS RESERVED

Manufactured in the United States of America on acid-free paper
17 16 15 14 13   5 4 3 2 1
First Edition

Typeset in Palatino LT Std and HelveticaNeue LT Std.

American Psychiatric Publishing
A Division of American Psychiatric Association
1000 Wilson Boulevard
Arlington, VA 22209-3901
www.appi.org

Library of Congress Cataloging-in-Publication Data
Black, Donald W., 1956– author.
    DSM-5 guidebook : the essential companion to the Diagnostic and statistical manual of mental disorders, fifth edition / Donald W. Black, Jon E. Grant. — First edition.
        p. ; cm.
    Includes bibliographical references and index.
    ISBN 978-1-58562-465-2 (pbk. : alk. paper)
    I. Grant, Jon E., author. II. American Psychiatric Association, issuing body.
III. Diagnostic and statistical manual of mental disorders. 5th ed. Complemented by (work): IV. Title.
    [DNLM: 1. Diagnostic and statistical manual of mental disorders. 5th ed. 2. Mental Disorders—classification. 3. Mental Disorders—diagnosis. WM 15]
    RC455.2.C4
    616.89′075—dc23   2013047640
British Library Cataloguing in Publication Data
A CIP record is available from the British Library.

Contents

About the Authors ix

Preface xi

Acknowledgments xv

Introduction xvii

1 The March to DSM-5 1

2 Use of DSM-5 and Major Changes From DSM-IV 9

3 Neurodevelopmental Disorders 29

    Intellectual Disabilities 32

    Communication Disorders 36

    Autism Spectrum Disorder 40

    Attention-Deficit/Hyperactivity Disorder 44

    Specific Learning Disorder 49

    Motor Disorders 51

    Other Neurodevelopmental Disorders 57

4 Schizophrenia Spectrum and Other Psychotic Disorders 61

5 Mood Disorders 89

    Bipolar and Related Disorders 90

    Depressive Disorders 103

6 Anxiety Disorders. 123

7 Obsessive-Compulsive and Related Disorders. 147

8 Trauma- and Stressor-Related Disorders 169

9 Dissociative Disorders. 191

10 Somatic Symptom and Related Disorders. 201

11 Feeding and Eating Disorders. 217

12 Elimination Disorders. 233

13 Sleep-Wake Disorders 239

    Breathing-Related Sleep Disorders 252

    Circadian Rhythm Sleep-Wake Disorders 257

    Parasomnias 260

14 Sexual Dysfunctions, Gender Dysphoria, and
Paraphilic Disorders. 273

    Sexual Dysfunctions 275

    Gender Dysphoria 283

    Paraphilic Disorders 286

15 Disruptive, Impulse-Control, and
Conduct Disorders. 295

16 Substance-Related and Addictive Disorders. 311

    Alcohol-Related Disorders 316

    Caffeine-Related Disorders 323

    Cannabis-Related Disorders 325

    Hallucinogen-Related Disorders 330

    Inhalant-Related Disorders 336

    Opioid-Related Disorders 338

Sedative-, Hypnotic-, or Anxiolytic-
Related Disorders 343

Stimulant-Related Disorders 348

Tobacco-Related Disorders 353

Other (or Unknown) Substance–
Related Disorders 356

Non-Substance-Related Disorders 356

17 Neurocognitive Disorders 359

Delirium 360

Major and Mild Neurocognitive Disorders 366

18 Personality Disorders 389

General Personality Disorder 391

Cluster A Personality Disorders 394

Cluster B Personality Disorders 397

Cluster C Personality Disorders 400

Other Personality Disorders 403

**19 Medication-Induced Movement Disorders and
Other Conditions That May Be a Focus of
Clinical Attention. 407**

Medication-Induced Movement Disorders and
Other Adverse Effects of Medication 408

Other Conditions That May Be a Focus of
Clinical Attention 413

20 Assessment Measures 433

**21 Alternative DSM-5 Model for
Personality Disorders 449**

General Criteria for Personality Disorder 452

Specific Personality Disorders 457

22 **Conditions for Further Study**. **469**

References 483

Appendix: DSM-5 Classification 489

Index 519

About the Authors

Donald W. Black, M.D. is Professor, Director of Residency Training, and Vice Chair for Education in the Department of Psychiatry at the University of Iowa Roy J. and Lucille A. Carver College of Medicine in Iowa City, Iowa.

Jon E. Grant, M.D., M.P.H., J.D., is Professor in the Department of Psychiatry and Behavioral Neuroscience at the University of Chicago Pritzker School of Medicine in Chicago, Illinois.

Disclosure of Competing Interests

Dr. Black reports receiving research grants from AstraZeneca and Psyadon Pharmaceuticals.

Dr. Grant reports receiving research grants from the National Center for Responsible Gambling, National Institute on Drug Abuse, Psyadon Pharmaceuticals and Transept Pharmaceuticals. He also reports royalties from American Psychiatric Publishing, Oxford University Press, McGraw-Hill, and W.W. Norton.

Preface

This guidebook serves as a companion to the *Diagnostic and Statistical Manual of Mental Disorders*, 5th Edition (DSM-5; American Psychiatric Association 2013). DSM has long been used as the psychiatric diagnostic system in the United States and elsewhere, and DSM-5 follows in the grand tradition of its predecessors. For many mental health practitioners, however, the method of psychiatric diagnostic classification is daunting. Because DSM-5 is large, totaling 947 pages (not including the classification listing and preface), many users will find it intimidating. Many will think, "Where do I begin? How will I ever understand and use the criteria?" Also, users of DSM-IV-TR (American Psychiatric Association 2000) will wonder how DSM-5 differs. These are some of the bread-and-butter issues we tackle in this guidebook.

Our goal with this book is not to recapitulate DSM-5. Rather, we aim to provide a user-friendly guide for fellow psychiatrists, psychologists, and other mental health practitioners, as well as other interested persons. We begin with the premise that users first and foremost want to know how DSM-5 differs from its immediate predecessor, DSM-IV-TR, in terms of its overall organization, the many diagnostic categories, and the diagnostic criteria themselves. In addressing these issues, we describe the rationale behind the reorganization and the many changes to the criteria. We strongly encourage readers to obtain a copy of DSM-5 and to study the diagnostic categories that are particularly relevant to their practice needs, while understanding that such a large—and, to some, unwieldy—book is not easily learned or digested.

In many ways this guidebook is an "owner's manual" to help practitioners incorporate DSM-5 into their practice. The book was written to teach clinicians how to use the revised diagnostic criteria. We explain the overall metastructure (i.e., organization) of DSM-5, its many diagnostic categories (including several new ones), and the diagnostic criteria for major disorders. We focus on the most important diagnoses and provide detailed descriptions of their criteria. In doing so, we place the criteria into context and provide a contrast to the prior edition. We believe *DSM-5 Guidebook* provides a blueprint to the many changes in the manual and practical information on the use of the many diagnostic categories and their codes.

To summarize, our goals in this guidebook are to

1. Provide an overview of diagnostic classification so as to place DSM-5 and its predecessors into historical perspective.
2. Review the development of DSM-5, and its innovations, its overall structure, and the major changes from DSM-IV (and DSM-IV-TR).
3. Discuss each major diagnostic category, associated diagnoses, and the criteria to clarify their meaning and facilitate understanding of the differential diagnostic process.

4. Explain the various components that constitute a complete DSM-5 diagnosis, including the use of dimensional scales described in Section III.

Diagnosis is fundamental to the practice of psychiatry and psychology. For many clinicians, the process of formulating a diagnosis takes years to master; however, it is an essential process for mental health practitioners to learn and in which to gain expertise. The introduction of operational diagnostic criteria in DSM-III (American Psychiatric Association 1980) greatly facilitated the process by making diagnosis far more reliable than it had been previously, and much less subject to the particular views and biases of the clinician. The two of us were both trained in the post–DSM-III era. To us, the use of criteria-based diagnoses is second nature.

DSM-5 is transformative in several respects (Kupfer and Regier 2011; Kupfer et al. 2013). The road to DSM-5 began in 1999, and its publication in 2013 was the culmination of a lengthy and labor-intensive process, reviewed in Chapter 1, "The March to DSM-5." The journey involved the efforts of many experts who carefully reviewed the literature, collected new data, and performed targeted analyses of existing data. DSM-5's predecessor, DSM-IV, was published in 1994 (American Psychiatric Association 1994), with a text revision in 2000 (DSM-IV-TR). For all intents and purposes, the DSM-5 criteria have been 19 years in the making. Not only have the diagnostic criteria been revised and updated, but chapter placement has changed. New categories have been introduced, and others have been consolidated. Many new disorders are included, and the multiaxial diagnostic scheme has been eliminated. Many dimensional assessments have been added to help clinicians better describe the patient's symptoms and functioning.

Symbolic of the transformation is that, unlike prior editions, DSM-5 has been discussed as a "living document." A future longer-term goal is to update DSM-5 in response to scientific advances *as they occur.* This is reflected in the decision to use an Arabic rather than a Roman numeral in the title—DSM-5 rather than DSM-V—so that future changes can be easily designated (e.g., DSM-5.1, DSM-5.2).

Make no mistake: DSM-5 is not inerrant. Those unfamiliar with the diagnostic process—and even some who are—consider the criteria with the same reverence they might apply to passages in such books as the Bible or Talmud. Others may see the diagnostic process as a cookbook in which each ingredient (i.e., criterion) is essential and any deviation invariably leads to fallen soufflé. We remind readers that DSM-5—or for that matter any diagnostic manual—cannot be used without applying clinical judgment. This is the critical element missing from any manual and not easily learned in the absence of training and practice. Will a psychiatrist tell a patient he is not depressed just because he fails to meet a diagnostic threshold? Is a psychotic patient whose symptoms fail to meet each criterion for schizophrenia less ill? Overly strict adherence to the rules (i.e., criteria) can get in the way of appropriate clinical care, and clinicians must be mindful of each patient's needs, not the sometimes arbitrary requirements of a coding system.

We have approached this guidebook informed by our day-to-day work as clinicians and researchers. We provide no insider detail about the workings of the DSM-5 Task Force or its many work groups because we have no personal knowledge of them.

In this respect, we write as outsiders tasked with explaining how the criteria sets are appropriately used in clinical and research settings. A disclaimer: What we have written reflects our views and not those of the DSM-5 Task Force or the American Psychiatric Association (APA). Neither of us served in any of the work groups. We did not edit and are not responsible for any of the content of DSM-5. Nonetheless, we are not uninformed about psychiatric diagnosis, or about the needs of our fellow practitioners or of trainees, because each of us serves as a faculty member at a major academic psychiatry department. Each of us has extensive experience educating residents, medical students, and other learners in the arcane rules of psychiatric diagnosis, a process that seems mysterious and impossibly difficult to the uninitiated, though routine (and even fun) from our perspective.

For perspective, both DSM-III and DSM-IV were met with criticism from all sides and yet emerged as healthy and influential documents. The APA Assembly approved DSM-5 in November 2012 without recommending changes, and the document was later unanimously accepted by the APA Board of Trustees. DSM-5 Task Force Co-Chairs David J. Kupfer, M.D., and Darrel A. Regier, M.D., M.P.H., deserve enormous credit for shepherding the process and keeping it on task, if not on schedule. Although we provide, in the introduction, an overview of the process that led to DSM-5, we make no attempt to provide a more detailed history of the process. That will be left to others. Already, many volumes have been published presenting early views on the process of revision, as well as the goals and objectives for DSM-5.

Let us review the structure of this guidebook. In the introduction, we briefly review the history of psychiatric diagnostic classification. Then, in Chapter 1, we focus on the march to DSM-5. Chapter 2 provides a crosswalk from DSM-IV to DSM-5, focusing on the major changes but not the many minor edits. In Chapters 3–19, we review the major diagnostic categories and specific diagnoses and their criteria to provide clarity to their assessment. Dimensional scales embedded in DSM-5 are discussed in Chapter 20, and an alternative model for personality disorders is presented in Chapter 21. Proposed disorders under consideration are reviewed in Chapter 22. A list of references and an appendix with the DSM-5 classification follow.

We believe this guidebook will appeal to a wide audience of practicing psychiatrists, psychologists, psychiatric nurses, social workers, and mental health professionals who wish to know how to implement DSM-5 in their ongoing practices. We expect that institutional audiences will include solo and small practices, health maintenance organizations, insurance providers, hospitals, libraries, academic institutions, medical school courses, and residency training programs. Students, residents, and office staff will also benefit from the guidebook, which will help them to better understand how DSM-5 diagnoses fit into current mental health practice. It is our hope that many will find this book useful for training health professionals of all stripes in the use of DSM-5.

Acknowledgments

When approached about writing this book, we jumped at the opportunity. The two of us are clinicians and educators highly interested in psychiatric classification and assessment. Although we are both university-based psychiatrists and researchers, we have been influenced by years of routine clinical care in all types of settings: academic medical centers, freestanding mental health clinics, correctional and forensic settings, and so on. Between us, we have more than 45 years of clinical experience that we bring to this effort.

Our task was greatly facilitated by using the official Web site (www.dsm5.org)—available to all persons—as well as by accessing DSM-5 drafts, which the American Psychiatric Association graciously provided us. Much of our work involved a straightforward comparison of DSM-5 with its predecessors (particularly DSM-IV and DSM-IV-TR), allowing us to show where changes have been made and why. We are grateful to the DSM-5 Task Force and work groups, and their many members and consultants. More than 1,000 persons were involved in creating DSM-5. The monumental task took countless hours by colleagues who gave freely of their time to craft a book that takes our field into the future.

In writing the guidebook, we were enormously influenced by our own experiences in providing patient care, as well as our years of work in teaching medical students and residents in psychiatric interviewing techniques and assessment methods. We are also sensitive to the needs that researchers have to systematically collect diagnostic data. We believe DSM-5 will be a major stimulant to research, as scientists retool their approach and incorporate new and reformulated criteria sets into their assessments.

Our practice style and knowledge base were also shaped by our training experiences. One of us (D.W.B.) trained in the psychiatry department at the University of Iowa. Under the leadership of the late George Winokur, M.D., the department was a member of the "invisible college" of neo-Kraepelinians, whose members were responsible for the first useful criteria sets in psychiatry—the Feighner criteria and, later, the Research Diagnostic Criteria, both of which were the intellectual forerunners to DSM-III, as we discuss in more detail in the Introduction. The other (J.E.G.) trained at the University of Minnesota, whose psychiatry department was led for a time by another member of the "invisible college," Paula Clayton, M.D. These experiences led us to appreciate the value of evidence-based operational criteria for both clinical and research use.

We are indebted to the staff at American Psychiatric Publishing. In particular, we are grateful to Robert E. Hales, M.D., who helped shape the book's vision and scope, and John McDuffie, who provided needed encouragement and support. In addition to the editorial staff, we wish to thank the many important mentors who have influenced us in our careers, including Nancy Andreasen, M.D., Raymond Crowe, M.D., Russell Noyes, M.D., William Coryell, M.D., Bruce Pfohl, M.D., Suck Won Kim, M.D., Katharine Phillips, M.D., Larry Price, M.D., and Steve Rasmussen, M.D. Robert Spitzer, M.D., a friend and colleague who led both the DSM-III and DSM-III-R Task Forces, has been an inspiration. Special thanks go to Susan Schultz, M.D., a University of Iowa colleague known for her good cheer. As text editor for DSM-5, she was especially knowledgeable about the manual.

We are also grateful to the countless patients with whom we have worked in Iowa, Minnesota, and elsewhere, who have taught us much of what we know about their disorders. They are the true teachers.

Introduction

Science is the systematic classification of experience.

George Henry Lewes, *The Physical Basis of Mind*, 1877

Fourteen years in development, the *Diagnostic and Statistical Manual of Mental Disorders*, 5th Edition (DSM-5; American Psychiatric Association 2013), is a landmark publication that sets an international standard for psychiatric diagnosis and classification. Published by the American Psychiatric Association (APA), DSM-5 follows a noble tradition set by its predecessors, beginning with the first edition (DSM-I), which appeared in 1952 (American Psychiatric Association 1952). DSM provides a compendium of all officially recognized diagnoses used in psychiatry and specifies the symptoms that must be present. The development of DSM was the product of the first systematic effort to create an official classification scheme for psychiatric disorders in the United States. Psychiatry is the only specialty in medicine that has consistently and comprehensively formalized the diagnostic processes for the disorders within its domain.

To those of us in psychiatry, the use of DSM is second nature, having been embedded in our training and clinical experience. Colleagues outside the field, however, may wonder what the fuss is about. Why be concerned with DSM? Why indeed. Simply put, DSM provides a common language to those among us who conduct research on and/or treat individuals with psychiatric disorders. Perhaps one of its most important missions is to help ensure consistency in the definition of mental disorders for clinicians in the United States and elsewhere. Developed for trained mental health professionals, DSM is widely used beyond the confines of psychiatry. Among its many users are researchers, administrators, civil servants, attorneys, and others. When used as intended, DSM requires clinical expertise and training. An important limitation is that it does not provide treatment information. Because psychiatry lacks specific laboratory diagnostic tests and confirmed etiologies for most disorders, diagnosis relies largely on the patient's symptoms and history. For that reason, it is essential that diagnostic criteria be precise and clear.

The psychiatric profession regularly reviews and revises DSM in response to new research findings. Science has rapidly advanced, particularly in the past two decades, contributing to the many changes in DSM-5. In the 1990s we experienced the so-called Decade of the Brain, followed by the Human Genome Project. We have since entered the Decade of the Mind. This explosion of knowledge in neuroscience and behavioral sciences has greatly expanded our understanding of mental disorders, including their prevalence and risk factors, brain structure and function, and the influence of genes and environment. Advances in technology have provided new tools that enable the investigation of mental disorders in ways not previously possible. In response to new knowledge, the classification of mental disorders—and their diagnostic criteria—must evolve.

Historical Considerations

The classification of mental illnesses had its start more than two millennia ago, when these conditions were first recognized as discrete illnesses. Perhaps the oldest medical document in evidence, the Ebers Papyrus (probably composed about 1550 B.C.), contains references to specific syndromes such as depression. Biblical writing also contains descriptions of people who suffered from major mental illnesses; for example, in 1 Samuel, Saul is portrayed as falling into a serious depression for which he is treated with soothing music.

Psychiatry owes a great deal to Hippocrates, who developed the first classification of mental illnesses. This schema included epilepsy, mania (excitement), melancholia, and paranoia, as well as toxic deliria (mental confusion accompanied by fever), and hysteria (sudden episodes of somatic illness). Hippocrates and his followers believed mental illnesses were due to imbalances in quantities of body fluids. Melancholia, for example, was due to an excess of black bile, and other abnormalities arose from incorrect balances between other fluids, or "humors" (blood, phlegm, and yellow bile). Humoral theories of mental illness persisted into the Middle Ages, and even today influence our understanding of personality types.

During the European Renaissance and the Enlightenment, systems of classification of disease were often patterned after those found in nature. In the sixteenth century, Paracelsus (1493–1541) developed a classification based on etiologies, including disorders caused by poisons, by phases of the moon, and by hereditary diseases. Thomas Sydenham (1624–1689) was a leading proponent of the notion of discrete and uniform disease categories. He offered detailed descriptions of the neuroses and hysteria. Contemporaries Carolus Linnaeus (1707–1778) and François Boissier de Sauvages (1706–1767) attempted to apply the taxonomic methods of biology to medical and psychiatric illnesses with categories based on observed signs and symptoms. Boissier de Sauvage's system listed more than two thousand diseases, arranged into classes, orders, and genera. Jean-Étienne-Dominique Esquirol (1772–1840), like his mentor Philippe Pinel (1745-1826), emphasized precise clinical description of mental illnesses and avoided speculation about causation. (He is known also for coining the word *hallucination*.)

A tension between paradigms based on observation and theory continued into the nineteenth century. The establishment of asylums allowed more prolonged and intensive observation of patients than had previously been possible. Autopsies were increasingly common and widely accepted, as attempts were made to identify a physical basis for psychiatric symptoms. Emil Kraepelin (1856–1926) aimed to develop a classification of mental disorders that emphasized the importance of symptoms, course and outcome. He is perhaps best known for separating manic-depressive illness from *dementia praecox.* The latter was renamed *schizophrenia* ("splitting of the mind") by Eugen Bleuler (1857–1939) to recognize the cognitive impairment that occurs and emphasize certain symptoms he felt were fundamental to the disorder, such as affective flattening and disturbances of association (i.e., peculiar and distorted thinking). Kraepelin's careful attention to symptoms and course in delineating syndromes later provided the basic conceptual framework for DSM-III (American Psychiatric Association 1980).

Beyond these historical trends, there was a growing need to develop classification systems for statistical, epidemiological, and reporting purposes. The initial reason for developing a classification of mental disorders in the United States was to collect statistical information for the census. For the 1880 census, seven categories of mental illnesses were listed: mania, melancholia, monomania, paresis, dementia, dipsomania, and epilepsy. The increasing role of government in health care created a greater push for diagnostic uniformity in the period, and the first standard psychiatric classification was produced in the United States in 1918 by the American Medico-Psychological Association, forerunner of the APA. Published as the *Statistical Manual for the Use of Institutions for the Insane*, it listed 22 disorders and was primarily used to gather uniform statistics from mental institutions (Shorter 1997).

Development of DSM

In 1927 the New York Academy of Medicine spearheaded a movement to develop a nationally accepted standard nomenclature of disease. The following year, a conference was organized that included participants from the government and all the medical specialties, including psychiatry (represented by the APA). Published in 1933 by the American Medical Association as *A Standard Classified Nomenclature of Disease*, the manual contained 24 major psychiatric categories that were strongly influenced by the sixth edition of Kraepelin's (1899) *Lehrbuch der Psychiatrie*.

In response to challenges faced by the military in the 1940s, and the need for more suitable diagnostic categories to describe psychiatric problems faced by combatants, the U.S. Army and Navy each developed their own classification system. Meanwhile, the Veterans Administration created its own system to incorporate outpatient presentations of World War II veterans. The situation with psychiatric nomenclature had led to considerable confusion, and at least four different systems—the Standard and those of the U.S. Army, the U.S. Navy, and the Veterans Administration—were in place. Some agencies used one system for clinical use, another for disability ratings, and a third for statistical reporting. The sixth revision of the *Manual of International Statistical Classification of Diseases, Injuries, and Causes of Death* (ICD-6), developed in 1948 by the World Health Organization (WHO), was not entirely satisfactory to American psychiatrists, so the APA chose to develop its own manual.

The APA Committee on Nomenclature and Statistics set to work on a single national system of classification of mental illnesses, which led to the publication in 1952 of the first edition of the *Diagnostic and Statistical Manual of Mental Disorders* (DSM-I). Relatively compact at 132 pages, DSM-I was the first official manual of mental disorders to focus on clinical utility for classification. Definitions were relatively simple and consisted of brief prototypical descriptions. Most disorders were "reactions" reflecting the influence of Adolf Meyer and his psychobiological approach to psychiatry, which hypothesized that disorders were types of reaction patterns that are exaggerations or aberrations of, or substitutions for, normal, healthy, and adaptable ways of living. For example, manic-depressive illness was defined in DSM-I as follows:

> **Manic Depressive Reactions:** These groups comprise the psychotic reactions which fundamentally are marked by severe mood swings and a tendency to remission and re-currence. Various accessory symptoms such as illusions, delusions, and hallucinations may be added to the fundamental affective alteration. Manic depressive reaction is synonymous with the term manic depressive psychosis. The reaction will be further classified in to the appropriate one of the following types: manic, depressed, or other. (American Psychiatric Association 1952, p. 25)

To encourage consistency internationally, WHO sponsored a revision that appeared as ICD-8 in 1967 (World Health Organization 1967). The APA contributed to ICD-8 and also published DSM-II (American Psychiatric Association 1968) the following year. Among the several changes in DSM-II, the most striking was the omission of the term *reaction* from diagnoses. The names of several disorders were changed, and the manual encouraged users to record multiple psychiatric diagnoses (listed in order of importance) and associated physical conditions, which presaged the development of the multiaxial diagnostic scheme of DSM-III.

In 1974 the APA created a task force to produce a revised version of DSM to coincide with the publication of ICD-9 (World Health Organization 1977). Robert Spitzer, head of the evaluation unit at the New York State Psychiatric Institute and consultant for the DSM-II revision, was appointed to lead the group. Spitzer had a strong interest in diagnosis and classification and was influenced by like-minded psychiatrists at Washington University in St. Louis who, in 1972, had published the *Feighner criteria,* named after first author—and psychiatric resident—John Feighner (Feighner et al. 1972). This was psychiatry's first attempt to develop operationalized diagnostic criteria. (*Operational* in this sense means taking something—in this case a diagnosis—and breaking it down into its component parts so they can be taught and mastered.)

Although the attempt was relatively modest (resulting in criteria for 15 psychiatric illnesses plus a residual category for individuals with undiagnosed symptoms), the Feighner criteria created a firestorm of interest. The expectation of Eli Robins, Samuel Guze, George Winokur, and other leaders of the St. Louis group was that each clinical syndrome would ultimately be validated by coherence in its clinical picture, separation (or "delimitation") from other disorders, common prognosis and outcome, genetic aggregation in families, and further differentiation by future laboratory tests (which now include neuroimaging, molecular genetics, neuropsychological testing, and so forth).

Spitzer and colleagues developed the Research Diagnostic Criteria (RDC) for use in the longitudinal Collaborative Study on the Psychobiology of Depression supported by the National Institute of Mental Health (Endicott and Spitzer 1978). Both the Feighner criteria and the RDC contributed to the intellectual ferment that led to DSM-III. The fact that one-third of DSM-III Task Force members trained at Washington University was evidence of the influence of the "invisible college" of neo-Kraepelinians, as they came to be known, who helped usher in an era of careful, systematic assessment and classification.

Published in 1980, DSM-III created a sensation. A hefty tome that came in at 494 pages, DSM-III was a reflection of the increased emphasis on empirical data in psychiatric practice and research. It was the first effort by a medical specialty to provide a comprehensive and detailed diagnostic manual in which all disorders were defined by specific criteria so that the methods for making a psychiatric diagnosis were relatively clear. Great care was taken in preparing the criteria. Detailed drafts were written, opinions were obtained from 550 clinicians, and results were subjected to field tests of more than 12,000 patients. Furthermore, DSM-III was published in coordination with the development of the ninth revision of the ICD.

In addition to the inclusion of diagnostic criteria, the other major innovation of DSM-III was the introduction of a multiaxial classification system. Five axes were described:

I. Clinical syndromes and "conditions not attributable to a mental disorder that are the focus of attention and treatment"
II. Personality disorders and specific developmental disorders
III. Physical disorders
IV. Severity of psychosocial stressors
V. Highest level of adaptive functioning in the last year

DSM-III relied less than its predecessors on psychoanalytic concepts, and its descriptive approach was meant to be neutral ("atheoretical") with regard to etiology. This approach was taken because task force members felt that the inclusion of etiological theories would present an "obstacle to use of the manual by clinicians of varying theoretical orientations since it would not be possible to present all reasonable etiologic theories for each disorder" (American Psychiatric Association 1980, p. 7).

Another major goal of DSM-III was to improve upon the poor reliability that had plagued previous systems. Because of their vagueness and imprecision, definitions in DSM-I and DSM-II did not facilitate communication between clinicians and often failed to distinguish one disorder from another. Research investigations had made clear that different clinicians using DSM-I or DSM-II would give different diagnoses to the same patient. DSM-III Task Force members agreed that the specific diagnostic criteria would be as objective as possible and be based on existing research data rather than expert opinion whenever possible. *Reliability,* a biometric concept, refers to the ability of two observers to agree on what they see. It is measured by a variety of statistical methods, such as percent agreement, correlation coefficients, or the kappa statistic, which corrects for chance agreement. The reliability of DSM-III was assessed in field trials and found to be relatively good, particularly for schizophrenia and major affective disorders. DSM-III included a definition for mental disorders that has been incorporated in all subsequent editions, albeit with wording changes:

> In DSM-III each of the mental disorders is conceptualized as a clinically significant behavioral or psychological syndrome or pattern that occurs in an individual and that is typically associated with either a painful symptom (distress) or impairment in one or more important areas of functioning (disability). In addition, there is an inference that

there is a behavioral, psychological, or biological dysfunction, and that the disturbance is not only in the relationship between the individual and society. (When the disturbance is limited to conflict between the individual and society, this may represent social deviance, which may or may not be commendable, but is not by itself a mental disorder.) (American Psychiatric Association 1980, p. 6)

A revision to DSM-III, DSM-III-R (American Psychiatric Association 1987), was published in 1987. Its purpose was to remedy some of the inconsistencies identified in DSM-III pending the production of a fourth version (DSM-IV; American Psychiatric Association 1994) to coincide with the tenth revision of the ICD (World Health Organization 1992). Several new disorders were added (e.g., body dysmorphic disorder), and others were deleted or subsumed within other categories (e.g., ego-dystonic homosexuality).

The APA created a task force in May 1988 to begin work on DSM-IV. Because early drafts of the mental disorders section of ICD-10 were quite different from the descriptions in ICD-9 and DSM-III-R, it seemed crucial for the groups working on DSM-IV and ICD-10 (then in the works) to have an opportunity for discussion and mutual influence. The APA had concluded that work on DSM-IV and ICD-10 should be coordinated. As a result, DSM-IV was technically compatible with ICD-10, although there were a number of specific differences, and coding in DSM-IV remained tied to that in ICD-9. Thirteen work groups were established, each responsible for a section of the classification.

DSM-IV was published in 1994, and its development involved systematic reviews of the literature, secondary data analyses of previously collected data, and analyses of primary data collected through 12 field trials. Changes were conservative and driven by evidence whenever possible rather than expert consensus. The goal was to balance historical precedent, new data, and the needs required for compatibility with ICD-10. Frances et al. (1990) observed that the "first priority [is] that it be a useful guide to clinical practice" (p. 1441). A major change from previous versions was the inclusion of a clinical significance criterion for almost half of all the categories, which required that symptoms cause "clinically significant distress or impairment in social, occupational, or other important areas of functioning." Several new disorders were introduced (e.g., acute stress disorder, bipolar II disorder, Asperger's disorder), and others were deleted or subsumed by other categories (e.g., cluttering, passive-aggressive personality disorder). Even more extensive field trials and reliability studies were done for DSM-IV than for DSM-III or DSM-III-R, and they are summarized in the DSM-IV sourcebooks.

A text revision was published in 2000 (DSM-IV-TR; American Psychiatric Association 2000). Its purpose was to correct errors and to add new information not available in 1994. No changes were made in the diagnostic criteria, nor were disorders added or deleted. The path to DSM-5 began even before DSM-IV-TR was published, and this story is told next in Chapter 1, "The March to DSM-5."

The various DSM editions—their lengths and the number of disorders contained—are compared in Table 1.

TABLE 1. DSMs from 1952 to 2013

Edition	Year of publication	Number of disorders	Number of pages
DSM-I	1952	106	132
DSM-II	1968	182	119
DSM-III	1980	265	494
DSM-III-R	1987	292	567
DSM-IV	1994	297	886
DSM-IV-TR	2000	297	943
DSM-5	2013	157[a]	947

[a]Not including other specified and unspecified disorders.

CHAPTER 1

The March to DSM-5

The process to develop DSM-5 (called DSM-V during much of its development) began in 1999, five years after the publication of DSM-IV. Steven E. Hyman, M.D., then director of the National Institute of Mental Health (NIMH), Steven M. Mirin, M.D., then president of the American Psychiatric Association (APA), and David J. Kupfer, M.D., who chaired the APA Committee on Psychiatric Diagnosis and Assessment, met and agreed that the APA and NIMH should work together to expand the scientific basis for psychiatric diagnosis and classification.

As described by Regier et al. (2011), issues included

1. The basic definition of mental illness.
2. The option of adding dimensional criteria to disorders.
3. The possible separation of impairment and diagnostic assessments.
4. The need to address various expressions of an illness across the life span.
5. The need to address various expressions of mental disorders as conditioned by gender and culture.

A conference was convened later that year, cosponsored by both organizations, to develop research priorities. Participants included experts in epidemiology and genetics, neuroscience, cognitive and behavioral science, child and adult development, and disability assessment. To encourage thinking "outside the box," those closely involved in the development of DSM-IV were not included. Participants recognized the need for a series of white papers to guide future research and promote further discussion covering overarching topic areas that cut across many psychiatric disorders. Work groups were created for developmental issues, gaps in the current diagnostic system, disability and impairment, neuroscience, nomenclature, and cross-cultural issues.

Darrel A. Regier, M.D., M.P.H., was recruited from NIMH in 2000 to serve as director of the APA's American Psychiatric Institute for Research and Education (APIRE) and to coordinate the development of DSM-5. Additional conferences were held to set the DSM-5 research agenda, to propose planning work group membership, and to hold face-to-face meetings. These groups, which included liaisons from the National

Institutes of Health (NIH) and the international psychiatric community, developed a series of white papers, published in *A Research Agenda for DSM-V* (Kupfer et al. 2002). A second series of white papers, titled *Age and Gender Considerations in Psychiatric Diagnosis,* was later commissioned by the APA and published in 2007 (Narrow et al. 2007).

In 2002, APIRE and Director Regier worked with leaders of the World Health Organization (WHO) and the World Psychiatric Association to develop a grant from NIMH to implement a series of research planning conferences that aimed to focus on the scientific evidence for revisions of specific diagnostic areas. With Regier as principal investigator, a $1.1 million cooperative agreement grant was awarded with joint support from NIMH, the National Institute on Drug Abuse, and the National Institute on Alcohol Abuse and Alcoholism.

The multiyear grant (2003–2008) supported 13 international conferences. For each, participants wrote papers addressing specific diagnostic questions, and from these papers and conference proceedings a research agenda was developed. More than 100 scientific articles were written that were later compiled into monographs. A consistent recommendation was the need for better integration of categorical and dimensional assessment criteria (Helzer et al. 2008). DSM-IV Task Force members had considered the feasibility of using dimensional measures to assess disorder thresholds and rate severity. Instead, language regarding "clinically significant distress or impairment" was incorporated into DSM-IV for all disorders, but the only dimensional component consisted of Axis V (of the multiaxial diagnostic scheme), which provided for the assessment of global functioning.

The DSM-5 Task Force was created in 2006 by APA President Steven S. Sharfstein, M.D., and APA Medical Director James H. Scully Jr., M.D., with Dr. Kupfer as chair and Dr. Regier as vice-chair. Additional members were appointed to the task force, including the chairs of the 13 diagnostic work groups that were responsible for reviewing the research and literature on which to base their recommendations.

The APA Board of Trustees established principles of appointment that required limits on investments and income that could be received from the pharmaceutical industry, mandated that no more than two representatives from any university could participate in the task force or in the same work group, and required a vetting and review process by a subcommittee of the board. Work group chairs, together with Drs. Kupfer and Regier, recommended to the successive APA presidents (Drs. Pedro Ruiz and Carolyn Robinowitz) nominees viewed as leading experts in their field. Task force members were announced in July 2007 and work group members in May 2008.

The DSM-5 Task Force had four guiding principles:

1. Give priority to clinical utility; that is, any changes to the criteria or organization of the manual had to be useful to clinicians.
2. Use research evidence accumulated since the publication of DSM-IV as a guide for making changes.
3. Maintain historical continuity with previous editions, particularly DSM-III and DSM-IV.
4. Do not establish a priori any limits on changes proposed by work groups.

Task force members respected precedent and understood that any changes to the manual would potentially affect clinical care, disorder prevalence, research protocols, and coding and billing practices. Diagnostic advances would be made through a careful and transparent process involving detailed literature reviews, secondary analyses of existing data sets, and primary analyses of newly collected data.

The task force was assigned the responsibility of addressing conceptual issues through six study groups (distinct from the work groups), each delegated to guide the overall development of revisions for one of the following specific diagnostic areas:

1. *Diagnostic spectra and DSM/ICD harmonization:* This group assessed the spectra of syndromes across existing diagnostic boundaries, made recommendations for the overall structure of DSM categories, and identified 11 potential criteria for testing the validity of mental disorder diagnoses, representing an expansion beyond the original five validating criteria proposed by Robins and Guze (1970).
2. *Life span developmental approaches:* This group focused on the different expressions of mental disorders that might emerge at progressive ages in human developmental life stages.
3. *Gender and cross-cultural issues:* This group was established to assess the different expression of symptom equivalence of mental disorders mediated by gender and culture.
4. *Psychiatric/general medical interface:* This group was formed to address approaches that would facilitate a better interface between general medical and mental disorder approaches to diagnosis.
5. *Impairment and disability:* This group was formed to address the development of global impairment and disability assessment strategies.
6. *Diagnostic assessment instruments:* This group considered the need to address measurement and assessment issues.

Last, a seventh study group was established to review secondary data analyses proposed for funding by the APA to assess the evidence base for proposed revisions.

Work groups met regularly via conference calls and convened in person twice annually. An initial task for the groups was to address how DSM-IV did or did not work well or otherwise failed to meet clinicians' needs. For example, work groups evaluated how to better assess symptom severity and how to handle the problem of multiple comorbidities. Other aims included reducing "not otherwise specified" diagnoses (seen as overused and problematic) and improving diagnostic criteria that lacked precision. The work groups also aimed to better specify treatment targets to help clinicians identify symptoms that could be addressed in treatment. Additionally, the DSM-5 Task Force focused on how best to include assessment of common symptoms not addressed within the diagnostic criteria for a specific illness (e.g., symptoms of insomnia that may be experienced by a patient with schizophrenia).

In addition, the work groups were asked to do the following:

1. Clarify the boundaries between mental disorders to reduce confusion of disorders with each other and to help guide effective treatment

2. Consider "cross-cutting" symptoms (those that commonly occur across different diagnoses)
3. Demonstrate the strength of research for the recommendations on as many evidence levels as possible
4. Clarify the boundaries between specific mental disorders and normal psychological functioning

Revisions to the diagnostic criteria were developed by each work group based on a review of research evidence, targeted data analyses, and expert consensus. Summaries of major work group issues were posted on the DSM-5 developmental Web site, and comments from public and professional colleagues were sought. The final phase of DSM-5 development included interactions between the study groups and the diagnostic work groups.

One goal was to establish a framework for an evolution of the diagnostic system that would advance clinical practice and facilitate ongoing testing of the diagnostic criteria. The task force concluded that an important advance would be to incorporate simple dimensional measures for assessing syndromes both within and across broad diagnostic categories (Regier 2007).

DSM-V or DSM-5?

One goal of the task force was to designate DSM-5 as a "living" document, meaning that future changes could be made rapidly in response to scientific advances. Task force members concluded that the ability to respond in a rapid and nimble fashion was best captured by the use of the Arabic numeral rather than the Roman numerals that have been used since DSM-II was published in 1968—hence, DSM-5 rather than DSM-V. Because technology allows immediate dissemination of information worldwide, Roman numerals were considered too limiting, especially considering that future text revisions appeared likely. For example, a "TR" designation (as in DSM-IV-TR) can only be applied once. For simplicity, future changes prior to the manual's next complete revision can be designated as DSM-5.1, DSM-5.2, and so forth.

Dimensional Assessment

A challenge in accurately diagnosing mental disorders is having the ability to fully assess a range of symptoms and other factors in patients. Since DSM-III, disorders have been described and arranged by category, with a specific list of criteria for each mental disorder. With this categorical system, a person either had a symptom or did not, and having a certain number of symptoms was required for a diagnosis to be made. If this number was not met, the disorder was not diagnosed.

The use of criteria represented a vast improvement over the previous guidelines available to diagnose patients with mental disorders, but categorical approaches do not always fit with the reality of the range of symptoms that people experience. For example, persons with schizophrenia often have other symptoms that do not fit the criteria for diagnosing schizophrenia (e.g., depression, anxiety). Because diagnostic criteria require a yes/no decision by the clinician, in most cases there is no method in DSM-IV to account for the severity of the disorder, nor an easy way to determine if the patient is improving with treatment.

Work groups were asked to consider ways to incorporate a simple method to enable clinicians to capture the symptoms and severity of mental disorders with dimensional measures that would allow clinicians to systematically evaluate patients on a full range of symptoms. Dimensional assessments allow clinicians to rate the presence and the severity of the symptoms (e.g., as *very severe, severe, moderate,* or *mild*). This rating can be used to track a patient's progress with treatment and can serve as a means to note improvements even when symptoms remain. Work groups also were asked to examine the available scientific evidence and determine appropriate dimensional assessments for the specific illnesses under review, and provide clinicians with specific guidance on their use. Dimensional assessments are discussed in Chapter 20, "Assessment Measures."

Diagnostic Reliability and Field Trials

DSM-5 Task Force members understood the need for diagnostic reliability. *Reliability* refers to the certainty with which it can be predicted that different clinicians will apply the same diagnosis to the same patient. While diagnostic reliability is rarely if ever absolute in any field of medicine, it has enormous importance. If two clinicians give a patient two different diagnoses, one of them is probably wrong. Methods of testing reliability were developed for DSM-5 to give a more accurate picture of real-world clinical reliability than did field trials for previous editions (Kraemer et al. 2010, 2012). Reliability was assessed through a series of field trials; the process included the examination of specific diagnostic criteria as well as overarching changes applicable across disorders, such as the integration of dimensional measures and diagnostic severity scales.

The field trials utilized two designs. In the first, a large-scale design implemented across 11 academic medical centers, approximately 2,000 patients were seen. In the second design, which was created for solo and small group clinicians in routine clinical practice settings, around 1,450 patients were seen. The designs provided an opportunity to examine the reliability, clinical utility, and feasibility of proposed changes both in high-volume research practice settings and in everyday clinical care settings. Diagnostic interviews were conducted by psychiatrists and other mental health practitioners, all of whom were expected to use the manual in their daily care of patients. Interviews were naturalistic and did not employ structured interviews, in order to replicate what clinicians do every day.

In field trials for prior editions of DSM, the main method used to measure reliability was *interrater testing,* in which two or more raters review the same patient material at the same time. The design accounts for the "noise" of clinical inconsistency but does not account for differences in the way patients with the same condition may present or the fact that the same patient can present differently on different days. For that reason, interrater reliability testing is likely to render a score that may not reflect clinical reality. *Test-retest reliability* was examined in the DSM-5 field trials. This design requires that the same patients be observed separately by two or more raters within an interval during which the clinical condition of the patients is unlikely to have changed, and a kappa statistic is calculated.

Innovations of the field trials included random patient selection with few exclusion criteria; use of clinicians not selected on the basis of special expertise in the disorders being evaluated; application of the entire DSM-5 system in each evaluation (rather than focusing on one diagnosis at a time); and instructions to participating clinicians that they make diagnoses according to their usual practice, not on the basis of a standardized diagnostic interview (rarely used in clinical practice). These changes were made to test with optimal fidelity diagnostic criteria intended for real-world clinicians treating real patients.

Preliminary results of the field trials were presented at the 2012 American Psychiatric Association annual meeting. DSM-5 criteria were at least adequately reliable for most of the disorder studies, while dimensional ratings fared better. Kappa values from tests conducted in the academic centers were in the "excellent" range for the following: autism spectrum disorder, 0.69; posttraumatic stress disorder, 0.67; attention-deficit/hyperactivity disorder, 0.61; and major neurocognitive disorder, 0.78. The following disorders were in the "good" range: bipolar I disorder, 0.54; schizophrenia, 0.46; schizoaffective disorder, 0.50; mild traumatic brain injury, 0.46; and borderline personality disorder, 0.58. Other disorders fared less well: generalized anxiety disorder, 0.20, and major depressive disorder, 0.32. Although attenuated psychosis syndrome fared reasonably well (0.46), the 95% confidence interval extended to zero, suggesting a failed trial.

Although kappa values reported for DSM-III and DSM-IV were better (e.g., 0.59 for major depressive disorder), patient samples were very different in those earlier field trials in that patients with psychiatric comorbidities had been excluded.

Final Approval

The proposed revisions to DSM-5 had a rigorous and multistage review prior to final approval by the APA Board of Trustees. Throughout 2011 and 2012, proposed changes continued to undergo revision with input from APA members and others via three postings on the DSM-5 developmental Web site. Field trial data was analyzed, discussed, and integrated into proposals during the review process. A scientific review committee was charged with reviewing the science validating the evidence for revisions. A peer review process took place in which hundreds of expert reviewers considered the clinical and public health risks and benefits of making changes from DSM-IV. The APA Assembly, its governing body, debated DSM-5 and voted to approve the new manual at their annual fall meeting in November 2012.

Last, there was an overall review by the DSM-5 Task Force, which sent final recommendations along with all supporting data to the APA's Board of Trustees for a final review. The final draft was approved by the board in December 2012 and thereafter submitted to American Psychiatric Publishing, a division of the APA. The official release of DSM-5 was set for the 166th Annual Meeting of the APA in San Francisco, May 18–22, 2013.

Controversies Involving DSM-5

The revision process was not without controversy, but this must be placed in perspective: all prior DSM editions were accompanied by considerable public consternation, and DSM-5 was no exception. A steady drumbeat of criticism began early, both within the field and among the public at large.

The main concerns from various critics were that the DSM-5 process lacked openness and transparency; that decisions were made capriciously and did not follow the evidence; that no independent scientific review was done; that rates of reliability were unacceptably low; that prevalence rates would increase because the thresholds for important categories (e.g., attention-deficit/hyperactivity disorder, mild neurocognitive disorder, disruptive mood dysregulation disorder) were too loose; and that many task force and work group members had conflicts of interest.

Allegations of conflict of interest were spurred in part by an article in an online journal that implied that the DSM-5 financial disclosure policy had not resulted in a reduction of conflicts (Cosgrove and Krimsky 2012). The article drew comparisons with the DSM-IV process (for which there were few stringent requirements to disclose) and suggested there was an increase in conflicts among DSM-5 Task Force and work group members. The APA responded that the data show 72% of task force and work group members had no relationship with the pharmaceutical industry in 2011. Of the remaining 28%, 12% reported grant support only, 10% reported paid consultations, and 7% reported receiving honoraria.

Several diagnostic categories received special criticism. One major concern was the introduction of the autism spectrum disorder diagnosis, in which five DSM-IV-TR diagnoses (autistic disorder, Asperger's disorder, childhood disintegrative disorder, Rett's disorder, and pervasive developmental disorder not otherwise specified) were consolidated. Interest groups led by those wanting to preserve Asperger's disorder were concerned new criteria would relegate individuals with this disorder to the diagnostic hinterlands. The decision to remove the "bereavement exclusion" for major depressive disorder was criticized by persons who claimed the change would turn normal bereavement into a mental disorder. The DSM-5 attenuated psychosis syndrome was harshly criticized by some who were motivated by the concern that the diagnosis would unfairly stigmatize persons for no reason other than that they might be considered odd by others or because of their family history, and that it is not possible to reliably identify persons likely to develop psychosis; furthermore, because there are no proven treatments for the proposed disorder, the diagnosis would merely increase off-label use of antipsychotics in a futile attempt to treat it. (The Psychotic Disorders Work Group later recommended placing attenuated psychosis syndrome in Section III, "Conditions for Further Study.") Likewise, disruptive mood dysregulation disorder was criticized for labeling irritable children with a mental disorder that would also increase off-label use of antipsychotics.

Finally, special fire was reserved for the entire personality disorders chapter (further discussed in Chapter 18). In addition to recommending that the number of disorders be reduced from 10 to 6, the Personality and Personality Disorders Work Group recommended revamping the diagnostic criteria for the remaining disorders, while incorporating a complex scheme to rate up to five personality trait domains and 25 facets. Critics pointed out that the new criteria were so complex as to be unworkable for busy clinicians, and that an already marginalized group of patients would only be further marginalized by clinicians who ignored the new criteria. The fact that two work group members resigned in 2012 further fueled the fire. In the end, the APA Board of Trustees voted to include the DSM-IV personality disorder criteria in Section II and place the proposed model in Section III.

Despite these many challenges, the task force and 13 work groups pressed on, and, although the initial timetable could not be followed (the initial plan was for release in 2012), DSM-5 emerged hale and hearty, and probably much improved because of the intense interest (and input) from clinicians and researchers, as well as the public.

Summary

The process that led to DSM-5 began 14 years ago, and was very much like the process that led to its predecessors—DSM-III, DSM-III-R, and DSM-IV—by involving the active participation of psychiatric leaders and of hundreds of practicing psychiatrists and psychologists. The process was labor intensive, was open and transparent, and had multiple layers of review. The task force had declared from the outset that DSM-5 should be transformative, and it held forth on that pledge, creating a 947-page document (not including the classification listing and preface) that has introduced dimensional assessment in a more fundamental way than its predecessors, has introduced many new diagnoses, has consolidated many others, and has eliminated some. To the extent possible, changes were based on the best scientific evidence, analyses of existing databases, and new data from field trials.

CHAPTER 2

Use of DSM-5 and Major Changes From DSM-IV

DSM-5 represents a significant departure from its predecessors, as indicated by changes to specific categories and disorders as well as its overall organization (its metastructure). The manual was reorganized in response to recommendations made by the Diagnostic Spectra and DSM/ICD Harmonization Study Group, convened by the American Psychiatric Association to consider ways in which disorders might be organized and whether advances in neuroscience, brain imaging, and genetics might suggest a framework for arranging disorders by more than common symptoms. What emerged from those discussions is reflected by the reorganization of the 19 major diagnostic classes in DSM-5 (Table 2–1).

The pattern of chapter placement in DSM-5 reflects scientific advances in the understanding of psychiatric disorders and of the presumed etiological and pathophysiological relationships among them (Andrews et al. 2009). These changes were made to facilitate a more comprehensive diagnosis and treatment approach. Rather than ordering the diagnostic classes as presented in DSM-IV, developers of the new manual arranged them in a developmental life span fashion. DSM-5 begins with neurodevelopmental disorders, often diagnosed in infancy and early childhood, and progresses through diagnostic areas more commonly diagnosed in adulthood, such as sleep-wake disorders.

Within each diagnostic class, specific disorders are arranged so that those typically diagnosed in childhood are listed first. This revised ordering also represents an attempt to place close to one another those diagnostic areas that appear related. For example, the specific class bipolar and related disorders has been created and placed immediately after schizophrenia spectrum and other psychotic disorders. Another example is the placement of dissociative disorders between the category trauma- and stressor-related disorders and the somatic symptom and related disorders. Dissociative disorders are thought by many to be strongly influenced by traumatic events and have traditionally been considered to overlap with somatizing disorders. Conversion disorder, for instance, has long been thought to represent a form of dissociation.

TABLE 2–1.	DSM-5 diagnostic classes

Neurodevelopmental disorders

Schizophrenia spectrum and other psychotic disorders

Bipolar and related disorders

Depressive disorders

Anxiety disorders

Obsessive-compulsive and related disorders

Trauma- and stressor-related disorders

Dissociative disorders

Somatic symptom and related disorders

Feeding and eating disorders

Elimination disorders

Sleep-wake disorders

Sexual dysfunctions

Gender dysphoria

Disruptive, impulse-control, and conduct disorders

Substance-related and addictive disorders

Neurocognitive disorders

Personality disorders

Paraphilic disorders

Other mental disorders

DSM-5 includes three major sections:

- Section I covers historical material and describes the development of DSM-5, as well as its organization and use.
- Section II presents the criteria sets for the 19 major diagnostic classes, plus other mental disorders. Also included in this section are medication-induced movement disorders and other adverse effects of medication, and other conditions that may be a focus of clinical attention (V and Z codes).
- Section III includes assessment measures, a cultural formulation, an alternative DSM-5 model for personality disorders, and criteria sets for conditions for further study.

The Appendix contains highlights of changes from DSM-IV to DSM-5, a technical glossary, a glossary of cultural concepts of distress, listings of disorders in both alphabetical and numerical (by code) order, and a listing of advisors and field trial participants involved in the development of DSM-5.

The conditions for further study, in Section III, were proposed for DSM-5 but had insufficient support from the relevant work group(s) for inclusion as disorders. With additional study, some of these conditions may be elevated to full disorder status in the future. They are described in Chapter 22, "Conditions for Further Study."

Several new diagnostic classes and disorders are included in DSM-5. The task force was aware that the number of new diagnoses had increased at a rapid rate in prior editions, which fueled speculation by both clinicians and critics about the motivations behind the additions. Because it is easier to add disorders than to remove them, the DSM-5 Task Force set a high bar for inclusion.

Using DSM-5

DSM-5 is large and complex, but users should not allow these features to intimidate them. Those new to DSM can begin by examining the lists of classes and diagnoses and studying the guidelines for its use. First-time users should focus on those areas most appropriate to the kind of work in which they regularly engage, rather than trying to master the entire manual. People may wish to carry the pocket edition of DSM-5 (*Desk Reference to the Diagnostic Criteria From DSM-5*), which includes the classification and diagnostic criteria only, or use its online counterpart, from which they can easily download needed criteria sets. Users are encouraged to become familiar with the criteria for a few common conditions (e.g., major depressive disorder, schizophrenia) and even to memorize a few that they use frequently. The system is too vast to commit all of it to memory, however, and clinicians should not feel reluctant to refer back to the criteria when evaluating a patient's symptoms and making a diagnosis.

The diagnostic process is a crucial step in any patient evaluation and contributes to developing a comprehensive formulation and treatment plan. Although a description of the patient evaluation is beyond the scope of this book, as part of the evaluation process, the clinician assesses the patient's chief complaint and conducts a detailed inquiry about the current illness, past psychiatric and medical history, and family and social history. With this information, data from the mental status examination, and laboratory data in some instances, the clinician can develop a differential diagnosis and circle in on a provisional diagnosis. It is not unusual for the diagnostic process to continue as additional information is gathered, and for the clinician to revise his or her initial impression.

Purpose of Diagnosis

Critics may downplay or belittle the significance of a psychiatric diagnosis, but the diagnostic process is fundamental to the clinician's role and paves the way to treatment selection. Some concern is understandable because the process sometimes relies on educated (or subjective) judgments and varying skill levels. Some critics deride a psychiatric diagnosis as a "label," yet that characterization trivializes the process and ignores the important functions that a diagnosis serves.

A psychiatric diagnosis helps to clarify the complex clinical phenomena characteristic of mental illness. The broad array of emotional, cognitive, and behavioral abnormalities can manifest in various ways, and diagnostic categories impose order on this chaos. Diagnoses make mental illnesses easier to understand for professionals in training, as well as patients, families, and friends of people with psychiatric disorders. They also facilitate communication among clinicians because the DSM-5 categories serve as a form of professional shorthand. Diagnoses also help predict what lies ahead for a patient because many psychiatric disorders have a characteristic course and outcome. The diagnosis alerts the patient's caregivers to potential problems and complications that may arise. The diagnosis can also serve as a wake-up call to patients and can lead them to seek help. Additionally, diagnoses are important to psychiatric researchers, helping them assemble groups of persons with similar symptoms and problems. This research allows investigators to determine incidence and prevalence, risk factors, and causes of various diagnoses. Diagnoses are also used as the basis for treatment selection by the U.S. Food and Drug Administration and for devising clinical practice guidelines.

Mental Disorder Definition

DSM-III was the first DSM edition to include an overall definition of *mental disorder*, reproduced in the introduction to this book. This definition has been revised for DSM-5. Although no definition can capture all aspects of all disorders, each disorder identified in Section II must meet the DSM-5 definition of a mental disorder:

> A mental disorder is a syndrome characterized by clinically significant disturbance in an individual's cognition, emotion regulation, or behavior that reflects a dysfunction in the psychological, biological, or developmental processes underlying mental functioning. Mental disorders are usually associated with significant distress or disability in social, occupational, or other important activities. An expectable or culturally approved response to a common stressor or loss, such as the death of a loved one, is not a mental disorder. Socially deviant behavior (e.g., political, religious, or sexual) and conflicts that are primarily between the individual and society are not mental disorders unless the deviance or conflict results from a dysfunction in the individual, as described above. (p. 20)

The diagnosis of a mental disorder is not equivalent to a need for treatment, which involves complex clinical decisions that consider symptom severity, subjective distress associated with the symptoms, disability related to the symptoms, and other factors (e.g., psychiatric symptoms complicating medical conditions). Clinicians may encounter individuals whose presentation does not meet full criteria for a mental disorder but demonstrates a clear need for treatment or care. Access to care should not be limited just because a person does not show all symptoms of a diagnosis.

DSM-5 makes clear that this definition was developed for clinical, public health, and research purposes, and that the inclusion of diagnostic categories such as gambling disorder and pedophilic disorder does not imply that such conditions meet legal or other nonmedical definitions of mental disease, mental disorder, mental defect, or mental disability. Additional information is usually required beyond that contained in the DSM-5 diagnostic criteria to make legal judgments on such issues as criminal responsibility, eligibility for disability compensation, and competency.

Recording a DSM-5 Diagnosis

Clinicians are encouraged to make multiple diagnoses when necessary to fully describe the patient's condition. DSM-III and DSM-IV encouraged the coding of multiple diagnoses. The DSM-5 Task Force and work groups were alert to concerns about multiple diagnoses and reestablished diagnostic hierarchies for several conditions to lessen this necessity (e.g., in the dissociative disorders chapter, the diagnosis dissociative identity disorder trumps dissociative amnesia and other diagnoses in the class). Nonetheless, clinicians need to be alert to all of the patient's symptoms and respond accordingly. With regard to the personality disorders, the clinician may wish to refer to the scales that assess personality trait domains and facets found in Section III of DSM-5 to more fully describe the patient's condition.

DSM-5 distinguishes between *principal diagnosis* and *reason for visit*. The former refers to the condition chiefly responsible for a patient's hospital stay, whereas the latter is the condition that prompted an outpatient visit, especially when more than one diagnosis is given. The principal diagnosis or reason for visit is indicated by listing it first, and the remaining disorders are listed in order of focus of attention or treatment. When the principal diagnosis or reason for visit is a mental disorder due to another medical condition (e.g., psychotic disorder due to malignant lung neoplasm), ICD coding rules require that the etiological medical condition be listed first. In most cases, the disorder listed as the principal diagnosis or the reason for visit is followed by the qualifying phrase "(principal diagnosis)" or "(reason for visit)." For example, if an outpatient with HIV disease seeks care for symptoms related to a mild neurocognitive disorder related to HIV, "HIV infection" is listed first, followed by "mild neurocognitive disorder due to HIV infection (reason for visit)."

If the clinician does not have sufficient information to allow a firm diagnosis, the clinician may indicate this uncertainty by recording "(provisional)" following the diagnosis. For example, the clinical presentation may support the diagnosis of schizophrenia but the patient is unable to provide adequate history to confirm. Sometimes it is difficult to tease apart the patient's principal diagnosis or reason for visit, particularly when multiple conditions (e.g., both schizophrenia and an alcohol use disorder) appear to have occasioned the hospital stay or clinic visit.

Several examples follow of how a clinician might record a diagnostic impression following an evaluation. In these examples, the ICD-9-CM code is listed first, followed in parentheses by the corresponding ICD-10-CM code:

> **Example 1:** A 25-year-old man is brought to the emergency room by family members for bizarre behavior including making threats of harm, muttering obscenities, and talking to himself. His bizarre behavior appears motivated by paranoid delusions. Family members report that he drinks nearly daily to intoxication and that he smokes cigarettes nearly nonstop. He has had several prior hospitalizations for similar reasons and has been diagnosed with schizophrenia. His DSM-5 diagnoses are:
>
> > **295.90 (F20.9)** Schizophrenia (principal diagnosis)
> > **303.90 (F10.20)** Alcohol use disorder, moderate
> > **305.1 (F17.200)** Tobacco use disorder, severe
>
> **Example 2:** A 65-year-old man is brought to the clinic by his worried spouse. She reports that he has been diagnosed with lung cancer, which his doctors believe has metastasized to his brain. He hears "voices" that tell him not to trust family members. He has become very suspicious and has threatened family members who he believes are planning to kill him. There is no psychiatric history. His DSM-5 diagnoses are:

162.9 (C34.90) Malignant lung neoplasm
293.81 (F06.2) Psychosis due to malignant lung neoplasm (provisional)

Example 3: A 27-year-old woman presents to the clinic for treatment of intrusive thoughts about a recent rape and recurrent nightmares. Prior to her recent symptoms, she reports having experienced overwhelming anxiety in social situations. She also reports a history of deliberate self-harm by cutting, relationship difficulties, and abandonment fears. Her DSM-5 diagnoses are:

309.81 (F43.10) Posttraumatic stress disorder (reason for visit)
300.23 (F40.10) Social anxiety disorder
301.83 (F60.3) Borderline personality disorder

Those familiar with prior DSM editions know that the manual is for the diagnosis of mental disorders and does *not* include treatment guidelines. Nonetheless, accurate diagnosis is the first step in providing appropriate treatment for any medical condition, and mental disorders are no exception. For that reason, DSM-5 is the starting point for clinicians as they begin by conducting a comprehensive assessment of their patient. Furthermore, DSM-5 can be helpful in monitoring the effectiveness of treatment because the many dimensional assessments included in the manual can help by measuring severity and change in response to treatment. Despite the absence of treatment information, DSM-5 provides a wealth of information about diagnostic classes and disorders that learners from all backgrounds will find useful. These are detailed in Table 2–2.

TABLE 2–2.   Useful information in DSM-5 regarding each diagnosis

---

Recording procedures (where applicable)

Subtypes and/or specifiers (where applicable)

Diagnostic features

Associated features supporting diagnosis

Prevalence

Development and course

Risk and prognostic factors

Culture-related diagnostic issues

Gender-related diagnostic issues

Diagnostic markers

Suicide risk

Functional consequences

Differential diagnosis

Comorbidity

DSM-5 Coding

Coding is an essential but underappreciated DSM feature. It is used in utilization review, in gathering statistics for public health purposes, and in making decisions regarding billings and collections. Readers may be surprised that the official coding system in the United States is not DSM-5 but rather the *International Classification of Diseases, Ninth Revision, Clinical Modification* (ICD-9-CM), released by the World Health Organization in 1978. This is the result of a treaty obligation to report health statistics using the ICD system. DSM-5 and ICD-9-CM use the same codes, which range from 290 to 319. (DSM codes form a subset of the ICD-9-CM system, which ranges to 999.) Some DSM-5 disorders are assigned the same ICD code, which is unavoidable because the selection of diagnostic codes in DSM-5 is limited to those already included in ICD-9-CM. It was expected that DSM-5 and its new counterpart, ICD-10-CM, would become available at the same time (May 2013), so that both would employ the same new codes. However, because implementation of ICD-10-CM is delayed to October 2014, DSM-5 uses ICD-9-CM codes. Nonetheless, ICD-10-CM codes are shown parenthetically in DSM-5, but they should not be used until the official implementation occurs.

The ICD-9-CM code is a three- to five-digit number in front of the name of a DSM-5 disorder; the code precedes the name of the disorder in the classification and accompanies the criteria set for each disorder. For some diagnoses, such as intellectual disability (intellectual developmental disorder)—formerly called *mental retardation*—the appropriate code depends on further specification and is listed *following* the criteria for the disorder. The names of some disorders are followed by alternative terms in parentheses—for example, persistent depressive disorder (dysthymia)—which in most cases are older terms for the disorder.

For each DSM disorder, an ICD-9-CM code is selected that most closely matches the symptoms of the disorder. For example, the ICD-9-CM code for depressive neurosis is assigned to DSM-5 persistent depressive disorder because that ICD-9-CM concept comes closest to matching the DSM-5 concept. If a category is not reflected in ICD-9-CM, the convention is to assign an "other" code. These are available throughout ICD-9-CM to accommodate the addition of new disorders. For example, with bipolar II disorder, which was new to DSM-IV, the code 296.89 was selected, which corresponds to "other bipolar disorder" in ICD-9-CM. For DSM-5 the same general rule applies to new diagnoses: a code is selected by 1) examining the existing system and finding a category that best corresponds to the condition in question or 2) assigning an "other" code. Even though the newly assigned DSM code may not be a precise conceptual match for the existing ICD-9-CM entity, from a practical perspective it does not matter because insurance companies usually accept and pay for most ICD-9-CM codes unless the code is specifically excluded by the insurer.

Some disorders have a three-digit code, although most have four or five digits. Certain diagnostic codes have a blank in place of a digit(s). In these cases, the user must insert a specific digit in place of the blank to indicate either a subtype or a level of severity. Subtypes and specifiers are provided for increased specificity. *Subtypes* define mutually exclusive and jointly exhaustive subgroupings within a diagnosis and are indicated by the instruction "specify whether" in the criteria set. For example, delusional disorder is subtyped based on the content of the delusions, with seven subtypes provided (e.g., erotomanic type).

In contrast, *specifiers* are not intended to be mutually exclusive or jointly exhaustive and are indicated with the instruction "specify" or "specify if" in the criteria set (e.g., for obsessive-compulsive disorder, the clinician is asked to specify if tic related). Specifiers provide an opportunity to define a more homogeneous subgrouping of individuals with the disorder who share certain features (e.g., major depressive disorder with melancholic features). Although a fifth digit is sometimes assigned to code a subtype or specifier, a majority of subtypes and most specifiers in DSM-5 *cannot* be coded in the ICD-9-CM system and are indicated only by including the subtype or specifier after the name of the disorder (e.g., social anxiety disorder, performance only).

Indicating Diagnostic Certainty

DSM-5 allows various ways for clinicians to specify level of diagnostic certainty, as shown in the following examples:

V/Z codes: Information is insufficient to know whether a presenting problem is attributable to a mental disorder (e.g., academic problem, partner-relational problem).

300.9 (F99) Unspecified mental disorder: Symptoms of a mental disorder are present, but sufficient information is unavailable to make a more specific diagnosis.

298.9 (F29) Unspecified schizophrenia spectrum and other psychotic disorder: The patient is having a psychotic episode, but further diagnostic specification is not possible.

Specific diagnosis (provisional): Enough information is available to make a "working" diagnosis, but the clinician wishes to indicate a significant level of diagnostic uncertainty by recording "(provisional)" following the diagnosis.

Specific diagnosis: The clinician has sufficient information to be confident of the diagnosis.

"Other Specified" and "Unspecified" Categories

In DSM-5, "other specified" and "unspecified" categories generally cover the same range of conditions as the "not otherwise specified" sections in DSM-IV. The "other specified" disorder category allows clinicians to communicate the specific reason that the presentation does not meet the criteria for any specific category, followed by the specific reason. For example, with an individual having one or more hypomanic episodes yet whose symptoms have never met full criteria for a major depressive or manic episode, a clinician could record "other specified bipolar and related disorder, with hypomanic episode without prior major depressive episode." If the clinician chooses not to specify the reason the criteria are not met for a specific disorder, then the category "unspecified bipolar and related disorder" is used. The unspecified category is also used when there is insufficient information to make a more specific diagnosis.

Demise of the Multiaxial System

The multiaxial diagnostic system, a familiar part of the diagnostic process, has been discontinued. Opinions about the value of the multiaxial system have sharply divided psychiatrists over the past three decades, many of whom considered it unhelpful and burdensome. Many simply ignored the system. The multiaxial diagnostic system was first included in DSM-III and involved the creation of five *axes*, each of which assessed a different domain of information, as reviewed in the Introduction to this book. The purpose of the multiaxial system, as pointed out in DSM-III (American Psychiatric Association 1980), was to ensure that "every case [was] assessed on each of several 'axes,' each of which refers to a different class of information" (p. 23). The multiaxial scheme continued mostly unchanged up through DSM-IV-TR.

One goal in developing the multiaxial diagnostic system was to ensure that personality disorders and mental retardation (now intellectual disability [intellectual developmental disorder]) were appropriately recognized and were not overlooked by clinicians whose attention was focused on the more florid disorders that were the presenting problems. Also, medical illnesses were known to be highly comorbid with psychiatric disorders and were often missed or ignored. The system also was meant to ensure that clinicians paid attention to psychosocial factors that may have played a role in the initiation or exacerbation of the psychiatric disorder. Axis V provided a way to rate a patient's global functioning, something often not captured in a diagnosis.

From the outset, critics disdained the artificial separation of Axis I and Axis II disorders, pointing to the lack of a fundamental distinction among these disorders, and decrying the fact that Axis II only further marginalized personality disorders and mental retardation. Third-party payers took advantage of this situation and often declined payment if Axis II disorders were coded as the primary problem. Furthermore, in many situations, there was no clear distinction between Axis I and Axis II (e.g., Axis I social anxiety disorder and Axis II avoidant personality disorder). Axis III was never used consistently, and often the distinction between Axis I and Axis III disorders was confusing or artificial. Axes IV and V were criticized as arbitrary and unreliable. Despite the fact that the Global Assessment of Functioning (GAF) Scale was derived from the widely used Global Assessment Scale (Endicott et al. 1976), there was little reason to believe the scale was used reliably by clinicians unfamiliar with rating scales. Further, GAF Scale scores were used arbitrarily by third-party payers to deny care when the score was either too high (meaning the patient was functioning too well to need treatment) or too low (meaning the patient was too ill to benefit from treatment). Finally, no other diagnostic system uses a multiaxial system, which placed DSM in conflict with the rest of medicine.

These concerns led the DSM-5 Task Force to end the multiaxial system. Clinicians no longer need to artificially separate conditions formerly listed on Axes I through III. Instead of Axis IV, clinicians can specify one or more of the V/Z code conditions ("Other Conditions That May Be a Focus of Clinical Attention"). In place of Axis V, clinicians can use the self-administered World Health Organization Disability Assessment Schedule 2.0, contained in Section III and briefly described in Chapter 20, "Assessment Measures," later in this book.

Overview of Changes to Each Diagnostic Category

This section provides an overview of the major changes made in each diagnostic category. They are described in more detail in Chapters 3–19 of this book.

Neurodevelopmental Disorders

Neurodevelopmental disorders is a reformulation of the DSM-IV chapter "Disorders Usually First Diagnosed in Infancy, Childhood, or Adolescence." There have been several major changes. First, the **mental retardation** diagnosis has been replaced by **intellectual disability (intellectual developmental disorder).** There is no longer a reliance on IQ as the determinant for inclusion in the category. Instead, subtypes are used to classify severity of the individual's disorder as mild, moderate, severe, or profound, while adaptive functioning is given greater emphasis. The arbitrary reliance on IQ was considered limiting because it does not take into account the different domains of functioning (social, conceptual/intellectual, practical) that allow a more nuanced view of the person with an intellectual deficit.

Another major change was the creation of an omnibus category, **autism spectrum disorder,** for pervasive developmental disorders. Consolidated into this category are the following DSM-IV diagnoses: **autistic disorder, Rett's disorder, childhood disintegrative disorder, Asperger's disorder,** and **pervasive developmental disorder not otherwise specified.** The change was prompted by research showing that the disorders were not as discrete and independent as once thought, and that clinicians had difficulty distinguishing them. All persons formerly diagnosed with each of these disorders should have their presentation covered by the new category, and its subtleties should be adequately addressed by the severity specifiers.

With **attention-deficit/hyperactivity disorder,** examples have been added to the criterion items to facilitate application across the life span, and the age at onset of inattentive or hyperactive-impulsive symptoms description has been changed from before age 7 years to before age 12 years. Subtypes have been replaced with presentation specifiers, and the comorbid diagnosis with autism spectrum disorder is now allowed.

The **communication disorders** are newly named from DSM-IV phonological disorder and stuttering, while **specific learning disorder** combines DSM-IV diagnoses of reading disorder, mathematics disorder, disorder of written expression, and learning disorder not otherwise specified.

Other changes to the class include moving **conduct disorder** to a new chapter, "Disruptive, Impulse-Control, and Conduct Disorders." **Elimination disorders (enuresis** and **encopresis)** now have their own chapter. The **feeding disorders (pica, rumination disorder,** and **avoidant/restrictive food intake disorder** [replacing and extending feeding disorder of infancy or early childhood]) have been combined with the eating disorders for a more comprehensive chapter titled "Feeding and Eating Disorders." **Separation anxiety disorder** and **selective mutism** have been moved to the chapter "Anxiety Disorders," while **reactive attachment disorder** has been moved to the chapter "Trauma- and Stressor-Related Disorders" because of its relationship with parental neglect.

Schizophrenia Spectrum and Other Psychotic Disorders

Disorders are now generally arranged along a gradient from least to most severe. **Schizotypal personality disorder** has been listed in this chapter because it is considered part of the schizophrenia spectrum, although the criteria and discussion remain in the chapter on personality disorders. The criteria for **delusional disorder** are mostly unchanged, but the adjective *nonbizarre* has been removed (Criterion A), and the somatic subtype has been edited to ensure that those who are delusional regarding a "physical defect" are more appropriately diagnosed with **body dysmorphic disorder** (moved to the chapter "Obsessive-Compulsive and Related Disorders"). **Shared psychotic disorder** has been dropped because the diagnosis was infrequently used and presentations that qualified for the diagnosis generally met criteria for another psychotic disorder. With **schizophrenia,** the special treatment given bizarre delusions and special types of hallucinations has been eliminated. Further, schizophrenia subtypes have been discontinued. Although these subtypes had a lengthy history, clinical utility and predictive validity were poor. **Schizoaffective disorder** has been changed to provide more guidance to clinicians regarding the total duration of mood symptoms. Instead of requiring that they last a "substantial portion of the total duration of the active and residual periods of the illness" (as in DSM-IV), DSM-5 requires that mood symptoms be present for the "majority of the total duration of the active and residual portions of the illness." Criteria for **catatonia** are described, and the disorder may be diagnosed with a specifier (for depressive, bipolar, and psychotic disorders, including schizophrenia), in the context of a known medical illness, or as an unspecified diagnosis.

Bipolar and Related Disorders

The mood disorders of DSM-IV have been divided into **bipolar and related disorders** and **depressive disorders,** each with its own chapter. Greater emphasis has been given to changes in activity and energy in the context of mania/hypomania, with the goal of improving the likelihood of early identification. Criteria for **bipolar I disorder, most recent episode mixed,** have been dropped, and instead the specifier "with mixed features" has been added that can be applied to episodes of mania/hypomania when depressive features are present and to episodes of depression in the context of both **major depressive disorder** and **bipolar disorder** lifetime diagnoses when features of hypomania are present. A "with anxious distress" specifier has also been delineated.

Depressive Disorders

Disruptive mood dysregulation disorder and **premenstrual dysphoric disorder** are new diagnoses. The former was added to address concerns about the potential overdiagnosis and overtreatment of bipolar disorder in children, whereas the latter was moved from DSM-IV Appendix B, "Criteria Sets and Axes Provided for Further Study," and given full disorder status. **Persistent depressive disorder** is new and replaces both DSM-IV dysthymia and chronic major depressive disorder. The coexistence within a major depressive episode of at least three manic symptoms insufficient to satisfy criteria for manic episode is now acknowledged by the specifier "with mixed features."

The exclusion applied to depressive symptoms lasting less than 2 months following the death of a loved one in DSM-IV (i.e., the so-called bereavement exclusion) has been omitted, and bereavement is now acknowledged as a severe psychosocial stressor that can precipitate a major depressive episode. The authors of DSM-5 felt that the evidence did not support the separation of loss of a loved one from other stressors in terms of its likelihood of precipitating a major depressive episode.

Anxiety Disorders

Obsessive-compulsive disorder, posttraumatic stress disorder, and **acute stress disorder** have been moved from the "Anxiety Disorders" chapter to other chapters. **Separation anxiety disorder** and **selective mutism** have been moved to "Anxiety Disorders" from "Disorders Usually First Diagnosed in Infancy, Childhood, or Adolescence." For **specific phobia** and **social anxiety disorder (social phobia)** diagnoses, changes include deletion of the requirement that individuals over age 18 years recognize their anxiety as excessive or unreasonable. Instead, the anxiety must be out of proportion to the actual danger or threat, after sociocultural contextual factors are taken into account. The 6-month duration, which was limited to individuals younger than 18 years, has been extended to all ages. This change is expected to minimize the overdiagnosis of transient fears. **Panic disorder** and **agoraphobia** have been unlinked; each is now its own diagnosis, and their co-occurrence is now coded as two diagnoses. **Panic attacks** can now be used as a specifier for any mental disorder and some medical conditions. The **specific phobia** types are now listed as specifiers. With **social anxiety disorder,** the "generalized" specifier has been dropped and replaced with a "performance only" specifier. Finally, for **separation anxiety disorder,** the wording has been changed to more adequately represent the expression of separation anxiety symptoms in adulthood.

Obsessive-Compulsive and Related Disorders

This new chapter brings together disorders related to **obsessive-compulsive disorder.** Other disorders include **body dysmorphic disorder, hoarding disorder, trichotillomania (hair-pulling disorder), excoriation (skin-picking) disorder, substance/medication-induced obsessive-compulsive and related disorder,** and **obsessive-compulsive and related disorder due to another medical condition. Body dysmorphic disorder** was moved from the somatoform disorders class. **Hoarding** was listed as a symptom of obsessive-compulsive personality disorder in DSM-IV (Criterion 5), but research evidence shows it to be a distinct condition. **Trichotillomania (hair-pulling disorder)** was moved from the DSM-IV chapter "Impulse-Control Disorders Not Elsewhere Classified," and **excoriation (skin-picking) disorder** is new. An insight specifier for **obsessive-compulsive disorder** allows clinicians to be more precise about the person's level of insight: good or fair, poor, and absent insight/delusional beliefs. Analogous specifiers have been included for **body dysmorphic disorder** and **hoarding disorder.** A tic-related specifier has been added for **obsessive-compulsive disorder** because the presence of a comorbid tic may have important clinical implications. A muscle dysmorphia specifier reflects the importance of making this distinction in individuals with **body dysmorphic disorder.**

Trauma- and Stressor-Related Disorders

This chapter brings together disorders that result from exposure to trauma or to a stressor and includes **reactive attachment disorder, disinhibited social engagement disorder, posttraumatic stress disorder, acute stress disorder,** and **adjustment disorders.** With **posttraumatic stress disorder,** the stressor criterion (Criterion A) is now more explicit with regard to events that qualify as "traumatic" experiences. Also, DSM-IV Criterion A2 (subjective reaction) has been eliminated. Whereas there were three major symptom clusters in DSM-IV—reexperiencing, avoidance/numbing, and arousal—there are now four because the avoidance/numbing cluster has been divided into two clusters: persistent avoidance and persistent negative alterations in cognitions and mood. This latter category, which retains most of the DSM-IV numbing symptoms, also includes new or reconceptualized symptoms such as persistent emotional states. The final cluster—marked alterations in arousal and reactivity—retains most of the DSM-IV arousal symptoms. It also includes irritable behavior and angry outbursts, and reckless or self-destructive behavior. Posttraumatic stress disorder is now developmentally sensitive in that diagnostic thresholds have been lowered for children and adolescents. Furthermore, separate criteria have been added for children age 6 years or younger with this disorder. Dissociative symptoms are no longer required (as in DSM-IV) for the diagnosis of **acute stress disorder. Adjustment disorders** now require distress *and/or* impairment for the diagnosis, rather than either distress *or* impairment.

Dissociative Disorders

Derealization is included in the name and symptom structure of what previously was called **depersonalization disorder** (now **depersonalization/derealization disorder**). **Dissociative fugue** has become a specifier of **dissociative amnesia** rather than a separate diagnosis. The criteria for **dissociative identity disorder** have been changed to indicate that symptoms of disruption of identity may be reported as well as observed, and that gaps in the recall of events may occur for everyday and not just traumatic events. Also, experiences of pathological possession in some cultures have been included as part of the description of identity disruption.

Somatic Symptom and Related Disorders

This chapter has been reorganized and renamed. Because of the considerable overlap among DSM-IV somatoform disorders, as well as a lack of clarity about their boundaries, the new diagnosis **somatic symptom disorder** replaces **somatization disorder, hypochondriasis, pain disorder,** and **undifferentiated somatoform disorder.** Most persons previously diagnosed with somatization disorder will now receive the diagnosis **somatic symptom disorder,** but only if they have excessive thoughts, feelings, and behaviors in addition to their somatic symptoms. People with high health anxiety but no somatic symptoms now receive a DSM-5 diagnosis of **illness anxiety disorder,** which is new. **Psychological factors affecting other medical conditions** is a new mental disorder in DSM-5, having formerly been listed in the DSM-IV chapter "Other Conditions That May Be a Focus of Clinical Attention." This condition and **factitious disorder** are placed with the somatic symptom and related disorders because somatic symptoms are predominant in each. Criteria for **conversion disorder (functional neurological symptom disorder)** have been changed to emphasize the essential importance of the neurological examination and in recognition that relevant psychological factors may not be demonstrable at the time of diagnosis. **Body dysmorphic disorder** was moved to the chapter "Obsessive-Compulsive and Related Disorders."

Feeding and Eating Disorders

Pica and **rumination disorder** have been moved from the DSM-IV chapter "Disorders Usually First Diagnosed in Infancy, Childhood, or Adolescence" because these two conditions involve disturbed feeding behaviors. Feeding disorder of infancy or early childhood has been renamed **avoidant/restrictive food intake disorder,** and the criteria have been expanded to allow the diagnosis to be used in adults who restrict their food intake but whose presentation does not meet criteria for one of the eating disorders. The criteria for **anorexia nervosa** are conceptually unchanged except that the requirement for amenorrhea has been eliminated. The wording of Criterion A has been clarified, and guidance regarding how to judge whether an individual is at or below a significantly low weight is provided in the text. Criterion B has been expanded to include not only expressed intense fear of weight gain or of becoming fat, but also persistent behavior that interferes with weight gain. The only change for **bulimia nervosa** is a reduction of the required minimum average frequency of binge eating and of inappropriate compensatory behavior from twice a week to once weekly. **Binge-eating disorder** is a new diagnosis; it was included in Appendix B of DSM-IV. The criteria have been changed such that the minimum average frequency of binge eating required is once weekly over the past 3 months, identical to the frequency criterion for bulimia nervosa.

Elimination Disorders

The elimination disorders **encopresis** and **enuresis** are conditions most often first diagnosed in childhood. They were previously included in the chapter "Disorders Usually First Diagnosed in Infancy, Childhood, or Adolescence," but they now have their own chapter.

Sleep-Wake Disorders

DSM-5 has removed **sleep disorder related to another medical disorder** and **sleep disorder related to a general medical condition,** and instead greater specification of coexisting conditions is provided for each sleep-wake disorder. The diagnosis primary insomnia has been renamed **insomnia disorder** to avoid the differentiation between primary and secondary insomnia. DSM-5 also distinguishes **narcolepsy** from other forms of hypersomnolence (**hypersomnolence disorder**). Throughout the class, pediatric and developmental criteria and text have been integrated where existing science and considerations of clinical utility support such integration. **Breathing-related sleep disorders** are divided into three relatively distinct disorders: **obstructive sleep apnea hypopnea, central sleep apnea,** and **sleep-related hypoventilation.** The types of **circadian rhythm sleep-wake disorders** are expanded to include **advanced sleep phase type** and **irregular sleep-wake type,** whereas **jet lag type** has been removed. **Rapid eye movement sleep behavior disorder** and **restless legs syndrome** are now independent disorders.

Sexual Dysfunctions

Gender-specific sexual dysfunctions have been added, and women's sexual desire and arousal disorders have been combined in one disorder, **female sexual interest/ arousal disorder.** All of the sexual dysfunctions (except **substance/medication-induced sexual dysfunction, other specified sexual dysfunction,** and **unspecified sexual dysfunction**), now require a minimum duration of approximately 6 months and more precise severity criteria. This will help distinguish transient sexual difficulties from more persistent sexual dysfunction. Vaginismus and dyspareunia have been merged into **genito-pelvic pain/penetration disorder,** because the two disorders were difficult to distinguish. **Sexual aversion disorder** was rarely used and has been deleted. There are now only two subtypes for sexual dysfunctions: **lifelong** versus **acquired,** and, for most of the dysfunctions, **generalized** versus **situational.**

Gender Dysphoria

Gender dysphoria is a new diagnostic class, having been moved from the DSM-IV chapter "Sexual and Gender Identity Disorders." The new name (from DSM-IV gender identity disorder) reflects a change by emphasizing the phenomenon of gender incongruence rather than cross-gender identification. For gender dysphoria in adolescents and adults, a more detailed and specific set of symptoms has been added. The previous Criterion A (cross-gender identification) and Criterion B (aversion toward one's gender) are merged because there was no supporting evidence to separate the two. The wording "the other sex" has been replaced by "the other gender." *Gender* instead of *sex* is used throughout because the concept *sex* is inadequate when referring to people with a disorder of sex development. In the child criteria, "strong desire to be of the other gender" replaces the previous "repeatedly stated desire to be…the other sex," to capture the situation of some children who, in a coercive environment, may not verbalize the desire to be of another gender. For **gender dysphoria in children,** Criterion A1 ("a strong desire to be of the other gender or an insistence that one is the other gender") is now necessary (but not sufficient), which makes the diagnosis more restrictive and conservative. Subtyping on the basis of sexual orientation has been removed because the distinction was no longer felt to be clinically useful. A posttransition specifier has been added to identify individuals who have undergone at least one cross-sex medical procedure or treatment regimen to support the new gender assignment.

Disruptive, Impulse-Control, and Conduct Disorders

This chapter brings together disorders characterized by problems with the self-regulation of emotions and behaviors and largely replaces the DSM-IV chapter "Impulse-Control Disorders Not Elsewhere Classified." The chapter includes **oppositional defiant disorder, intermittent explosive disorder, conduct disorder, antisocial personality disorder** (which is described in the chapter on personality disorders), **pyromania,** and **kleptomania.** DSM-5 has removed the exclusionary criterion of DSM-IV that allowed for the diagnosis of **oppositional defiant disorder** only if the criteria for **conduct disorder** were not met. The criteria for **conduct disorder** include a descriptive features specifier for individuals whose symptoms meet full criteria but who also present with limited prosocial emotions. The primary change in **intermittent explosive disorder** is the type of aggressive outbursts that should be considered: DSM-IV required physical aggression, whereas in DSM-5 verbal aggression or non-destructive/noninjurious physical aggression also meets the criterion. Furthermore, a minimum age of 6 years (or equivalent developmental level) is now required.

Substance-Related and Addictive Disorders

This chapter has been expanded to include **gambling disorder.** The inclusion of this disorder reflects increasing evidence that some behaviors, such as gambling, activate the same reward system as do substances and have effects similar to those of drugs of abuse. *Importantly, the distinction is no longer made between abuse and dependence.* These two former diagnoses are merged into a single **substance use disorder** because the distinction between abuse and dependence was often arbitrary, of limited utility, and frequently confusing. Within substance use disorders, the DSM-IV recurrent substance-related legal problems criterion has been deleted, and a new criterion—craving, or a strong desire or urge to use a substance—has been added. Severity of the disorder is specified on the basis of the number of symptoms present. **Caffeine withdrawal** and **cannabis withdrawal** are new, the former having been included in DSM-IV Appendix B, "Criteria Sets and Axes Provided for Further Study."

Neurocognitive Disorders

The DSM-IV diagnoses **dementia** and **amnestic disorder** are subsumed under the new diagnosis **major neurocognitive disorder,** although the word *dementia* is not precluded for use in the subtypes where it is standard. Notably, DSM-5 recognizes a less severe level of cognitive impairment, **mild neurocognitive disorder,** which is a new disorder that permits the diagnosis of less disabling syndromes that may nonetheless be the focus of concern and treatment. Diagnostic criteria are provided for both major and mild neurocognitive disorders, and these are followed by diagnostic criteria for the different etiological subtypes (e.g., major or mild neurocognitive disorder due to Alzheimer's disease).

Personality Disorders

The personality disorders class is no longer coded on Axis II since the multiaxial system has been discontinued. The criteria in Section II have not changed from those in DSM-IV. An alternative approach to the diagnosis of personality disorders was developed for DSM-5, and subsequently designated for further study, and can be found in Section III of the manual (see Chapter 21, "Alternative DSM-5 Model for Personality Disorders"). Other changes to the diagnostic class include moving **personality change due to another medical condition** from the DSM-IV chapter "Delirium, Dementia, Amnestic, and Other Cognitive Disorders."

Paraphilic Disorders

Paraphilic disorders were previously placed in the DSM-IV chapter "Sexual and Gender Identity Disorders." In DSM-5, course specifiers "in a controlled environment" and "in remission" have been added to the diagnostic criteria sets for all **paraphilic disorders** (except pedophilic disorder). The specifiers are added to indicate important changes in an individual's status. In DSM-5, paraphilias are not ipso facto mental disorders: "A *paraphilic disorder* is a paraphilia that is currently causing distress or impairment to the individual or a paraphilia whose satisfaction has entailed personal harm, or risk of harm, to others. A paraphilia is a necessary but not a sufficient condition for having a paraphilic disorder, and a paraphilia by itself does not necessarily justify or require clinical intervention" (American Psychiatric Association 2013, pp. 685–686).

Other Conditions

DSM-5 includes additional categories for important conditions and problems that are not considered mental disorders. These include **medication-induced movement disorders and other adverse effects of medication** (e.g., tardive dyskinesia, antidepressant discontinuation syndrome) and **other conditions that may be a focus of clinical attention** (V/Z code diagnoses). The latter have the potential to cause great distress to patients or their family members. Although common, the V/Z code diagnoses are underutilized.

Conditions for Further Study

Placing "Conditions for Further Study" in Section III of DSM-5 ensures that interested investigators are discussing and researching the same condition for possible inclusion in future DSM editions. Proposed criteria sets for conditions for further study were first included in DSM-III-R as a way to promote the collection of new data that could be used to validate new disorders. Few proposed conditions have achieved full disorder status, but this method allows the scientific process to determine the outcome. Some of the proposed conditions in DSM-5 are **attenuated psychosis syndrome, persistent complex bereavement disorder,** and **Internet gaming disorder.**

"Another Medical Condition"

Careful readers of DSM-5 will note that the wording has been changed regarding the universal exclusion of medical conditions in the differential diagnostic process. In DSM-IV, the wording used was "general medical condition." In DSM-5, the wording is "another medical condition." In both cases, before a diagnosis can be made, a medical condition must be excluded as a cause of the symptoms. The change of wording in DSM-5 helps to emphasize that psychiatric disorders are *medical* and that as part of the differential diagnostic process, clinicians need to exclude other medical conditions as the cause. This should help learners understand that mental disorders have physical causes.

KEY POINTS

- DSM-5 has three sections: I, which presents historical material and describes the manual's organization and use; II, which presents the criteria sets for the 19 major diagnostic classes, plus other mental disorders, medication-induced movement disorders and other adverse effects of medication, and other conditions that may be a focus of clinical attention (V/Z codes); and III, which provides assessment measures, a cultural formulation, an alternative DSM-5 model for personality disorders, and conditions for further study.

- The overall organization (metastructure) has changed to better reflect the relatedness of various classes. Chapters are arranged in a developmental life span fashion, starting with neurodevelopmental disorders and progressing through diagnostic areas more commonly diagnosed in adulthood.

- The multiaxial diagnostic scheme has been discontinued.

- The following diagnostic classes have been added in response to clinical need and scientific advances:
  - Trauma- and stressor-related disorders
  - Obsessive-compulsive and related disorders
  - Disruptive, impulse-control, and conduct disorders

- Several classes have been substantially revised, renamed, or reorganized:
  - Neurodevelopmental disorders
  - Somatic symptom and related disorders
  - Substance-related and addictive disorders
  - Neurocognitive disorders

- Several classes have been divided or consolidated:
  - Mood disorders were separated into two chapters: "Bipolar and Related Disorders" and "Depressive Disorders."
  - Sexual and gender identity disorders were separated into three chapters: "Sexual Dysfunctions," "Gender Dysphoria," and "Paraphilic Disorders."
  - Elimination disorders have been removed from the DSM-IV chapter "Disorders Usually First Diagnosed in Infancy, Childhood, or Adolescence" and now have their own chapter.
  - Feeding disorders have been removed from the DSM-IV chapter "Disorders Usually First Diagnosed in Infancy, Childhood, or Adolescence" and are combined with the eating disorders.

- Some disorders have been moved to different chapters:
  - Schizotypal personality disorder is now dually listed in "Schizophrenia Spectrum and Other Psychotic Disorders" and "Personality Disorders."
  - Antisocial personality disorder is now dually listed in "Disruptive, Impulse-Control, and Conduct Disorders" and "Personality Disorders."
  - Separation anxiety disorder and selective mutism have been moved from the DSM-IV chapter "Disorders Usually First Diagnosed in Infancy, Childhood, or Adolescence" to "Anxiety Disorders."
  - Body dysmorphic disorder and trichotillomania (hair-pulling disorder) have been moved to "Obsessive-Compulsive and Related Disorders."
  - Reactive attachment disorder has been moved to "Trauma- and Stressor-Related Disorders."
  - Pica and rumination disorder are now in "Feeding and Eating Disorders."
  - Gambling disorder is now in "Substance-Related and Addictive Disorders."
- The following new disorders have been added based on clinical need and scientific advances:
  - Avoidant/restrictive food intake disorder
  - Binge-eating disorder
  - Caffeine withdrawal
  - Cannabis withdrawal
  - Depersonalization/derealization disorder
  - Disruptive mood dysregulation disorder
  - Excoriation (skin-picking) disorder
  - Genito-pelvic pain/penetration disorder
  - Hoarding disorder
  - Illness anxiety disorder
  - Mild neurocognitive disorder
  - Premenstrual dysphoric disorder

CHAPTER 3

Neurodevelopmental Disorders

Intellectual Disabilities

	Intellectual Disability (Intellectual Developmental Disorder)
317 (F70)	Mild
318.0 (F71)	Moderate
318.1 (F72)	Severe
318.2 (F73)	Profound
315.8 (F88)	Global Developmental Delay
319 (F79)	Unspecified Intellectual Disability (Intellectual Developmental Disorder)

Communication Disorders

315.32 (F80.2)	Language Disorder
315.39 (F80.0)	Speech Sound Disorder
315.35 (F80.81)	Childhood-Onset Fluency Disorder (Stuttering)
315.39 (F80.89)	Social (Pragmatic) Communication Disorder
307.9 (F80.9)	Unspecified Communication Disorder

Autism Spectrum Disorder

299.00 (F84.0)	Autism Spectrum Disorder

Attention-Deficit/Hyperactivity Disorder

	Attention-Deficit/Hyperactivity Disorder
314.01 (F90.2)	Combined Presentation
314.00 (F90.0)	Predominantly Inattentive Presentation
314.01 (F90.1)	Predominantly Hyperactive/Impulsive Presentation
314.01 (F90.8)	Other Specified Attention-Deficit/Hyperactivity Disorder
314.01 (F90.9)	Unspecified Attention-Deficit/Hyperactivity Disorder

Specific Learning Disorder

	Specific Learning Disorder
315.00 (F81.0)	With Impairment in Reading
315.2 (F81.81)	With Impairment in Written Expression
315.1 (F81.2)	With Impairment in Mathematics

Motor Disorders
315.4 (F82)   Developmental Coordination Disorder
307.3 (F98.4)   Stereotypic Movement Disorder
                   Tic Disorders
307.23 (F95.2)   Tourette's Disorder
307.22 (F95.1)   Persistent (Chronic) Motor or Vocal Tic Disorder
307.21 (F95.0)   Provisional Tic Disorder
307.20 (F95.8)   Other Specified Tic Disorder
307.20 (F95.9)   Unspecified Tic Disorder

Other Neurodevelopmental Disorders
315.8 (F88)   Other Specified Neurodevelopmental Disorder
315.9 (F89)   Unspecified Neurodevelopmental Disorder

This chapter is a reformulation of the DSM-IV chapter "Disorders Usually First Diagnosed in Infancy, Childhood, or Adolescence." The category was first included in DSM-III, which brought together intellectual disorders (under the rubric "mental retardation"), attention-deficit/hyperactivity disorder, conduct disorder, anxiety disorders of childhood, eating disorders, stereotypic movement disorders, and several other disorders. This represented an advance over the earlier editions, in which intellectual disorders were recognized but other childhood-onset disorders received little attention. In DSM-I, childhood disorders were subsumed within the categories mental deficiency, transient situational personality disturbances, adjustment reaction of infancy, adjustment reaction of adolescence, and adjustment reaction of childhood. The latter included such conditions as habit disturbances (i.e., nail biting, thumb sucking, enuresis, masturbation, tantrums, tics, habit spasms, somnambulism, overactivity, and phobias).

The term *mental retardation* was introduced in DSM-II (American Psychiatric Association 1968) to replace *mental deficiency*, and the category was expanded to include the variety of physical, infectious, and other causes of retardation. The category "behavior disorders of childhood and adolescence" was introduced to group together disorders "occurring in childhood and adolescence that are more stable, internalized, and resistant to treatment than *Transient situational disturbances* but less so than the *Psychoses, Neuroses,* and *Personality disorders*" (pp. 49–50). Included were hyperkinetic reaction, withdrawing reaction, overanxious reaction, runaway reaction, unsocialized aggressive reaction, and group delinquent reaction.

The authors of DSM-III brought together the intellectual, behavioral, emotional, physical, and developmental disorders that have their origins in infancy, childhood, or adolescence. An important contribution was the introduction of the *pervasive developmental disorders,* whose most prominent example was infantile autism and which had been recognized in one form or another for decades but never formally classified. Also new was the multiaxial system, in which mental retardation was coded on Axis II. As discussed in Chapter 2, "Use of DSM-5 and Major Changes From DSM-IV," the multiaxial system has been omitted from DSM-5. DSM-III-R and DSM-IV made further changes (e.g., creating a new chapter for eating disorders), but the category of early developing disorders remained largely unchanged.

Several major changes are highlighted in this chapter. First, its placement as the first class in DSM-5 is a reflection of the manual's metastructure and its emphasis on the developmental trajectory of disorders. Second, the term *mental retardation* has been replaced by *intellectual disability (intellectual developmental disorder)*. The revised diagnosis will capture those individuals formerly diagnosed with mental retardation, but there is no longer a reliance on IQ as the determinant for inclusion in the category. Instead, subtypes are used to classify the individual as having a mild, moderate, severe, or profound level of severity. The Neurodevelopmental Disorders Work Group considered the term *mental retardation* to be stigmatizing and no longer helpful. Further, the term *intellectual disability* reflects wording adopted into U.S. law in 2010 (Rosa's Law), and the term is used in professional journals and has been endorsed by some patient advocacy groups. The term *intellectual developmental disorder* is consistent with language proposed for ICD-11. Another concern expressed by the work group was the arbitrary reliance on IQ as the defining feature of intellectual disability, because it does not take into account the different domains of functioning (social, conceptual/intellectual, practical) that allow a more nuanced view of the person with an intellectual deficit.

Another major change in DSM-5 was the decision to create an omnibus category, autism spectrum disorder, that consolidates the DSM-IV categories autistic disorder, Rett's disorder, childhood disintegrative disorder, Asperger's disorder, and pervasive developmental disorder not otherwise specified. The change was prompted by research showing that the disorders were not as discrete and independent as once believed, and that clinicians had difficulty distinguishing them. All persons formerly included in each of these disorders should fit the new category, and its subtleties should be adequately captured by severity specifiers. This change has been criticized by clinicians, their patients, and the patients' parents. Parents expressed concern that the revised categories might leave their child unable to qualify for educational or other benefits, whereas individuals with Asperger's disorder who had developed a sense of identity felt disenfranchised.

Other changes to the class include moving oppositional defiant disorder and conduct disorder to the chapter "Disruptive, Impulse-Control, and Conduct Disorders." Elimination disorders (encopresis and enuresis) now have their own chapter, and the feeding disorders (pica, rumination disorder, and feeding disorder of infancy or early childhood) have combined with the eating disorders for a more comprehensive chapter on disturbed eating behaviors. Separation anxiety disorder and selective mutism have been moved to the "Anxiety Disorders" chapter. Reactive attachment disorder has been moved to the "Trauma- and Stressor-Related Disorders" chapter because of its clear relationship with social neglect.

The communication disorders include language disorder, speech sound disorder, childhood-onset fluency disorder (stuttering), and social (pragmatic) communication disorder. The term *learning disorder* has been changed to *specific learning disorder,* and the previous types of learning disorders (reading disorder, mathematics disorder, and disorder of written expression) are no longer included. They are now presented as a single disorder with coded specifiers for deficits in reading, writing, and mathematics. Finally, other specified and unspecified attention-deficit/hyperactivity disorder diagnoses have been added (Table 3–1).

TABLE 3–1.	DSM-5 neurodevelopmental disorders

Intellectual disabilities
 Intellectual disability (intellectual developmental disorder)
 Global developmental delay
 Unspecified intellectual disability (intellectual developmental disorder)
Communication disorders
 Language disorder
 Speech sound disorder (previously phonological disorder)
 Childhood-onset fluency disorder (stuttering)
 Social (pragmatic) communication disorder
 Unspecified communication disorder
Autism spectrum disorder
Attention-deficit/hyperactivity disorder
 Attention-deficit/hyperactivity disorder
 Other specified attention-deficit/hyperactivity disorder
 Unspecified attention-deficit/hyperactivity disorder
Specific learning disorder
Motor disorders
 Developmental coordination disorder
 Stereotypic movement disorder
 Tourette's disorder
 Persistent (chronic) motor or vocal tic disorder
 Provisional tic disorder
 Other specified tic disorder
 Unspecified tic disorder
Other neurodevelopmental disorders
 Other specified neurodevelopmental disorder
 Unspecified neurodevelopmental disorder

INTELLECTUAL DISABILITIES

Intellectual Disability (Intellectual Developmental Disorder)

The essential features of intellectual disability (intellectual developmental disorder) are deficits in general mental abilities (Criterion A) and impairment in everyday adaptive functioning in comparison to the individual's age-, gender-, and socioculturally matched peers (Criterion B), with onset in the developmental period (Criterion C).

Individuals with intellectual developmental disorder may also have difficulties in managing their behavior and emotions, in interpersonal relationships, and in maintaining motivation in the learning process.

The diagnosis is based on both clinical assessment and standardized testing of intelligence. *Intelligence* has been defined as a general mental ability that involves reasoning, problem solving, planning, thinking abstractly, comprehending complex ideas, judgment, academic learning, and learning from experience, as applied in academic learning and social understanding, as well as practical understanding and manipulation of objects. IQ is typically measured using standardized tests. With such tests, the category of intellectual disorder is considered to be about two standard deviations or more below the population mean, including a margin for measurement error (generally +5 points). On tests with a standard deviation of 15 and a mean of 100, this involves a score of 65–75. Clinical training and judgment are needed to interpret test results and assess intellectual performance. Factors other than intellectual developmental disorders, such as associated cultural background, native language, and communication disorders, may limit performance.

Intellectual developmental disorders are common (about 1%–2% of the general population), more so in boys than girls. These disorders almost certainly result from a final common pathway produced by a variety of factors that injure the brain and affect its normal development. Down syndrome is the most common chromosomal cause of mental retardation, whereas fragile X syndrome is probably the most common heritable form of intellectual disability. Inborn errors of metabolism (e.g., Tay-Sachs disease) account for a small percentage of cases. Other factors include maternal malnutrition or substance abuse; exposure to mutagens such as radiation; maternal illnesses such as diabetes, toxemia, or rubella; and maternal abuse and neglect. Perinatal and early postnatal factors also may contribute, such as traumatic deliveries that cause brain injury or malnutrition during infancy or early childhood.

Several important changes have been made to this category in DSM-5. The name was changed to *intellectual disability (intellectual developmental disorder)* from *mental retardation*, a term that is no longer used internationally or in U.S. federal legislation. The name *intellectual developmental disorder* was chosen to be consistent with DSM-5 as a classification of *disorders* and to harmonize this diagnosis with the proposed ICD-11. In DSM-5, IQ test scores and standard deviations from the mean on those tests, which were included in the diagnostic criteria for mental retardation in DSM-IV, have been moved to the body of the text and are not contained within the criteria. However, DSM-5 continues to specify that standardized psychological testing must be included in the assessment of persons with these disorders, consistent with the American Association on Intellectual and Developmental Disabilities (AAIDD) definition, but that psychological testing should accompany clinical assessment. With the elimination of the multiaxial classification in DSM-5, intellectual developmental disorder is no longer relegated to Axis II. Removing IQ ranges from the criteria means that IQ can no longer be used inappropriately to define a person's overall ability. Cognitive profiles are generally more useful than a single Full Scale IQ score for describing intellectual abilities, and clinical training and judgment are required for interpretation of test results.

Both AAIDD and DSM-5 define *intellectual functioning* as a general mental ability that involves reasoning, problem solving, planning, abstract thinking, comprehension of complex ideas, judgment, academic learning, and learning from experience. In DSM-5, the definition is applied to reasoning in three contexts: academic learning (conceptual domain), social understanding (social domain), and practical understanding (practical domain). A wide range of skills are contained within the three domains of adaptive behavior. The conceptual domain involves skills used to solve problems in language, reading, writing, math, reasoning, knowledge, and memory, among others. The social domain involves awareness of others' experiences, empathy, interpersonal communication skills, friendship abilities, social judgment, and self-regulation. The practical domain involves self-management across life settings, including personal care, job responsibilities, money management, recreation, managing one's behavior, and organizing school and work tasks.

With the inclusion of severity levels (mild, moderate, severe, profound) in DSM-5, the focus is on adaptive functioning rather than IQ. Adaptive functioning deficits are now required. *Adaptive functioning* refers to how well an individual copes with the common tasks of everyday life in three general domains (i.e., conceptual, social, and practical), and how well an individual meets the standards of personal independence and social responsibility expected for someone of a similar age, sociocultural background, and community setting in one or more aspects of daily life activities, such as communication, social participation, functioning at school or work, or personal independence at home or in community settings. For an individual with intellectual disability (intellectual developmental disorder), adaptive behavior limitations result in the need for ongoing support in school, work, or independent life.

Diagnostic Criteria for Intellectual Disability (Intellectual Developmental Disorder)

Intellectual disability (intellectual developmental disorder) is a disorder with onset during the developmental period that includes both intellectual and adaptive functioning deficits in conceptual, social, and practical domains. The following three criteria must be met:

A. Deficits in intellectual functions, such as reasoning, problem solving, planning, abstract thinking, judgment, academic learning, and learning from experience, confirmed by both clinical assessment and individualized, standardized intelligence testing.

B. Deficits in adaptive functioning that result in failure to meet developmental and sociocultural standards for personal independence and social responsibility. Without ongoing support, the adaptive deficits limit functioning in one or more activities of daily life, such as communication, social participation, and independent living, across multiple environments, such as home, school, work, and community.

C. Onset of intellectual and adaptive deficits during the developmental period.

Note: The diagnostic term *intellectual disability* is the equivalent term for the ICD-11 diagnosis of *intellectual developmental disorders.* Although the term *intellectual disability* is used throughout this manual, both terms are used in the title to clarify relationships with other classification systems. Moreover, a federal statute in the United

States (Public Law 111-256, Rosa's Law) replaces the term *mental retardation* with *intellectual disability,* and research journals use the term *intellectual disability.* Thus, *intellectual disability* is the term in common use by medical, educational, and other professions and by the lay public and advocacy groups.

Specify current severity (see Table 1 in DSM-5, pp. 34–36):

> 317 (F70)   **Mild**
>
> 318.0 (F71) **Moderate**
>
> 318.1 (F72) **Severe**
>
> 318.2 (F73) **Profound**

Criteria A and B

Deficits in intellectual functions and impairment in adaptive functioning are both required in order for the diagnosis. For example, intellectual developmental disorder would not be recognized in an individual with an IQ score lower than 70 in the absence of significant deficits in adaptive functioning. The person must also have significant impairment in adaptive functioning (i.e., how well the person copes with the common tasks of everyday life and meets the standards of personal independence in social responsibility expected for someone of a similar age, sociocultural background, and community setting). Adaptive behavior reflects performance in academic, social, and practical settings in spite of intellectual ability, education, motivation, personality features, social and vocational opportunity, and coexisting medical conditions or mental disorders. When adaptive functioning is impaired, performance is limited and participation is restricted in one or more aspects of daily life activities, such as communication, social participation, and independent living, at home or in community settings.

Criterion C

Onset during the developmental period refers to recognition and diagnosis before adolescence.

Global Developmental Delay

Global developmental delay is a new diagnosis and allows the clinician to note cases in which evidence clearly indicates significant intellectual or general developmental delay or disability, but clinical severity level cannot be reliably assessed. The diagnosis is reserved for individuals under the age of 5 years.

Global Developmental Delay	315.8 (F88)

This diagnosis is reserved for individuals *under* the age of 5 years when the clinical severity level cannot be reliably assessed during early childhood. This category is diagnosed when an individual fails to meet expected developmental milestones in several areas of intellectual functioning, and applies to individuals who are unable to undergo systematic assessments of intellectual functioning, including children who are too young to participate in standardized testing. This category requires reassessment after a period of time.

Unspecified Intellectual Disability (Intellectual Developmental Disorder)

The diagnosis unspecified intellectual disability (intellectual developmental disorder) is used in persons over age 5 years who have significant intellectual or general developmental delay or disability and who cannot be reliably assessed.

Unspecified Intellectual Disability (Intellectual Disability Disorder)	319 (F79)

This category is reserved for individuals *over* the age of 5 years when assessment of the degree of intellectual disability (intellectual developmental disorder) by means of locally available procedures is rendered difficult or impossible because of associated sensory or physical impairments, as in blindness or prelingual deafness; locomotor disability; or presence of severe problem behaviors or co-occurring mental disorder. This category should only be used in exceptional circumstances and requires reassessment after a period of time.

COMMUNICATION DISORDERS

The communication disorders are characterized by difficulties in language, speech, and communication. While not traditionally considered mental disorders, they can cause distress and impair functioning in important life domains and are important for purposes of differential diagnosis. The communication disorders include language disorder (which combines the DSM-IV categories expressive and mixed receptive-expressive language disorders), speech sound disorder (previously phonological disorder), and childhood-onset fluency disorder (previously stuttering). Social (pragmatic) communication disorder is a newly defined condition involving persistent difficulties in the social uses of verbal and nonverbal communication. DSM-IV *learning disorder* has been changed to *specific learning disorder,* and the previous types of learning disorders (reading disorder, mathematics disorder, and disorder of written expression) are no longer included. Instead, specifiers are used to describe the individual's impairment.

Language Disorder

The essential feature of language disorder is a persistent disturbance in the acquisition and use of spoken language, written language, or sign language that is due to deficits in comprehension or production (Criterion A). Language abilities are substantially and quantifiably below those expected for age, significantly interfering with socialization, effective communication, academic achievement, or occupational performance (Criterion B). Regional variations in language (e.g., dialects) do not constitute a language disorder. Symptom onset is in the early developmental period (Criterion C). Other disorders (e.g., intellectual disability [intellectual developmental disorder], hearing impairment, motor dysfunction) must be ruled out as a cause of the language difficulties (Criterion D).

Diagnostic Criteria for Language Disorder   315.32 (F80.2)

A. Persistent difficulties in the acquisition and use of language across modalities (i.e., spoken, written, sign language, or other) due to deficits in comprehension or production that include the following:

1. Reduced vocabulary (word knowledge and use).
2. Limited sentence structure (ability to put words and word endings together to form sentences based on the rules of grammar and morphology).
3. Impairments in discourse (ability to use vocabulary and connect sentences to explain or describe a topic or series of events or have a conversation).

B. Language abilities are substantially and quantifiably below those expected for age, resulting in functional limitations in effective communication, social participation, academic achievement, or occupational performance, individually or in any combination.

C. Onset of symptoms is in the early developmental period.

D. The difficulties are not attributable to hearing or other sensory impairment, motor dysfunction, or another medical or neurological condition and are not better explained by intellectual disability (intellectual developmental disorder) or global developmental delay.

Speech Sound Disorder

Speech sound disorder is characterized by persistent difficulties in speech production that are developmentally inappropriate and involve articulation, fluency, and voice production in its various aspects. This disorder often coexists with language disorder, intellectual disability (intellectual developmental disorder), and neurological conditions such as Landau-Kleffner syndrome.

Diagnostic Criteria for Speech Sound Disorder   315.39 (F80.0)

A. Persistent difficulty with speech sound production that interferes with speech intelligibility or prevents verbal communication of messages.

B. The disturbance causes limitations in effective communication that interfere with social participation, academic achievement, or occupational performance, individually or in any combination.

C. Onset of symptoms is in the early developmental period.

D. The difficulties are not attributable to congenital or acquired conditions, such as cerebral palsy, cleft palate, deafness or hearing loss, traumatic brain injury, or other medical or neurological conditions.

Childhood-Onset Fluency Disorder (Stuttering)

Childhood-onset fluency disorder (stuttering) is characterized by a disturbance in the normal fluency and time patterning of speech that is inappropriate for age. The disturbance can manifest as frequent repetitions or prolongations of sounds or syllables or other types of speech dysfluencies, such as sound and syllable repetitions, broken words (e.g., pauses within a word), audible or silent blocking (e.g., filled or unfilled pauses in speech), or circumlocutions (e.g., word substitutions to avoid problematic words). The disturbance interferes with academic or occupational achievement or with social communication. Stuttering can also cause humiliation and embarrassment and lead individuals to avoid situations that may be associated with speech, such as using a telephone. The disorder usually occurs by age 6 years, although most recover from the dysfluency. Stress and anxiety can exacerbate the disorder.

Diagnostic Criteria for Childhood-Onset Fluency Disorder (Stuttering)   315.35 (F80.81)

A. Disturbances in the normal fluency and time patterning of speech that are inappropriate for the individual's age and language skills, persist over time, and are characterized by frequent and marked occurrences of one (or more) of the following:

   1. Sound and syllable repetitions.
   2. Sound prolongations of consonants as well as vowels.
   3. Broken words (e.g., pauses within a word).
   4. Audible or silent blocking (filled or unfilled pauses in speech).
   5. Circumlocutions (word substitutions to avoid problematic words).
   6. Words produced with an excess of physical tension.
   7. Monosyllabic whole-word repetitions (e.g., "I-I-I-I see him").

B. The disturbance causes anxiety about speaking or limitations in effective communication, social participation, or academic or occupational performance, individually or in any combination.

C. The onset of symptoms is in the early developmental period. (**Note:** Later-onset cases are diagnosed as 307.0 [F98.5] adult-onset fluency disorder.)

D. The disturbance is not attributable to a speech-motor or sensory deficit, dysfluency associated with neurological insult (e.g., stroke, tumor, trauma), or another medical condition and is not better explained by another mental disorder.

Social (Pragmatic) Communication Disorder

Social (pragmatic) communication disorder is new to DSM-5. This is a disorder of children who have difficulty with the pragmatic aspects of social communication, including comprehension, formulation, and discourse comprehension, affecting idiomatic and nonliteral language inferences in narrative texts and conversation (Bishop 2000). This disorder is unexpected given a child's relatively intact vocabulary and sentence abilities. Research suggests that such children exhibit socially inappropriate behavior but do not have autism spectrum disorder (Bishop and Norbury 2002). Thus, the pragmatic difficulties they experience constitute a fundamentally different form of language impairment. Children with this condition display common difficulties in social communication but not repetitive behaviors or restricted interests consistent with autism spectrum disorder. Autism spectrum disorder needs to be ruled out, as do attention-deficit/hyperactivity disorder, social anxiety disorder, and intellectual disability (intellectual developmental disorder).

Diagnostic Criteria for Social (Pragmatic) Communication Disorder   315.39 (F80.89)

A. Persistent difficulties in the social use of verbal and nonverbal communication as manifested by all of the following:

1. Deficits in using communication for social purposes, such as greeting and sharing information, in a manner that is appropriate for the social context.
2. Impairment of the ability to change communication to match context or the needs of the listener, such as speaking differently in a classroom than on a playground, talking differently to a child than to an adult, and avoiding use of overly formal language.
3. Difficulties following rules for conversation and storytelling, such as taking turns in conversation, rephrasing when misunderstood, and knowing how to use verbal and nonverbal signals to regulate interaction.
4. Difficulties understanding what is not explicitly stated (e.g., making inferences) and nonliteral or ambiguous meanings of language (e.g., idioms, humor, metaphors, multiple meanings that depend on the context for interpretation).

B. The deficits result in functional limitations in effective communication, social participation, social relationships, academic achievement, or occupational performance, individually or in combination.

C. The onset of the symptoms is in the early developmental period (but deficits may not become fully manifest until social communication demands exceed limited capacities).

D. The symptoms are not attributable to another medical or neurological condition or to low abilities in the domains of word structure and grammar, and are not better explained by autism spectrum disorder, intellectual disability (intellectual developmental disorder), global developmental delay, or another mental disorder.

Unspecified Communication Disorder

Unspecified Communication Disorder	307.9 (F80.9)

This category applies to presentations in which symptoms characteristic of communication disorder that cause clinically significant distress or impairment in social, occupational, or other important areas of functioning predominate but do not meet the full criteria for communication disorder or for any of the disorders in the neurodevelopmental disorders diagnostic class. The unspecified communication disorder category is used in situations in which the clinician chooses *not* to specify the reason that the criteria are not met for communication disorder or for a specific neurodevelopmental disorder, and includes presentations in which there is insufficient information to make a more specific diagnosis.

AUTISM SPECTRUM DISORDER

Autism Spectrum Disorder

Autism was described by Leo Kanner (1948) as a syndrome of social communication deficits combined with repetitive and stereotyped behaviors and as having an onset in early childhood. In DSM-III, the disorder was called "infantile autism" and was listed as one of several pervasive developmental disorders. In DSM-III-R and DSM-IV, other related disorders were included in the category, including Rett's disorder, childhood disintegrative disorder, Asperger's disorder, and pervasive developmental disorder not otherwise specified. DSM-5 now replaces all of these diagnoses with a single diagnosis, autism spectrum disorder. Autism spectrum disorder is considered a neurodevelopmental disorder. Although present from infancy or early childhood, the disorder may not be detected until later because of minimal social demands and support from parents or caregivers in early years.

For DSM-5, the diagnosis has been reconceptualized as a "spectrum" that includes all of the various disorders previously distinguished in DSM-IV. The essential features of autism spectrum disorder are persistent deficits in reciprocal social communication, in nonverbal communicative behaviors used for social interaction, and in developing, managing, and understanding relationships (Criterion A) and restricted, repetitive patterns of behavior, interests, or activities (Criterion B). Distinctions among the pervasive developmental disorders were inconsistent over time, variable across sites, and often associated with severity, language level, or intelligence rather than features of the disorder. The Neurodevelopmental Disorders Work Group considered various options and concluded that because autism is defined by a common set of behaviors, it is best represented as a single diagnostic category adapted to the individual's clinical presentation by inclusion of clinical specifiers (e.g., severity, intellectual impairment, language impairment) and associated features (e.g., known genetic disorders, epilepsy, intellectual disability). For example, an individual formerly diagnosed with Asperger's disorder can now be diagnosed with autism spectrum disorder, without intellectual impairment and without accompanying structural language impairment.

The work group made other changes to the category. The three domains in DSM-IV (social interaction, communication, repetitive/stereotyped behaviors) have become two: 1) social-communication and social-interactive deficits and 2) restricted, repetitive behaviors, interests, and activities. Research shows that deficits in communication and social behaviors are inseparable and best considered as a single set of symptoms with contextual and environmental specificities. Also, delays in language acquisition are neither unique nor universal, and are more accurately considered as a factor that influences the clinical symptoms of autism spectrum disorder rather than as a feature that defines the diagnosis. Requiring that both criteria be met improves specificity of diagnosis without impairing sensitivity.

Diagnostic Criteria for Autism Spectrum Disorder   299.00 (F84.0)

A. Persistent deficits in social communication and social interaction across multiple contexts, as manifested by the following, currently or by history (examples are illustrative, not exhaustive; see DSM-5 text):

1. Deficits in social-emotional reciprocity, ranging, for example, from abnormal social approach and failure of normal back-and-forth conversation; to reduced sharing of interests, emotions, or affect; to failure to initiate or respond to social interactions.

2. Deficits in nonverbal communicative behaviors used for social interaction, ranging, for example, from poorly integrated verbal and nonverbal communication; to abnormalities in eye contact and body language or deficits in understanding and use of gestures; to a total lack of facial expressions and nonverbal communication.

3. Deficits in developing, maintaining, and understanding relationships, ranging, for example, from difficulties adjusting behavior to suit various social contexts; to difficulties in sharing imaginative play or in making friends; to absence of interest in peers.

Specify current severity:
Severity is based on social communication impairments and restricted, repetitive patterns of behavior (see Table 2 in DSM-5, p. 52).

B. Restricted, repetitive patterns of behavior, interests, or activities, as manifested by at least two of the following, currently or by history (examples are illustrative, not exhaustive; see DSM-5 text):

1. Stereotyped or repetitive motor movements, use of objects, or speech (e.g., simple motor stereotypies, lining up toys or flipping objects, echolalia, idiosyncratic phrases).

2. Insistence on sameness, inflexible adherence to routines, or ritualized patterns of verbal or nonverbal behavior (e.g., extreme distress at small changes, difficulties with transitions, rigid thinking patterns, greeting rituals, need to take same route or eat same food every day).

3. Highly restricted, fixated interests that are abnormal in intensity or focus (e.g., strong attachment to or preoccupation with unusual objects, excessively circumscribed or perseverative interests).

4. Hyper- or hyporeactivity to sensory input or unusual interest in sensory aspects of the environment (e.g., apparent indifference to pain/temperature, adverse response to specific sounds or textures, excessive smelling or touching of objects, visual fascination with lights or movement).

Specify current severity:

Severity is based on social communication impairments and restricted, repetitive patterns of behavior (see Table 2 in DSM-5, p. 52).

C. Symptoms must be present in the early developmental period (but may not become fully manifest until social demands exceed limited capacities, or may be masked by learned strategies in later life).

D. Symptoms cause clinically significant impairment in social, occupational, or other important areas of current functioning.

E. These disturbances are not better explained by intellectual disability (intellectual developmental disorder) or global developmental delay. Intellectual disability and autism spectrum disorder frequently co-occur; to make comorbid diagnoses of autism spectrum disorder and intellectual disability, social communication should be below that expected for general developmental level.

Note: Individuals with a well-established DSM-IV diagnosis of autistic disorder, Asperger's disorder, or pervasive developmental disorder not otherwise specified should be given the diagnosis of autism spectrum disorder. Individuals who have marked deficits in social communication, but whose symptoms do not otherwise meet criteria for autism spectrum disorder, should be evaluated for social (pragmatic) communication disorder.

Specify if:

With or without accompanying intellectual impairment

With or without accompanying language impairment

Associated with a known medical or genetic condition or environmental factor (**Coding note:** Use additional code to identify the associated medical or genetic condition.)

Associated with another neurodevelopmental, mental, or behavioral disorder (**Coding note:** Use additional code[s] to identify the associated neurodevelopmental, mental, or behavioral disorder[s].)

With catatonia (refer to the criteria for catatonia associated with another mental disorder, DSM-5, pp. 119–120, for definition) (**Coding note:** Use additional code 293.89 [F06.1] catatonia associated with autism spectrum disorder to indicate the presence of the comorbid catatonia.)

Criterion A

The essential feature of autism spectrum disorder is persistent impairment in reciprocal social communication and social interaction across multiple contexts. This
symptom is pervasive and sustained. Manifestations depend in part on age, intellectual level, and language ability, as well as on individual differences in personality and
other factors, such as treatment history and current support. For many with this disorder, language will be affected (e.g., speech may be absent or its onset delayed).
Communication may be impaired even when formal skills, including vocabulary and
grammar, are intact. Deficits in social-emotional reciprocity are clearly evident, and
young children with the disorder may show little or no initiation of social interaction
and no sharing of emotions. An early feature is poor or absent eye contact.

Criterion B

This criterion requires the child to have restricted, repetitive patterns of behavior, interests, or activities. For example, the child may prefer rigid routines and insist that
things be done in the same way. The child may have a narrow and intense focus on
particular topics, such as train schedules. The child may exhibit stereotyped or repetitive behaviors, such as hand flapping or finger flicking. Excessive adherence to routines and restricted patterns of behavior may be manifested as resistance to change or
ritualized patterns of verbal or nonverbal behavior, such as repetitive questioning.
Highly restricted, fixated interests tend to be abnormal in intensity and/or focus (e.g.,
preoccupation with vacuum cleaners). Interests and routines may relate to high or
low levels of reactivity to sensory input, as shown by extreme responses to specific
sounds or textures, excessive smelling or touching of objects, fascination with lights
or spinning objects, and sometimes apparent indifference to pain, heat, or cold.

Criteria C, D, and E

Symptoms begin early in life and limit or cause impairments in social, occupational,
or other critical areas of functioning. The stage at which functional impairment becomes apparent varies by individual and his or her environment. Core diagnostic features are evident in the developmental period, but intervention, compensation, and
current supports may mask difficulties at later stages of the disorder.

Autism spectrum disorder needs to be differentiated from intellectual disability
(intellectual developmental disorder) and global developmental delay, because the
latter conditions can be associated with communication difficulties. The distinction may
be particularly difficult in young children. The determination may rest on whether
the communication and interaction are significantly impaired relative to the developmental level of the individual's nonverbal skills, in which case the diagnosis of autism
spectrum disorder is likely.

Children with an autism spectrum disorder may have relatively obvious problems early in life. Within the first 3–6 months, parents may note that their child does
not develop a normal pattern of smiling or responding to cuddling. The first clear
sign of abnormality is usually in the area of language. As the child grows older, he or

she does not progress through developmental milestones, such as learning to say words and speak sentences, and seems aloof, withdrawn, and detached. Instead of developing patterns of relating warmly to his or her parents, the child may instead engage in self-stimulating behavior, such as rocking or head banging. Eventually, it becomes clear that something is severely wrong, and the features of the disorder continue to become more apparent over time as these children fail to develop normal verbal and interpersonal communication.

In young children, lack of social and communication abilities may hamper learning, especially that associated with social interactions. In the home, insistence on routines and aversion to change, as well as sensory sensitivities, may interfere with eating and sleeping and make routine care (e.g., haircuts, dental appointments) extremely difficult. In adulthood, rigidity and difficulty with novelty may limit independence even in highly intelligent people with autism spectrum disorder.

ATTENTION-DEFICIT/HYPERACTIVITY DISORDER

Attention-Deficit/Hyperactivity Disorder

Attention-deficit/hyperactivity disorder (ADHD) was first acknowledged in DSM-II as a hyperkinetic reaction of childhood (or adolescence), characterized by overactivity, restlessness, distractibility, and short attention span. DSM-III provided operational diagnostic criteria and emphasized deficits in attention, impulsivity, and hyperactivity, but included a category for those without hyperactivity. In DSM-IV, the criteria were revised to focus on two broad groups of symptoms: 1) difficulty focusing and maintaining attention and 2) hyperactivity and impulsivity. The criteria required that at least 12 of 18 symptoms (6 from the domain of attention and 6 from the domain of hyperactivity-impulsivity) be present for at least 6 months, with onset before age 7 years. Subtypes could be used to specify whether the presentation was predominantly inattentive, predominantly hyperactive-impulsive, or mixed. Several changes have been made to the diagnosis in DSM-5. First, age at onset has been changed from onset of impairing symptoms by age 7 to onset of symptoms by age 12. Research has shown that estimates of onset by age 7 years are unreliable and that few clinical differences exist between children identified as having onset by age 7 versus those with later onset in terms of course, severity, outcome, or treatment response (Applegate et al. 1997). Subtypes have been replaced with presentation specifiers that map directly to the prior subtypes. Examples used in the criterion items have been changed to accommodate a life span relevance of each symptom and to improve clarity (Matte et al. 2012). Symptom threshold for adults age 17 years or older was reduced to five (from six for those younger than 17 years) both for inattention and for hyperactivity and impulsivity. The change was prompted by research showing that individuals tend to have fewer symptoms of ADHD in adulthood than in childhood. Finally, in response to data showing that ADHD and autism spectrum disorder can coexist, a comorbid diagnosis with autism spectrum disorder is now allowed. This change brings the ADHD criteria into harmony with the revised criteria for autism spectrum disorder.

Diagnostic Criteria for Attention-Deficit/Hyperactivity Disorder

A. A persistent pattern of inattention and/or hyperactivity-impulsivity that interferes with functioning or development, as characterized by (1) and/or (2):

1. **Inattention:** Six (or more) of the following symptoms have persisted for at least 6 months to a degree that is inconsistent with developmental level and that negatively impacts directly on social and academic/occupational activities:

   Note: The symptoms are not solely a manifestation of oppositional behavior, defiance, hostility, or failure to understand tasks or instructions. For older adolescents and adults (age 17 and older), at least five symptoms are required.

   a. Often fails to give close attention to details or makes careless mistakes in schoolwork, at work, or during other activities (e.g., overlooks or misses details, work is inaccurate).

   b. Often has difficulty sustaining attention in tasks or play activities (e.g., has difficulty remaining focused during lectures, conversations, or lengthy reading).

   c. Often does not seem to listen when spoken to directly (e.g., mind seems elsewhere, even in the absence of any obvious distraction).

   d. Often does not follow through on instructions and fails to finish schoolwork, chores, or duties in the workplace (e.g., starts tasks but quickly loses focus and is easily sidetracked).

   e. Often has difficulty organizing tasks and activities (e.g., difficulty managing sequential tasks; difficulty keeping materials and belongings in order; messy, disorganized work; has poor time management; fails to meet deadlines).

   f. Often avoids, dislikes, or is reluctant to engage in tasks that require sustained mental effort (e.g., schoolwork or homework; for older adolescents and adults, preparing reports, completing forms, reviewing lengthy papers).

   g. Often loses things necessary for tasks or activities (e.g., school materials, pencils, books, tools, wallets, keys, paperwork, eyeglasses, mobile telephones).

   h. Is often easily distracted by extraneous stimuli (for older adolescents and adults, may include unrelated thoughts).

   i. Is often forgetful in daily activities (e.g., doing chores, running errands; for older adolescents and adults, returning calls, paying bills, keeping appointments).

2. **Hyperactivity and impulsivity:** Six (or more) of the following symptoms have persisted for at least 6 months to a degree that is inconsistent with developmental level and that negatively impacts directly on social and academic/occupational activities:

   Note: The symptoms are not solely a manifestation of oppositional behavior, defiance, hostility, or a failure to understand tasks or instructions. For older adolescents and adults (age 17 and older), at least five symptoms are required.

   a. Often fidgets with or taps hands or feet or squirms in seat.

   b. Often leaves seat in situations when remaining seated is expected (e.g., leaves his or her place in the classroom, in the office or other workplace, or in other situations that require remaining in place).

    c. Often runs about or climbs in situations where it is inappropriate. (**Note:** In adolescents or adults, may be limited to feeling restless.)

    d. Often unable to play or engage in leisure activities quietly.

    e. Is often "on the go," acting as if "driven by a motor" (e.g., is unable to be or uncomfortable being still for extended time, as in restaurants, meetings; may be experienced by others as being restless or difficult to keep up with).

    f. Often talks excessively.

    g. Often blurts out an answer before a question has been completed (e.g., completes people's sentences; cannot wait for turn in conversation).

    h. Often has difficulty waiting his or her turn (e.g., while waiting in line).

    i. Often interrupts or intrudes on others (e.g., butts into conversations, games, or activities; may start using other people's things without asking or receiving permission; for adolescents and adults, may intrude into or take over what others are doing).

B. Several inattentive or hyperactive-impulsive symptoms were present prior to age 12 years.

C. Several inattentive or hyperactive-impulsive symptoms are present in two or more settings (e.g., at home, school, or work; with friends or relatives; in other activities).

D. There is clear evidence that the symptoms interfere with, or reduce the quality of, social, academic, or occupational functioning.

E. The symptoms do not occur exclusively during the course of schizophrenia or another psychotic disorder and are not better explained by another mental disorder (e.g., mood disorder, anxiety disorder, dissociative disorder, personality disorder, substance intoxication or withdrawal).

Specify whether:

314.01 (F90.2) Combined presentation: If both Criterion A1 (inattention) and Criterion A2 (hyperactivity-impulsivity) are met for the past 6 months.

314.00 (F90.0) Predominantly inattentive presentation: If Criterion A1 (inattention) is met but Criterion A2 (hyperactivity-impulsivity) is not met for the past 6 months.

314.01 (F90.1) Predominantly hyperactive/impulsive presentation: If Criterion A2 (hyperactivity-impulsivity) is met and Criterion A1 (inattention) is not met for the past 6 months.

Specify if:

In partial remission: When full criteria were previously met, fewer than the full criteria have been met for the past 6 months, and the symptoms still result in impairment in social, academic, or occupational functioning.

Specify current severity:

Mild: Few, if any, symptoms in excess of those required to make the diagnosis are present, and symptoms result in no more than minor impairments in social or occupational functioning.

Moderate: Symptoms or functional impairment between "mild" and "severe" are present.

Severe: Many symptoms in excess of those required to make the diagnosis, or several symptoms that are particularly severe, are present, or the symptoms result in marked impairment in social or occupational functioning.

Criterion A

The essential feature of ADHD is a persistent pattern of inattention (Criterion A1) and/or hyperactivity-impulsivity (Criterion A2) sufficiently severe that it interferes with functioning or development. *Inattention* refers to problems with the following: staying on task, being persistent, focusing, being organized, planning, and following through. *Hyperactivity* is manifested as excessive motor activity, such as running about or climbing, or excessive fidgeting, tapping, or squirming, in situations where it is not appropriate. Hyperactivity may not be continuous, but overactivity may occur very frequently.

Criterion B

This item requires that several symptoms of ADHD have an onset before age 12 years because it is difficult to reliably establish precise childhood onset retrospectively (Kieling et al. 2010). For adolescents or young adults, a longitudinal perspective should indicate that the condition had its roots during childhood and is not of recent onset.

Criterion C

This item requires that several symptoms of ADHD appear in two or more settings. Although potentially costly and time consuming, and while not a requirement for diagnosis, the text recommends consulting informants (e.g., parents, teachers, employers) who have seen the individual across various settings. For children, teacher rating scales can provide valuable and adjunctive information as to expectations for normative patterns of behavior.

Criterion D

In children, ADHD can impair school performance. In adults, worse occupational performance and attendance, higher probability of unemployment, interpersonal conflict, and reduced self-esteem are common. Children with ADHD are about twice as likely as children without a disorder to experience an injury requiring medical attention, presumably due to their impulsivity and inattention. Inadequate self-application to tasks that require sustained effort is often interpreted by others as laziness, a poor sense of responsibility, and oppositional behavior. Family relationships are often characterized by resentment and antagonism, especially because variability in the person's symptomatic status often leads others to believe that the troublesome behavior is willful.

Criterion E

Other mental disorders need to be ruled out as a cause for the symptoms. ADHD shares symptoms of inattention with both anxiety disorders and major depression. Individuals with ADHD are inattentive due to daydreaming or their attraction to external stimuli or new activities. ADHD should be readily distinguished from the inattention due to worry, rumination, and internal stimuli seen with anxiety disorders or major depression. Young people with bipolar disorder may have increased activity, but the activity is episodic, varying with mood and goal-directed behavior. ADHD should not be confused with mania. Disruptive mood dysregulation disorder is characterized by consistent moodiness, irritability, and intolerance of frustration, but impulsivity and disorganized attention are not part of the condition.

In some adults, distinguishing ADHD from various personality disorders (e.g., antisocial, borderline, narcissistic) may be difficult. These disorders tend to share the features of disorganization, social intrusiveness, emotional dysregulation, and cognitive dysregulation. However, ADHD is not characterized by fears of abandonment, self-injury, extreme ambivalence, or other features of severe personality disorders. Lastly, ADHD is not diagnosed if the symptoms of inattention and hyperactivity occur exclusively during the course of a psychotic disorder.

Other Specified Attention-Deficit/ Hyperactivity Disorder and Unspecified Attention-Deficit/Hyperactivity Disorder

Other specified ADHD and unspecified ADHD are residual categories for those presentations of ADHD that do not fit within the more specific diagnostic category.

Other Specified Attention-Deficit/Hyperactivity Disorder   314.01 (F90.8)

This category applies to presentations in which symptoms characteristic of attention-deficit/hyperactivity disorder that cause clinically significant distress or impairment in social, occupational or other important areas of functioning predominate but do not meet the full criteria for attention-deficit/hyperactivity disorder or any of the disorders in the neurodevelopmental disorders diagnostic class. The other specified attention-deficit/hyperactivity disorder category is used in situations in which the clinician chooses to communicate the specific reason that the presentation does not meet the criteria for attention-deficit/hyperactivity disorder or any specific neurodevelopmental disorder. This is done by recording "other specified attention-deficit/hyperactivity disorder" followed by the specific reason (e.g., "with insufficient inattention symptoms").

Unspecified Attention-Deficit/Hyperactivity Disorder 314.01 (F90.9)

This category applies to presentations in which symptoms characteristic of attention-deficit/hyperactivity disorder that cause clinically significant distress or impairment in social, occupational, or other important areas of functioning predominate but do not meet the full criteria for attention-deficit/hyperactivity disorder or any of the disorders in the neurodevelopmental disorders diagnostic class. The unspecified attention-deficit/hyperactivity disorder category is used in situations in which the clinician chooses *not* to specify the reason that the criteria are not met for attention-deficit/hyperactivity disorder or for a specific neurodevelopmental disorder, and includes presentations in which there is insufficient information to make a more specific diagnosis.

SPECIFIC LEARNING DISORDER

Specific Learning Disorder

Specific learning disorder is characterized by persistent difficulties in learning and using academic skills, with onset during the developmental period. Specific learning disorder is a clinical diagnosis based on a synthesis of the person's medical, developmental, educational, and family history; the history of the learning difficulty and its manifestation; the impact on academic, occupational, or social functioning; observations as the person reads or solves age- or grade-level material; school reports; and scores from individual standardized educational or neuropsychological testing. This diagnosis replaces reading disorder, mathematics disorder, and disorder of written expression. Instead, these disorders are now included in a single diagnosis with coded specifiers for impairments in reading, written expression, and mathematics. The reason for the change was widespread concern among clinicians and researchers that DSM-IV's three independent learning disorders lacked validity. This change is particularly important given that most children with a specific learning disorder manifest deficits in more than one area. With the reclassification of these conditions as a single disorder, separate specifiers can be used to code the specific deficits present in each of the three areas as well as current severity. Specific types of reading disorders are widely described as *dyslexia*, while specific types of mathematics deficits are described as *dyscalculia*.

The essential feature is a persistent problem in learning or using academic skills as quickly or as accurately as peers during the developmental period (Criterion A). Thus, the individual's academic skills are well below the average range for his or her age, gender-based peers, and cultural group (Criterion B). The clinical expression of the specific learning difficulties occurs during the school-age years, and therefore these difficulties may not be apparent until demands on the affected skills exceed the individual's abilities (Criterion C). The learning difficulties cannot be accounted for by intellectual difficulties, uncorrected visual or auditory problems, psychosocial adversity, poor proficiency in the language of academic instruction, or inadequate educational instruction (Criterion D).

Diagnostic Criteria for Specific Learning Disorder

A. Difficulties learning and using academic skills, as indicated by the presence of at least one of the following symptoms that have persisted for at least 6 months, despite the provision of interventions that target those difficulties:

1. Inaccurate or slow and effortful word reading (e.g., reads single words aloud incorrectly or slowly and hesitantly, frequently guesses words, has difficulty sounding out words).
2. Difficulty understanding the meaning of what is read (e.g., may read text accurately but not understand the sequence, relationships, inferences, or deeper meanings of what is read).
3. Difficulties with spelling (e.g., may add, omit, or substitute vowels or consonants).
4. Difficulties with written expression (e.g., makes multiple grammatical or punctuation errors within sentences; employs poor paragraph organization; written expression of ideas lacks clarity).
5. Difficulties mastering number sense, number facts, or calculation (e.g., has poor understanding of numbers, their magnitude, and relationships; counts on fingers to add single-digit numbers instead of recalling the math fact as peers do; gets lost in the midst of arithmetic computation and may switch procedures).
6. Difficulties with mathematical reasoning (e.g., has severe difficulty applying mathematical concepts, facts, or procedures to solve quantitative problems).

B. The affected academic skills are substantially and quantifiably below those expected for the individual's chronological age, and cause significant interference with academic or occupational performance, or with activities of daily living, as confirmed by individually administered standardized achievement measures and comprehensive clinical assessment. For individuals age 17 years and older, a documented history of impairing learning difficulties may be substituted for the standardized assessment.

C. The learning difficulties begin during school-age years but may not become fully manifest until the demands for those affected academic skills exceed the individual's limited capacities (e.g., as in timed tests, reading or writing lengthy complex reports for a tight deadline, excessively heavy academic loads).

D. The learning difficulties are not better accounted for by intellectual disabilities, uncorrected visual or auditory acuity, other mental or neurological disorders, psychosocial adversity, lack of proficiency in the language of academic instruction, or inadequate educational instruction.

Note: The four diagnostic criteria are to be met based on a clinical synthesis of the individual's history (developmental, medical, family, educational), school reports, and psychoeducational assessment.

Coding note: Specify all academic domains and subskills that are impaired. When more than one domain is impaired, each one should be coded individually according to the following specifiers.

Specify if:

315.00 (F81.0) With impairment in reading:

Word reading accuracy

Reading rate or fluency

Reading comprehension

Note: *Dyslexia* is an alternative term used to refer to a pattern of learning difficulties characterized by problems with accurate or fluent word recognition, poor decoding, and poor spelling abilities. If dyslexia is used to specify this particular pattern of difficulties, it is important also to specify any additional difficulties that are present, such as difficulties with reading comprehension or math reasoning.

315.2 (F81.81) With impairment in written expression:

Spelling accuracy

Grammar and punctuation accuracy

Clarity or organization of written expression

315.1 (F81.2) With impairment in mathematics:

Number sense

Memorization of arithmetic facts

Accurate or fluent calculation

Accurate math reasoning

Note: *Dyscalculia* is an alternative term used to refer to a pattern of difficulties characterized by problems processing numerical information, learning arithmetic facts, and performing accurate or fluent calculations. If dyscalculia is used to specify this particular pattern of mathematic difficulties, it is important also to specify any additional difficulties that are present, such as difficulties with math reasoning or word reasoning accuracy.

Specify current severity:

Mild: Some difficulties learning skills in one or two academic domains, but of mild enough severity that the individual may be able to compensate or function well when provided with appropriate accommodations or support services, especially during the school years.

Moderate: Marked difficulties learning skills in one or more academic domains, so that the individual is unlikely to become proficient without some intervals of intensive and specialized teaching during the school years. Some accommodations or supportive services at least part of the day at school, in the workplace, or at home may be needed to complete activities accurately and efficiently.

Severe: Severe difficulties learning skills, affecting several academic domains, so that the individual is unlikely to learn those skills without ongoing intensive individualized and specialized teaching for most of the school years. Even with an array of appropriate accommodations or services at home, at school, or in the workplace, the individual may not be able to complete all activities efficiently.

MOTOR DISORDERS

Developmental Coordination Disorder

The essential feature of developmental coordination disorder is a marked impairment in the developmental acquisition and execution of skills requiring motor coordination (Criterion A). Manifestations vary with age and stage of development. For example, younger children may display delays and clumsiness in achieving developmental motor milestones such as crawling, sitting, and walking, or in acquiring and using motor skills or tasks such as negotiating stairs, pedaling bicycles, buttoning shirts, and using zippers. Older children may display difficulties with motor aspects of assembling puzzles or building models.

Developmental coordination disorder is diagnosed when the impairment significantly and persistently interferes with the performance of or participation in daily activities in family, social, school, or community life (Criterion B). These include activities such as getting dressed, eating meals with appropriate utensils, engaging in physical games with peers, and participating in exercise activities at school. Typically, the child's ability to perform these actions is impaired, and there is a marked slowness in their execution. Consequences of this disorder can include reduced participation in team play and sports, low self-esteem and sense of self-worth, and emotional or behavioral problems. For adolescents and adults, impairment in fine motor skills and motor speed may affect performance in the workplace or school setting. Onset is in the early developmental period (Criterion C).

Developmental coordination disorder must be distinguished from other medical conditions that may produce coordination problems, such as cerebral palsy or muscular dystrophy, visual impairment, or intellectual disability (intellectual developmental disorder) (Criterion D).

Diagnostic Criteria for Developmental Coordination Disorder   315.4 (F82)

A. The acquisition and execution of coordinated motor skills is substantially below that expected given the individual's chronological age and opportunity for skill learning and use. Difficulties are manifested as clumsiness (e.g., dropping or bumping into objects) as well as slowness and inaccuracy of performance of motor skills (e.g., catching an object, using scissors or cutlery, handwriting, riding a bike, or participating in sports).

B. The motor skills deficit in Criterion A significantly and persistently interferes with activities of daily living appropriate to chronological age (e.g., self-care and self-maintenance) and impacts academic/school productivity, prevocational and vocational activities, leisure, and play.

C. Onset of symptoms is in the early developmental period.

D. The motor skills deficits are not better explained by intellectual disability (intellectual developmental disorder) or visual impairment and are not attributable to a neurological condition affecting movement (e.g., cerebral palsy, muscular dystrophy, degenerative disorder).

Stereotypic Movement Disorder

Stereotypic movement disorder is characterized by repetitive, seemingly driven, and apparently purposeless motor behavior (Criterion A) that interferes with social, academic, and other activities or results in self-injury (Criterion B). The disorder has an onset in the early developmental period (Criterion C). The behaviors are not attributable to the physiological effects of a substance or a neurological condition, and are not better explained by another neurodevelopmental or mental disorder (e.g., a compulsion as in obsessive-compulsive disorder, a tic as in a tic disorder, a stereotypy that is part of autism spectrum disorder, or hair pulling as in trichotillomania) (Criterion D). Typical movements include hand waving, rocking, playing with hands, fiddling with fingers, twirling objects, head banging, self-biting, and hitting various parts of one's own body. These behaviors may cause permanent and disabling tissue damage and may sometimes be life threatening.

Changes have been made in the criteria for DSM-5. Because the term *nonfunctional* (DSM-IV Criterion A) may be inaccurate, the wording "apparently purposeless" has been substituted. Because there is no evidence that the disorder must persist for 4 weeks or longer, that criterion (DSM-IV Criterion F) has been eliminated.

Diagnostic Criteria for Stereotypic Movement Disorder   307.3 (F98.4)

A. Repetitive, seemingly driven, and apparently purposeless motor behavior (e.g., hand shaking or waving, body rocking, head banging, self-biting, hitting own body).

B. The repetitive motor behavior interferes with social, academic, or other activities and may result in self-injury.

C. Onset is in the early developmental period.

D. The repetitive motor behavior is not attributable to the physiological effects of a substance or neurological condition and is not better explained by another neurodevelopmental or mental disorder (e.g., trichotillomania [hair-pulling disorder], obsessive-compulsive disorder).

Specify if:

With self-injurious behavior (or behavior that would result in an injury if preventive measures were not used)

Without self-injurious behavior

Specify if:

Associated with a known medical or genetic condition, neurodevelopmental disorder, or environmental factor (e.g., Lesch-Nyhan syndrome, intellectual disability [intellectual developmental disorder], intrauterine alcohol exposure)

Coding note: Use additional code to identify the associated medical or genetic condition, or neurodevelopmental disorder.

Specify current severity:

Mild: Symptoms are easily suppressed by sensory stimulus or distraction.

Moderate: Symptoms require explicit protective measures and behavioral modification.

Severe: Continuous monitoring and protective measures are required to prevent serious injury.

Tic Disorders

Tic disorders are characterized by the presence of clinically significant tics and differ mainly with respect to duration and type. The inclusion of five tic disorders—Tourette's disorder, persistent (chronic) motor or vocal tic disorder, provisional tic disorder, other specified tic disorder, and unspecified tic disorder—represents an expansion from the four listed in DSM-IV (Walkup et al. 2010). The latter two diagnoses were added based on research suggesting that tics may result from the effect of certain substances (e.g., cocaine) or medical conditions (e.g., Huntington's disease).

Tourette's Disorder

Tourette's disorder is characterized by stereotypical but nonrhythmic motor movements and vocalizations. The vocal tics can be socially offensive, such as loud grunting or barking noises or shouted words, which may be obscenities. The individual is aware that he or she is producing the vocal tics and is able to exert a mild degree of control over them, but ultimately must submit to them. Because people with Tourette's disorder are aware that their tics are socially inappropriate, they find the tics embarrassing. Motor tics occurring in Tourette's disorder are also often odd or offensive behaviors, such as tongue protrusion, sniffing, hopping, squatting, blinking, or nodding. Because most of the general public is unaware of the nature of Tourette's disorder, the behavior is seen as inappropriate or bizarre.

Diagnostic Criteria for Tourette's Disorder   307.23 (F95.2)

Note: A tic is a sudden, rapid, recurrent, nonrhythmic motor movement or vocalization.

A. Both multiple motor and one or more vocal tics have been present at some time during the illness, although not necessarily concurrently.

B. The tics may wax and wane in frequency but have persisted for more than 1 year since first tic onset.

C. Onset is before age 18 years.

D. The disturbance is not attributable to the physiological effects of a substance (e.g., cocaine) or another medical condition (e.g., Huntington's disease, postviral encephalitis).

Criterion A

The definition of a tic has been made consistent for all tic disorders. The term *stereotyped* has been removed to make it less likely that individuals with stereotypic movement disorder will be diagnosed with a tic disorder.

Criterion B

The maximum tic-free interval (DSM-IV Criterion B) was eliminated because there are no data to suggest that tic-free periods of more than 3 months do *not* constitute a chronic course. Also, tic-free intervals are more difficult to assess because they require the patient to recall offset of symptoms, and this may lead to unreliability in diagnosis. DSM-5 maintains that tics must have persisted for more than 1 year, as in DSM-IV, but it clarifies that the 12-month duration of symptoms is since first tic onset. The phrase "usually in bouts" was eliminated because this feature of tics is not critical to diagnosis.

Criteria C and D

The tics must be present before age 18 years. This requirement helps distinguish Tourette's disorder from other causes of tics that occur later in life, such as Huntington's disease or postviral encephalitis. Stimulant medication use as an example of a substance-induced movement disorder is not consistent with the evidence base and has been eliminated. Cocaine has been substituted as an example.

Persistent (Chronic) Motor or Vocal Tic Disorder

The essential feature of persistent (chronic) motor or vocal tic disorder is the presence of either motor tics or vocal tics, but not both. This disorder differs from Tourette's disorder, for which diagnosis requires *both* multiple motor tics and one or more vocal tics. The other features are the same as for Tourette's disorder, such as onset before age 18 years. Other disorders, such as Huntington's disease, need to be ruled out as causes. The diagnosis cannot be made if the criteria for Tourette's disorder have ever been met. The other characteristics are generally the same as for Tourette's disorder except that the severity of the symptoms and the functional impairment are usually much less. Persistent (chronic) motor or vocal tic disorder and Tourette's disorder may be genetically related. Clinicians can specify whether the disorder is "with motor tics only" or "with vocal tics only."

Diagnostic Criteria for Persistent (Chronic) Motor or Vocal Tic Disorder   307.22 (F95.1)

Note: A tic is a sudden, rapid, recurrent, nonrhythmic motor movement or vocalization.

A. Single or multiple motor or vocal tics have been present during the illness, but not both motor and vocal.

B. The tics may wax and wane in frequency but have persisted for more than 1 year since first tic onset.

C. Onset is before age 18 years.

D. The disturbance is not attributable to the physiological effects of a substance (e.g., cocaine) or another medical condition (e.g., Huntington's disease, postviral encephalitis).

E. Criteria have never been met for Tourette's disorder.

Specify if:
With motor tics only
With vocal tics only

Criteria A and B

The definition of a tic has been made consistent with that used in the other tic disorders. The changes to Criterion B for persistent (chronic) motor or vocal tic disorder are identical to those for Tourette's disorder.

Criteria C and D

Onset must occur before age 18. This requirement helps separate the disorder from other causes of tics that occur later in life, such as Huntington's disease or postviral encephalitis. Stimulant medication use as an example of a substance-induced movement disorder has been removed. Cocaine has been substituted as an example.

Provisional Tic Disorder

The provisional tic disorder diagnosis represents a modification of transient tic disorder in DSM-IV. The DSM-IV criteria were difficult to use because individuals with current tic symptoms of less than 1 year's duration would be diagnosed as having transient tics when the tics were actually present. Given the need for a diagnostic category for persons with tics of less than 1 year's duration, the transient tic disorder category has been renamed *provisional tic disorder.*

Diagnostic Criteria for Provisional Tic Disorder   307.21 (F95.0)

Note: A tic is a sudden, rapid, recurrent, nonrhythmic motor movement or vocalization.

A. Single or multiple motor and/or vocal tics.

B. The tics have been present for less than 1 year since first tic onset.

C. Onset is before age 18 years.

D. The disturbance is not attributable to the physiological effects of a substance (e.g., cocaine) or another medical condition (e.g., Huntington's disease, postviral encephalitis).

E. Criteria have never been met for Tourette's disorder or persistent (chronic) motor or vocal tic disorder.

Criteria A, B, C, and D

The definition of a tic has been made consistent with that used in the other tic disorders. No evidence suggests that the 4-week threshold described in DSM-IV was valid or useful, so it has been omitted. Onset must occur before age 18; this helps separate the disorder from other causes of tics that occur later in life, such as Huntington's disease or postviral encephalitis. Stimulant medication use as an example of a substance-induced movement disorder has been removed. Cocaine has been substituted as an example.

Other Specified Tic Disorder and Unspecified Tic Disorder

Other specified tic disorder is a diagnosis used when an impairing tic disorder is present, but the full criteria for a specific tic disorder or any of the disorders in the neurodevelopmental disorders diagnostic class are not met. Unspecified tic disorder is used when the above conditions are present, but the clinician chooses not to specify the reason that the criteria are not met for a specific disorder, and includes presentations in which there is insufficient information to make a more specific diagnosis. These two diagnoses replace DSM-IV's tic disorder not otherwise specified.

Other Specified Tic Disorder   307.20 (F95.8)

This category applies to presentations in which symptoms characteristic of a tic disorder that cause clinically significant distress or impairment in social, occupational, or other important areas of functioning predominate but do not meet the full criteria for a tic disorder or any of the disorders in the neurodevelopmental disorders diagnostic class. The other specified tic disorder category is used in situations in which the clinician chooses to communicate the specific reason that the presentation does not meet the criteria for a tic disorder or any specific neurodevelopmental disorder. This is done by recording "other specified tic disorder" followed by the specific reason (e.g., "with onset after age 18 years").

Unspecified Tic Disorder   307.20 (F95.9)

This category applies to presentations in which symptoms characteristic of a tic disorder that cause clinically significant distress or impairment in social, occupational, or other important areas of functioning predominate but do not meet the full criteria for a tic disorder or for any of the disorders in the neurodevelopmental disorders diagnostic class. The unspecified tic disorder category is used in situations in which the clinician chooses *not* to specify the reason that the criteria are not met for a tic disorder or for a specific neurodevelopmental disorder, and includes presentations in which there is insufficient information to make a more specific diagnosis.

OTHER NEURODEVELOPMENTAL DISORDERS

Other Specified Neurodevelopmental Disorder and Unspecified Neurodevelopmental Disorder

These categories apply to presentations in which symptoms characteristic of a neurodevelopmental disorder are present and impairing but do not meet the full criteria for any of the disorders in the neurodevelopmental disorders diagnostic class. The other specified neurodevelopmental disorder category is used when the clinician chooses to communicate the reason that the presentation does not meet the criteria. The unspecified neurodevelopmental disorder category is used when the clinician chooses not to specify the reason, or there is insufficient information to make a more specific diagnosis.

Other Specified Neurodevelopmental Disorder   315.8 (F88)

This category applies to presentations in which symptoms characteristic of a neuro-developmental disorder that cause impairment in social, occupational, or other important areas of functioning predominate but do not meet the full criteria for any of the disorders in the neurodevelopmental disorders diagnostic class. The other specified neurodevelopmental disorder category is used in situations in which the clinician chooses to communicate the specific reason that the presentation does not meet the criteria for any specific neurodevelopmental disorder. This is done by recording "other specified neurodevelopmental disorder" followed by the specific reason (e.g., "neuro-developmental disorder associated with prenatal alcohol exposure").

An example of a presentation that can be specified using the "other specified" designation is the following:

Neurodevelopmental disorder associated with prenatal alcohol exposure: Neurodevelopmental disorder associated with prenatal alcohol exposure is characterized by a range of developmental disabilities following exposure to alcohol in utero.

Unspecified Neurodevelopmental Disorder   315.9 (F89)

This category applies to presentations in which symptoms characteristic of a neuro-developmental disorder that cause impairment in social, occupational, or other important areas of functioning predominate but do not meet the full criteria for any of the disorders in the neurodevelopmental disorders diagnostic class. The unspecified neurodevelopmental disorder category is used in situations in which the clinician chooses *not* to specify the reason that the criteria are not met for a specific neurodevelopmental disorder, and includes presentations in which there is insufficient information to make a more specific diagnosis (e.g., in emergency room settings).

KEY POINTS

- The chapter on neurodevelopmental disorders is a reformulation of the DSM-IV chapter "Disorders Usually First Diagnosed in Infancy, Childhood, or Adolescence."

- Mental retardation has been renamed *intellectual disability (intellectual developmental disorder).* Severity is determined on the basis of adaptive functioning rather than an IQ score, though diagnostic criteria emphasize the need to assess cognitive capacity.

- The communication disorders are newly named and include language disorder (which combines expressive and mixed receptive-expressive language disorders), speech sound disorder (previously phonological disorder), and childhood-onset fluency disorder (previously stuttering). Social (pragmatic) communication disorder is new and describes persistent difficulties in the social uses of verbal and nonverbal communication.

- Autism spectrum disorder is a new diagnosis that now subsumes DSM-IV autistic disorder, Rett's disorder, childhood disintegrative disorder, Asperger's disorder, and pervasive developmental disorder not otherwise specified. Work group members believed that there was little validity to the specific diagnoses and that clinicians had difficulty distinguishing them.

- With attention-deficit/hyperactivity disorder, examples have been added to the criterion items to enhance use of these items across the life span. Age at onset has been changed from before age 7 years to before age 12 years. A comorbid diagnosis with autism spectrum disorder is now allowed. Last, the symptom threshold has been changed for adults, with a cutoff of five symptoms instead of the six required for younger persons, both for inattention and for hyperactivity and impulsivity.

- DSM-IV learning disorder has been changed to *specific learning disorder.* The previous types of learning disorders (reading disorder, mathematics disorder, and disorder of written expression) have been combined, and specifiers are now used to describe the individual's impairment.

- With tic disorders, the maximum tic-free interval (DSM-IV Criterion B) was eliminated because there are no scientific data to suggest that tic-free periods of more than 3 months do *not* constitute a chronic course.

Schizophrenia Spectrum and Other Psychotic Disorders

301.22 (F21)	Schizotypal (Personality) Disorder (see also "Personality Disorders")
297.1 (F22)	Delusional Disorder
298.8 (F23)	Brief Psychotic Disorder
295.40 (F20.81)	Schizophreniform Disorder
295.90 (F20.9)	Schizophrenia
295.70 (F25._)	Schizoaffective Disorder
	Substance/Medication-Induced Psychotic Disorder
	Psychotic Disorder Due to Another Medical Condition
293.89 (F06.1)	Catatonia Associated With Another Mental Disorder (Catatonia Specifier)
293.89 (F06.1)	Catatonic Disorder Due to Another Medical Condition
293.89 (F06.1)	Unspecified Catatonia
298.8 (F28)	Other Specified Schizophrenia Spectrum and Other Psychotic Disorder
298.9 (F29)	Unspecified Schizophrenia Spectrum and Other Psychotic Disorder

The diagnostic class schizophrenia spectrum and other psychotic disorders comprises schizophrenia and related disorders, other major psychoses, and disorders with subthreshold psychoses (Table 4–1). All are unified by the presence of one or more of the following five domains of psychopathology: delusions, hallucinations, disorganized thinking, grossly disorganized or catatonic behavior, and negative symptoms. Whereas the first four domains are examples of psychosis, negative symptoms are characterized by the absence of something that should be present, such as fluency and spontaneity of verbal expression. The term *psychosis* holds different meanings, but beginning with DSM-III, the term has had a more restricted definition that requires the person to experience a break with reality. In the psychoanalytic era, the term was often used to describe persons who were severely ill and functionally impaired but had a broad range of problems and symptoms.

61

TABLE 4–1.   DSM-5 schizophrenia spectrum and other psychotic disorders

Schizotypal (personality) disorder (see Chapter 18, "Personality Disorders")

Delusional disorder

Brief psychotic disorder

Schizophreniform disorder

Schizophrenia

Schizoaffective disorder

Substance/medication-induced psychotic disorder

Psychotic disorder due to another medical condition

Catatonia associated with another mental disorder (catatonia specifier)

Catatonic disorder due to another medical condition

Unspecified catatonia

Other specified schizophrenia spectrum and other psychotic disorder

Unspecified schizophrenia spectrum and other psychotic disorder

Schizophrenia is arguably the most disabling of the psychoses, yet other psychotic disorders are also important to recognize and diagnose. These include delusional disorder, brief psychotic disorder, schizophreniform disorder, and schizoaffective disorder. The chapter also includes psychoses that are attributable to other medical conditions or are induced by substances or medications. Catatonic disorder due to another medical condition has been moved to this chapter and is used for those cases in which the disorder is medically induced. Unspecified catatonia is new to DSM-5. Other specified and unspecified schizophrenia spectrum and other psychotic disorders constitute residual categories that are used to describe psychotic symptoms that do not fit into any of the better-defined categories.

All psychotic disorders are included in this chapter of DSM-5 except those related to bipolar disorder, depressive disorders, or a neurocognitive disorder. This organization should help facilitate the differential diagnosis of psychotic disorders.

Several important changes have been made to this class. The most basic change involves overall chapter organization. Disorders are now arranged along a gradient from least to most severe. Severity is defined by the level, number, and duration of psychotic signs and symptoms. DSM-5 cautions users to diagnose more severe conditions once the lesser conditions are ruled out. Clinicians know (and trainees learn) that for many individuals the diagnostic process may take months or even years because signs and symptoms evolve gradually. For example, a young man evaluated for social withdrawal and magical thinking may have symptoms that initially meet criteria for schizotypal personality disorder, but several years later he may develop frank delusions and hallucinations that meet criteria for schizophrenia. At the same time, the clinician needs to have ruled out alternative explanations, such as a substance use disorder or another medical condition, in order to arrive at the best diagnosis.

Schizotypal personality disorder is included in this chapter because of its membership in the schizophrenia spectrum, but criteria and text are found with the personality disorders (see Chapter 18, "Personality Disorders"). The criteria for delusional disorder are mostly unchanged, but the adjective *nonbizarre* has been removed (Criterion A), and the somatic subtype has been edited to ensure that those who are delusional regarding a "physical defect" are more appropriately diagnosed with body dysmorphic disorder, now placed in the chapter "Obsessive-Compulsive and Related Disorders" (see Chapter 7). In DSM-IV, body dysmorphic disorder was included with the somatoform disorders.

Shared psychotic disorder has been eliminated because the diagnosis was infrequently used and persons whose symptoms met criteria for the diagnosis generally also met criteria for some other psychotic disorder (e.g., delusional disorder). The essence of shared psychotic disorder is the transmission of delusional beliefs from one person to another. In the past, these rare cases were called *folie à deux*, a French term for "double insanity."

Clinicians will no longer record schizophrenia subtypes. Although the paranoid, disorganized, catatonic, undifferentiated, and residual subtypes have a lengthy history that predates DSM-I (McGlashan and Fenton 1994), there was little evidence to support either their clinical utility or their predictive validity (Helmes and Landmark 2003). Because the course of schizophrenia is highly variable, the subtypes had little stability, so that at various stages of illness it was not unusual for a person's symptoms to meet criteria for different subtypes. For example, a person's symptoms may have met the criteria for disorganized subtype early in the illness and then met criteria for the paranoid subtype and, eventually, the residual subtype later in the course of the illness.

The criteria for schizoaffective disorder have been modified to provide more guidance to clinicians regarding the total duration of mood symptoms. Instead of requiring that mood symptoms last a "substantial portion of the total duration of the active and residual periods of the illness" (as in DSM-IV [American Psychiatric Association 1994]), DSM-5 requires that they be present for a "majority of the total duration of the active and residual portions of the illness." The change was prompted by the low reliability of the criterion and its limited clinical utility.

The Psychotic Disorders Work Group had debated the possible inclusion of attenuated psychosis syndrome. The syndrome is a collection of symptoms associated with a high probability of the person developing schizophrenia. The impetus to include this condition was that it would help to identify those likely to develop schizophrenia, thereby allowing early clinical attention and treatment. The decision was made to include this syndrome in Section III, in "Conditions for Further Study" (see Chapter 22) but include it as an example of an other specified schizophrenia spectrum and other psychotic disorder.

Schizotypal (Personality) Disorder

Schizotypal personality disorder is included in this chapter because of its presence within the the schizophrenia specturum. Criteria and text for the disorder are found in the chapter on personality disorders (see Chapter 18).

Delusional Disorder

Delusional disorder is a diagnosis used in individuals who have persistent delusions but relatively normal psychosocial functioning apart from the ramifications of the delusions and who exhibit behavior that is not obviously odd or bizarre. First included in DSM-III under the rubric "paranoid disorder," the name was changed to delusional (paranoid) disorder in DSM-III-R because while delusions are the primary symptoms, the term *paranoid* has many other meanings.

Delusional disorders have a long history. Kraepelin distinguished paranoia from *dementia praecox* and used the diagnosis for persons with systematized delusions (but no hallucinations) and a prolonged course without recovery but not leading to mental deterioration. Traditionally, the diagnosis has been used for persons who have nonbizarre (i.e., possible but not plausible) delusions but whose functioning is relatively well preserved, without the deterioration in functioning seen in persons with schizophrenia and schizoaffective disorder. Because these individuals experience their delusional beliefs as ego-syntonic (i.e., consistent with their own expectations, sense of self, and sense of reality in general), their insight is poor and they generally have little interest in seeking treatment.

In DSM-5, a number of changes have been made to the diagnosis. The adjective *nonbizarre* has been removed from Criterion A. One reason is that "bizarreness" is often hard to judge, especially across different cultures (Cermolacce et al. 2010). Another reason behind the change is more practical and stems in part from a change in the definition of schizophrenia, in which the special treatment of bizarre delusions has been deleted from Criterion A. With this change, the presence of a single bizarre delusion no longer satisfies Criterion A for schizophrenia. Removing the term *nonbizarre* from the criteria for delusional disorder was necessary to allow a place within the delusional disorder category for the rare individual with a single bizarre delusion. The work group found little justification for differential treatment of delusions based on whether they are bizarre or nonbizarre. The addition of the "with bizarre content" specifier allows for the recording of the nature of the delusion and permits continuity with DSM-IV. This specifier is used when the delusions are thought to be clearly implausible.

Criterion E has been added to rule out other mental disorders, including body dysmorphic disorder and obsessive-compulsive disorder. In addition, the somatic subtype has been edited to delete the phrase "some physical defect." Both changes will help ensure that those who are delusional regarding a "physical defect" are more appropriately diagnosed with body dysmorphic disorder, which is now included with the new diagnostic class obsessive-compulsive and related disorders (see Chapter 7). The work group felt that this change was necessary because people with body dysmorphic disorder—delusional or not—have a course of illness similar to those with obsessive-compulsive disorder, and tend to respond to selective serotonin reuptake inhibitor medications. The changes help to distinguish delusional disorder from body dysmorphic disorder, with absent insight/delusional beliefs, and obsessive-compulsive disorder, with absent insight/delusional beliefs.

Diagnostic Criteria for Delusional Disorder　　　**297.1** (F22)

A. The presence of one (or more) delusions with a duration of 1 month or longer.

B. Criterion A for schizophrenia has never been met.

　Note: Hallucinations, if present, are not prominent and are related to the delusional theme (e.g., the sensation of being infested with insects associated with delusions of infestation).

C. Apart from the impact of the delusion(s) or its ramifications, functioning is not markedly impaired, and behavior is not obviously bizarre or odd.

D. If manic or major depressive episodes have occurred, these have been brief relative to the duration of the delusional periods.

E. The disturbance is not attributable to the physiological effects of a substance or another medical condition and is not better explained by another mental disorder, such as body dysmorphic disorder or obsessive-compulsive disorder.

Specify whether:

　Erotomanic type: This subtype applies when the central theme of the delusion is that another person is in love with the individual.

　Grandiose type: This subtype applies when the central theme of the delusion is the conviction of having some great (but unrecognized) talent or insight or having made some important discovery.

　Jealous type: This subtype applies when the central theme of the individual's delusion is that his or her spouse or lover is unfaithful.

　Persecutory type: This subtype applies when the central theme of the delusion involves the individual's belief that he or she is being conspired against, cheated, spied on, followed, poisoned or drugged, maliciously maligned, harassed, or obstructed in the pursuit of long-term goals.

　Somatic type: This subtype applies when the central theme of the delusion involves bodily functions or sensations.

　Mixed type: This subtype applies when no one delusional theme predominates.

　Unspecified type: This subtype applies when the dominant delusional belief cannot be clearly determined or is not described in the specific types (e.g., referential delusions without a prominent persecutory or grandiose component).

Specify if:

　With bizarre content: Delusions are deemed bizarre if they are clearly implausible, not understandable, and not derived from ordinary life experiences (e.g., an individual's belief that a stranger has removed his or her internal organs and replaced them with someone else's organs without leaving any wounds or scars).

Specify if:

The following course specifiers are only to be used after a 1-year duration of the disorder:

　First episode, currently in acute episode: First manifestation of the disorder meeting the defining diagnostic symptom and time criteria. An *acute episode* is a time period in which the symptom criteria are fulfilled.

　First episode, currently in partial remission: *Partial remission* is a time period during which an improvement after a previous episode is maintained and in which the defining criteria of the disorder are only partially fulfilled.

First episode, currently in full remission: *Full remission* is a period of time after a previous episode during which no disorder-specific symptoms are present.

Multiple episodes, currently in acute episode

Multiple episodes, currently in partial remission

Multiple episodes, currently in full remission

Continuous: Symptoms fulfilling the diagnostic symptom criteria of the disorder are remaining for the majority of the illness course, with subthreshold symptom periods being very brief relative to the overall course.

Unspecified

Specify current severity:

Severity is rated by a quantitative assessment of the primary symptoms of psychosis, including delusions, hallucinations, disorganized speech, abnormal psychomotor behavior, and negative symptoms. Each of these symptoms may be rated for its current severity (most severe in the last 7 days) on a 5-point scale ranging from 0 (not present) to 4 (present and severe). (See Clinician-Rated Dimensions of Psychosis Symptom Severity in Chapter 20, "Assessment Measures," this volume.)

Note: Diagnosis of delusional disorder can be made without using this severity specifier.

Criterion A

Delusional disorder requires the presence of delusions for a minimum of 1 month. DSM-IV specified that the delusions were nonbizarre. Although the term *nonbizarre* has been deleted, the spirit of the disorder as involving persons with nonbizarre delusions remains, as indicated by the various subtypes. Individuals with schizophrenia often have very bizarre delusions not possible in real life. For example, we have had patients claim they are being controlled by radio transmitters implanted in their brains (although with rapidly developing technology, that situation may be possible in the future).

Criterion B

Excluding symptoms that meet Criterion A of schizophrenia has helped to separate delusional disorder from schizophrenia. People with schizophrenia have other psychotic symptoms (hallucinations; disorganized speech; grossly abnormal behavior, including catatonia) in addition to negative symptoms. Although individuals with delusional disorder may have tactile and olfactory hallucinations that relate to their delusion, they are otherwise free of those symptoms common to persons with schizophrenia (e.g., auditory hallucinations). For example, individuals with delusional disorder, somatic type, may have delusions of being infested with parasites and report feeling them moving about under their skin. (This particular delusion has been referred to as *delusional parasitosis* and is more commonly seen by dermatologists.)

Criterion C

People with delusional disorder do not behave in an obviously odd or bizarre fashion. This is an important distinction from people with schizophrenia, who often act in strange ways, such as muttering to themselves, wearing dirty or inappropriate clothing, or accosting strangers. The purpose of this criterion is to ensure that delusional disorder is restricted to persons who, apart from their delusion or its ramifications, are able to function. That said, the behavior of some persons is greatly influenced by their delusions, and this can be reflected in their actions. For example, a person in love with a television actress may attempt to contact the person, or in rare cases may stalk her. A person who thinks his wife is unfaithful may read her private e-mail or monitor her daily activities in an attempt to catch her with the paramour.

Criterion D

If persons with delusional disorder have had concurrent mood episodes, these episodes must have been relatively brief. The goal is to separate delusional disorder from psychotic forms of major depressive disorder. Individuals with the latter may develop delusions in the context of suffering severe depression, but these delusions tend to have depressive content, such as believing oneself to have committed a sinful act or to have lost all of one's savings. If the delusions occur exclusively during the course of the depressive illness, the diagnosis is a mood disorder with psychotic features.

Individuals with delusional disorder often have significant depressive symptoms. The clinician may feel that the symptoms merit an independent diagnosis of major depressive disorder or other specified or unspecified depressive disorder (or if there is a bipolar course, other specified or unspecified bipolar and related disorder). Schizoaffective disorder is another diagnostic possibility if the delusions are long-standing and the mood disorder is severe.

Criterion E

This criterion excludes delusional disorders attributable to the physiological effects of a substance or another medical condition or are better explained by another mental disorder. Delusions can result from a variety of medical illnesses, certain medical treatments or medications (e.g., corticosteroids), and use of drugs of abuse (e.g., stimulants). This criterion requires ruling out neurocognitive disorders, such as a dementia, as well as traumatic brain injuries or a convulsive disorder. Also, certain forms of body dysmorphic disorder and obsessive-compulsive disorder are relatively severe and are associated with delusions (e.g., when an individual believes his normal-appearing nose is ugly and misshapen). Even when the belief reaches delusional proportions, the diagnosis body dysmorphic disorder is more appropriate than delusional disorder.

Subtypes and Specifiers

Subtypes are used to indicate the specific theme the disorder has taken, such as erotomania or grandiosity. Bizarreness, course of the disorder, and current severity can also be specified.

Brief Psychotic Disorder

Brief psychotic disorder is a diagnosis used for relatively brief episodes of psychosis lasting at least 1 day but less than 1 month. The disorder is relatively uncommon and occurs in persons who otherwise have not experienced a decline in their day-to-day functioning or who display signs that in retrospect suggest the prodrome of schizophrenia. Further, the psychotic symptoms associated with this diagnosis tend to be brought on by stressful situations or acute mood changes. In the past, this diagnosis was often referred to as a reactive, hysterical, or psychogenic psychosis. The diagnosis is essentially unchanged from DSM-IV except for minor editing and the addition of the specifiers for catatonia and current severity.

Some individuals report new-onset psychotic symptoms that last minutes to hours and that therefore do not qualify for the diagnosis. These symptoms can occur in persons with borderline personality disorder or schizotypal personality disorder; in these cases no additional diagnosis is necessary. Otherwise, when these short-lived symptoms occur, and they are not attributable to a medication, a drug of abuse, or another medical condition, the diagnosis other specified or unspecified schizophrenia spectrum and other psychotic disorder may be appropriate.

Diagnostic Criteria for Brief Psychotic Disorder   298.8 (F23)

A. Presence of one (or more) of the following symptoms. At least one of these must be (1), (2), or (3):

1. Delusions.
2. Hallucinations.
3. Disorganized speech (e.g., frequent derailment or incoherence).
4. Grossly disorganized or catatonic behavior.

Note: Do not include a symptom if it is a culturally sanctioned response.

B. Duration of an episode of the disturbance is at least 1 day but less than 1 month, with eventual full return to premorbid level of functioning.

C. The disturbance is not better explained by major depressive or bipolar disorder with psychotic features or another psychotic disorder such as schizophrenia or catatonia, and is not attributable to the physiological effects of a substance (e.g., a drug of abuse, a medication) or another medical condition.

Specify if:

With marked stressor(s) (brief reactive psychosis): If symptoms occur in response to events that, singly or together, would be markedly stressful to almost anyone in similar circumstances in the individual's culture.

Without marked stressor(s): If symptoms do not occur in response to events that, singly or together, would be markedly stressful to almost anyone in similar circumstances in the individual's culture.

With postpartum onset: If onset is during pregnancy or within 4 weeks postpartum.

Specify if:

With catatonia (refer to the criteria for catatonia associated with another mental disorder, DSM-5, pp. 119–120, for definition)

Coding note: Use additional code 293.89 (F06.1) catatonia associated with brief psychotic disorder to indicate the presence of the comorbid catatonia.

Specify current severity:

Severity is rated by a quantitative assessment of the primary symptoms of psychosis, including delusions, hallucinations, disorganized speech, abnormal psychomotor behavior, and negative symptoms. Each of these symptoms may be rated for its current severity (most severe in the last 7 days) on a 5-point scale ranging from 0 (not present) to 4 (present and severe). (See Clinician-Rated Dimensions of Psychosis Symptom Severity in Chapter 20, "Assessment Measures," this volume.)

Note: Diagnosis of brief psychotic disorder can be made without using this severity specifier.

Criterion A

Psychotic symptoms must be present, and the Criterion A list for brief psychotic disorder replicates that for schizophrenia *except* that negative symptoms are not included; these usually occur over long periods of time and do not generally present acutely. The diagnosis does not apply when the psychotic symptoms appear to have developed in response to culturally sanctioned activities, such as *Qigong*, a Chinese health-enhancing practice that can reportedly lead to transient psychosis. This is an important consideration, because psychotic-like phenomena are reported to occur during extended religious or ceremonial rituals in several non-Western cultures.

Criterion B

The disturbance lasts at least 1 day but less than 1 month. If the duration is longer, the person will presumably qualify for another diagnosis, such as schizophreniform disorder.

Criterion C

The language has been edited for consistency within DSM-5, but otherwise this criterion is unchanged from DSM-IV. Mood disorders, other psychotic disorders, medical conditions, and the physiological effects of substances need to be ruled out as a cause of the disturbance.

Specifiers

When the disorder occurs in response to stressors, the clinician can use the specifier "with marked stressor(s)." If brief psychotic disorder occurs within 4 weeks postpartum, the "with postpartum onset" specifier is appropriate. Typically, women with postpartum onset generally develop symptoms within 1–2 weeks of delivery. Symptoms can include disorganized speech, misperceptions, labile mood, confusion, and hallucinations. Frequently referred to as "postpartum psychosis," the disorder tends to arise in otherwise normally functioning individuals. The disorder should be distinguished from the "baby blues," which occurs in many new mothers and may last for a few days after delivery but is not considered pathologic. The new specifier "with catatonia" can be used when the full syndrome is present. Current severity can be specified as well.

Schizophreniform Disorder

The term *schizophreniform* was used by Gabriel Langfeldt (1939) to describe acute psychoses that were reactive and occurred in persons with relatively normal personalities. Such cases were referred to as "acute schizophrenic episodes" in DSM-II. Schizophreniform disorder was formally recognized in DSM-III as one of several psychotic disorders not elsewhere classified. The diagnosis is used for symptoms of schizophrenia that last at least 1 month but less than 6 months. Once the symptoms have lasted 6 months or longer, the diagnosis changes to schizophrenia, even if only residual symptoms remain (e.g., blunted affect).

The validity of schizophreniform disorder has been debated. Some individuals diagnosed with this disorder develop schizophrenia, whereas others develop a mood disorder or schizoaffective disorder. Persons with schizophreniform disorder have a relatively better prognosis than those diagnosed with schizophrenia at first encounter.

Diagnostic Criteria for Schizophreniform Disorder   295.40 (F20.81)

A. Two (or more) of the following, each present for a significant portion of time during a 1-month period (or less if successfully treated). At least one of these must be (1), (2), or (3):

   1. Delusions.
   2. Hallucinations.
   3. Disorganized speech (e.g., frequent derailment or incoherence).
   4. Grossly disorganized or catatonic behavior.
   5. Negative symptoms (i.e., diminished emotional expression or avolition).

B. An episode of the disorder lasts at least 1 month but less than 6 months. When the diagnosis must be made without waiting for recovery, it should be qualified as "provisional."

C. Schizoaffective disorder and depressive or bipolar disorder with psychotic features have been ruled out because either 1) no major depressive or manic episodes have occurred concurrently with the active-phase symptoms, or 2) if mood episodes have occurred during active-phase symptoms, they have been present for a minority of the total duration of the active and residual periods of the illness.

D. The disturbance is not attributable to the physiological effects of a substance (e.g., a drug of abuse, a medication) or another medical condition.

Specify if:

   With good prognostic features: This specifier requires the presence of at least two of the following features: onset of prominent psychotic symptoms within 4 weeks of the first noticeable change in usual behavior or functioning; confusion or perplexity; good premorbid social and occupational functioning; and absence of blunted or flat affect.

Without good prognostic features: This specifier is applied if two or more of the above features have not been present.

Specify if:

With catatonia (refer to the criteria for catatonia associated with another mental disorder, DSM-5, pp. 119–120, for definition).

> **Coding note:** Use additional code 293.89 (F06.1) catatonia associated with schizophreniform disorder to indicate the presence of the comorbid catatonia.

Specify current severity:

Severity is rated by a quantitative assessment of the primary symptoms of psychosis, including delusions, hallucinations, disorganized speech, abnormal psychomotor behavior, and negative symptoms. Each of these symptoms may be rated for its current severity (most severe in the last 7 days) on a 5-point scale ranging from 0 (not present) to 4 (present and severe). (See Clinician-Rated Dimensions of Psychosis Symptom Severity in Chapter 20, "Assessment Measures," this volume.)

Note: Diagnosis of schizophreniform disorder can be made without using this severity specifier.

The criteria require that the individual's symptoms meet schizophrenia Criterion A (psychotic symptoms), as well as schizophrenia Criteria D and E (which require that other mental disorders, substances of abuse, and other medical disorders have been ruled out as a cause of the disorder). Because the individual would have new-onset symptoms, alternative explanations need to be ruled out during a comprehensive evaluation.

The clinician should specify whether the individual has good prognostic features, such as acute onset, confusion or perplexity, good premorbid functioning, and absence of a flattened affect—all of which are symptoms identified in research studies as correlating with good prognosis. Catatonic features should be specified if present. Current severity can also be specified.

Schizophrenia

In DSM-5, schizophrenia is defined by a group of characteristic symptoms, such as delusions, hallucinations, and negative symptoms (i.e., diminished emotional expression or avolition); deterioration in social, occupational, or interpersonal functioning; and continuous signs of the disturbance for at least 6 months. No symptoms are specific—or pathognomonic—to schizophrenia, complicating the task of establishing the proper boundaries for the disorder.

Kraepelin (1919) is generally credited for producing the first coherent definition of schizophrenia, which he called *dementia praecox*. His conceptualization was of an early-onset illness characterized by psychotic symptoms with a chronic and deteriorating course. He was also instrumental in separating dementia praecox from manic-depressive illness, which had its onset throughout life and had a more episodic course.

Kraepelin's emphasis on psychotic symptoms and a deteriorating course helped to identify a relatively narrow group of severely ill patients with chronic symptoms and poor prognosis.

Dementia praecox was eventually renamed *schizophrenia* by Bleuler (1950) in 1911 to emphasize the cognitive impairment that occurs, which he saw as a "splitting" of the psychic processes. Bleuler maintained that certain symptoms were fundamental to the illness, including affective blunting, disturbance of association (i.e., peculiar and distorted thinking), autism, and indecisiveness (ambivalence). He de-emphasized course and regarded delusions and hallucinations as accessory symptoms because they could occur in other disorders. Bleuler's ideas earned acceptance and guided the practice of generations of American and European psychiatrists who were taught the importance of Bleuler's fundamental symptoms ("the four A's"). Because these symptoms were imprecise, they defined a much more heterogeneous group of patients, often much less ill than those identified by Kraepelin, and contributed to an increasingly broad concept of schizophrenia.

The ideas of Kurt Schneider (1959) helped reshape the concept of schizophrenia into that of a relatively severe psychotic disorder, bringing it back to the original ideas of Kraepelin. He described "first-rank" psychotic symptoms that he believed were relatively specific and that thus helped to discriminate schizophrenia from other disorders. These symptoms included thought insertion, thought withdrawal, thought broadcasting, voices communicating with (or about) the person, and delusions of being externally controlled (i.e., delusions of passivity). Schneider's description of schizophrenia emphasized the presence of one or more of these psychotic symptoms and was cross-sectional in its definition of the illness. Although later research suggested that these "Schneiderian" symptoms were not particularly specific (Nordgaard et al. 2008), Schneider's ideas gained prominence and influenced DSM-III, DSM-III-R, and DSM-IV with their special treatment of "bizarre" delusions and certain hallucinations.

With DSM-5, modest changes have been made in the criteria for schizophrenia. The main change has been to eliminate the special status of Schneiderian first-rank symptoms, including bizarre delusions and certain hallucinations such as voices conversing. The recommendation was also made to eliminate schizophrenia subtypes. Work group members agreed that the classic subtypes provided a poor description of the heterogeneity of the disorder and had low diagnostic stability, with only the paranoid and undifferentiated subtypes being used with any frequency.

Diagnostic Criteria for Schizophrenia   **295.90** (F20.9)

A. Two (or more) of the following, each present for a significant portion of time during a 1-month period (or less if successfully treated). At least one of these must be (1), (2), or (3):

   1. Delusions.
   2. Hallucinations.

3. Disorganized speech (e.g., frequent derailment or incoherence).
4. Grossly disorganized or catatonic behavior.
5. Negative symptoms (i.e., diminished emotional expression or avolition).

B. For a significant portion of the time since the onset of the disturbance, level of functioning in one or more major areas, such as work, interpersonal relations, or self-care, is markedly below the level achieved prior to the onset (or when the onset is in childhood or adolescence, there is failure to achieve expected level of interpersonal, academic, or occupational functioning).

C. Continuous signs of the disturbance persist for at least 6 months. This 6-month period must include at least 1 month of symptoms (or less if successfully treated) that meet Criterion A (i.e., active-phase symptoms) and may include periods of prodromal or residual symptoms. During these prodromal or residual periods, the signs of the disturbance may be manifested by only negative symptoms or by two or more symptoms listed in Criterion A present in an attenuated form (e.g., odd beliefs, unusual perceptual experiences).

D. Schizoaffective disorder and depressive or bipolar disorder with psychotic features have been ruled out because either 1) no major depressive or manic episodes have occurred concurrently with the active-phase symptoms, or 2) if mood episodes have occurred during active-phase symptoms, they have been present for a minority of the total duration of the active and residual periods of the illness.

E. The disturbance is not attributable to the physiological effects of a substance (e.g., a drug of abuse, a medication) or another medical condition.

F. If there is a history of autism spectrum disorder or a communication disorder of childhood onset, the additional diagnosis of schizophrenia is made only if prominent delusions or hallucinations, in addition to the other required symptoms of schizophrenia, are also present for at least 1 month (or less if successfully treated).

Specify if:
The following course specifiers are only to be used after a 1-year duration of the disorder and if they are not in contradiction to the diagnostic course criteria.

First episode, currently in acute episode: First manifestation of the disorder meeting the defining diagnostic symptom and time criteria. An *acute episode* is a time period in which the symptom criteria are fulfilled.

First episode, currently in partial remission: *Partial remission* is a period of time during which an improvement after a previous episode is maintained and in which the defining criteria of the disorder are only partially fulfilled.

First episode, currently in full remission: *Full remission* is a period of time after a previous episode during which no disorder-specific symptoms are present.

Multiple episodes, currently in acute episode: Multiple episodes may be determined after a minimum of two episodes (i.e., after a first episode, a remission and a minimum of one relapse).

Multiple episodes, currently in partial remission

Multiple episodes, currently in full remission

Continuous: Symptoms fulfilling the diagnostic symptom criteria of the disorder are remaining for the majority of the illness course, with subthreshold symptom periods being very brief relative to the overall course.

Unspecified

Specify if:

> **With catatonia** (refer to the criteria for catatonia associated with another mental disorder, DSM-5, pp. 119–120, for definition).
>
> > **Coding note:** Use additional code 293.89 (F06.1) catatonia associated with schizophrenia to indicate the presence of the comorbid catatonia.

Specify current severity:

> Severity is rated by a quantitative assessment of the primary symptoms of psychosis, including delusions, hallucinations, disorganized speech, abnormal psychomotor behavior, and negative symptoms. Each of these symptoms may be rated for its current severity (most severe in the last 7 days) on a 5-point scale ranging from 0 (not present) to 4 (present and severe). (See Clinician-Rated Dimensions of Psychosis Symptom Severity in Chapter 20, "Assessment Measures," this volume.)
>
> **Note:** Diagnosis of schizophrenia can be made without using this severity specifier.

Criterion A

At least one of the two required symptoms must be delusions, hallucinations, or disorganized speech. These three are core "positive symptoms" that are diagnosed with high reliability and might reasonably be considered necessary for a diagnosis of schizophrenia. In DSM-IV, only one characteristic symptom was required if it was a bizarre delusion or "first-rank" hallucination. Because bizarre delusions and first-rank hallucinations have little diagnostic specificity and their reliability is poor (Bell et al. 2006), these "positive symptoms" are now treated like any other with regard to their diagnostic implication: as with other characteristic symptoms, two Criterion A symptoms need to be present for a diagnosis of schizophrenia. This change also eliminates the possibility that an individual with only catatonia and negative symptoms will receive a diagnosis of schizophrenia.

To better describe the nature of the affective abnormality in schizophrenia, the fifth characteristic type of symptoms in Criterion A—negative symptoms—has been changed from "affective flattening, alogia, or avolition" (as in DSM-IV) to "diminished emotional expression or avolition." This change to emphasize restricted affect should help clarify and more accurately describe the individual's presentation.

Criterion B

Schizophrenia involves impairment in one or more major areas of functioning. Typically, functioning is clearly below prior levels of achievement, or, if the disturbance begins in childhood or adolescence, the expected level of functioning is not attained.

Criterion C

Signs of the disturbance must persist continuously for at least 6 months. During at least 1 month of that time, symptoms must meet Criterion A (active-phase symptoms). Prodromal symptoms often proceed the active phase, and residual symptoms may follow.

Some prodromal and residual symptoms are mild or subthreshold forms of hallucinations or delusions. Individuals may express a variety of unusual or odd beliefs that are not of delusional proportions; these are often referred to as "magical thinking" or "ideas of reference." The individual may report having unusual perceptual experiences, such as sensing the presence of an unseen person. The person's speech may be generally understandable but vague or digressive, while his or her behavior may be unusual but not grossly disorganized, such as muttering to oneself in public. Negative symptoms are common in the prodromal and residual phases and can be severe.

Criterion D

Although mood symptoms and mood episodes are common and may be concurrent with active-phase symptoms, individuals with schizophrenia must have delusions or hallucinations in the absence of mood episodes, or the total duration of the mood episodes must be present for only a minority of the total duration of the active and residual periods of the illness. Otherwise, schizoaffective disorder may be the more appropriate diagnosis.

Criterion E

Before making a diagnosis of schizophrenia, the clinician must rule out a wide variety of medical conditions that can present with psychotic symptoms, and must exclude drug-induced psychoses and psychoses attributable to delirium or other medical conditions (e.g., epilepsy, brain tumors, inflammatory brain disorders).

Criterion F

If the individual has a history of autism spectrum disorder or a communication disorder of childhood onset, the additional diagnosis of schizophrenia is made only if prominent delusions or hallucinations, and the other required symptoms of schizophrenia, have been present for at least 1 month (or less if successfully treated).

Specifiers

Multiple specifiers are provided to better describe the individual's course of illness. Catatonia may be specified if the full syndrome is present. Catatonic behaviors that may have previously led to the diagnosis of a catatonic subtype of schizophrenia are now covered in Criterion A4, which involves the presence of "grossly disorganized or catatonic behavior." The following additional diagnostic categories should be considered if the individual's symptoms are predominantly catatonic: catatonia associated with another mental disorder, catatonic disorder due to another medical condition, and unspecified catatonia.

Schizoaffective Disorder

Schizoaffective is a term first used by Jacob Kasanin (1933) to describe a small group of severely ill patients with a mix of psychotic and mood symptoms. In DSM-5, the hallmark of schizoaffective disorder is the presence of either a major depressive or a manic mood episode concurrent with psychotic symptoms that meet schizophrenia Criterion A, such as hallucinations, delusions, disorganized speech, grossly disorganized or catatonic behavior, or negative symptoms. Additionally, mood symptoms must be a *prominent* feature of the condition and not a minor aspect. Other causes of these symptoms, including other medical conditions, substances of abuse, and medications, must be ruled out. The symptoms typically present together, or sometimes in an alternating fashion; psychotic symptoms may be mood-congruent or mood-incongruent.

Although schizoaffective disorder has long filled an important role in psychiatric practice, the diagnosis has suffered from low reliability. This situation began in 1980 when the diagnosis was included in DSM-III but had no operational criteria. Instead, two clinical vignettes were described in which the diagnosis was used. Criteria were introduced in DSM-III-R, and these continued mostly unchanged through DSM-IV. The criteria indicated that the mood symptoms had to be present for a "substantial portion of the total duration" of the illness; however, little guidance was given to help clinicians judge how long the duration of the mood symptoms should be relative to the duration of the illness. This gap has now been addressed: a major mood episode must be present for the majority of the total duration of the active and residual portions of the illness (i.e., the time since Criterion A has been met). This change should help clarify the boundaries of the disorder by providing guidance to the clinician about the proportion of time the patient experiences a mood syndrome.

Diagnostic Criteria for Schizoaffective Disorder

A. An uninterrupted period of illness during which there is a major mood episode (major depressive or manic) concurrent with Criterion A of schizophrenia.
   Note: The major depressive episode must include Criterion A1: Depressed mood.
B. Delusions or hallucinations for 2 or more weeks in the absence of a major mood episode (depressive or manic) during the lifetime duration of the illness.
C. Symptoms that meet criteria for a major mood episode are present for the majority of the total duration of the active and residual portions of the illness.
D. The disturbance is not attributable to the effects of a substance (e.g., a drug of abuse, a medication) or another medical condition.

Specify whether:
   295.70 (F25.0) Bipolar type: This subtype applies if a manic episode is part of the presentation. Major depressive episodes may also occur.
   295.70 (F25.1) Depressive type: This subtype applies if only major depressive episodes are part of the presentation.

Specify if:
   With catatonia (refer to the criteria for catatonia associated with another mental disorder, DSM-5, pp. 119–120, for definition).
      Coding note: Use additional code 293.89 (F06.1) catatonia associated with schizoaffective disorder to indicate the presence of the comorbid catatonia.

Specify if:

The following course specifiers are only to be used after a 1-year duration of the disorder and if they are not in contradiction to the diagnostic course criteria.

First episode, currently in acute episode: First manifestation of the disorder meeting the defining diagnostic symptom and time criteria. An *acute episode* is a time period in which the symptom criteria are fulfilled.

First episode, currently in partial remission: *Partial remission* is a time period during which an improvement after a previous episode is maintained and in which the defining criteria of the disorder are only partially fulfilled.

First episode, currently in full remission: *Full remission* is a period of time after a previous episode during which no disorder-specific symptoms are present.

Multiple episodes, currently in acute episode: Multiple episodes may be determined after a minimum of two episodes (i.e., after a first episode, a remission and a minimum of one relapse).

Multiple episodes, currently in partial remission

Multiple episodes, currently in full remission

Continuous: Symptoms fulfilling the diagnostic symptom criteria of the disorder are remaining for the majority of the illness course, with subthreshold symptom periods being very brief relative to the overall course.

Unspecified

Specify current severity:

Severity is rated by a quantitative assessment of the primary symptoms of psychosis, including delusions, hallucinations, disorganized speech, abnormal psychomotor behavior, and negative symptoms. Each of these symptoms may be rated for its current severity (most severe in the last 7 days) on a 5-point scale ranging from 0 (not present) to 4 (present and severe). (See Clinician-Rated Dimensions of Psychosis Symptom Severity in Chapter 20, "Assessment Measures," this volume.)

Note: Diagnosis of schizoaffective disorder can be made without using this severity specifier.

Criterion A

The presence of psychotic and mood symptoms is the essence of schizoaffective disorder. There must be an uninterrupted period in which major depressive or manic symptoms must be concurrent with Criterion A (of schizophrenia) psychotic symptoms. In fact, for many if not most individuals, the actual duration of the symptom overlap is a matter of months or years, not days or weeks.

Criterion B

An important change in DSM-5 is that psychotic symptoms have to be present for 2 or more weeks in the absence of a major mood episode (depressive or manic) "during the lifetime duration of the illness" rather than "during the same period of illness" as in DSM-IV. This change was prompted by the goal of making explicit that the diagnosis of schizoaffective disorder is based on the assessment of psychotic and mood symptoms during the lifetime duration of the illness. DSM-IV implied that a "period of illness" could refer, at a minimum, to a single *episode* of illness lasting at least 1 month (to meet Criterion A) or, at a maximum, to the *lifetime duration* of the illness. To increase reliability, the authors of DSM-IV restricted the diagnosis to a given episode. This resulted in a person's receiving a diagnosis of schizoaffective disorder, schizophreniform disorder, schizophrenia, or even a psychotic mood disorder at various times during the illness.

Criterion C

The DSM-IV phrase "substantial portion of the total duration of the active and residual periods of the illness" has been replaced with "majority of the total duration of the active and residual portions, of the illness." The change was necessary because of the low reliability of the criterion and its limited clinical utility. Furthermore, the relative proportion of mood and psychotic symptoms can change over time, and clinicians and researchers often used different thresholds when applying this criterion. Researchers in several large studies had set the figure at 30% for total duration of their mood episodes (relative to the total duration of psychosis), but after examining field trial data the Psychotic Disorders Work Group recommended a threshold set at ≥50% as indicated by the word *majority.* Also new to DSM-5, Criterion C requires the assessment of mood symptoms not only during a current period of illness but over the entire course of a psychotic illness. If the mood symptoms are present for only a relatively brief period of time, the diagnosis is schizophrenia rather than schizoaffective disorder. When deciding whether an individual meets Criterion C, the clinician should review the total duration of psychotic illness (i.e., both active and residual symptoms) and determine when significant mood symptoms (untreated or in need of treatment with antidepressant and/or mood-stabilizing medication) accompanied the psychotic symptoms. This requires historical information and clinical judgment. For example, an individual with a 4-year history of active and residual symptoms of schizophrenia develops depressive and manic episodes that, taken together, do not occupy more than 1 year during the 4-year history of psychotic illness. This presentation would not meet Criterion C. The diagnosis in this example is schizophrenia, with the additional diagnosis of major depressive disorder to indicate the superimposed depressive episode.

Criterion D

Medical illnesses, medications, and drugs of abuse need to be ruled out as a cause of the disturbance.

Subtypes and Specifiers

The clinician may indicate whether the presentation includes a manic episode (bipolar type) or whether only major depressive episodes occur (depressive type). The presence of catatonia may be specified, as may course and current severity.

Substance/Medication-Induced Psychotic Disorder

The essential feature of substance/medication-induced psychotic disorder is that the delusions or hallucinations (Criterion A) are judged to be causally related to the effects of a substance or medication because they have developed during or soon after substance intoxication or withdrawal, or following exposure to a medication (Criterion B). Last, the disturbance is not better explained by an independent psychotic disorder (Criterion C). The criteria have been edited for clarity and readability but are otherwise unchanged from DSM-IV. The diagnosis is used when the symptoms are in *excess* of those associated with an intoxication or withdrawal syndrome. For example, because hallucinations can occur during an alcohol withdrawal delirium, an additional diagnosis of a substance-induced psychotic disorder is not appropriate.

The diagnosis is common among persons who abuse substances, as well as in hospitals and clinics, where medications are often the cause of induced psychotic symptoms. The initiation of the disorder varies considerably depending on the substance and its pharmacological properties. For example, smoking a high dose of cocaine may produce psychosis within minutes, but days or weeks of high doses of alcohol or sedatives may be required to produce psychosis. Hallucinations may occur in any modality, but in the absence of a delirium they are often auditory. Alcohol-induced psychotic disorder usually occurs only after heavy prolonged use (generally years) in individuals with an alcohol use disorder. Stimulant medications are known to produce persecutory delusions, which may develop rapidly following the use of the stimulant (e.g., amphetamine, methamphetamine). Induced psychotic disorders usually resolve when the offending agent is withdrawn, although in some cases they can persist for weeks or months even when the person is treated with antipsychotic medications.

The diagnostic code recorded depends on the class of the substance. Further specifications include whether the symptoms had an onset during intoxication or withdrawal, and current severity.

Diagnostic Criteria for Substance/Medication-Induced Psychotic Disorder

A. Presence of one or both of the following symptoms:

1. Delusions.
2. Hallucinations.

B. There is evidence from the history, physical examination, or laboratory findings of both (1) and (2):

1. The symptoms in Criterion A developed during or soon after substance intoxication or withdrawal or after exposure to a medication.
2. The involved substance/medication is capable of producing the symptoms in Criterion A.

C. The disturbance is not better explained by a psychotic disorder that is not sub-stance/medication-induced. Such evidence of an independent psychotic disorder could include the following:

> The symptoms preceded the onset of the substance/medication use; the symp-toms persist for a substantial period of time (e.g., about 1 month) after the ces-sation of acute withdrawal or severe intoxication; or there is other evidence of an independent non-substance/medication-induced psychotic disorder (e.g., a history of recurrent non-substance/medication-related episodes).

D. The disturbance does not occur exclusively during the course of a delirium.

E. The disturbance causes clinically significant distress or impairment in social, oc-cupational, or other important areas of functioning.

Note: This diagnosis should be made instead of a diagnosis of substance intoxication or substance withdrawal only when the symptoms in Criterion A predominate in the clinical picture and when they are sufficiently severe to warrant clinical attention.

Coding note: The ICD-9-CM and ICD-10-CM codes for the [specific substance/med-ication]-induced psychotic disorders are indicated in the table below. Note that the ICD-10-CM code depends on whether or not there is a comorbid substance use dis-order present for the same class of substance. If a mild substance use disorder is co-morbid with the substance-induced psychotic disorder, the 4th position character is "1," and the clinician should record "mild [substance] use disorder" before the sub-stance-induced psychotic disorder (e.g., "mild cocaine use disorder with cocaine-in-duced psychotic disorder"). If a moderate or severe substance use disorder is comorbid with the substance-induced psychotic disorder, the 4th position character is "2," and the clinician should record "moderate [substance] use disorder" or "severe [substance] use disorder," depending on the severity of the comorbid substance use disorder. If there is no comorbid substance use disorder (e.g., after a one-time heavy use of the substance), then the 4th position character is "9," and the clinician should record only the substance-induced psychotic disorder.

		ICD-10-CM		
	ICD-9-CM	With use disorder, mild	With use disorder, moderate or severe	Without use disorder
Alcohol	291.9	F10.159	F10.259	F10.959
Cannabis	292.9	F12.159	F12.259	F12.959
Phencyclidine	292.9	F16.159	F16.259	F16.959
Other hallucinogen	292.9	F16.159	F16.259	F16.959
Inhalant	292.9	F18.159	F18.259	F18.959
Sedative, hypnotic, or anxiolytic	292.9	F13.159	F13.259	F13.959
Amphetamine (or other stimulant)	292.9	F15.159	F15.259	F15.959
Cocaine	292.9	F14.159	F14.259	F14.959
Other (or unknown) substance	292.9	F19.159	F19.259	F19.959

Specify if (see Table 16–1 in the chapter "Substance-Related and Addictive Disorders" for diagnoses associated with substance class):

    With onset during intoxication: If the criteria are met for intoxication with the substance and the symptoms develop during intoxication.

    With onset during withdrawal: If the criteria are met for withdrawal from the substance and the symptoms develop during, or shortly after, withdrawal.

Specify current severity:

    Severity is rated by a quantitative assessment of the primary symptoms of psychosis, including delusions, hallucinations, abnormal psychomotor behavior, and negative symptoms. Each of these symptoms may be rated for its current severity (most severe in the last 7 days) on a 5-point scale ranging from 0 (not present) to 4 (present and severe). (See Clinician-Rated Dimensions of Psychosis Symptom Severity in Chapter 20, "Assessment Measures," this volume.)

    Note: Diagnosis of substance/medication-induced psychotic disorder can be made without using this severity specifier.

Criterion A

In DSM-IV, if a person realized that his or her hallucinations were substance or medication induced, the hallucinations were not counted toward this diagnosis, but this no longer applies.

Criterion B

The delusions and/or hallucinations must have developed "during or soon after" substance intoxication or withdrawal or after other exposure to a medication, and the substance/medication involved must be "capable" of producing the psychosis. This language is more specific than in DSM-IV, which used the phrase "etiologically related."

Criteria C, D, and E

This criterion outlines situations that cast doubt on a putative relationship between the use of a substance and the psychosis. For example, if the symptoms were present before the onset of substance or medication use, it is likely the psychosis is not substance induced. Delirium has been excluded as a cause of the psychosis, in which case the delirium would be separately coded. The disturbance must cause clinically significant distress or impairment.

Psychotic Disorder Due to Another Medical Condition

This diagnosis is relatively unchanged from DSM-IV except for the addition of Criterion E to acknowledge the presence of significant distress or impairment. In addition, there must be evidence that the disorder is the direct pathophysiological consequence of another medical condition, and the disorder must not occur exclusively in the course of a delirium (otherwise the diagnosis is delirium). The code used is based on whether delusions or hallucinations are the predominant symptom. Further, the name of the medical disorder is included in the name of the mental disorder (e.g., psychotic disorder due to malignant lung neoplasm). Current severity can also be recorded.

Diagnostic Criteria for Psychotic Disorder Due to a Another Medical Condition

---

A. Prominent hallucinations or delusions.
B. There is evidence from the history, physical examination, or laboratory findings that the disturbance is the direct pathophysiological consequence of another medical condition.
C. The disturbance is not better explained by another mental disorder.
D. The disturbance does not occur exclusively during the course of a delirium.
E. The disturbance causes clinically significant distress or impairment in social, occupational, or other important areas of functioning.

Specify whether:

Code based on predominant symptom:

293.81 (F06.2) With delusions: If delusions are the predominant symptom.

293.82 (F06.0) With hallucinations: If hallucinations are the predominant symptom.

Coding note: Include the name of the other medical condition in the name of the mental disorder (e.g., 293.81 [F06.2] psychotic disorder due to malignant lung neoplasm, with delusions). The other medical condition should be coded and listed separately immediately before the psychotic disorder due to the medical condition (e.g., 162.9 [C34.90] malignant lung neoplasm; 293.81 [F06.2] psychotic disorder due to malignant lung neoplasm, with delusions).

Specify current severity:

Severity is rated by a quantitative assessment of the primary symptoms of psychosis, including delusions, hallucinations, abnormal psychomotor behavior, and negative symptoms. Each of these symptoms may be rated for its current severity (most severe in the last 7 days) on a 5-point scale ranging from 0 (not present) to 4 (present and severe). (See Clinician-Rated Dimensions of Psychosis Symptom Severity in Chapter 20, "Assessment Measures," this volume.)

Note: Diagnosis of psychotic disorder due to another medical condition can be made without using this severity specifier.

Catatonia Associated With Another Mental Disorder (Catatonia Specifier)

Catatonia associated with another mental disorder (catatonia specifier) may be used when criteria are met for catatonia during the course of a neurodevelopmental, psychotic, bipolar, depressive, or other mental disorder. The catatonia specifier is appropriate when the clinical picture is characterized by marked psychomotor disturbance and involves at least 3 of the 12 diagnostic features listed in Criterion A.

While catatonia occurs in over one-third of schizophrenia cases, the majority of catatonia cases occur in patients with a mood disorder. For this reason, catatonia was added as an episode specifier for the major mood disorders in DSM-IV. Catatonic symptoms need to be recognized because they have prognostic and treatment implications. The presence of neuroleptic malignant syndrome should be ruled out because of the serious nature of its complications.

The name of the associated mental disorder should be included when recording the name of the disorder (e.g., catatonia associated with schizoaffective disorder).

Diagnostic Criteria for Catatonia Associated With Another Mental Disorder (Catatonia Specifier)   293.89 (F06.1)

A. The clinical picture is dominated by three (or more) of the following symptoms:

1. Stupor (i.e., no psychomotor activity; not actively relating to environment).
2. Catalepsy (i.e., passive induction of a posture held against gravity).
3. Waxvy flexibility (i.e., slight, even resistance to positioning by examiner).
4. Mutism (i.e., no, or very little, verbal response [exclude if known aphasia]).
5. Negativism (i.e., opposition or no response to instructions or external stimuli).
6. Posturing (i.e., spontaneous and active maintenance of a posture against gravity).
7. Mannerism (i.e., odd, circumstantial caricature of normal actions).
8. Stereotypy (i.e., repetitive, abnormally frequent, non-goal-directed movements).
9. Agitation, not influenced by external stimuli.
10. Grimacing.
11. Echolalia (i.e., mimicking another's speech).
12. Echopraxia (i.e., mimicking another's movements).

Coding note: Indicate the name of the associated mental disorder when recording the name of the condition (i.e., 293.89 [F06.1] catatonia associated with major depressive disorder). Code first the associated mental disorder (e.g., neurodevelopmental disorder, brief psychotic disorder, schizophreniform disorder, schizophrenia, schizoaffective disorder, bipolar disorder, major depressive disorder, or other mental disorder) (e.g., 295.70 [F25.1] schizoaffective disorder, depressive type; 293.89 [F06.1] catatonia associated with schizoaffective disorder).

Catatonic Disorder Due to Another Medical Condition

Catatonic disorder due to another medical condition has been moved from the DSM-IV chapter "Mental Disorders Due to a General Medical Condition." Catatonia has generally been viewed as a subtype of schizophrenia, as reflected in DSM-IV, but research has shown that catatonic symptoms can result from several medical disorders. For that reason, catatonic disorder due to a general medical condition was added as a new category in DSM-IV. The criteria for this disorder have changed to reflect greater specificity in the symptoms and impairment caused by the condition.

Diagnostic Criteria for Catatonic Disorder Due to Another Medical Condition 293.89 (F06.1)

A. The clinical picture is dominated by three (or more) of the following symptoms:
   1. Stupor (i.e., no psychomotor activity; not actively relating to environment).
   2. Catalepsy (i.e., passive induction of a posture held against gravity).
   3. Waxy flexibility (i.e., slight, even resistance to positioning by examiner).
   4. Mutism (i.e., no, or very little, verbal response [**Note:** not applicable if there is an established aphasia]).
   5. Negativism (i.e., opposition or no response to instructions or external stimuli).
   6. Posturing (i.e., spontaneous and active maintenance of a posture against gravity).
   7. Mannerism (i.e., odd, circumstantial caricature of normal actions).
   8. Stereotypy (i.e., repetitive, abnormally frequent, non-goal-directed movements).
   9. Agitation, not influenced by external stimuli.
   10. Grimacing.
   11. Echolalia (i.e., mimicking another's speech).
   12. Echopraxia (i.e., mimicking another's movements).
B. There is evidence from the history, physical examination, or laboratory findings that the disturbance is the direct pathophysiological consequence of another medical condition.
C. The disturbance is not better explained by another mental disorder (e.g., a manic episode).
D. The disturbance does not occur exclusively during the course of a delirium.
E. The disturbance causes clinically significant distress or impairment in social, occupational, or other important areas of functioning.

Coding note: Include the name of the medical condition in the name of the mental disorder (e.g., 293.89 [F06.1]) catatonic disorder due to hepatic encephalopathy). The other medical condition should be coded and listed separately immediately before the catatonic disorder due to the medical condition (e.g., 572.2 [K71.90] hepatic encephalopathy; 293.89 [F06.1] catatonic disorder due to hepatic encephalopathy).

Criterion A

This criterion requires the presence of 3 or more of 12 symptoms typical for catatonia. In DSM-IV, the criteria were unclear as to how many symptoms were required.

Criteria B and C

Because catatonic symptoms have been associated with a variety of medical disorders, medical conditions apart from the disorder in question need to be ruled out as a cause. This entails a detailed medical workup to rule out neurological, infectious, and other potential causes of the symptoms. For example, before concluding that the catatonia resulted from a herpes-related encephalopathy, the clinician should rule out brain tumors and other mass lesions.

Catatonic symptoms can occur in the context of other major mental disorders, such as mania, and these disorders need to be ruled out as well.

Criteria D and E

If the symptoms occur only in the context of a delirium, then delirium is the appropriate diagnosis. This criterion is new to DSM-5 and specifies that the symptoms cause significant distress or impairment in social, occupational, and other important areas of functioning.

Unspecified Catatonia

Catatonic syndromes can occur within the context of many other disorders, including psychotic disorders, depressive and bipolar disorders, and general medical conditions. In DSM-5, catatonia is no longer listed as a specific subtype of schizophrenia, but the text recognizes catatonic disorder as being due to another medical condition, as a specifier for a psychotic disorder or a depressive or bipolar disorder, or as an unspecified catatonia.

Unspecified Catatonia

This category applies to presentations in which symptoms characteristic of catatonia cause clinically significant distress or impairment in social, occupational, or other important areas of functioning but either the nature of the underlying mental disorder or other medical condition is unclear, full criteria for catatonia are not met, or there is insufficient information to make a more specific diagnosis (e.g., in emergency room settings).

Coding note: Code first **781.99 (R29.818)** other symptoms involving nervous and musculoskeletal systems, followed by **293.89 (F06.1)** unspecified catatonia.

The diagnosis unspecified catatonia may be used when individuals with catatonic symptoms have clinically significant distress or impairment but the nature of the underlying mental disorder or other medical condition is unclear, the full criteria for catatonic disorder are not met, or there is insufficient information to make a more specific diagnosis.

Other Specified Schizophrenia Spectrum and Other Psychotic Disorder and Unspecified Schizophrenia Spectrum and Other Psychotic Disorder

Other specified and unspecified schizophrenia spectrum and other psychotic disorders are residual categories for individuals whose symptoms do not fit within one of the more specific categories. The categories replace DSM-IV's psychotic disorder not otherwise specified.

Other specified schizophrenia spectrum and other psychotic disorder can be used in situations in which an individual has symptoms characteristic of a spectrum disorder that cause distress or impairment but that do not meet full criteria for a more specific disorder. In this case, the clinician chooses to communicate the reason that individual's symptoms do not meet the criteria. Specific examples are given in DSM-5 to describe situations in which this diagnosis may be appropriate. The category unspecified schizophrenia spectrum and other psychotic disorder is used when the clinician chooses not to specify the reason that criteria are not met for a more specific disorder, or when there is insufficient information to make a more specific diagnosis.

Other Specified Schizophrenia Spectrum and Other Psychotic Disorder   298.8 (F28)

This category applies to presentations in which symptoms characteristic of a schizophrenia spectrum and other psychotic disorder that cause clinically significant distress or impairment in social, occupational, or other important areas of functioning predominate but do not meet the full criteria for any of the disorders in the schizophrenia spectrum and other psychotic disorders diagnostic class. The other specified schizophrenia spectrum and other psychotic disorder category is used in situations in which the clinician chooses to communicate the specific reason that the presentation does not meet the criteria for any specific schizophrenia spectrum and other psychotic disorder. This is done by recording "other specified schizophrenia spectrum and other psychotic disorder" followed by the specific reason (e.g., "persistent auditory hallucinations").

Examples of presentations that can be specified using the "other specified" designation include the following:

1. **Persistent auditory hallucinations** occurring in the absence of any other features.
2. **Delusions with significant overlapping mood episodes:** This includes persistent delusions with periods of overlapping mood episodes that are present for a substantial portion of the delusional disturbance (such that the criterion stipulating only brief mood disturbance in delusional disorder is not met).

3. **Attenuated psychosis syndrome:** This syndrome is characterized by psychotic-like symptoms that are below a threshold for full psychosis (e.g., the symptoms are less severe and more transient, and insight is relatively maintained).
4. **Delusional symptoms in partner of individual with delusional disorder:** In the context of a relationship, the delusional material from the dominant partner provides content for delusional belief by the individual who may not otherwise entirely meet criteria for delusional disorder.

Unspecified Schizophrenia Spectrum and Other Psychotic Disorder   298.9 (F29)

This category applies to presentations in which symptoms characteristic of a schizophrenia spectrum and other psychotic disorder that cause clinically significant distress or impairment in social, occupational, or other important areas of functioning predominate but do not meet the full criteria for any of the disorders in the schizophrenia spectrum and other psychotic disorders diagnostic class. The unspecified schizophrenia spectrum and other psychotic disorder category is used in situations in which the clinician chooses *not* to specify the reason that the criteria are not met for a specific schizophrenia spectrum and other psychotic disorder, and includes presentations in which there is insufficient information to make a more specific diagnosis (e.g., in emergency room settings).

Clinician-Rated Dimensions of Psychosis Symptom Severity

The Clinician-Rated Dimensions of Psychosis Symptom Severity is available to help the clinician make detailed assessments of individuals across important domains, including hallucinations, delusions, disorganized speech, abnormal psychomotor behavior, negative symptoms, impaired cognition, depression, and mania. This instrument is described in Chapter 20, "Assessment Measures."

KEY POINTS

- Chapter organization has changed so that schizophrenia spectrum and other psychotic disorders are arranged along a gradient from least to most severe. Severity is defined by the level, number, and duration of psychotic signs and symptoms.
- Schizotypal personality disorder has been included in the schizophrenia spectrum, but the criteria and text remain in the personality disorders chapter. Evidence has accumulated since its initial description in DSM-III confirming its close etiological relationship with schizophrenia and other psychotic disorders.

- In the criteria for delusional disorder, the adjective *nonbizarre* has been removed (Criterion A), and the somatic subtype has been edited to ensure that individuals with a delusion regarding a physical defect are more appropriately diagnosed with body dysmorphic disorder.

- The diagnosis shared psychotic disorder has been eliminated because it was infrequently used and persons with the diagnosis generally had symptoms that met criteria for some other psychotic disorder (e.g., delusional disorder).

- With schizophrenia, bizarre delusions and "first-rank" hallucinations are no longer accorded special treatment. Further, clinicians will no longer record schizophrenia subtypes; despite historical precedent, there is scant research evidence supporting their clinical utility or predictive validity.

- The criteria for schizoaffective disorder now clarify that mood symptoms must constitute the "majority of the total duration of the active and residual portions of the illness." The change was necessary because of the low reliability and limited clinical utility of the wording in DSM-IV.

CHAPTER 5

Mood Disorders

Bipolar and Related Disorders
Bipolar I Disorder
296.89 (F31.81) Bipolar II Disorder
301.13 (F34.0) Cyclothymic Disorder
Substance/Medication-Induced Bipolar and Related Disorder
293.83 (F06.3_) Bipolar and Related Disorder Due to Another Medical Condition
296.89 (F31.89) Other Specified Bipolar and Related Disorder
296.80 (F31.9) Unspecified Bipolar and Related Disorder

Depressive Disorders
296.99 (F34.8) Disruptive Mood Dysregulation Disorder
Major Depressive Disorder, Single Episode
Major Depressive Disorder, Recurrent Episode
300.4 (F34.1) Persistent Depressive Disorder (Dysthymia)
625.4 (N94.3) Premenstrual Dysphoric Disorder
Substance/Medication-Induced Depressive Disorder
293.83 (F06.3_) Depressive Disorder Due to Another Medical Condition
311 (F32.8) Other Specified Depressive Disorder
311 (F32.9) Unspecified Depressive Disorder

The major change in DSM-5 regarding mood disorders is that the DSM-IV chapter of that name has been divided into two separate chapters: one for bipolar and related disorders and the other for depressive disorders. Both diagnostic classes are reviewed in this chapter.

Mood disorders are highly prevalent, have high morbidity, and are associated with early mortality and suicide. They are among the world's most disabling illnesses, as documented in *The Global Burden of Disease* (Murray and Lopez 1996). Characterized by prominent and prolonged disturbances of mood generally inappropriate to the individual's life situation, depression and mania are considered the primary syndromes. Many symptoms occur in individuals with mood disorder, including insomnia, suicidal thoughts, anorexia, and feelings of being a burden to others in individuals with depression, and euphoria, irritability, decreased need for sleep, and hyperactivity in individuals with mania. In DSM-III, these conditions were collectively referred to as *affective disorders,* but they were renamed mood disorders for DSM-III-R. The term *mood disorder* is more appropriate because *affect* refers to fluctuating mood changes in emotional expression, whereas *mood* refers to more sustained and pervasive feeling states.

The mood disorders have been divided in many different ways over the years in attempts to identify the best classification scheme. Although that goal has been elusive, research and clinical experience both show that the fundamental symptoms of mood disorders are depressed mood, elevated mood, or an admixture of the two.

Despite having a limited number of disorders, the two DSM-5 mood disorder chapters are lengthy because of all the specifiers that can be used to provide greater detail about an individual's illness. These allow the clinician to record whether the current or most recent episode is manic, hypomanic, or depressed; whether the mood disorder is accompanied by anxious distress; whether there are mixed features, melancholic features, atypical features, psychotic features, or catatonia; whether there is rapid cycling; whether there is a peripartum onset; or whether there is a seasonal pattern.

Because mood symptoms are not specific to these diagnostic classes and are found in many other psychiatric disorders, differential diagnosis is complicated. For example, manic/hypomanic symptoms commonly occur in individuals with neurocognitive disorders or in those with schizophrenia spectrum and other psychotic disorders, whereas depression is found to some extent in individuals with disorders as wide ranging as adjustment disorders, anxiety disorders, and personality disorders. Mood symptoms are sometimes masked as complaints about insomnia, fatigue, or unexplained pain, which can further complicate the differential diagnosis.

Historically, mood disorders are among the oldest recognized psychiatric syndromes, and have been included in nearly all diagnostic classification systems through the centuries. Both depressive and bipolar conditions were included within the same category in DSM-I ("manic depressive reaction") and DSM-II ("manic-depressive illness"). All were classified as psychoses except one: mood syndromes precipitated by stressful life experience. Later, unipolar and bipolar disorders were separated in response to research showing that individuals with manic episodes have a fundamentally different course and outcome than those who experience only depression. These new concepts were reflected in the Feighner criteria (Feighner et al. 1972), the Research Diagnostic Criteria (Spitzer et al. 1975), and DSM-III. This fundamental distinction has been fully accepted by psychiatric clinicians and researchers.

We begin with a review of the DSM-5 chapter on bipolar and related disorders, which include those disorders listed in Table 5–1.

BIPOLAR AND RELATED DISORDERS

This diagnostic class recognizes disorders characterized by marked oscillations in mood, activity, and behavior. The classic form of bipolar disorder was described by Kraepelin as an illness that was episodic and nondeteriorating, in contrast to schizophrenia. Research evidence has confirmed the existence of a milder form of the disorder, which was

TABLE 5–1. DSM-5 bipolar and related disorders

Bipolar I disorder

Bipolar II disorder

Cyclothymic disorder

Substance/medication-induced bipolar and related disorder

Bipolar and related disorder due to another medical condition

Other specified bipolar and related disorder

Unspecified bipolar and related disorder

listed in DSM-III as an atypical bipolar disorder and given its own category, bipolar II disorder, in DSM-IV. In DSM-5, bipolar and related disorders are placed between the chapters on schizophrenia spectrum and other psychotic disorders and the depressive disorders in recognition of their place in bridging these diagnostic classes.

Several changes were made in the criteria for DSM-5, with the goal of improving specificity and sensitivity of the bipolar diagnoses. One objective was to reduce the delay from the onset of first symptoms to correct diagnosis. Because of misdiagnosis, people with bipolar disorder often receive inappropriate treatments, such as antidepressant pharmacotherapy in the absence of mood stabilizers, and thus are exposed to the risk of cycle acceleration or hypomanic/manic switches, mixed states, and suicidal behaviors. Improving diagnostic precision is expected to increase recognition of bipolarity among people presenting with depressed mood and increase the probability of their receiving early treatment.

The Mood Disorders Work Group added the phrase "persistently increased goal-directed activity or energy" to Criterion A for both mania and hypomania. This addition should make explicit the requirement that this hallmark symptom of bipolar I or II disorder needs to be present for the diagnosis to be made. The work group also recommended deleting the diagnosis of bipolar I disorder, mixed type, which required the criteria for mania and major depressive episode to be met simultaneously. Instead, a "with mixed features" specifier has been added that can be applied to mania or hypomania when depressive features are present. The requirement that both full syndromes be present was difficult to employ and had the potential to lead clinicians to ignore important mood symptoms that failed to meet full diagnostic threshold (Cassano et al. 2004; Goldberg et al. 2009).

Another change is that mania or hypomania that emerges during antidepressant treatment (a medication, electroconvulsive therapy) but persists at full syndromal level beyond the physiological effect of that treatment is now considered sufficient evidence for a diagnosis of bipolar disorder.

In summary, these changes reflect refinements aimed at improving the recognition and treatment of bipolar disorders by encouraging the clinician to observe and record symptoms reflecting increased activity and mixed forms of mania/hypomania and depression to consider in treatment decisions and future patient follow-up. Additionally, people with substance-induced conditions that persist beyond the action of a medication or substance will now receive a bipolar diagnosis.

Manic Episode

Diagnostic Criteria for Manic Episode

For a diagnosis of bipolar I disorder, it is necessary to meet the following criteria for a manic episode. The manic episode may have been preceded by and may be followed by hypomanic or major depressive episodes.

A. A distinct period of abnormally and persistently elevated, expansive, or irritable mood and abnormally and persistently increased activity or energy, lasting at least 1 week and present most of the day, nearly every day (or any duration if hospitalization is necessary).

B. During the period of mood disturbance and increased energy or activity, three (or more) of the following symptoms (four if the mood is only irritable) are present to a significant degree and represent a noticeable change from usual behavior:

1. Inflated self-esteem or grandiosity.
2. Decreased need for sleep (e.g., feels rested after only 3 hours of sleep).
3. More talkative than usual or pressure to keep talking.
4. Flight of ideas or subjective experience that thoughts are racing.
5. Distractibility (i.e., attention too easily drawn to unimportant or irrelevant external stimuli), as reported or observed.
6. Increase in goal-directed activity (either socially, at work or school, or sexually) or psychomotor agitation (i.e., purposeless non-goal-directed activity).
7. Excessive involvement in activities that have a high potential for painful consequences (e.g., engaging in unrestrained buying sprees, sexual indiscretions, or foolish business investments).

C. The mood disturbance is sufficiently severe to cause marked impairment in social or occupational functioning or to necessitate hospitalization to prevent harm to self or others, or there are psychotic features.

D. The episode is not attributable to the physiological effects of a substance (e.g., a drug of abuse, a medication, other treatment) or to another medical condition.
   Note: A full manic episode that emerges during antidepressant treatment (e.g., medication, electroconvulsive therapy) but persists at a fully syndromal level beyond the physiological effect of that treatment is sufficient evidence for a manic episode and, therefore, a bipolar I diagnosis.

Note: Criteria A–D constitute a manic episode. At least one lifetime manic episode is required for the diagnosis of bipolar I disorder.

Criterion A

The phrase "persistently increased goal-directed activity or energy" has been added to ensure that changes in both mood and activity level are appropriately recognized. Increased activity or energy is a core symptom of mania and hypomania. This change is prompted by the concern that mild mania, hypomania, and subthreshold bipolar features are often unrecognized or misdiagnosed as major depressive disorder when level of activity is not taken into account (Angst et al. 2011, 2012). Furthermore, because the clinician is often seeing the individual in the depressive state and attempting to assess mania retrospectively, it may be easier for the individual to recall periods of increased activity than changes in mood that may be more subtle and ego-syntonic. The addition of "persistently increased goal-directed activity or energy" will increase specificity of the application of this diagnosis.

The wording has also been changed to acknowledge that these symptoms are present "most of the day, nearly every day." This helps clinicians distinguish mania (and hypomania) from borderline personality disorder and the mood swings that people with this condition typically report (i.e., very short-lived, usually involving a change from feeling normal to suddenly feeling angry or depressed, and tending to occur in response to a psychosocial stressor).

Criterion B

The wording "increased energy or activity" has been added to this criterion to emphasize the importance of this symptom in distinguishing mania and hypomania. In addition, the wording "and represent a noticeable change from usual behavior" was added to emphasize that mania and hypomania represent a change from the person's usual behavior, and constitute a distinct mood or mood state. Clearly, manic changes represent an alteration in conduct and behavior that is not normal for the individual, and that is usually observable to others, especially family members distressed by the changes noted in their loved one. Three or more of seven classic manic symptoms are required for the diagnosis (four if the mood is only irritable).

Criterion C

This criterion is simplified from DSM-IV Criterion D. Mania is clearly impairing. Although mild forms may be tolerated (and perhaps even desirable in some situations), full-blown mania can be disastrous to the individual's personal and professional life, particularly when the individual makes bad decisions about his or her personal life (e.g., infidelity, sexual promiscuity) or business (e.g., major purchases, personnel decisions). Delusions and/or hallucinations (e.g., believing one is wealthy, has a special religious mission, knows famous persons) may further influence a person's behavior.

Criterion D

This criterion requires that the mania not be induced by a substance (e.g., drug of abuse, medication, other treatment). There are many drugs that have been associated with manic symptoms and need to be ruled out (e.g., stimulants, corticosteroids). The notation that mania resulting from antidepressant treatment (e.g., medication, electroconvulsive therapy) and persisting "at a fully syndromal level beyond the physiological effect of that treatment is sufficient evidence for a manic episode and, therefore, a bipolar I diagnosis" is new to DSM-5. By contrast, in DSM-IV, "manic-like episodes" that were "clearly caused by somatic antidepressant treatment" were not to be counted toward a bipolar I diagnosis.

Specifiers

In DSM-5, the "with mixed features" specifier for mania, hypomania, and depressive episodes has replaced the criteria in DSM-IV for bipolar I disorder, most recent episode mixed. The criteria were often considered confusing, and therefore persons with depressive symptoms may have been ignored and their symptoms unrecognized. Because a substantial proportion of individuals with bipolar disorder (and persons whose symptoms meet criteria for a major depressive episode) also describe an admixture of depressive (or manic) symptoms that are insufficient in number to meet the DSM-IV definition of a mixed episode, the significance of the symptoms went unnoticed or the symptoms were altogether ignored. The presence of mixed symptoms is important to recognize because it has been associated with course (earlier onset), greater number of episodes, higher likelihoods of alcohol abuse and suicide attempts, greater likelihood of rapid cycling, and greater likelihood of a lifetime diagnosis of bipolar disorder.

Hypomanic Episode

The criteria for hypomanic episode describe a mild form of mania that may be seen either in the course of bipolar I disorder or as a regular part of bipolar II disorder.

Diagnostic Criteria for Hypomanic Episode

A. A distinct period of abnormally and persistently elevated, expansive, or irritable mood and abnormally and persistently increased activity or energy, lasting at least 4 consecutive days and present most of the day, nearly every day.

B. During the period of mood disturbance and increased energy and activity, three (or more) of the following symptoms (four if the mood is only irritable) have persisted, represent a noticeable change from usual behavior, and have been present to a significant degree:

  1. Inflated self-esteem or grandiosity.
  2. Decreased need for sleep (e.g., feels rested after only 3 hours of sleep).
  3. More talkative than usual or pressure to keep talking.
  4. Flight of ideas or subjective experience that thoughts are racing.
  5. Distractibility (i.e., attention too easily drawn to unimportant or irrelevant external stimuli), as reported or observed.
  6. Increase in goal-directed activity (either socially, at work or school, or sexually) or psychomotor agitation.
  7. Excessive involvement in activities that have a high potential for painful consequences (e.g., engaging in unrestrained buying sprees, sexual indiscretions, or foolish business investments).

C. The episode is associated with an unequivocal change in functioning that is uncharacteristic of the individual when not symptomatic.

D. The disturbance in mood and the change in functioning are observable by others.

E. The episode is not severe enough to cause marked impairment in social or occupational functioning or to necessitate hospitalization. If there are psychotic features, the episode is, by definition, manic.

F. The episode is not attributable to the physiological effects of a substance (e.g., a drug of abuse, a medication, other treatment).

Note: A full hypomanic episode that emerges during antidepressant treatment (e.g., medication, electroconvulsive therapy) but persists at a fully syndromal level beyond the physiological effect of that treatment is sufficient evidence for a hypomanic episode diagnosis. However, caution is indicated so that one or two symptoms (particularly increased irritability, edginess, or agitation following antidepressant use) are not taken as sufficient for diagnosis of a hypomanic episode, nor necessarily indicative of a bipolar diathesis.

Note: Criteria A–F constitute a hypomanic episode. Hypomanic episodes are common in bipolar I disorder but are not required for the diagnosis of bipolar I disorder.

The criteria for hypomanic episode are mostly unchanged from DSM-IV other than the added phrase "persistently increased activity or energy" in Criterion A, and the added requirement that the changes be present "most of the day, nearly every day," also in Criterion A. Also new is the notation indicating that a hypomanic episode can result from antidepressant therapy, but that if only one or two symptoms are present, the diagnosis is not justified.

Major Depressive Episode

See "Depressive Disorders" later in this chapter for criteria for and discussion of major depressive episode.

Bipolar I Disorder

DSM-5 no longer includes six separate criteria sets for bipolar I disorder as in DSM-IV. Emphasis is now given to the use of specifiers, as previously noted.

Diagnostic Criteria for Bipolar I Disorder

A. Criteria have been met for at least one manic episode (Criteria A–D under "Manic Episode" above).

B. The occurrence of the manic and major depressive episode(s) is not better explained by schizoaffective disorder, schizophrenia, schizophreniform disorder, delusional disorder, or other specified or unspecified schizophrenia spectrum and other psychotic disorder.

Coding and Recording Procedures
The diagnostic code for bipolar I disorder is based on type of current or most recent episode and its status with respect to current severity, presence of psychotic features, and remission status. Current severity and psychotic features are only indicated if full

criteria are currently met for a manic or major depressive episode. Remission specifiers are only indicated if the full criteria are not currently met for a manic, hypomanic, or major depressive episode. Codes are as follows:

Bipolar I disorder	Current or most recent episode manic	Current or most recent episode hypomanic*	Current or most recent episode depressed	Current or most recent episode unspecified**
Mild (DSM-5, p. 154)	296.41 (F31.11)	NA	296.51 (F31.31)	NA
Moderate (DSM-5, p. 154)	296.42 (F31.12)	NA	296.52 (F31.32)	NA
Severe (DSM-5, p. 154)	296.43 (F31.13)	NA	296.53 (F31.4)	NA
With psychotic features*** (DSM-5, p. 152)	296.44 (F31.2)	NA	296.54 (F31.5)	NA
In partial remission (DSM-5, p. 154)	296.45 (F31.73)	296.45 (F31.71)	296.55 (F31.75)	NA
In full remission (DSM-5, p. 154)	296.46 (F31.74)	296.46 (F31.72)	296.56 (F31.76)	NA
Unspecified	296.40 (F31.9)	296.40 (F31.9)	296.50 (F31.9)	NA

*Severity and psychotic specifiers do not apply; code 296.40 (F31.0) for cases not in remission.
**Severity, psychotic, and remission specifiers do not apply. Code 296.7 (F31.9).
***If psychotic features are present, code the "with psychotic features" specifier irrespective of episode severity.

In recording the name of a diagnosis, terms should be listed in the following order: bipolar I disorder, type of current or most recent episode, severity/psychotic/remission specifiers, followed by as many specifiers without codes as apply to the current or most recent episode.

Specify:
   With anxious distress (DSM-5, p. 149)
   With mixed features (DSM-5, pp. 149–150)
   With rapid cycling (DSM-5, pp. 150–151)
   With melancholic features (DSM-5, p. 151)
   With atypical features (DSM-5, pp. 151–152)
   With mood-congruent psychotic features (DSM-5, p. 152)
   With mood-incongruent psychotic features (DSM-5, p. 152)
   With catatonia (DSM-5, p. 152). **Coding note:** Use additional code 293.89 (F06.1).
   With peripartum onset (DSM-5, pp. 152–153)
   With seasonal pattern (DSM-5, pp. 153–154)

Bipolar II Disorder

Criteria for bipolar II disorder are relatively unchanged from DSM-IV except for minor editing. Emphasis is placed on the use of specifiers, as noted earlier in the chapter.

Diagnostic Criteria for Bipolar II Disorder   **296.89** (F31.81)

For a diagnosis of bipolar II disorder, it is necessary to meet the criteria for a current or past hypomanic episode *and* the following criteria for a current or past major depressive episode.

A. Criteria have been met for at least one hypomanic episode (Criteria A–F under "Hypomanic Episode"; see p. 94) and at least one major depressive episode (Criteria A–C under "Major Depressive Episode"; see pp. 108–109).

B. There has never been a manic episode.

C. The occurrence of the hypomanic episode(s) and major depressive episode(s) is not better explained by schizoaffective disorder, schizophrenia, schizophreniform disorder, delusional disorder, or other specified or unspecified schizophrenia spectrum and other psychotic disorder.

D. The symptoms of depression or the unpredictability caused by frequent alternation between periods of depression and hypomania causes clinically significant distress or impairment in social, occupational, or other important areas of functioning.

Coding and Recording Procedures

Bipolar II disorder has one diagnostic code: 296.89 (F31.81). Its status with respect to current severity, presence of psychotic features, course, and other specifiers cannot be coded but should be indicated in writing (e.g., 296.89 [F31.81] bipolar II disorder, current episode depressed, moderate severity, with mixed features; 296.89 [F31.81] bipolar II disorder, most recent episode depressed, in partial remission).

Specify current or most recent episode:

 Hypomanic
 Depressed

Specify if:

 With anxious distress (DSM-5, p. 149)
 With mixed features (DSM-5, pp. 149–150)
 With rapid cycling (DSM-5, pp. 150–151)
 With mood-congruent psychotic features (DSM-5, p. 152)
 With mood-incongruent psychotic features (DSM-5, p. 152)
 With catatonia (DSM-5, p. 152). **Coding note:** Use additional code 293.89 (F06.1).
 With peripartum onset (DSM-5, pp. 152–153)
 With seasonal pattern (DSM-5, pp. 153–154): Applies only to the pattern of major depressive episodes.

Specify course if full criteria for a mood episode are not currently met:

 In partial remission (DSM-5, p. 154)
 In full remission (DSM-5, p. 154)

Specify severity if full criteria for a mood episode are currently met:
Mild (DSM-5, p. 154)
Moderate (DSM-5, p. 154)
Severe (DSM-5, p. 154)

Cyclothymic Disorder

The individual with cyclothymic disorder has mild swings between the two poles of depression and hypomania. In the hypomanic phase, the person appears to be high but not so high as to be socially or professionally incapacitated. In the depressed phase, the individual has symptoms of depression, but not severe enough to meet criteria for a full major depressive episode. Thus, the individual with cyclothymic disorder tends to swing from high to low and may have chronic mild mood instability.

The disorder was first included in DSM-III and was derived from DSM-II (American Psychiatric Association 1968) cyclothymic personality, described as a "behavior pattern [that is] manifested by recurring and alternating periods of depression and elation" (p. 42). The move to the mood disorders chapter ("Affective Disorders" in DSM-III) was made based on evidence that cyclothymic disorder was related to bipolar disorder; for example, some individuals will develop manic episodes, whereas others will develop major depressive episodes, and therefore meet criteria for either a bipolar I or II disorder.

The DSM-5 criteria for cyclothymia are mostly unchanged from DSM-IV, but have been edited for clarity. The major change has been to indicate that during the 2-year period hypomanic and depressive symptoms have been present for "at least half the time." This is in addition to the existing requirement (in DSM-IV) that individuals could not be without symptoms for "more than 2 months at a time." The new wording provides greater guidance to clinicians, and reinforces the concept of cyclothymia being a relatively chronic and persistent mood disorder.

Diagnostic Criteria for Cyclothymic Disorder   **301.13** (F34.0)

A. For at least 2 years (at least 1 year in children and adolescents) there have been numerous periods with hypomanic symptoms that do not meet criteria for a hypomanic episode and numerous periods with depressive symptoms that do not meet criteria for a major depressive episode.
B. During the above 2-year period (1 year in children and adolescents), the hypomanic and depressive periods have been present for at least half the time and the individual has not been without the symptoms for more than 2 months at a time.
C. Criteria for a major depressive, manic, or hypomanic episode have never been met.
D. The symptoms in Criterion A are not better explained by schizoaffective disorder, schizophrenia, schizophreniform disorder, delusional disorder, or other specified or unspecified schizophrenia spectrum and other psychotic disorder.
E. The symptoms are not attributable to the physiological effects of a substance (e.g., a drug of abuse, a medication) or another medical condition (e.g., hyperthyroidism).

F. The symptoms cause clinically significant distress or impairment in social, occupa-
    tional, or other important areas of functioning.

Specify if:
    With anxious distress (see DSM-5, p. 149)

Substance/Medication-Induced Bipolar and Related Disorder

The criteria for substance/medication-induced bipolar disorder derive from those for
DSM-IV substance-induced mood disorder but are specific to bipolar disorder. These
criteria are patterned after those for manic episode except that the bipolar disorder is
induced by a substance of abuse or a medication.

Diagnostic Criteria for Substance/Medication-Induced Bipolar and Related Disorder

A. A prominent and persistent disturbance in mood that predominates in the clinical picture
    and is characterized by elevated, expansive, or irritable mood, with or without depressed
    mood, or markedly diminished interest or pleasure in all, or almost all, activities.
B. There is evidence from the history, physical examination, or laboratory findings of both
    (1) and (2):
    1. The symptoms in Criterion A developed during or soon after substance intoxica-
        tion or withdrawal or after exposure to a medication.
    2. The involved substance/medication is capable of producing the symptoms in
        Criterion A.
C. The disturbance is not better explained by a bipolar or related disorder that is not
    substance/medication-induced. Such evidence of an independent bipolar or relat-
    ed disorder could include the following:

    The symptoms precede the onset of the substance/medication use; the symp-
    toms persist for a substantial period of time (e.g., about 1 month) after the ces-
    sation of acute withdrawal or severe intoxication; or there is other evidence
    suggesting the existence of an independent non-substance/medication-in-
    duced bipolar and related disorder (e.g., a history of recurrent non-substance/
    medication-related episodes).

D. The disturbance does not occur exclusively during the course of a delirium.
E. The disturbance causes clinically significant distress or impairment in social, oc-
    cupational, or other important areas of functioning.

Coding note: The ICD-9-CM and ICD-10-CM codes for the [specific substance/medica-
tion]-induced bipolar and related disorders are indicated in the table below. Note that the
ICD-10-CM code depends on whether or not there is a comorbid substance use disorder
present for the same class of substance. If a mild substance use disorder is comorbid with
the substance-induced bipolar and related disorder, the 4th position character is "1," and
the clinician should record "mild [substance] use disorder" before the substance-induced

bipolar and related disorder (e.g., "mild cocaine use disorder with cocaine-induced bipolar and related disorder"). If a moderate or severe substance use disorder is comorbid with the substance-induced bipolar and related disorder, the 4th position character is "2," and the clinician should record "moderate [substance] use disorder" or "severe [substance] use disorder," depending on the severity of the comorbid substance use disorder. If there is no comorbid substance use disorder (e.g., after a one-time heavy use of the substance), then the 4th position character is "9," and the clinician should record only the substance-induced bipolar and related disorder.

		ICD-10-CM		
	ICD-9-CM	With use disorder, mild	With use disorder, moderate or severe	Without use disorder
Alcohol	291.89	F10.14	F10.24	F10.94
Phencyclidine	292.84	F16.14	F16.24	F16.94
Other hallucinogen	292.84	F16.14	F16.24	F16.94
Sedative, hypnotic, or anxiolytic	292.84	F13.14	F13.24	F13.94
Amphetamine (or other stimulant)	292.84	F15.14	F15.24	F15.94
Cocaine	292.84	F14.14	F14.24	F14.94
Other (or unknown) substance	292.84	F19.14	F19.24	F19.94

Specify if (see Table 16–1 in the chapter "Substance-Related and Addictive Disorders" for diagnoses associated with substance class):
   With onset during intoxication: If the criteria are met for intoxication with the substance and the symptoms develop during intoxication.
   With onset during withdrawal: If criteria are met for withdrawal from the substance and the symptoms develop during, or shortly after, withdrawal.

Clinicians should note the potential for confusing this disorder with a bipolar I or II disorder that emerges during antidepressant treatment. In substance/medication-induced bipolar and related disorder, the symptoms are clearly associated with the ingestion of a substance and do *not* persist beyond the physiological effect of that treatment. The opposite occurs in bipolar I or II disorder, in that a manic/hypomanic episode emerging *during* antidepressant treatment (medication, electroconvulsive therapy) and persisting at the full syndromal level for a *substantial period of time* after the cessation of acute withdrawal or severe intoxication is evidence of bipolarity.

Bipolar and Related Disorder Due to Another Medical Condition

The criteria for bipolar and related disorder due to another medical condition are patterned after the DSM-IV criteria for mood disorder due to a general medical condition but are specific to bipolar disorder. In this case, the manic or hypomanic episode has been attributed to a medical condition.

Diagnostic Criteria for Bipolar and Related Disorder Due to Another Medical Condition

---

A. A prominent and persistent period of abnormally elevated, expansive, or irritable mood and abnormally increased activity or energy that predominates in the clinical picture.
B. There is evidence from the history, physical examination, or laboratory findings that the disturbance is the direct pathophysiological consequence of another medical condition.
C. The disturbance is not better explained by another mental disorder.
D. The disturbance does not occur exclusively during the course of a delirium.
E. The disturbance causes clinically significant distress or impairment in social, occupational, or other important areas of functioning, or necessitates hospitalization to prevent harm to self or others, or there are psychotic features.

Coding note: The ICD-9-CM code for bipolar and related disorder due to another medical condition is **293.83,** which is assigned regardless of the specifier. The ICD-10-CM code depends on the specifier (see below).

Specify if:
(F06.33) With manic features: Full criteria are not met for a manic or hypomanic episode.
(F06.33) With manic- or hypomanic-like episode: Full criteria are met except Criterion D for a manic episode or except Criterion F for a hypomanic episode.
(F06.34) With mixed features: Symptoms of depression are also present but do not predominate in the clinical picture.

Coding note: Include the name of the other medical condition in the name of the mental disorder (e.g., 293.83 [F06.33] bipolar disorder due to hyperthyroidism, with manic features). The other medical condition should also be coded and listed separately immediately before the bipolar and related disorder due to the medical condition (e.g., 242.90 [E05.90] hyperthyroidism; 293.83 [F06.33] bipolar disorder due to hyperthyroidism, with manic features).

Other Specified Bipolar and Related Disorder and Unspecified Bipolar and Related Disorder

The diagnoses other specified bipolar and related disorder and unspecified bipolar and related disorder are residual categories that replace DSM-IV's bipolar disorder not otherwise specified.

The category other specified bipolar and related disorder is used for individuals with symptoms characteristic of a bipolar or related disorder that cause distress or impairment but do not meet the full criteria for a more specific disorder. In this case, the clinician chooses to communicate the reason that the presentation does not meet full criteria. Clinicians are encouraged to record the specific reason (e.g., short-duration hypomanic episodes [2-3 days] and major depressive episodes).

The category unspecified bipolar and related disorder is used when characteristic symptoms are present that cause distress or impairment but these symptoms do not meet full criteria for a more specific disorder, and the clinician chooses not to communicate the reason criteria for a more specific disorder are not met, or there is insufficient information to make a more specific diagnosis.

Other Specified Bipolar and Related Disorder   296.89 (F31.89)

This category applies to presentations in which symptoms characteristic of a bipolar and related disorder that cause clinically significant distress or impairment in social, occupational, or other important areas of functioning predominate but do not meet the full criteria for any of the disorders in the bipolar and related disorders diagnostic class. The other specified bipolar and related disorder category is used in situations in which the clinician chooses to communicate the specific reason that the presentation does not meet the criteria for any specific bipolar and related disorder. This is done by recording "other specified bipolar and related disorder" followed by the specific reason (e.g., "short-duration cyclothymia").

Examples of presentations that can be specified using the "other specified" designation include the following:

1. **Short-duration hypomanic episodes (2–3 days) and major depressive episodes:** A lifetime history of one or more major depressive episodes in individuals whose presentation has never met full criteria for a manic or hypomanic episode but who have experienced two or more episodes of short-duration hypomania that meet the full symptomatic criteria for a hypomanic episode but that only last for 2–3 days. The episodes of hypomanic symptoms do not overlap in time with the major depressive episodes, so the disturbance does not meet criteria for major depressive episode, with mixed features.

2. **Hypomanic episodes with insufficient symptoms and major depressive episodes:** A lifetime history of one or more major depressive episodes in individuals whose presentation has never met full criteria for a manic or hypomanic episode but who have experienced one or more episodes of hypomania that do not meet full symptomatic criteria (i.e., at least 4 consecutive days of elevated mood and one or two of the other symptoms of a hypomanic episode, or irritable mood and two or three of the other symptoms of a hypomanic episode). The episodes of hypomanic symptoms do not overlap in time with the major depressive episodes, so the disturbance does not meet criteria for major depressive episode, with mixed features.

3. **Hypomanic episode without prior major depressive episode:** One or more hypomanic episodes in an individual whose presentation has never met full criteria for a major depressive episode or a manic episode. If this occurs in an individual with an established diagnosis of persistent depressive disorder (dysthymia), both diagnoses can be concurrently applied during the periods when the full criteria for a hypomanic episode are met.

4. **Short-duration cyclothymia (less than 24 months):** Multiple episodes of hypomanic symptoms that do not meet criteria for a hypomanic episode and multiple episodes of depressive symptoms that do not meet criteria for a major depressive
episode that persist over a period of less than 24 months (less than 12 months for
children or adolescents) in an individual whose presentation has never met full criteria for a major depressive, manic, or hypomanic episode and does not meet criteria for any psychotic disorder. During the course of the disorder, the hypomanic or
depressive symptoms are present for more days than not, the individual has not been
without symptoms for more than 2 months at a time, and the symptoms cause clinically significant distress or impairment.

Unspecified Bipolar and Related Disorder   296.80 (F31.9)

This category applies to presentations in which symptoms characteristic of a bipolar and
related disorder that cause clinically significant distress or impairment in social, occupational, or other important areas of functioning predominate but do not meet the full criteria for any of the disorders in the bipolar and related disorders diagnostic class. The
unspecified bipolar and related disorder category is used in situations in which the clinician chooses *not* to specify the reason that the criteria are not met for a specific bipolar
and related disorder, and includes presentations in which there is insufficient information
to make a more specific diagnosis (e.g., in emergency room settings).

DEPRESSIVE DISORDERS

The DSM-5 depressive disorders are listed in Table 5–2. There are two new diagnoses:
disruptive mood dysregulation disorder and premenstrual dysphoric disorder. A new
specifier to indicate the presence of mixed symptoms has been added across the depressive disorders. The core criterion items applied to the diagnosis major depressive disorder, as well as its 2-week duration, are unchanged from DSM-IV, although minor
editing changes have been made. The Mood Disorders Work Group concluded that the
major depressive disorder criteria, which were introduced in DSM-III and which had
accumulated considerable research support, have held up well over the past 30 years.

One important change is the omission of the so-called bereavement exclusion.
This change led to unwanted controversy whereby critics claimed it would medicalize the normal process of bereavement. In DSM-IV, major depressive episode Criterion E required that the symptoms be "not better accounted for by Bereavement."
This exclusion applied to symptoms lasting less than 2 months following the death of
a loved one. The change for DSM-5 was made because evidence does not support the
separation of loss of a loved one from other stressors in terms of its likelihood of precipitating a major depressive episode or in terms of the relative likelihood that the
symptoms will remit spontaneously. Bereavement is a severe psychosocial stressor
known to precipitate major depressive episodes in vulnerable persons. Typically, when

TABLE 5–2.	DSM-5 depressive disorders

Disruptive mood dysregulation disorder

Major depressive disorder, single episode

Major depressive disorder, recurrent episode

Persistent depressive disorder (dysthymia)

Premenstrual dysphoric disorder

Substance/medication-induced depressive disorder

Depressive disorder due to another medical condition

Other specified depressive disorder

Unspecified depressive disorder

that happens, the depression begins soon after the loss. Although bereavement may be painful, most persons do not develop a major depressive episode. Those who do, however, typically experience more suffering, feel worthless, and may have suicidal ideation. General medical health can suffer, as can interpersonal and work function. These individuals can be at risk for "complicated grief," characterized by ruminating about the deceased person, seeking proximity to the deceased person, and striving to avoid experiences that trigger reminders of loss. Furthermore, bereavement-related depression has most of the characteristics of a major depressive episode; that is, it is most likely to occur in individuals with past personal and family history of a major depressive episode, is genetically influenced, and is associated with similar personality characteristics, patterns of comorbidity, and outcome. Finally, the symptoms associated with a bereavement-related major depressive disorder respond to antidepressant medication. Depending on the particular circumstances, the clinician observing a full depressive syndrome in an individual within the first 2 months following the death of a loved one can elect to observe rather than initiate treatment.

The coexistence within a major depressive episode of at least three manic/hypomanic symptoms insufficient to satisfy criteria for a manic/hypomanic episode is now acknowledged with the specifier "with mixed features." This change recognizes findings from family and follow-up studies that show that the presence of mixed features in an episode of major depressive disorder increases the likelihood that the illness falls within the bipolar spectrum. The presence of a full manic syndrome within a depressive episode will continue to be an exclusion criterion for a depressive disorder diagnosis, and individuals with this pattern will be considered to have a bipolar disorder.

The addition of *disruptive mood dysregulation disorder* and *premenstrual dysphoric disorder* has generated controversy, although of a different order of magnitude than that pertaining to the bereavement exclusion. Disruptive mood dysregulation disorder was created in part to address concerns about the possible overdiagnosis of bipolar disorder in children younger than 12 years who display persistent irritability and frequent episodes of extreme behavioral dyscontrol (Axelson et al. 2006). On the other hand, premenstrual dysphoric disorder was moved from Appendix B of DSM-IV ("Criteria Sets and Axes Provided for Further Study") to become a stand-alone diagnosis following a careful literature review.

There has been some controversy about the premenstrual dysphoric disorder diagnosis through the years. Some groups have felt that a disorder that focuses on the menstrual cycle may "pathologize" normal reproductive functioning. Others have believed that the disorder serves to stigmatize women's health, and perhaps implies that women would not be able to perform needed activities during the premenstrual phase of the cycle. Because the disorder is common and problematic, work group members concluded that it would be inappropriate *not* to acknowledge the condition or encourage clinicians to recognize the disorder and offer appropriate treatment.

Persistent depressive disorder (dysthymia) is new to DSM-5 and merges DSM-IV-defined chronic major depressive disorder and dysthymic disorder. Major depressive disorder may precede persistent depressive disorder, and major depressive episodes may occur during persistent depressive disorder. There is no longer a requirement that the disturbance not occur exclusively during the course of a chronic psychotic disorder, such as schizophrenia or delusional disorder (DSM-IV Criterion F). This change allows clinicians to diagnose persistent depressive disorder in persons with one of these psychotic conditions.

In summary, the depressive disorders chapter reflects refinements aimed at improving the recognition and treatment of these conditions by encouraging the clinician to record and consider specifiers that allow coverage of important information not conveyed by the categorical diagnoses themselves. New diagnoses have been added that address problems that are common and have been inadequately covered in DSM, yet are associated with significant distress and impairment, and merit recognition and special clinical management.

Disruptive Mood Dysregulation Disorder

The diagnosis of disruptive mood dysregulation disorder will help fill an important gap for children with mood dysregulation characterized by chronic, severe persistent irritability. In the past 20 years, there has been a 40-fold increase in the number of youth diagnosed with bipolar disorder. Research, however, shows that children with disruptive mood dysregulation disorder have a different outcome, gender ratio, and family history than those with bipolar disorder. Furthermore, they do not go on to develop manic or hypomanic episodes. While impaired, these children often have symptoms that meet criteria for other disruptive behavior disorders, anxiety disorders, and attention-deficit/hyperactivity disorder. The Childhood and Adolescent Disorders Work Group concluded that the best fit was with the depressive disorders.

Initially, the work group considered naming the disorder "temper dysregulation disorder" but in response to feedback chose to name it "disruptive mood dysregulation disorder." Because most of the children who meet criteria for this new disorder will also meet criteria for oppositional defiant disorder (due to overlapping symptoms), the work group decided that youth who meet criteria for both disorders should be assigned only the diagnosis of disruptive mood dysregulation disorder. This avoids the problem of having artificial comorbidity due to overlapping criteria.

Diagnostic Criteria for Disruptive Mood
Dysregulation Disorder   **296.99** (F34.8)

A. Severe recurrent temper outbursts manifested verbally (e.g., verbal rages) and/or behaviorally (e.g., physical aggression toward people or property) that are grossly out of proportion in intensity or duration to the situation or provocation.

B. The temper outbursts are inconsistent with developmental level.

C. The temper outbursts occur, on average, three or more times per week.

D. The mood between temper outbursts is persistently irritable or angry most of the day, nearly every day, and is observable by others (e.g., parents, teachers, peers).

E. Criteria A–D have been present for 12 or more months. Throughout that time, the individual has not had a period lasting 3 or more consecutive months without all of the symptoms in Criteria A–D.

F. Criteria A and D are present in at least two of three settings (i.e., at home, at school, with peers) and are severe in at least one of these.

G. The diagnosis should not be made for the first time before age 6 years or after age 18 years.

H. By history or observation, the age at onset of Criteria A–E is before 10 years.

I. There has never been a distinct period lasting more than 1 day during which the full symptom criteria, except duration, for a manic or hypomanic episode have been met.

   Note: Developmentally appropriate mood elevation, such as occurs in the context of a highly positive event or its anticipation, should not be considered as a symptom of mania or hypomania.

J. The behaviors do not occur exclusively during an episode of major depressive disorder and are not better explained by another mental disorder (e.g., autism spectrum disorder, posttraumatic stress disorder, separation anxiety disorder, persistent depressive disorder [dysthymia]).

   Note: This diagnosis cannot coexist with oppositional defiant disorder, intermittent explosive disorder, or bipolar disorder, though it can coexist with others, including major depressive disorder, attention-deficit/hyperactivity disorder, conduct disorder, and substance use disorders. Individuals whose symptoms meet criteria for both disruptive mood dysregulation disorder and oppositional defiant disorder should only be given the diagnosis of disruptive mood dysregulation disorder. If an individual has ever experienced a manic or hypomanic episode, the diagnosis of disruptive mood dysregulation disorder should not be assigned.

K. The symptoms are not attributable to the physiological effects of a substance or to another medical or neurological condition.

Criteria A and B

This item notes that the child has "severe recurrent *temper outbursts*…that are grossly out of proportion in intensity or duration to the situation or provocation" (emphasis added). Because nearly all children have temper tantrums, this criterion is needed to help distinguish ordinary tantrums from outbursts that stand apart due to their severity and regularity. Furthermore, the outbursts are inconsistent with the situation, and most parents would see these as indicating the child is out of control. Also, the outbursts are manifested verbally and/or behaviorally, such as in a tantrum, and are not consistent with the child's developmental level (i.e., the child is outside the range of the "terrible twos").

Criteria C, D, and E

The requirement that temper outbursts occur three or more times per week is somewhat arbitrary, but the point is that the outbursts occur regularly and with some frequency. Between outbursts the child's mood is persistently irritable or angry "most of the day, nearly every day." In other words, the symptoms are not just a passing phase.

These symptoms have been present for 12 or more months, during which time the child has not had at least 3 consecutive months without all of the symptoms in Criteria A–D. This item also indicates that the symptoms do not represent a temporary phase, but are pervasive and lasting.

Criterion F

The symptoms occur in at least two settings, such as at home and school. Some children seem to turn symptoms on and off at will, and this criterion separates those children in whom the symptoms seem voluntary from those who seem less likely to be able to control themselves.

Criteria G and H

This diagnosis is not made before the child is age 6 years nor after the youth turns age 18 years (Criterion G). This criterion helps to establish that the temper outbursts are not attributable to a neurodevelopmental syndrome, in which the symptoms would likely have an earlier onset, and are not attributable to adult misbehavior from an antisocial personality disorder, which is not diagnosed in persons under age 18 years.

Onset is before age 10 years (Criterion H). Again, this criterion helps guard against using the diagnosis to justify a bipolar diagnosis, which generally has an onset during adolescence or beyond.

Criteria I, J, and K

Criterion I helps separate disruptive mood dysregulation disorder from bipolar disorder by excluding individuals with symptoms that meet the full criteria for a manic or hypomanic episode for more than 1 day. Also, the item recognizes, in a note, that some "developmentally appropriate" episodes of mood elevation can occur in the context of a highly positive event or its anticipation (e.g., a birthday party, a visit to an amusement park) and should not be confused with bipolar disorder.

Criteria J and K ensure that the temper outbursts do not occur exclusively during a major depressive episode and are not better explained by another mental disorder (e.g., autism spectrum disorder), and that the symptoms are not attributable to the physiological effects of a substance or to another medical or neurological condition.

It is further noted that disruptive mood dysregulation disorder cannot coexist with oppositional defiant disorder, intermittent explosive disorder, or bipolar disorder. On the other hand, it may coexist with some other mental disorders, such as major depressive disorder, attention-deficit/hyperactivity disorder, conduct disorder, and substance use disorders.

If the child's symptoms meet criteria for both disruptive mood dysregulation disorder and oppositional defiant disorder, the former diagnosis trumps the latter. Research shows that most children with disruptive mood dysregulation disorder will also have a presentation that meets criteria for oppositional defiant disorder, but the reverse is not true. Only about 15% of children with oppositional defiant disorder will have symptoms that also meet criteria for disruptive mood dysregulation disorder.

Major Depressive Episode

The syndrome major depressive episode described in DSM-III continues in DSM-5 nearly unchanged apart from editing changes, except for the bereavement exclusion and several new specifiers to help clinicians better describe an individual's episode (see "Depressive Disorders" introduction above). Major depressive disorder is the codable disorder for people with one or more major depressive episodes. Major depressive disorders are coded based on whether only a single major depressive episode has occurred or the episodes are recurrent.

Diagnostic Criteria for Major Depressive Episode

A. Five (or more) of the following symptoms have been present during the same 2-week period and represent a change from previous functioning; at least one of the symptoms is either (1) depressed mood or (2) loss of interest or pleasure.
Note: Do not include symptoms that are clearly attributable to another medical condition.

1. Depressed mood most of the day, nearly every day, as indicated by either subjective report (e.g., feels sad, empty, hopeless) or observation made by others (e.g., appears tearful). (**Note:** In children and adolescents, can be irritable mood.)
2. Markedly diminished interest or pleasure in all, or almost all, activities most of the day, nearly every day (as indicated by either subjective account or observation).
3. Significant weight loss when not dieting or weight gain (e.g., a change of more than 5% of body weight in a month), or decrease or increase in appetite nearly every day. (**Note:** In children, consider failure to make expected weight gain.)
4. Insomnia or hypersomnia nearly every day.
5. Psychomotor agitation or retardation nearly every day (observable by others, not merely subjective feelings of restlessness or being slowed down).
6. Fatigue or loss of energy nearly every day.
7. Feelings of worthlessness or excessive or inappropriate guilt (which may be

     delusional) nearly every day (not merely self-reproach or guilt about being sick).

    8. Diminished ability to think or concentrate, or indecisiveness, nearly every day (either by subjective account or as observed by others).

    9. Recurrent thoughts of death (not just fear of dying), recurrent suicidal ideation without a specific plan, or a suicide attempt or a specific plan for committing suicide.

B. The symptoms cause clinically significant distress or impairment in social, occupational, or other important areas of functioning.

C. The episode is not attributable to the physiological effects of a substance or to another medical condition.

Note: Criteria A–C represent a major depressive episode.

Note: Responses to a significant loss (e.g., bereavement, financial ruin, losses from a natural disaster, a serious medical illness or disability) may include the feelings of intense sadness, rumination about the loss, insomnia, poor appetite, and weight loss noted in Criterion A, which may resemble a depressive episode. Although such symptoms may be understandable or considered appropriate to the loss, the presence of a major depressive episode in addition to the normal response to a significant loss should also be carefully considered. This decision inevitably requires the exercise of clinical judgment based on the individual's history and the cultural norms for the expression of distress in the context of loss.[1]

D. The occurrence of the major depressive episode is not better explained by schizoaffective disorder, schizophrenia, schizophreniform disorder, delusional disorder, or other specified and unspecified schizophrenia spectrum and other psychotic disorders.

E. There has never been a manic episode or a hypomanic episode.

    Note: This exclusion does not apply if all of the manic-like or hypomanic-like episodes are substance-induced or are attributable to the physiological effects of another medical condition.

---

[1]In distinguishing grief from a major depressive episode (MDE), it is useful to consider that in grief the predominant affect is feelings of emptiness and loss, while in MDE it is persistent depressed mood and the inability to anticipate happiness or pleasure. The dysphoria in grief is likely to decrease in intensity over days to weeks and occurs in waves, the so-called pangs of grief. These waves tend to be associated with thoughts or reminders of the deceased. The depressed mood of MDE is more persistent and not tied to specific thoughts or preoccupations. The pain of grief may be accompanied by positive emotions and humor that are uncharacteristic of the pervasive unhappiness and misery characteristic of MDE. The thought content associated with grief generally features a preoccupation with thoughts and memories of the deceased, rather than the self-critical or pessimistic ruminations seen in MDE. In grief, self-esteem is generally preserved, whereas in MDE feelings of worthlessness and self-loathing are common. If self-derogatory ideation is present in grief, it typically involves perceived failings vis-à-vis the deceased (e.g., not visiting frequently enough, not telling the deceased how much he or she was loved). If a bereaved individual thinks about death and dying, such thoughts are generally focused on the deceased and possibly about "joining" the deceased, whereas in MDE such thoughts are focused on ending one's own life because of feeling worthless, undeserving of life, or unable to cope with the pain of depression.

Coding and Recording Procedures

The diagnostic code for major depressive disorder is based on whether this is a single or recurrent episode, current severity, presence of psychotic features, and remission status. Current severity and psychotic features are only indicated if full criteria are currently met for a major depressive episode. Remission specifiers are only indicated if the full criteria are not currently met for a major depressive episode. Codes are as follows:

Severity/course specifier	Single episode	Recurrent episode*
Mild (DSM-5, p. 188)	296.21 (F32.0)	296.31 (F33.0)
Moderate (DSM-5, p. 188)	296.22 (F32.1)	296.32 (F33.1)
Severe (DSM-5, p. 188)	296.23 (F32.2)	296.33 (F33.2)
With psychotic features** (DSM-5, p. 186)	296.24 (F32.3)	296.34 (F33.3)
In partial remission (DSM-5, p. 188)	296.25 (F32.4)	296.35 (F33.41)
In full remission (DSM-5, p. 188)	296.26 (F32.5)	296.36 (F33.42)
Unspecified	296.20 (F32.9)	296.30 (F33.9)

*For an episode to be considered recurrent, there must be an interval of at least 2 consecutive months between separate episodes in which criteria are not met for a major depressive episode. The definitions of specifiers are found on the indicated pages.
**If psychotic features are present, code the "with psychotic features" specifier irrespective of episode severity.

In recording the name of a diagnosis, terms should be listed in the following order: major depressive disorder, single or recurrent episode, severity/psychotic/remission specifiers, followed by as many of the following specifiers without codes that apply to the current episode.

Specify:
   With anxious distress (DSM-5, p. 184)
   With mixed features (DSM-5, pp. 184–185)
   With melancholic features (DSM-5, p. 185)
   With atypical features (DSM-5, pp. 185–186)
   With mood-congruent psychotic features (DSM-5, p. 186)
   With mood-incongruent psychotic features (DSM-5, p. 186)
   With catatonia (DSM-5, p. 186). **Coding note:** Use additional code 293.89 (F06.1).
   With peripartum onset (DSM-5, pp. 186–187)
   With seasonal pattern (recurrent episode only) (DSM-5, pp. 187–188)

Criterion A

This item specifies that five or more of nine depressive symptoms must be present for a diagnosis of major depressive episode to be given, and at least one must be criterion A1 (depressed mood) or A2 (loss of interest or pleasure). This list has remained unchanged since DSM-III-R and contains the classic depressive symptoms recognized for centuries. Although individual symptoms are common in the general population, the fact that they cluster together over a minimum of 2 weeks to form the syndrome sets the diagnosis apart. It is important for clinicians to note that each item must be present during the 2-week period before it is counted as "present." Some symptoms that may have been present before the onset of the episode count only if they become appreciably worse during the episode. For example, some individuals have chronic insomnia that would otherwise not count unless it worsens as part of the depressive illness.

The most important symptoms are depressed mood (Criterion A1) and loss of interest or pleasure (criterion A2), and one of the two is required. Some depressed individuals will have lost the ability to describe their emotions (alexithymia) or to feel that they are depressed; others have trouble acknowledging depressed mood for cultural or other reasons. In almost all cases, the person will be able to admit to loss of interest or pleasure. Criterion A8 can be vexing because many disorders can cause poor concentration. Many individuals with mild or early forms of dementia will report memory impairment and difficulty concentrating. That said, the most important cause of these symptoms is depression and not dementia.

Suicidal thoughts or behaviors (criterion A9) are the most worrisome of the depressive symptoms, and once these are ascertained, the clinician will need to explore this symptom at greater length to determine the individual's degree of suicidality and the urgency of medical intervention.

Clinicians should note that there must be an interval of at least 2 months in which criteria are *not* met for two major depressive episodes to be considered separate and independent episodes.

Criterion B

Originally Criterion C in DSM-IV, this criterion states that depressive symptoms must cause "clinically significant distress or impairment in social, occupational, or other important areas of functioning." This criterion, added to the diagnosis in DSM-IV, is supplemented by the specifiers of mild, moderate, and severe. Although depression is perceived by most as distressing, the social and occupational impairment may manifest in a variety of ways. The individual may have poor job performance due to impaired concentration or being overly tired and therefore being inefficient at work. He or she may take too many sick days or not show up. In the social arena, the person may ignore friendships and become withdrawn; irritability may drive off remaining friends. Families may suffer because the person ignores household tasks due to lack of motivation. In severe cases, individuals may become preoccupied with thoughts of death or dying, or develop suicidal plans; some will attempt (or complete) suicide.

Criterion C

Alternative explanations for the syndrome must be eliminated during the process of differential diagnosis. Substances of abuse, medications, and other medical conditions need to be ruled out. Alcohol and other drugs are known to induce depression; in such cases, the appropriate diagnosis is substance/medication-induced depressive disorder. Likewise, medical conditions such as hypothyroidism are associated with depression and need to be ruled out as the cause; in these cases, the more appropriate diagnosis is depressive disorder due to another medical condition. These conditions will have important treatment implications.

Criterion D

The depression is not better explained by schizoaffective disorder and is not superimposed on schizophrenia, schizophreniform disorder, delusional disorder, or other specified or unspecified schizophrenia spectrum and other psychotic disorder. All of these disorders may be accompanied to some extent by the presence of depression.

Criterion E

The individual has never had a manic or a hypomanic episode. This criterion is important because it helps to separate major depressive disorder from bipolar disorder. This distinction is fundamental to the mood disorders and has important treatment implications. That said, for individuals with subsyndromal manic or hypomanic symptoms, the specifier "with mixed features" is available.

Major Depressive Disorder, Single Episode

Specifiers

The specifiers allow the clinician to describe the individual's illness in great detail, including recording whether the mood disorder is accompanied by anxious distress; whether there are mixed features, melancholic features, atypical features, psychotic features, or catatonia; and whether the depression had a peripartum onset or has a seasonal pattern. Clinicians can rate the major depressive episode as mild, moderate, or severe and as with or without psychotic features.

The DSM-IV specifier "with postpartum onset" has been changed to "with peripartum onset." This change acknowledges that half of major depressive episodes occur *prior* to delivery. The specifier is appropriate for when a major depressive episode develops during pregnancy or during the 4 weeks following delivery.

Major Depressive Disorder, Recurrent Episode

For a major depressive disorder to be considered recurrent, there must be an interval of at least 2 consecutive months between separate episodes in which criteria are not met for a major depressive episode.

Persistent Depressive Disorder (Dysthymia)

Persistent depressive disorder (dysthymia) is a chronic and persistent disturbance in mood present for at least 2 years (or at least 1 year for children and adolescents) and characterized by relatively typical depressive symptoms, such as anorexia, insomnia, decreased energy, low self-esteem, difficulty concentrating, and feelings of hopelessness. The diagnosis merges DSM-IV-defined chronic major depressive disorder and dysthymic disorder. Clinicians had trouble distinguishing the two disorders, and consolidating the disorders will make it easier to identify individuals with chronic and persistent depression.

Dysthymic disorder was introduced in DSM-III and was referred to parenthetically as depressive neurosis. Individuals with a persistent depressive disorder often develop relatively more severe major depressive episodes. When the major depressive episode clears, these individuals subsequently return to their chronic state of dysthymia. The coexistence of both mild and severe forms of depression is sometimes referred to as "double depression" because both disorders are coded.

The criteria for persistent depressive disorder are mostly unchanged from those for DSM-IV dysthymic disorder. The most important difference affects Criterion D. DSM-IV specified the *absence* of any major depressive episode in the first 2 years of the disturbance. The Mood Disorders Work Group was concerned that clinicians were unable to reliably distinguish dysthymic disorder from chronic major depressive disorder. Many clinicians were confused about the differences and tended to ignore one or the other diagnosis. Part of the confusion stems from the fact that patients are asked to recall information that most individuals are unable to retrieve. That is, does the patient recall having had in that 2-year period (that could have been decades in the past) any symptom-free periods longer than 2 months in duration, or having had 2 weeks or more in which he or she had symptoms that met criteria for a major depressive episode (in which case the patient would receive the diagnosis major depressive disorder). These changes should help clinicians distinguish these disorders more reliably. Research also showed that there were few differences among individuals with dysthymic disorder and those with chronic major depressive disorder in symptoms, family history, or treatment response (Klein et al. 2004; McCullough et al. 2000).

Diagnostic Criteria for Persistent Depressive Disorder (Dysthymia)   300.4 (F34.1)

This disorder represents a consolidation of DSM-IV-defined chronic major depressive disorder and dysthymic disorder.

A. Depressed mood for most of the day, for more days than not, as indicated by either subjective account or observation by others, for at least 2 years.

Note: In children and adolescents, mood can be irritable and duration must be at least 1 year.

B. Presence, while depressed, of two (or more) of the following:

1. Poor appetite or overeating.
2. Insomnia or hypersomnia.
3. Low energy or fatigue.
4. Low self-esteem.

    5. Poor concentration or difficulty making decisions.

    6. Feelings of hopelessness.

C. During the 2-year period (1 year for children or adolescents) of the disturbance, the individual has never been without the symptoms in Criteria A and B for more than 2 months at a time.

D. Criteria for a major depressive disorder may be continuously present for 2 years.

E. There has never been a manic episode or a hypomanic episode, and criteria have never been met for cyclothymic disorder.

F. The disturbance is not better explained by a persistent schizoaffective disorder, schizophrenia, delusional disorder, or other specified or unspecified schizophrenia spectrum and other psychotic disorder.

G. The symptoms are not attributable to the physiological effects of a substance (e.g., a drug of abuse, a medication) or another medical condition (e.g., hypothyroidism).

H. The symptoms cause clinically significant distress or impairment in social, occupational, or other important areas of functioning.

Note: Because the criteria for a major depressive episode include four symptoms that are absent from the symptom list for persistent depressive disorder (dysthymia), a very limited number of individuals will have depressive symptoms that have persisted longer than 2 years but will not meet criteria for persistent depressive disorder. If full criteria for a major depressive episode have been met at some point during the current episode of illness, they should be given a diagnosis of major depressive disorder. Otherwise, a diagnosis of other specified depressive disorder or unspecified depressive disorder is warranted.

Specify if:

    With anxious distress (DSM-5, p. 184)

    With mixed features (DSM-5, pp. 184–185)

    With melancholic features (DSM-5, p. 185)

    With atypical features (DSM-5, pp. 185–186)

    With mood-congruent psychotic features (DSM-5, p. 186)

    With mood-incongruent psychotic features (DSM-5, p. 186)

    With peripartum onset (DSM-5, pp. 186–187)

Specify if:

    In partial remission (DSM-5, p. 188)

    In full remission (DSM-5, p. 188)

Specify if:

    Early onset: If onset is before age 21 years.

    Late onset: If onset is at age 21 years or older.

Specify if (for most recent 2 years of persistent depressive disorder):

    With pure dysthymic syndrome: Full criteria for a major depressive episode have not been met in at least the preceding 2 years.

    With persistent major depressive episode: Full criteria for a major depressive episode have been met throughout the preceding 2-year period.

    With intermittent major depressive episodes, with current episode: Full criteria for a major depressive episode are currently met, but there have been periods of at least 8 weeks in at least the preceding 2 years with symptoms below the threshold for a full major depressive episode.

With intermittent major depressive episodes, without current episode: Full criteria for a major depressive episode are not currently met, but there has been one or more major depressive episodes in at least the preceding 2 years.

Specify current severity:
  Mild (DSM-5, p. 188)
  Moderate (DSM-5, p. 188)
  Severe (DSM-5, p. 188)

Premenstrual Dysphoric Disorder

The Mood Disorders Work Group recommended that premenstrual dysphoric disorder receive full disorder status in DSM-5. In DSM-IV, it was included in Appendix B and, if present, was coded as depressive disorder not otherwise specified. Since the disorder was initially proposed in DSM-III-R as late luteal phase dysphoric disorder, research evidence has accumulated and shown the disorder to be prevalent and to cause significant distress and impairment. The work group felt that information on the diagnosis, treatment, and validators of the disorder had matured to the point that the disorder qualified for inclusion as an independent diagnosis.

Clinical research and epidemiological studies have shown that many women experience symptoms that begin during the luteal phase of the menstrual cycle and terminate around the onset of menses. Additionally, these studies identified a subset of women (about 2% in the community) who suffer intermittently from severe symptoms associated with the luteal phase of the menstrual cycle. Women with these symptoms have not been adequately covered in DSM. Including premenstrual dysphoric disorder helps ensure that clinicians will recognize the syndrome and that women with the disorder will receive appropriate treatment.

Diagnostic Criteria for Premenstrual Dysphoric Disorder   625.4 (N94.3)

A. In the majority of menstrual cycles, at least five symptoms must be present in the final week before the onset of menses, start to *improve* within a few days after the onset of menses, and become *minimal* or absent in the week postmenses.

B. One (or more) of the following symptoms must be present:

  1. Marked affective lability (e.g., mood swings; feeling suddenly sad or tearful, or increased sensitivity to rejection).
  2. Marked irritability or anger or increased interpersonal conflicts.
  3. Marked depressed mood, feelings of hopelessness, or self-deprecating thoughts.
  4. Marked anxiety, tension, and/or feelings of being keyed up or on edge.

C. One (or more) of the following symptoms must additionally be present, to reach a total of *five* symptoms when combined with symptoms from Criterion B above.

  1. Decreased interest in usual activities (e.g., work, school, friends, hobbies).
  2. Subjective difficulty in concentration.

3. Lethargy, easy fatigability, or marked lack of energy.
4. Marked change in appetite; overeating; or specific food cravings.
5. Hypersomnia or insomnia.
6. A sense of being overwhelmed or out of control.
7. Physical symptoms such as breast tenderness or swelling, joint or muscle pain, a sensation of "bloating," or weight gain.

Note: The symptoms in Criteria A–C must have been met for most menstrual cycles that occurred in the preceding year.

D. The symptoms are associated with clinically significant distress or interference with work, school, usual social activities, or relationships with others (e.g., avoidance of social activities; decreased productivity and efficiency at work, school, or home).
E. The disturbance is not merely an exacerbation of the symptoms of another disorder, such as major depressive disorder, panic disorder, persistent depressive disorder (dysthymia), or a personality disorder (although it may co-occur with any of these disorders).
F. Criterion A should be confirmed by prospective daily ratings during at least two symptomatic cycles. (**Note:** The diagnosis may be made provisionally prior to this confirmation.)
G. The symptoms are not attributable to the physiological effects of a substance (e.g., a drug of abuse, a medication, other treatment) or another medical condition (e.g., hyperthyroidism).

Substance/Medication-Induced Depressive Disorder

Substance/medication-induced depressive disorder is diagnosed when an individual's depressive symptoms have clearly resulted from the effect of a substance or from its withdrawal. Such disorders occur commonly and have been associated with particular substances, with alcohol being perhaps the most common incitant. The disorder is also frequently observed in hospital and clinic populations. The diagnostic criteria are mostly unchanged from those for substance-induced mood disorder in DSM-IV except that Criterion A has been edited to reflect the focus on depressive symptoms, as is appropriate for this chapter. Coding depends on the substance implicated as inducing the disorder. The name of the substance is included in the name of the disorder (e.g., alcohol-induced depressive disorder).

Diagnostic Criteria for Substance/Medication-Induced Depressive Disorder

A. A prominent and persistent disturbance in mood that predominates in the clinical picture and is characterized by depressed mood or markedly diminished interest or pleasure in all, or almost all, activities.
B. There is evidence from the history, physical examination, or laboratory findings of both (1) and (2):

1. The symptoms in Criterion A developed during or soon after substance intoxication or withdrawal or after exposure to a medication.
2. The involved substance/medication is capable of producing the symptoms in Criterion A.

C. The disturbance is not better explained by a depressive disorder that is not substance/medication-induced. Such evidence of an independent depressive disorder could include the following:

The symptoms preceded the onset of the substance/medication use; the symptoms persist for a substantial period of time (e.g., about 1 month) after the cessation of acute withdrawal or severe intoxication; or there is other evidence suggesting the existence of an independent non-substance/medication-induced depressive disorder (e.g., a history of recurrent non-substance/medication-related episodes).

D. The disturbance does not occur exclusively during the course of a delirium.
E. The disturbance causes clinically significant distress or impairment in social, occupational, or other important areas of functioning.

Note: This diagnosis should be made instead of a diagnosis of substance intoxication or substance withdrawal only when the symptoms in Criterion A predominate in the clinical picture and when they are sufficiently severe to warrant clinical attention.

Coding note: The ICD-9-CM and ICD-10-CM codes for the [specific substance/medication]-induced depressive disorders are indicated in the table below. Note that the ICD-10-CM code depends on whether or not there is a comorbid substance use disorder present for the same class of substance. If a mild substance use disorder is comorbid with the substance-induced depressive disorder, the 4th position character is "1," and the clinician should record "mild [substance] use disorder" before the substance-induced depressive disorder (e.g., "mild cocaine use disorder with cocaine-induced depressive disorder"). If a moderate or severe substance use disorder is comorbid with the substance-induced depressive disorder, the 4th position character is "2," and the clinician should record "moderate [substance] use disorder" or "severe [substance] use disorder," depending on the severity of the comorbid substance use disorder. If there is no comorbid substance use disorder (e.g., after a one-time heavy use of the substance), then the 4th position character is "9," and the clinician should record only the substance-induced depressive disorder.

		ICD-10-CM		
	ICD-9-CM	With use disorder, mild	With use disorder, moderate or severe	Without use disorder
Alcohol	291.89	F10.14	F10.24	F10.94
Phencyclidine	292.84	F16.14	F16.24	F16.94
Other hallucinogen	292.84	F16.14	F16.24	F16.94
Inhalant	292.84	F18.14	F18.24	F18.94
Opioid	292.84	F11.14	F11.24	F11.94
Sedative, hypnotic, or anxiolytic	292.84	F13.14	F13.24	F13.94

		ICD-10-CM		
	ICD-9-CM	With use disorder, mild	With use disorder, moderate or severe	Without use disorder
Amphetamine (or other stimulant)	292.84	F15.14	F15.24	F15.94
Cocaine	292.84	F14.14	F14.24	F14.94
Other (or unknown) substance	292.84	F19.14	F19.24	F19.94

Specify if (see Table 16–1 in the chapter "Substance-Related and Addictive Disorders" for diagnoses associated with substance class):
   With onset during intoxication: If criteria are met for intoxication with the substance and the symptoms develop during intoxication.
   With onset during withdrawal: If criteria are met for withdrawal from the substance and the symptoms develop during, or shortly after, withdrawal.

Depressive Disorder Due to Another Medical Condition

Some people develop depressive symptoms that are attributable to a known medical disorder. These disorders are common, particularly in hospitals and consultation-liaison services. Many physical disorders, such as hypothyroidism, are known to induce depressive disorders. The DSM-5 criteria alert clinicians to the possibility that a person's depression is induced and that a search for a medical cause may be appropriate. For that reason, this diagnosis has important treatment implications.

The diagnosis may be further specified as with depressive features, with major depressive–like episode, or with mixed features. In recording the diagnosis, the name of the other medical condition should be included in the name of the disorder (e.g., depressive disorder due to hypothyroidism, with mixed features).

Diagnostic Criteria for Depressive Disorder Due to Another Medical Condition

A. A prominent and persistent period of depressed mood or markedly diminished interest or pleasure in all, or almost all, activities that predominates in the clinical picture.
B. There is evidence from the history, physical examination, or laboratory findings that the disturbance is the direct pathophysiological consequence of another medical condition.
C. The disturbance is not better explained by another mental disorder (e.g., adjustment disorder, with depressed mood, in which the stressor is a serious medical condition).
D. The disturbance does not occur exclusively during the course of a delirium.
E. The disturbance causes clinically significant distress or impairment in social, occupational, or other important areas of functioning.

Coding note: The ICD-9-CM code for depressive disorder due to another medical condition is **293.83,** which is assigned regardless of the specifier. The ICD-10-CM code depends on the specifier (see below).

Specify if:

(F06.31) With depressive features: Full criteria are not met for a major depressive episode.

(F06.32) With major depressive–like episode: Full criteria are met (except Criterion C) for a major depressive episode.

(F06.34) With mixed features: Symptoms of mania or hypomania are also present but do not predominate in the clinical picture.

Coding note: Include the name of the other medical condition in the name of the mental disorder (e.g., 293.83 [F06.31] depressive disorder due to hypothyroidism, with depressive features). The other medical condition should also be coded and listed separately immediately before the depressive disorder due to the medical condition (e.g., 244.9 [E03.9] hypothyroidism; 293.83 [F06.31] depressive disorder due to hypothyroidism, with depressive features).

Other Specified Depressive Disorder and Unspecified Depressive Disorder

These categories replace DSM-IV's depressive disorder not otherwise specified. The category other specified depressive disorder is used when symptoms characteristic of a depressive disorder are present and cause distress or impairment but do not meet the full criteria for a more specific disorder in the class, and when the clinician chooses to communicate the reason that the presentation does not meet full criteria. The clinician is encouraged to record the specific reason (e.g., recurrent brief depression, short-duration depressive episode [4–13 days], depressive episode with insufficient symptoms).

The category unspecified depressive disorder is used when the the full criteria for a more specific disorder are not met but symptoms cause clinically significant distress or impairment, and the clinician chooses not to specify the reason the criteria are not met, or there is insufficient information to make a more specific diagnosis.

Other Specified Depressive Disorder   311 (F32.8)

This category applies to presentations in which symptoms characteristic of a depressive disorder that cause clinically significant distress or impairment in social, occupational, or other important areas of functioning predominate but do not meet the full criteria for any of the disorders in the depressive disorders diagnostic class. The other specified depressive disorder category is used in situations in which the clinician chooses to communicate the specific reason that the presentation does not meet the criteria for any specific depressive disorder. This is done by recording "other specified depressive disorder" followed by the specific reason (e.g., "short-duration depressive episode").

Examples of presentations that can be specified using the "other specified" designation include the following:

1. **Recurrent brief depression:** Concurrent presence of depressed mood and at least four other symptoms of depression for 2–13 days at least once per month (not associated with the menstrual cycle) for at least 12 consecutive months in an individual whose presentation has never met criteria for any other depressive or bipolar disorder and does not currently meet active or residual criteria for any psychotic disorder.

2. **Short-duration depressive episode (4–13 days):** Depressed affect and at least four of the other eight symptoms of a major depressive episode associated with clinically significant distress or impairment that persists for more than 4 days, but less than 14 days, in an individual whose presentation has never met criteria for any other depressive or bipolar disorder, does not currently meet active or residual criteria for any psychotic disorder, and does not meet criteria for recurrent brief depression.

3. **Depressive episode with insufficient symptoms:** Depressed affect and at least one of the other eight symptoms of a major depressive episode associated with clinically significant distress or impairment that persist for at least 2 weeks in an individual whose presentation has never met criteria for any other depressive or bipolar disorder, does not currently meet active or residual criteria for any psychotic disorder, and does not meet criteria for mixed anxiety and depressive disorder symptoms.

Unspecified Depressive Disorder   311 (F32.9)

This category applies to presentations in which symptoms characteristic of a depressive disorder that cause clinically significant distress or impairment in social, occupational, or other important areas of functioning predominate but do not meet the full criteria for any of the disorders in the depressive disorders diagnostic class. The unspecified depressive disorder category is used in situations in which the clinician chooses *not* to specify the reason that the criteria are not met for a specific depressive disorder, and includes presentations for which there is insufficient information to make a more specific diagnosis (e.g., in emergency room settings).

KEY POINTS

- The mood disorders have been split into two chapters: "Bipolar and Related Disorders" and "Depressive Disorders."
- The wording "persistently increased goal-directed activity or energy" has been added to Criterion A for manic episode and hypomanic episode. This should make explicit the requirement that this hallmark symptom of bipolar I or II disorder needs to be present for the diagnosis to be made.

- The diagnosis of bipolar I disorder, most recent episode mixed, which required criteria for both mania and major depressive episode to be met simultaneously, has been deleted. Instead, a "with mixed features" specifier has been added that can be applied to a manic episode or a hypomanic episode when depressive features are present.

- With the depressive disorders, an important change is the omission of the bereavement exclusion that applied in DSM-IV to depressive symptoms lasting less than 2 months following the death of a loved one. This change was made because evidence does not support the separation of loss of a loved one from other stressors in terms of its likelihood of precipitating a major depressive episode.

- Disruptive mood dysregulation disorder is new to the depressive disorders and describes the presentation of children with persistent irritability and behavioral dyscontrol. This change should help reduce the problem of overdiagnosis of bipolar disorder in children and adolescents.

- Persistent depressive disorder (dysthymia) is new and merges DSM-IV-defined chronic major depressive disorder and dysthymic disorder. Clinicians had trouble distinguishing the two disorders.

- Premenstrual dysphoric disorder has been elevated to a stand-alone diagnosis. The diagnosis applies to the presentation of women who develop a cluster of depressive symptoms in association with their menstrual cycle.

CHAPTER 6

Anxiety Disorders

309.21 (F93.0)	Separation Anxiety Disorder
313.23 (F94.0)	Selective Mutism
300.29 (F40.2__)	Specific Phobia
300.23 (F40.10)	Social Anxiety Disorder (Social Phobia)
300.01 (F41.0)	Panic Disorder
	Panic Attack Specifier
300.22 (F40.00)	Agoraphobia
300.02 (F41.1)	Generalized Anxiety Disorder
	Substance/Medication-Induced Anxiety Disorder
293.84 (F06.4)	Anxiety Disorder Due to Another Medical Condition
300.09 (F41.8)	Other Specified Anxiety Disorder
300.00 (F41.9)	Unspecified Anxiety Disorder

Anxiety disorders are among the most prevalent psychiatric conditions worldwide. Research consistently shows them to be associated with increased psychiatric and physical morbidity, use of health care services, and psychosocial impairment. Necessity dictates that clinicians recognize and treat anxiety disorders without delay. Table 6–1 lists the DSM-5 anxiety disorders.

The word *anxiety* has been used to describe diverse phenomena, but in the clinical literature the term refers to the presence of fear or apprehension that is out of proportion to the situation. Anxiety was considered to play an important role in several conditions identified in the nineteenth century (Goodwin and Guze 1989). In the late nineteenth century, Da Costa wrote about an "irritable heart syndrome," characterized by chest pain, palpitations, and dizziness, a disorder thought to be due to a functional cardiac disturbance. He described the syndrome as occurring in a Civil War veteran, and later the syndrome was variously referred to as "soldier's heart," the "effort syndrome," or "neurocirculatory asthenia." At about the same time, Beard described *neurasthenia,* thought to be a disorder of nervous exhaustion. Freud later separated neurasthenia from cases affected mainly with anxiety symptoms under the name *anx-*

TABLE 6–1.	Anxiety disorders

Separation anxiety disorder

Selective mutism

Specific phobia

Social anxiety disorder (social phobia)

Panic disorder

Agoraphobia

Generalized anxiety disorder

Substance/medication-induced anxiety disorder

Anxiety disorder due to another medical condition

Other specified anxiety disorder

Unspecified anxiety disorder

iety neurosis. He described its clinical characteristics as including general irritability, anxious expectation, pangs of conscience, anxiety attacks, and phobias.

In DSM-I, the category psychoneurotic disorders constituted a distinct class in which anxiety was the chief characteristic. According to DSM-I, the anxiety "may be directly felt and expressed or…may be unconsciously and automatically controlled by the utilization of various psychological defense mechanisms" (p. 31). Several "reactions" were enumerated, including "anxiety reaction" and "phobic reaction"—disorders that continue to be recognized as anxiety disorders—and others that now fall into separate categories (i.e., dissociative reaction, obsessive compulsive reaction). In DSM-II, the category was renamed "neuroses" and the term *reaction* was eliminated, but the category was otherwise mostly unchanged.

DSM-III's all-encompassing changes led to a regrouping of some disorders and the creation of new disorders in which anxiety was either experienced as the predominant disturbance or experienced by the person as he or she attempted to master its symptoms (e.g., confronting a dreaded object or situation). The new diagnostic class, anxiety disorders, included panic disorder, agoraphobia, social phobia, simple phobia, generalized anxiety disorder, obsessive-compulsive disorder, and post-traumatic stress disorder (which was hyphenated until DSM-IV). Acute stress disorder was later added in DSM-IV. DSM-III-R, DSM-IV, and DSM-IV-TR otherwise remained true to DSM-III, except for minor changes in the criteria sets and some name changes (e.g., from simple phobia to specific phobia).

In DSM-5, the anxiety disorders chapter has remained largely faithful to its immediate predecessor, with several major exceptions. Obsessive-compulsive disorder now has its own chapter (see Chapter 7, "Obsessive-Compulsive and Related Disorders"). Post-traumatic stress disorder and acute stress disorder have been moved to "Trauma- and Stressor-Related Disorders" (see Chapter 8). These changes were made in response to scientific data showing that these disorders stand apart from the other anxiety disorders. The sequential order of the chapters in DSM-5 (i.e., the metastructure), however, reflects the close relationship among the disorders. Last, separation anxiety disorder and selective mutism are new to the chapter, having been formerly included in the DSM-IV chapter "Disorders Usually First Diagnosed in Infancy, Childhood, or Adolescence."

Other changes include the wording of criteria sets, which have been modified to 1) reflect the dysfunction underlying these disorders as intense, frequent, and chronic fear and anxiety; 2) separate the main constructs (e.g., situational triggers, cognitive ideation, intensity, frequency, duration); and 3) enhance consistency across the disorders. For specific phobia and social anxiety disorder, changes include deletion of the requirement that adults recognize that their anxiety is excessive or unreasonable. In addition, the minimum 6-month duration, which had been limited to individuals under age 18 years in DSM-IV, has been extended to all ages. The essential features of panic attacks remain unchanged, but the terminology for describing different types has been replaced with the terms *expected* or *unexpected*. Panic disorder and agoraphobia have been unlinked, and the criteria for agoraphobia have been extended to be consistent with criteria sets for the other disorders. With social anxiety disorder, the "generalized" specifier had been deleted and replaced with a "performance only" specifier.

Separation Anxiety Disorder

Separation anxiety disorder is a condition in which a person has excessive anxiety regarding separation from places or people to whom he or she has a strong emotional attachment. Included with the childhood disorders in DSM-III through DSM-IV-TR, separation anxiety disorder has now been moved because of research that links it to the anxiety disorders and the growing recognition that it occurs in adults. In fact, the lifetime estimate of separation anxiety disorder in childhood is 4.1%, whereas the rate among adults is 6.6%. Although about one-third of adults with separation anxiety disorder had it in childhood, the majority of adults had a first onset in adulthood. In children, the strong emotional attachment is likely to a parent; with adults, the attachment might be to a spouse or a friend.

Separation anxiety disorder should not be confused with separation anxiety that occurs as a normal stage of development for healthy, secure babies. Separation anxiety typically starts at around 8 months of age and increases until 13–15 months, when it begins to decline.

Diagnostic Criteria for Separation Anxiety Disorder   309.21 (F93.0)

A. Developmentally inappropriate and excessive fear or anxiety concerning separation from those to whom the individual is attached, as evidenced by at least three of the following:

  1. Recurrent excessive distress when anticipating or experiencing separation from home or from major attachment figures.
  2. Persistent and excessive worry about losing major attachment figures or about possible harm to them, such as illness, injury, disasters, or death.
  3. Persistent and excessive worry about experiencing an untoward event (e.g., getting lost, being kidnapped, having an accident, becoming ill) that causes separation from a major attachment figure.

4. Persistent reluctance or refusal to go out, away from home, to school, to work, or elsewhere because of fear of separation.
5. Persistent and excessive fear of or reluctance about being alone or without major attachment figures at home or in other settings.
6. Persistent reluctance or refusal to sleep away from home or to go to sleep without being near a major attachment figure.
7. Repeated nightmares involving the theme of separation.
8. Repeated complaints of physical symptoms (e.g., headaches, stomachaches, nausea, vomiting) when separation from major attachment figures occurs or is anticipated.

B. The fear, anxiety, or avoidance is persistent, lasting at least 4 weeks in children and adolescents and typically 6 months or more in adults.
C. The disturbance causes clinically significant distress or impairment in social, academic, occupational, or other important areas of functioning.
D. The disturbance is not better explained by another mental disorder, such as refusing to leave home because of excessive resistance to change in autism spectrum disorder; delusions or hallucinations concerning separation in psychotic disorders; refusal to go outside without a trusted companion in agoraphobia; worries about ill health or other harm befalling significant others in generalized anxiety disorder; or concerns about having an illness in illness anxiety disorder.

Criterion A

Although some separation anxiety is normal at various developmental phases, when the fear or anxiety is excessive and functionally impairing, this diagnosis may be appropriate. To increase the relevance to adults with separation anxiety disorder, terms have been added (e.g., addition of "work" in Criterion A4) or deleted (e.g., removal of "adults" in DSM-IV's Criterion A5 because attachment figures are not always adults; for adults, attachment figures can be partners, children, and so forth).

Criterion B

The duration is specified as typically lasting at least 6 months in adults (instead of the 4-week requirement in DSM-IV that has been retained in DSM-5 for children and adolescents) to minimize overdiagnosis of transient fears. A caveat permits shorter durations in cases of acute onset or exacerbation of severe symptoms.

Criteria C and D

Separation anxiety disorder is associated with significant impairment. People with the disorder may refuse to attend school or work, complain of somatic problems, and become socially isolated. Untreated, the disorder is associated with low educational attainment, unemployment, and either remaining unmarried or experiencing marital disruption. Because separation anxiety may occur in association with other mental disorders, the clinician needs to determine whether the person's symptoms meet full criteria for an independent diagnosis of separation anxiety disorder.

Selective Mutism

Selective mutism is characterized by the consistent failure to speak in specific social situations where speaking is expected despite being able to speak in other situations (e.g., at home). Originally named "elective mutism" in DSM-III, and renamed "selective mutism" for DSM-IV, the disorder was included with DSM-IV's "Disorders Usually First Diagnosed in Infancy, Childhood, or Adolescence." Selective mutism has been moved because of research that connects it with the anxiety disorders, and growing recognition that it continues into adulthood (or in rare cases begins in adulthood). Selective mutism is rare and most likely to manifest in young children.

Diagnostic Criteria for Selective Mutism   313.23 (F94.0)

A. Consistent failure to speak in specific social situations in which there is an expectation for speaking (e.g., at school) despite speaking in other situations.
B. The disturbance interferes with educational or occupational achievement or with social communication.
C. The duration of the disturbance is at least 1 month (not limited to the first month of school).
D. The failure to speak is not attributable to a lack of knowledge of, or comfort with, the spoken language required in the social situation.
E. The disturbance is not better explained by a communication disorder (e.g., childhood-onset fluency disorder) and does not occur exclusively during the course of autism spectrum disorder, schizophrenia, or another psychotic disorder.

Criterion A

When encountering individuals in specific social interactions, children and adults with selective mutism do not initiate speech or reciprocally respond when spoken to by others. These same individuals when seen at home, however, can interact normally. The diagnosis requires a *consistent* failure to speak in social situations.

Criterion B

Selective mutism is associated with significant impairment. Children with selective mutism often refuse to speak at school, leading to academic or educational impairment. As these children mature, they may face increasing social isolation, and in school settings, they suffer academic impairment because often they do not communicate appropriately with teachers regarding academic or personal needs.

Criterion C

Selective silence lasting less than a month (e.g., a child's being upset and refusing to talk for a few days) would not meet criteria for the diagnosis.

Criterion D

Children in families who have immigrated to a country where a different language is spoken may refuse to speak the new language because of lack of knowledge of the language. If comprehension of the new language is adequate but refusal to speak persists, a diagnosis of selective mutism would be warranted.

Criterion E

Although children with selective mutism generally have normal language skills, there may occasionally be an associated communication disorder. Selective mutism should be distinguished from speech disturbances that are better explained by a communication disorder, such as language disorder, speech sound disorder (previously phonological disorder), childhood-onset fluency disorder (stuttering), or pragmatic (social) communication disorder. Unlike selective mutism, the speech disturbance in these conditions is not restricted to a specific social situation. Individuals with autism spectrum disorder, schizophrenia or other psychotic disorders, or severe intellectual disability may have problems with social communication and be unable to speak appropriately in social situations. In contrast, selective mutism should be diagnosed only when a child has an established capacity to speak in some social situations (typically at home).

Specific Phobia

The term *phobia* refers to an excessive fear of a specific object, circumstance, or situation. Phobias are classified on the basis of the feared object or situation. Both specific phobia and social anxiety disorder (social phobia) require the development of intense anxiety, upon exposure to the feared object or situation. Both diagnoses also require that the fear or anxiety either interferes with functioning or causes marked distress.

Specific phobia includes the following specifiers: animal, natural environment, blood-injection-injury, situational, and other (for phobias that do not clearly fall into the previous four categories). The key feature for each stimulus type is that the fear or anxiety is limited to a specific object, both temporally and with respect to other objects. An individual with specific phobia becomes immediately frightened or anxious when presented with a feared object. This fear may relate to concern about harm from a feared object, concern about embarrassment, or fear of consequences related to exposure to the feared object. For example, individuals with blood-injection-injury phobia may be afraid of fainting on exposure to blood, and individuals with fear of heights may be afraid of becoming dizzy.

Specific phobia may involve fear of more than one object, particularly within a specific subcategory of phobia. For example, an individual with a phobia of insects may also have a phobia of mice, both phobias being classified as animal-type phobias. Quantifying the impairment associated with a specific phobia is sometimes difficult, because a comorbid disorder typically tends to cause more impairment than a specific phobia. Impairment associated with specific phobia typically restricts the social or professional activities of the individual.

Phobias have been recognized as incapacitating for more than 100 years. The prominent place of phobias in the history of modern mental health is indicated by the major role that case histories of patients with phobias played in the development of both psychoanalytic and cognitive therapies. The phobia category has undergone progressive refinement over the years. In DSM-III, phobias were regarded as a group of related but distinct conditions. Between DSM-III and DSM-IV, specific phobia was modified to include subcategories, based on research noting distinct physiology and demographics of the stimulus types.

Specific phobias are usually quite easily distinguished from other conditions because of the focused nature of the anxiety, both over time and with respect to objects or situations. The most difficult diagnostic issues involve differentiating specific phobia from other anxiety disorders.

Specific phobia exhibits a bimodal age at onset, with a childhood peak for animal phobia, natural environment phobia, and blood-injection-injury phobia and an early adulthood peak for other phobias, such as situational phobia. Because individuals with isolated specific phobias rarely present for treatment, research on the course of the disorder in the clinic is limited. Data suggest that most specific phobias that begin in childhood and persist into adulthood will continue to persist over many years. The severity of the condition when it persists into adulthood is thought to remain relatively constant, without the waxing and waning course of the disorder during childhood and adolescence or seen with other anxiety disorders.

Diagnostic Criteria for Specific Phobia

A. Marked fear or anxiety about a specific object or situation (e.g., flying, heights, animals, receiving an injection, seeing blood).

    Note: In children, the fear or anxiety may be expressed by crying, tantrums, freezing, or clinging.

B. The phobic object or situation almost always provokes immediate fear or anxiety.

C. The phobic object or situation is actively avoided or endured with intense fear or anxiety.

D. The fear or anxiety is out of proportion to the actual danger posed by the specific object or situation and to the sociocultural context.

E. The fear, anxiety, or avoidance is persistent, typically lasting for 6 months or more.

F. The fear, anxiety, or avoidance causes clinically significant distress or impairment in social, occupational, or other important areas of functioning.

G. The disturbance is not better explained by the symptoms of another mental disorder, including fear, anxiety, and avoidance of situations associated with panic-like symptoms or other incapacitating symptoms (as in agoraphobia); objects or situations related to obsessions (as in obsessive-compulsive disorder); reminders of traumatic events (as in posttraumatic stress disorder); separation from home or attachment figures (as in separation anxiety disorder); or social situations (as in social anxiety disorder).

Specify if:

Code based on the phobic stimulus:

300.29 (F40.218) Animal (e.g., spiders, insects, dogs).
300.29 (F40.228) Natural environment (e.g., heights, storms, water).

300.29 (F40.23x) Blood-injection-injury (e.g., needles, invasive medical procedures).

> **Coding note:** Select specific ICD-10-CM code as follows: **F40.230** fear of
> blood; **F40.231** fear of injections and transfusions; **F40.232** fear of other medi-
> cal care; or **F40.233** fear of injury.

300.29 (F40.248) Situational (e.g., airplanes, elevators, enclosed places).
300.29 (F40.298) Other (e.g., situations that may lead to choking or vomiting; in children, e.g., loud sounds or costumed characters).

Coding note: When more than one phobic stimulus is present, code all ICD-10-CM
codes that apply (e.g., for fear of snakes and flying, F40.218 specific phobia, animal,
and F40.248 specific phobia, situational).

Criteria A and B

There is marked fear or anxiety that is triggered by exposure to a specific stimulus.
The term *marked* has been operationalized as "intense." The phrase "fear or anxiety"
is used consistently across anxiety disorders. The phobic object or situation almost always provokes immediate fear or anxiety.

Criterion C

There are generally two responses to the fear or anxiety elicited by the stimulus. A person may avoid situations in which he or she is exposed to the stimulus, or the person
may expose himself or herself to the phobic object or situation and endure the fear or
anxiety. DSM-5 has added the descriptor "actively avoided" to minimize overdiagnosis of mild fears.

Criterion D

The fear or anxiety is out of proportion, or more intense than is deemed necessary,
given the actual danger that the object or situation poses—that is, the fear or anxiety
is greater than is deemed appropriate to the actual danger in the situation. Although
people with specific phobia often recognize their reactions as disproportionate to the
situation, they tend to overestimate the danger in their feared situations, and thus the
judgment of being out of proportion should not be made solely on the basis of self-
report. In DSM-IV, Criterion C required that the individual be aware that the fear or
anxiety was excessive, but stated that this requirement might not be present in children. Self-recognition has been removed because many adults deny that their fears
are out of proportion or excessive, and the notation that in children the feature many
be absent has been deleted. This criterion requires that the sociocultural context be
taken into account.

Criterion E

With the duration criterion "typically lasting for 6 months or more" (with text clarification that the cutoff should not be applied too rigidly), the overdiagnosis of transient fears and phobias should be minimized. DSM-IV included a duration criterion

(6 months or more) for children under age 18, but this is now extended to all age groups given the evidence that transient fears and phobias occur in adulthood.

Criterion F

The fear, anxiety, or avoidance needs to result in clinically significant distress or functional impairment. For example, a person who avoids the ferris wheel at a state fair because of fear of heights may still have a lovely day at the fair and pay little heed to how this fear affects the experience. Some people cope with their phobias by manipulating their environments (e.g., avoidance of zoos by a person who fears snakes). In these cases, the impairment would be minimal or nonexistent and the person's presentation would not qualify for the diagnosis. If the manipulation of the environment affects the person's work, for example, then it may cause significant interference.

Criterion G

Many disorders are characterized by avoidance (e.g., obsessive-compulsive disorder, agoraphobia). Specific phobia should be diagnosed only when avoidance is related to an object or situation and is not accounted for by another disorder.

Specifiers

The specifiers reflect the general categories of phobic stimulus. DSM-5 has removed reference to fears of contracting an illness in the "other" category because of the relatedness of such fears to obsessive-compulsive disorder and to hypochondriasis (which has been replaced, in DSM-5, by somatic symptom disorder and, in a minority of cases, illness anxiety disorder).

Social Anxiety Disorder (Social Phobia)

Social anxiety disorder involves fear of or anxiety about social situations, including situations that involve scrutiny or contact with strangers. Individuals with this disorder typically fear embarrassing themselves in social situations, such as while speaking in public or meeting new people. This disorder can involve specific fears or anxiety about performing certain activities, such as writing, eating, or speaking in front of others. It can also involve a vague, nonspecific fear of embarrassing oneself or feeling foolish. The clinician should recognize that many individuals exhibit at least some social anxiety or self-consciousness. Community studies suggest that roughly one-third of all people consider themselves to be more anxious than other people in social situations. Such anxiety becomes a disorder only when the anxiety either prevents the person from participating in desired activities or causes marked distress in such activities.

Diagnostic Criteria for Social Anxiety Disorder (Social Phobia)
300.23 (F40.10)

A. Marked fear or anxiety about one or more social situations in which the individual is exposed to possible scrutiny by others. Examples include social interactions (e.g., having a conversation, meeting unfamiliar people), being observed (e.g., eating or drinking), and performing in front of others (e.g., giving a speech).

Note: In children, the anxiety must occur in peer settings and not just during interactions with adults.

B. The individual fears that he or she will act in a way or show anxiety symptoms that will be negatively evaluated (i.e., will be humiliating or embarrassing; will lead to rejection or offend others).

C. The social situations almost always provoke fear or anxiety.

Note: In children, the fear or anxiety may be expressed by crying, tantrums, freezing, clinging, shrinking, or failing to speak in social situations.

D. The social situations are avoided or endured with intense fear or anxiety.

E. The fear or anxiety is out of proportion to the actual threat posed by the social situation and to the sociocultural context.

F. The fear, anxiety, or avoidance is persistent, typically lasting for 6 months or more.

G. The fear, anxiety, or avoidance causes clinically significant distress or impairment in social, occupational, or other important areas of functioning.

H. The fear, anxiety, or avoidance is not attributable to the physiological effects of a substance (e.g., a drug of abuse, a medication) or another medical condition.

I. The fear, anxiety, or avoidance is not better explained by the symptoms of another mental disorder, such as panic disorder, body dysmorphic disorder, or autism spectrum disorder.

J. If another medical condition (e.g., Parkinson's disease, obesity, disfigurement from burns or injury) is present, the fear, anxiety, or avoidance is clearly unrelated or is excessive.

Specify if:

Performance only: If the fear is restricted to speaking or performing in public.

Criteria A and B

These items cover the three contexts in which social anxiety disorder most commonly occurs: social interactions, being observed by others, and performing in front of others.

In Criterion B, *humiliation* and *embarrassment* have been brought under the broader phrase "negatively evaluated," which is the core fear in social anxiety disorder. The phrase "offend others" has been added to increase cultural sensitivity; in some cultures the underlying fear is the concern that one will make others uncomfortable.

Criterion C

This criterion highlights that social anxiety is a conditioned, stimulus response. In addition, the criterion clarifies that in children, fear and anxiety may present in a range of ways (e.g., tantrums).

Criterion D

Although some individuals with social anxiety disorder avoid the contexts that elicit their anxiety, others endure the anxiety-provoking environments even when the anxiety or fear is intense.

Criterion E

People with social anxiety disorder often have difficulty recognizing that their fear is excessive. Therefore, the clinician may be in a better position to judge this. Use of the phrase "out of proportion to the actual threat posed" is intended to operationalize what was meant by "excessive or unreasonable" in DSM-IV. Criterion C in DSM-IV included a note that self-recognition may be absent in children; this note has been deleted. Finally, the DSM-5 item reminds the clinician to take into account the "sociocultural context."

Criterion F

The DSM-IV requirement that the duration be 6 months or more in children under age 18 years has now been extended to all age groups, given the data that transient social anxieties can occur in adulthood as well. This duration criterion helps to minimize overdiagnosis of transient social anxiety.

Criteria G, H, I, and J

Most individuals experience some social anxiety at some point in their lives. Criterion G requires that the symptoms cause considerable impairment or distress. This criterion prevents the overdiagnosis of social anxiety disorder.

Many disorders are characterized by fear of social situations. Social anxiety disorder should be diagnosed only when the avoidance is not attributable to the effects of a substance or medication, is not better explained by another mental disorder, and is not related to another medical condition (Criteria H, I, and I).

Specifiers

Evidence suggests that the "performance only" specifier represents a subset of the larger social anxiety disorder group with different pathophysiological correlates and treatment response.

Panic Disorder

Panic disorder is characterized by a pattern of recurrent panic attacks accompanied by persistent worry or behavioral change. Therefore, individuals with panic disorder experience anxiety symptoms and functional impairment independent of the actual attack. The panic attacks occur spontaneously, arising without any trigger or environmental cue. There has been considerable interest in the relationship between panic disorder and agoraphobia. Although DSM-IV described panic disorder both with agoraphobia and without agoraphobia, this distinction is not included in DSM-5 because it was not meaningful. Panic disorder often co-occurs with a number of mental conditions beyond agoraphobia, particularly anxiety and depressive disorders.

Panic disorder was included in DSM-III and was recognized as a distinct entity. From DSM-III through DSM-IV-TR, panic disorder and agoraphobia were tightly linked. As conceptualized in DSM-IV, agoraphobia invariably involves at least some form of spontaneous crescendo anxiety, even if such episodes do not meet formal criteria for panic attacks. In the earlier versions of DSM and in ICD-10, agoraphobia is considered less closely linked to panic disorder.

Diagnostic Criteria for Panic Disorder   300.01 (F41.0)

A. Recurrent unexpected panic attacks. A panic attack is an abrupt surge of intense fear or intense discomfort that reaches a peak within minutes, and during which time four (or more) of the following symptoms occur:

   Note: The abrupt surge can occur from a calm state or an anxious state.

   1. Palpitations, pounding heart, or accelerated heart rate.
   2. Sweating.
   3. Trembling or shaking.
   4. Sensations of shortness of breath or smothering.
   5. Feelings of choking.
   6. Chest pain or discomfort.
   7. Nausea or abdominal distress.
   8. Feeling dizzy, unsteady, light-headed, or faint.
   9. Chills or heat sensations.
   10. Paresthesias (numbness or tingling sensations).
   11. Derealization (feelings of unreality) or depersonalization (being detached from oneself).
   12. Fear of losing control or "going crazy."
   13. Fear of dying.

   Note: Culture-specific symptoms (e.g., tinnitus, neck soreness, headache, uncontrollable screaming or crying) may be seen. Such symptoms should not count as one of the four required symptoms.

B. At least one of the attacks has been followed by 1 month (or more) of one or both of the following:

   1. Persistent concern or worry about additional panic attacks or their consequences (e.g., losing control, having a heart attack, "going crazy").
   2. A significant maladaptive change in behavior related to the attacks (e.g., behaviors designed to avoid having panic attacks, such as avoidance of exercise or unfamiliar situations).

C. The disturbance is not attributable to the physiological effects of a substance (e.g., a drug of abuse, a medication) or another medical condition (e.g., hyperthyroidism, cardiopulmonary disorders).

D. The disturbance is not better explained by another mental disorder (e.g., the panic attacks do not occur only in response to feared social situations, as in social anxiety disorder; in response to circumscribed phobic objects or situations, as in specific phobia; in response to obsessions, as in obsessive-compulsive disorder; in response to reminders of traumatic events, as in posttraumatic stress disorder; or in response to separation from attachment figures, as in separation anxiety disorder).

Criteria A and B

Panic disorder requires recurrent and "unexpected" panic attacks, at least one of which is associated with either persistent concern or worry about additional attacks, or changes in behavior related to the attacks. Examples are provided to help the clinician understand the functional impact of the attacks.

Criteria C and D

Panic disorder must be differentiated from medical conditions that produce similar symptoms. Panic attacks have been associated with a variety of endocrinological disorders, including both hypo- and hyperthyroid states, hyperparathyroidism, and pheochromocytomas. Episodic hypoglycemia can also produce panic symptoms. Seizure disorders, vestibular dysfunction, neoplasms, prescribed and illicit substances, and cardiac and pulmonary problems (e.g., arrhythmias, chronic obstructive pulmonary disease, asthma) can all result in panic symptoms. Clues to an underlying medical cause for panic symptoms include atypical features during panic attacks, such as ataxia, alterations in consciousness, or bladder dyscontrol; onset of panic disorder relatively late in life; or physical signs and symptoms indicating a medical condition.

Panic disorder also must be differentiated from a number of mental disorders, particularly other anxiety states. Differentiation from generalized anxiety disorder can sometimes be difficult, but classic panic attacks are characterized by rapid onset and short duration, in contrast to the anxiety associated with generalized anxiety disorder, which emerges and dissipates more slowly. Anxiety also frequently accompanies many other psychiatric disorders, including psychotic and mood disorders.

Panic Attack Specifier

A panic attack is a sudden episode of intense fear or discomfort lasting minutes to hours that triggers uncomfortable physical sensations. Panic attacks usually begin abruptly, peak within minutes, and can be frightening to the individual. When they occur, the person may believe he or she is losing control, having a heart attack, or even dying. Although many people have isolated panic attacks during stressful times, these attacks do not occur repeatedly. Panic attacks may occur in various psychopathological states.

Freud's description of anxiety neurosis was defined by the coexistence of a state of moderate and permanent anxiety and of anxiety attacks, whose manifestations were similar to today's panic attack. Anxiety neurosis was later subdivided into the acute anxiety attack (i.e., a panic attack) and a state of moderate and continuous anxiety (now referred to as generalized anxiety disorder). This distinction was included in the Research Diagnostic Criteria (Spitzer et al. 1975) and appeared a few years later in DSM-III.

Importantly, as stated in DSM-5, panic attacks can be noted as a specifier for any anxiety disorder as well as for other mental disorders (e.g., depressive disorders, posttraumatic stress disorder) and some medical conditions (e.g., cardiac, respiratory, vestibular, gastrointestinal). When the presence of a panic attack is identified, it should be documented with the specifier "with panic attacks" (e.g., posttraumatic stress disorder with panic attacks).

Panic Attack Specifier

Note: Symptoms are presented for the purpose of identifying a panic attack; however, panic attack is not a mental disorder and cannot be coded. Panic attacks can occur in the context of any anxiety disorder as well as other mental disorders (e.g., depressive disorders, posttraumatic stress disorder, substance use disorders) and some medical conditions (e.g., cardiac, respiratory, vestibular, gastrointestinal). When the presence of a panic attack is identified, it should be noted as a specifier (e.g., "posttraumatic stress disorder with panic attacks"). For panic disorder, the presence of panic attack is contained within the criteria for the disorder and panic attack is not used as a specifier.

An abrupt surge of intense fear or intense discomfort that reaches a peak within minutes, and during which time four (or more) of the following symptoms occur:
Note: The abrupt surge can occur from a calm state or an anxious state.

1. Palpitations, pounding heart, or accelerated heart rate.
2. Sweating.
3. Trembling or shaking.
4. Sensations of shortness of breath or smothering.
5. Feelings of choking.
6. Chest pain or discomfort.
7. Nausea or abdominal distress.
8. Feeling dizzy, unsteady, light-headed, or faint.
9. Chills or heat sensations.
10. Paresthesias (numbness or tingling sensations).
11. Derealization (feelings of unreality) or depersonalization (being detached from oneself).
12. Fear of losing control or "going crazy."
13. Fear of dying.

Note: Culture-specific symptoms (e.g., tinnitus, neck soreness, headache, uncontrollable screaming or crying) may be seen. Such symptoms should not count as one of the four required symptoms.

By itself, a panic attack is not a codable disorder. Episodes of abrupt fear occur in many situations. A healthy person might experience a panic attack when confronted with sudden extreme danger, and an individual with a phobia of heights might experience a panic attack when confronted with the feared situation. DSM-5 requires that panic attacks be listed as a specifier to the specific disorder with which they occur. The importance of the specifier is based on data demonstrating that panic attacks predict the severity of other forms of psychopathology. A person who meets at least four of the symptoms qualifies as having a panic attack. Data from the DSM-IV field trial confirmed that the four-symptom threshold is optimal.

Although the DSM-5 symptoms are unchanged from DSM-IV, they are now rank-ordered from most to least common. In addition, "heat sensations" replaces the DSM-IV symptom "hot flushes." The concluding note is included to increase clinician awareness of culture-based symptoms. For example, higher rates of paresthesias occur in African Americans, trembling in Caribbean Latinos, and depersonalization/derealization in Puerto Ricans.

Agoraphobia

Agoraphobia was first identified by Westphal in the late 19th century when he described people who feared public places (Goodwin and Guze 1989). DSM-III introduced and codified agoraphobia as a distinctive syndrome characterized by "marked fear and avoidance of being alone or in public places from which escape might be difficult or help not available in case of sudden incapacitations" (p. 226). In DSM-III-R, agoraphobia was specifically defined as a classically conditioned response to panic attacks. Although agoraphobia could be diagnosed in the absence of a history of panic attacks, such an occurrence was thought to be rare. Therefore, agoraphobia became conceptually linked to panic attacks, but was also seen explicitly and exclusively as a secondary complication. In DSM-IV, agoraphobia could be diagnosed only within the context of panic disorder or as the result of panic attacks or panic-like symptoms (i.e., agoraphobia was related to fear of developing panic symptoms such as dizziness or diarrhea). In community samples, however, the majority of people with agoraphobia never experienced panic attacks or panic-like symptoms or psychophysiological symptoms of other types that clearly preceded the onset of agoraphobic avoidance. In DSM-5, agoraphobia is a codable disorder independent of panic disorder or panic attacks (Wittchen et al. 2010).

Diagnostic Criteria for Agoraphobia   **300.22 (F40.00)**

A. Marked fear or anxiety about two (or more) of the following five situations:

   1. Using public transportation (e.g., automobiles, buses, trains, ships, planes).
   2. Being in open spaces (e.g., parking lots, marketplaces, bridges).
   3. Being in enclosed places (e.g., shops, theaters, cinemas).
   4. Standing in line or being in a crowd.
   5. Being outside of the home alone.

B. The individual fears or avoids these situations because of thoughts that escape might be difficult or help might not be available in the event of developing panic-like symptoms or other incapacitating or embarrassing symptoms (e.g., fear of falling in the elderly; fear of incontinence).

C. The agoraphobic situations almost always provoke fear or anxiety.

D. The agoraphobic situations are actively avoided, require the presence of a companion, or are endured with intense fear or anxiety.

E. The fear or anxiety is out of proportion to the actual danger posed by the agoraphobic situations and to the sociocultural context.

F. The fear, anxiety, or avoidance is persistent, typically lasting for 6 months or more.

G. The fear, anxiety, or avoidance causes clinically significant distress or impairment in social, occupational, or other important areas of functioning.

H. If another medical condition (e.g., inflammatory bowel disease, Parkinson's disease) is present, the fear, anxiety, or avoidance is clearly excessive.

I. The fear, anxiety, or avoidance is not better explained by the symptoms of another mental disorder—for example, the symptoms are not confined to specific phobia, situational type; do not involve only social situations (as in social anxiety disorder); and are not related exclusively to obsessions (as in obsessive-compulsive disorder), perceived defects or flaws in physical appearance (as in body dysmorphic disorder), reminders of traumatic events (as in posttraumatic stress disorder), or fear of separation (as in separation anxiety disorder).

Note: Agoraphobia is diagnosed irrespective of the presence of panic disorder. If an individual's presentation meets criteria for panic disorder and agoraphobia, both diagnoses should be assigned.

Criterion A

The person with agoraphobia must report fear or anxiety arising from at least two of the five general situations listed. The requirement of at least two such situations differentiates agoraphobia from a specific phobia, which may be limited to one particular situation. Also, the fear or anxiety is related exclusively to the situations and is not attributable to more generalized anxiety that the person experiences in multiple situations.

Criterion B

The diagnosis of agoraphobia requires the person to have a cognitive ideational component related to the fear or avoidance. This criterion emphasizes the motivation for the avoidance, such as fear that escape will be difficult. In addition, the cognitive aspect of agoraphobia can be associated with fear or avoidance of the situation because of thoughts that "help might not be available in the event of developing panic-like symptoms or other incapacitating or embarrassing symptoms (e.g., fear of falling in the elderly; fear of incontinence)," and thereby allows for the diagnosis in the absence of panic-like symptoms.

Criterion C

This criterion requires that the situations almost always provoke fear or anxiety and therefore raises the threshold for making the diagnosis. A single or even occasional event of avoiding situations due to fear would not qualify for the diagnosis.

Criterion D

DSM-5 includes the phrase "actively avoided" to minimize overdiagnosis of mild fears.

Criterion E

This criterion is new and is used to increase reliability and separation from normal fears. The criterion evokes clinician judgment (vs. self-recognition). For example, a person with a history of incontinence may refuse to leave home for long stretches of time, and that may be reasonable. If the person had only a single episode of incontinence and has refused to leave home for years, then that would be out of proportion to the fear.

Criterion F

To avoid overdiagnosis of transient fear or anxiety, the duration is indicated as typically for 6 months or more. This was previously not a requirement.

Criteria G, H, and I

The degree of impairment associated with agoraphobia can vary from only avoiding situations to being entirely housebound (Criterion G). This criterion is intended to increase separation of individuals with agoraphobia from those with mild or transient fears.

The core feature of agoraphobia is avoidance, a symptom that may be present in a number of other disorders. The clinician should rule out other medical conditions (e.g., inflammatory bowel disease) in which avoidance behavior may be present (Criterion H). Other mental disorders also need to be ruled out (e.g., obsessive-compulsive disorder) (Criterion I).

Generalized Anxiety Disorder

Generalized anxiety disorder is characterized by a pattern of frequent, persistent excessive anxiety and worry that is out of proportion to the impact of the event or circumstance that is the focus of the worry. Individuals with generalized anxiety disorder may not acknowledge the excessive nature of their worry, but they are bothered by their degree of worry. This pattern of worry occurs "more days than not for at least 6 months" (Criterion A). Individuals find it difficult to control this worry and report at least three of six somatic or cognitive symptoms (or one symptom for children).

Generalized anxiety disorder was first included in DSM-III, having been split off from anxiety neurosis. The disorder was originally considered a diagnosis of exclusion, because it could not be "attributable to another mental disorder." DSM-III also required a 1-month duration of symptoms, but concerns later arose about the low reliability of the diagnosis. In DSM-III-R, the duration was increased to 6 months and the symptom list was expanded. DSM-III-R also removed some of the hierarchical rules that had limited the diagnosis to individuals in whom the symptoms were not due to another disorder. Finally, in DSM-IV the list of associated symptoms was simplified from 18 to 6, of which individuals had to exhibit at least 3. More emphasis was placed on the pervasiveness of the worry, and the criteria were modified to accommodate childhood presentations. DSM-IV attempted to integrate the approach to worry across development. In DSM-5, the diagnosis is mostly unchanged from that in DSM-IV except for wording changes and a reorganization of the criteria.

Diagnostic Criteria for Generalized Anxiety Disorder   300.02 (F41.1)

A. Excessive anxiety and worry (apprehensive expectation), occurring more days than not for at least 6 months, about a number of events or activities (such as work or school performance).

B. The individual finds it difficult to control the worry.
C. The anxiety and worry are associated with three (or more) of the following six symptoms (with at least some symptoms having been present for more days than not for the past 6 months):

Note: Only one item is required in children.

1. Restlessness or feeling keyed up or on edge.
2. Being easily fatigued.
3. Difficulty concentrating or mind going blank.
4. Irritability.
5. Muscle tension.
6. Sleep disturbance (difficulty falling or staying asleep, or restless, unsatisfying sleep).

D. The anxiety, worry, or physical symptoms cause clinically significant distress or impairment in social, occupational, or other important areas of functioning.
E. The disturbance is not attributable to the physiological effects of a substance (e.g., a drug of abuse, a medication) or another medical condition (e.g., hyperthyroidism).
F. The disturbance is not better explained by another mental disorder (e.g., anxiety or worry about having panic attacks in panic disorder, negative evaluation in social anxiety disorder [social phobia], contamination or other obsessions in obsessive-compulsive disorder, separation from attachment figures in separation anxiety disorder, reminders of traumatic events in posttraumatic stress disorder, gaining weight in anorexia nervosa, physical complaints in somatic symptom disorder, perceived appearance flaws in body dysmorphic disorder, having a serious illness in illness anxiety disorder, or the content of delusional beliefs in schizophrenia or delusional disorder).

Criteria A and B

Generalized anxiety disorder is not the same as normal worry, and these criteria are intended to distinguish the two. Worries considered sufficient for the disorder must be excessive. An evaluation of the intensity, frequency, and focus of worries provides clues to whether the anxiety is excessive. The minimum duration requirement of 6 months is set high enough to distinguish generalized anxiety disorder from episodic or short-lived events that cause worry. Furthermore, the person finds it difficult to control the worry.

Criterion C

This item includes both somatic and cognitive aspects of generalized anxiety disorder. The requirement of three or more symptoms for adults and one for children is unchanged from DSM-IV.

Criterion D

This criterion establishes a threshold by which normal worry will not become pathologized. The requirement that the worry cause significant distress or impairment should prevent an individual from receiving this diagnosis unless the worry is severe.

Criteria E and F

Anxiety is a frequent symptom of substance use and of several medical conditions, which must be ruled out. Anxiety or worry is also a defining or associated feature of many mental disorders. Criterion F provides examples of worries covered by other diagnoses and thereby reserves the diagnosis of generalized anxiety disorder to those worries not covered by other conditions. An additional diagnosis of generalized anxiety disorder, however, may be appropriate when the worries extend beyond the specific symptoms of another disorder.

Substance/Medication-Induced Anxiety Disorder

For individuals with a substance/medication-induced anxiety disorder, clinically significant symptoms of panic, worry, phobia, or obsessions emerge in the context of prescribed or illicit substance use. The differential diagnosis requires that substance use and medications be ruled out as possible causes of anxiety before one of the other anxiety disorders is diagnosed. Clinicians should routinely document the substance use status of all patients and record all medications.

Clinicians should be particularly attuned to substance misuse when encountering an anxious individual. If misuse is present, the clinician must then determine whether it has any relationship to the ongoing anxiety symptoms. Although no definitive test exists to establish such a causal relationship, several factors can help confirm the diagnosis. These include the timing of the symptoms, the existing literature pertaining to the strength of the association between anxiety and the potential complicating factor, and signs or symptoms that are atypical of an anxiety disorder.

Onset of anxiety symptoms may occur during substance intoxication or withdrawal, and onset of such symptoms is indicated by use of specifiers. Anxiety is associated with multiple illicit substances (e.g., amphetamines, cocaine), alcohol, and caffeine. The diagnosis can also be made when the anxiety is associated with use of prescription drugs (e.g., anticholinergics, antidepressants, lithium). A diagnosis of substance-induced anxiety disorder rather than substance intoxication or withdrawal is appropriate when the anxiety symptoms predominate and are in excess of what is expected and warrant independent clinical attention.

Diagnostic Criteria for Substance/Medication-Induced Anxiety Disorder

A. Panic attacks or anxiety is predominant in the clinical picture.
B. There is evidence from the history, physical examination, or laboratory findings of both (1) and (2):
 1. The symptoms in Criterion A developed during or soon after substance intoxication or withdrawal or after exposure to a medication.
 2. The involved substance/medication is capable of producing the symptoms in Criterion A.

C. The disturbance is not better explained by an anxiety disorder that is not substance/medication-induced. Such evidence of an independent anxiety disorder could include the following:

> The symptoms precede the onset of the substance/medication use; the symptoms persist for a substantial period of time (e.g., about 1 month) after the cessation of acute withdrawal or severe intoxication; or there is other evidence suggesting the existence of an independent non-substance/medication-induced anxiety disorder (e.g., a history of recurrent non-substance/medication-related episodes).

D. The disturbance does not occur exclusively during the course of a delirium.

E. The disturbance causes clinically significant distress or impairment in social, occupational, or other important areas of functioning.

Note: This diagnosis should be made instead of a diagnosis of substance intoxication or substance withdrawal only when the symptoms in Criterion A predominate in the clinical picture and they are sufficiently severe to warrant clinical attention.

Coding note: The ICD-9-CM and ICD-10-CM codes for the [specific substance/medication]-induced anxiety disorders are indicated in the table below. Note that the ICD-10-CM code depends on whether or not there is a comorbid substance use disorder present for the same class of substance. If a mild substance use disorder is comorbid with the substance-induced anxiety disorder, the 4th position character is "1," and the clinician should record "mild [substance] use disorder" before the substance-induced anxiety disorder (e.g., "mild cocaine use disorder with cocaine-induced anxiety disorder"). If a moderate or severe substance use disorder is comorbid with the substance-induced anxiety disorder, the 4th position character is "2," and the clinician should record "moderate [substance] use disorder" or "severe [substance] use disorder," depending on the severity of the comorbid substance use disorder. If there is no comorbid substance use disorder (e.g., after a one-time heavy use of the substance), then the 4th position character is "9," and the clinician should record only the substance-induced anxiety disorder.

		ICD-10-CM		
	ICD-9-CM	With use disorder, mild	With use disorder, moderate or severe	Without use disorder
Alcohol	291.89	F10.180	F10.280	F10.980
Caffeine	292.89	F15.180	F15.280	F15.980
Cannabis	292.89	F12.180	F12.280	F12.980
Phencyclidine	292.89	F16.180	F16.280	F16.980
Other hallucinogen	292.89	F16.180	F16.280	F16.980
Inhalant	292.89	F18.180	F18.280	F18.980
Opioid	292.89	F11.188	F11.288	F11.988
Sedative, hypnotic, or anxiolytic	292.89	F13.180	F13.280	F13.980
Amphetamine (or other stimulant)	292.89	F15.180	F15.280	F15.980

		ICD-10-CM		
	ICD-9-CM	With use disorder, mild	With use disorder, moderate or severe	Without use disorder
Cocaine	292.89	F14.180	F14.280	F14.980
Other (or unknown) substance	292.89	F19.180	F19.280	F19.980

Specify if (see 16–1 in the chapter "Substance-Related and Addictive Disorders" for diagnoses associated with substance class):

With onset during intoxication: This specifier applies if criteria are met for intoxication with the substance and the symptoms develop during intoxication.

With onset during withdrawal: This specifier applies if criteria are met for withdrawal from the substance and the symptoms develop during, or shortly after, withdrawal.

With onset after medication use: Symptoms may appear either at initiation of medication or after a modification or change in use.

Anxiety Disorder Due to Another Medical Condition

Anxiety symptoms can develop in the context of identifiable medical syndromes. Endocrine conditions (e.g., hyperthyroidism, hypoglycemia), cardiovascular conditions (e.g., arrhythmia, congestive heart failure), respiratory diseases (e.g., chronic obstructive pulmonary disease, pneumonia), neurological conditions (e.g., neoplasms, encephalitis), and metabolic conditions (e.g., vitamin B_{12} deficiency) all may be associated with anxiety. If another medical condition is present and determined to be the direct physiological cause of the anxiety symptoms, then anxiety disorder due to another medical condition should be diagnosed. When recording the diagnosis, the clinician should include the name of the other medical condition within the name of the mental disorder (e.g., 293.84 [F06.4] anxiety disorder due to pheochromocytoma). The other medical condition should be coded and listed separately immediately before the anxiety disorder due to the medical condition (e.g., 227.0 [D35.00] pheochromocytoma; 293.84 [F06.4] anxiety disorder due to pheochromocytoma).

Diagnostic Criteria for Anxiety Disorder Due to Another Medical Condition   **293.84 (F06.4)**

A. Panic attacks or anxiety is predominant in the clinical picture.

B. There is evidence from the history, physical examination, or laboratory findings that the disturbance is the direct pathophysiological consequence of another medical condition.

C. The disturbance is not better explained by another mental disorder.

D. The disturbance does not occur exclusively during the course of a delirium.

E. The disturbance causes clinically significant distress or impairment in social, occupational, or other important areas of functioning.

Coding note: Include the name of the other medical condition within the name of the mental disorder (e.g., 293.84 [F06.4] anxiety disorder due to pheochromocytoma). The other medical condition should be coded and listed separately immediately before the anxiety disorder due to the medical condition (e.g., 227.0 [D35.00] pheochromocytoma; 293.84 [F06.4] anxiety disorder due to pheochromocytoma.

Other Specified Anxiety Disorder and Unspecified Anxiety Disorder

Because anxiety represents one of the most common psychiatric symptoms, it is not uncommon to encounter individuals who have impairment from anxiety but whose symptoms do not meet criteria for one of the specific anxiety disorders. These individuals are appropriately classified as having an other specified or unspecified anxiety disorder.

The categories replace DSM-IV's anxiety disorder not otherwise specified. Other specified anxiety disorder is used when symptoms characteristic of an anxiety disorder are present and cause distress or impairment but do not meet the full criteria for a more specific disorder in the class. The category is used when the clinician chooses to communicate the reason that the presentation does not meet full criteria. The clinician is encouraged to record the specific reason (e.g., limited-symptom attacks).

The category unspecified anxiety disorder is used when the individual's symptoms do not meet full criteria for a more specific disorder that causes distress or impairment, and the clinician chooses not to specify the reason the criteria are not met or there is insufficient information to make a more specific diagnosis.

Other Specified Anxiety Disorder   300.09 (F41.8)

This category applies to presentations in which symptoms characteristic of an anxiety disorder that cause clinically significant distress or impairment in social, occupational, or other important areas of functioning predominate but do not meet the full criteria for any of the disorders in the anxiety disorders diagnostic class. The other specified anxiety disorder category is used in situations in which the clinician chooses to communicate the specific reason that the presentation does not meet the criteria for any specific anxiety disorder. This is done by recording "other specified anxiety disorder" followed by the specific reason (e.g., "generalized anxiety not occurring more days than not").

Examples of presentations that can be specified using the "other specified" designation include the following:

1. **Limited-symptom attacks.**
2. **Generalized anxiety not occurring more days than not.**
3. *Khyâl cap* **(wind attacks):** See "Glossary of Cultural Concepts of Distress" in the Appendix to DSM-5.
4. *Ataque de nervios* **(attack of nerves):** See "Glossary of Cultural Concepts of Distress" in the Appendix to DSM-5.

Unspecified Anxiety Disorder 300.00 (F41.9)

This category applies to presentations in which symptoms characteristic of an anxiety disorder that cause clinically significant distress or impairment in social, occupational, or other important areas of functioning predominate but do not meet the full criteria for any of the disorders in the anxiety disorders diagnostic class. The unspecified anxiety disorder category is used in situations in which the clinician chooses *not* to specify the reason that the criteria are not met for a specific anxiety disorder, and includes presentations in which there is insufficient information to make a more specific diagnosis (e.g., in emergency room settings).

KEY POINTS

- The anxiety disorders class no longer includes obsessive-compulsive disorder, posttraumatic stress disorder, or acute stress disorder. Separation anxiety disorder and selective mutism have been added to the class. The wording of the former has been changed to more adequately represent the expression of separation anxiety symptoms in adulthood.

- For specific phobia and social anxiety disorder, changes to the criteria include deletion of the requirement that adults recognize their anxiety as excessive or unreasonable. Instead, the anxiety should be "out of proportion" to the actual danger or threat, after sociocultural factors are taken into account. The typical minimum 6-month duration, which was limited to individuals younger than age 18 years, has been extended to persons of all ages.

- The specific phobia criteria are reworded so that the chance of encountering the phobic stimulus is no longer a determinant of whether an individual receives the diagnosis. The different stimulus types of specific phobias (now specifiers) are mostly unchanged.

- With social anxiety disorder, the "generalized" specifier has been dropped and replaced with a "performance only" specifier.

- Panic disorder and agoraphobia have been unlinked. The specifier "with panic attacks" can be used for any anxiety disorder, other mental disorders, and some medical conditions.

CHAPTER 7

Obsessive-Compulsive and Related Disorders

300.3 (F42)   Obsessive-Compulsive Disorder
300.7 (F45.22) Body Dysmorphic Disorder
300.3 (F42)   Hoarding Disorder
312.39 (F63.2) Trichotillomania (Hair-Pulling Disorder)
698.4 (L98.1) Excoriation (Skin-Picking) Disorder
                   Substance/Medication-Induced Obsessive-Compulsive and Related
                   Disorder
294.8 (F06.8) Obsessive-Compulsive and Related Disorder Due to Another
                   Medical Condition
300.3 (F42)   Other Specified Obsessive-Compulsive and Related Disorder
300.3 (F42)   Unspecified Obsessive-Compulsive and Related Disorder

The chapter on obsessive-compulsive and related disorders is new to DSM-5 and brings together disorders previously classified in DSM-IV with the anxiety disorders (obsessive-compulsive disorder [OCD]), somatoform disorders (body dysmorphic disorder), and impulse-control disorders not elsewhere classified (trichotillomania). The chapter represents a departure from DSM-IV but shows continuity with the approach taken by the DSM-5 Task Force to group related disorders together. Relatedness is a fundamental concept underlying any classification system. The placement of these disorders in DSM-IV had been criticized because of the perceived failure to recognize the similarities among them. Evidence has accumulated showing the various disorders' relatedness to OCD in terms of shared phenomenology, patterns of familial aggregation, and etiological mechanisms (Hollander et al. 2011). With these disorders now grouped together, clinicians are encouraged to screen for these conditions and consider their overlap. Finally, the metastructure of DSM-5 is reflected by the placement of this chapter following the one on anxiety disorders.

The obsessive-compulsive and related disorders (Table 7–1) are unified by the presence of obsessions (recurrent and persistent intrusive and unwanted thoughts, urges, or images that lead to marked anxiety or distress) and/or compulsive rituals (repetitive behaviors or mental acts performed in a habitual or stereotyped manner) that cause significant functional impairment in important life domains. These disorders are relatively common, with OCD having a lifetime prevalence of 1.6%–3%, and the other disorders in this chapter having estimated prevalence rates ranging from 1% to 5%. OCD is one of the top causes of global disability according to the World Health Organization (2001).

TABLE 7–1.   DSM-5 obsessive-compulsive and related disorders

Obsessive-compulsive disorder

Body dysmorphic disorder

Hoarding disorder

Trichotillomania (hair-pulling disorder)

Excoriation (skin-picking) disorder

Substance/medication-induced obsessive-compulsive and related disorder

Obsessive-compulsive and related disorder due to another medical condition

Other specified obsessive-compulsive and related disorder

Unspecified obsessive-compulsive and related disorder

Hoarding—long considered a subtype of OCD—is now accorded its own diagnosis, in response to research showing that it has unique features, symptom patterns, and treatment response. Body dysmorphic disorder has been moved from the DSM-IV chapter "Somatoform Disorders" in recognition of its close relationship with OCD. Trichotillomania has been renamed "trichotillomania (hair-pulling disorder)" and has been moved from the DSM-IV chapter "Impulse-Control Disorders Not Elsewhere Classified." Excoriation (skin-picking) disorder, long considered an impulsive disorder similar to trichotillomania, is new (Stein et al. 2010).

Obsessive-Compulsive Disorder

The hallmark of OCD is the presence of obsessions and/or compulsions. *Obsessions* are recurrent and persistent ideas, thoughts, urges, or images that are experienced as intrusive and unwanted and that in most individuals cause marked anxiety or distress (e.g., fears of germs and contamination). *Compulsions* are repetitive and intentional behaviors or mental acts performed in response to obsessions or according to certain rules that must be applied rigidly (e.g., repetitive hand washing, ritualistic checking). Compulsions are meant to neutralize or reduce the person's discomfort or prevent a dreaded event or situation. The rituals are not connected in a realistic way to the event or situation or are clearly excessive. The specific definitions for obsessions and compulsions have treatment implications because each requires a different approach.

First described clinically by Esquirol (1838), OCD was considered a form of monomania, or partial insanity. Esquirol described how disturbed patients would ruminate on a central theme, giving it their full attention. Later, obsessive-compulsive symptoms were attributed to depression, but this gave way to their acceptance as a neurotic syndrome. Freud (1895/1962) drew upon his concepts of mental structure and described *obsessional neurosis,* a syndrome in which the person struggles with unacceptable impulses (obsessions) and attempts to control them through imperfect defenses that result in rituals (compulsions). Psychoanalytic ideas held sway until advances in neuroscience and learning theory led to a more useful reconceptualization of OCD. As for formal classification, DSM-I included "obsessive compulsive reaction," giving rise to "obsessive compulsive neurosis" in DSM-II:

> This disorder is characterized by the persistent intrusion of unwanted thoughts, urges, or actions that the patient is unable to stop. The thoughts may consist of single words or ideas, ruminations, or trains of thought often perceived by the patient as nonsensical. The actions vary from simple movements to complex rituals such as repeated hand washing. Anxiety and distress are often present either if the patient is prevented from completing his compulsive ritual or if he is concerned about being unable to control it himself. (p. 40)

The disorder was included in the Feighner criteria (Feighner et al. 1972), which became the basis for the DSM-III criteria. The criteria were slightly modified for DSM-III-R and DSM-IV. The DSM-5 criteria have been further refined to reflect the field's greater understanding of this disorder.

Diagnostic Criteria for Obsessive-Compulsive Disorder 300.3 (F42)

A. Presence of obsessions, compulsions, or both:

Obsessions are defined by (1) and (2):

1. Recurrent and persistent thoughts, urges, or images that are experienced, at some time during the disturbance, as intrusive and unwanted, and that in most individuals cause marked anxiety or distress.
2. The individual attempts to ignore or suppress such thoughts, urges, or images, or to neutralize them with some other thought or action (i.e., by performing a compulsion).

Compulsions are defined by (1) and (2):

1. Repetitive behaviors (e.g., hand washing, ordering, checking) or mental acts (e.g., praying, counting, repeating words silently) that the individual feels driven to perform in response to an obsession or according to rules that must be applied rigidly.
2. The behaviors or mental acts are aimed at preventing or reducing anxiety or distress, or preventing some dreaded event or situation; however, these behaviors or mental acts are not connected in a realistic way with what they are designed to neutralize or prevent, or are clearly excessive.
   Note: Young children may not be able to articulate the aims of these behaviors or mental acts.

B. The obsessions or compulsions are time-consuming (e.g., take more than 1 hour per day) or cause clinically significant distress or impairment in social, occupational, or other important areas of functioning.

C. The obsessive-compulsive symptoms are not attributable to the physiological effects of a substance (e.g., a drug of abuse, a medication) or another medical condition.

D. The disturbance is not better explained by the symptoms of another mental disorder (e.g., excessive worries, as in generalized anxiety disorder; preoccupation with appearance, as in body dysmorphic disorder; difficulty discarding or parting with possessions, as in hoarding disorder; hair pulling, as in trichotillomania [hair-pulling disorder]; skin picking, as in excoriation [skin-picking] disorder; stereotypies, as in stereotypic movement disorder; ritualized eating behavior, as in eating disorders; preoccupation with substances or gambling, as in substance-related and addictive disorders; preoccupation with having an illness, as in illness anxiety disorder; sexual urges or fantasies, as in paraphilic disorders; impulses, as in disruptive, impulse-control, and conduct disorders; guilty ruminations, as in major depressive disorder; thought insertion or delusional preoccupations, as in schizophrenia spectrum and other psychotic disorders; or repetitive patterns of behavior, as in autism spectrum disorder).

Specify if:

With good or fair insight: The individual recognizes that obsessive-compulsive disorder beliefs are definitely or probably not true or that they may or may not be true.

With poor insight: The individual thinks obsessive-compulsive disorder beliefs are probably true.

With absent insight/delusional beliefs: The individual is completely convinced that obsessive-compulsive disorder beliefs are true.

Specify if:

Tic-related: The individual has a current or past history of a tic disorder.

Criterion A

Instead of four features defining an obsession, as in DSM-IV, DSM-5 relies on two: 1) "recurrent and persistent thoughts, urges, or images that are experienced, at some time during the disturbance, as intrusive and unwanted, and that in most individuals cause marked anxiety or distress," and 2) attempts to "ignore or suppress such thoughts, urges, or images, or to neutralize them with some other thought or action."

Obsessions

Criterion A1. The wording of Criterion A1 has changed from "recurrent and persistent thoughts, *impulses,* or images" to "recurrent and persistent thoughts, *urges,* or images." Both *impulse* and *urge* capture the involuntary (losing control) nature of some obsessions. However, *impulse* indirectly refers to the notion of impulse-control disorders, which may complicate differential diagnosis. For example, someone with kleptomania may report recurrent impulses to steal, and so the criteria for OCD would potentially be met. The change in wording in this criterion, in addition to a larger exclusionary list in Criterion D, is aimed at preventing this misdiagnosis. Interestingly, *urge* was a descriptor used in DSM-II.

Additionally, the DSM-IV definition of *obsession* stated that the thoughts are "experienced, at some time during the disturbance, as intrusive and *inappropriate.*" In DSM-5, the last word has been changed to *unwanted*. Replacing *inappropriate* with *unwanted* attempts to address the difficulties in operationalizing the ego-dystonic quality of obsessional thoughts. In DSM-III, the term *ego-dystonic* was used to reflect the belief that obsessional thoughts are involuntary and regarded as senseless or repugnant. In DSM-III-R, *ego-dystonic* was replaced with *senseless*. In DSM-IV, *senseless* was dropped because the term could imply a loss of reality testing and thereby confuse OCD with psychoses. Also, the term *inappropriate* may have different definitions based on culture, gender, and age; use of the term *unwanted* in DSM-5 seeks to avoid these social and cultural differences that may complicate the diagnosis.

The final change in the DSM-5 definition of obsession is the addition of "in most individuals" before the phrase "cause marked anxiety or distress." Data from several large studies show that although most people with OCD experience at least moderate anxiety or distress from obsessional thoughts, not all obsessions generate marked anxiety or distress. In addition, some people who have experienced OCD for many years may not report the same level of anxiety or distress from their obsessions as they did at illness onset.

Criterion A2. Many DSM-5 disorders are characterized by repetitive thoughts or behaviors, and these must be distinguished from obsessions and compulsions. The statement that the person attempts to ignore or suppress the obsessive thoughts, urges, or images, or to neutralize them by performing a compulsion, provides a functional link between obsessions and compulsions. This link allows the clinician to distinguish the thoughts of OCD from those found in anxiety disorders such as generalized anxiety disorder *because* of the presence of compulsions. Although not everyone with OCD reports obsessions *and* compulsions, the vast majority (approximately 90%) do so.

In DSM-5, two DSM-IV criteria have been deleted from the definition of obsession: that the thoughts are not simply excessive worries about real-life problems (A2) and that the person recognizes that the thoughts are a product of his or her own mind (A4). These criteria were originally used to distinguish OCD from generalized anxiety disorder (e.g., a person worrying excessively about financial problems when out of work) and from psychotic disorders (e.g., when a person believes someone has inserted these thoughts into his or her head). In DSM-5, instead of being used to define an obsession, these criteria have been incorporated into Criterion D, which includes information about the differential diagnosis between OCD, generalized anxiety disorder, psychotic disorders, and other mental disorders.

Compulsions

Criterion A1. Compulsions are repetitive behaviors that a person feels driven to perform. The "feels driven" aspect of the behavior reflects that the behavior is not willed, purposeful, or intentional.

Criterion A2. The definition of compulsion requires that the person's motivation for the behavior be to reduce or prevent anxiety or distress associated with an obsessive thought. For example, a person may need to write a sentence over and over again as a means of reducing the anxiety associated with "just right" obsessions. Another example is when a person asks forgiveness multiple times to reduce the distress from an obsessive thought of violence. This requirement that the compulsion be designed to reduce anxiety or distress from an obsession helps to differentiate the behavior from repetitive behaviors seen in tics or stereotypies.

The requirement that the compulsive behavior be designed to reduce a negative feeling triggered by an obsessive thought also differentiates OCD from repetitive behaviors seen in impulsive or addictive disorders. The motivating drive behind impulsive or addictive behaviors is generally, although not exclusively, the pleasure or gratification associated with the behavior.

The second criterion further defines compulsive behaviors as those that are "not connected in a realistic way with what they are designed to neutralize or prevent, or are clearly excessive." For example, most people consider it advisable to check that the iron is unplugged and lights are off before leaving home. Checking once or twice is prudent, whereas checking multiple times is clearly excessive. The extremes, such as checking 30 times, are much easier to recognize than the "gray areas" of checking (e.g., four times).

Criterion B

DSM-IV's Criterion B has been deleted from DSM-5. It stated that during the course of illness, "the person has recognized that the obsessions or compulsions are excessive or unreasonable." Because *excessive* and *unreasonable* were not defined or operationalized, it was unclear how clinicians and researchers should interpret the terms.

DSM-5 Criterion B is a modified version of DSM-IV Criterion C. Given that most people have some obsessive thoughts or engage in repetitive behaviors, this criterion gives the clinician a general threshold for when thoughts or behaviors may be considered problematic and not normative. The time threshold should be considered an approximation for when these thoughts or behaviors have become excessive, which is why the phrase "take more than 1 hour per day" has been added as an example. Many people with OCD rationalize that their behavior is useful; they also may present with an apparent lack of concern over the behavior or lack insight regarding the impact of these symptoms on their lives. Ritualistic behaviors that consume more than 1 hour per day are not necessarily evidence of OCD. For example, a surgeon may wash her hands more than 1 hour each day, and yet this should not be taken as evidence of OCD.

Criterion C

This item mirrors DSM-IV Criterion E, with minor edits, and is intended to remind clinicians to distinguish OCD from obsessions or compulsions that occur in relation to substance use or a medical condition. For example, people who misuse stimulants (e.g., amphetamines) sometimes report compulsive skin picking. Likewise, individuals treated with dopaminergic medications (e.g., pramipexole) for Parkinson's disease often exhibit "punding" behaviors, which are repetitive mechanical tasks, such as sorting, collecting, or assembling/disassembling common items. An OCD diagnosis is not appropriate in these cases.

Criterion D

Many psychiatric disorders are characterized by recurrent, intrusive thoughts and/or repetitive behaviors. This criterion clarifies the instances in which the diagnosis of OCD would not be appropriate. DSM-5 has expanded the list of diagnoses with symptoms that may resemble those in OCD, to include disorders such as major depressive disorder, generalized anxiety disorder, illness anxiety disorder, impulse-control disorders, hoarding disorder, excoriation (skin-picking) disorder, and paraphilic disorders.

Specifiers

The subtyping of OCD has been expanded to allow clinicians to make a more detailed assessment of the individual and his or her disorder (Leckman et al. 2010). Instead of the single specifier "with poor insight," as in DSM-IV, DSM-5 includes a range of insight specifiers (good or fair, poor, absent), as well as a specifier of tic-related OCD. Because insight may fluctuate over time, the insight specifier has been changed to refer to the current presentation. The revised specifiers have the potential advantage of conveying the broad range of insight that can characterize OCD beliefs, including delusional beliefs. Insight may be associated with clinical presentation (e.g., greater OCD severity, higher rates of co-occurring depression) and treatment outcome (e.g., less robust treatment response to cognitive-behavioral therapy).

Research evidence provides support for the inclusion of a tic-related specifier. This OCD variant is highly familial with specific clinical characteristics (early onset, male predominance) and high rates of symmetry and exactness obsessions and of ordering and arranging compulsions, as well as sensory phenomena. Individuals with symptoms characteristic of this specifier may also benefit differentially from antipsychotic augmentation if treatment with a selective serotonin reuptake inhibitor does not sufficiently reduce the symptoms.

Body Dysmorphic Disorder

Body dysmorphic disorder requires both obsessional thoughts regarding perceived defects in appearance and, at some point, compulsive behaviors that develop in response to those thoughts. Body dysmorphic disorder and OCD have many similarities—symptoms, aspects of treatment response, comorbidities, and perhaps underlying pathophysiology. They also have important differences; for example, people with body dysmorphic disorder have poorer insight and are more likely to have suicidal ideation and co-occurring substance use disorders.

The condition has been referred to in the past as *dysmorphophobia*. Body dysmorphic disorder was included in DSM-III as an example of an atypical somatoform disorder and received full disorder status in DSM-III-R. DSM-IV continued to include body dysmorphic disorder with the somatoform disorders. The relocation of body dysmorphic disorder to the obsessive-compulsive and related disorders reflects research regarding its etiological relationship with OCD (Phillips et al. 2010).

Body dysmorphic disorder is relatively common, with prevalence rates in the general population of 0.7%–2.4%, although studies of clinical samples suggest higher rates: 3%–

16% among cosmetic surgery patients, 9%–15% among dermatology patients, 8%–12% among patients with OCD, and 39% among patients with anorexia nervosa.

Diagnostic Criteria for Body Dysmorphic Disorder   300.7 (F45.22)

A. Preoccupation with one or more perceived defects or flaws in physical appearance that are not observable or appear slight to others.
B. At some point during the course of the disorder, the individual has performed repetitive behaviors (e.g., mirror checking, excessive grooming, skin picking, reassurance seeking) or mental acts (e.g., comparing his or her appearance with that of others) in response to the appearance concerns.
C. The preoccupation causes clinically significant distress or impairment in social, occupational, or other important areas of functioning.
D. The appearance preoccupation is not better explained by concerns with body fat or weight in an individual whose symptoms meet diagnostic criteria for an eating disorder.

Specify if:

With muscle dysmorphia: The individual is preoccupied with the idea that his or her body build is too small or insufficiently muscular. This specifier is used even if the individual is preoccupied with other body areas, which is often the case.

Specify if:

Indicate degree of insight regarding body dysmorphic disorder beliefs (e.g., "I look ugly" or "I look deformed").

With good or fair insight: The individual recognizes that the body dysmorphic disorder beliefs are definitely or probably not true or that they may or may not be true.
With poor insight: The individual thinks that the body dysmorphic disorder beliefs are probably true.
With absent insight/delusional beliefs: The individual is completely convinced that the body dysmorphic disorder beliefs are true.

Criterion A

Persons with body dysmorphic disorder are preoccupied with the idea that some aspect or aspects of their appearance look abnormal. They may describe these areas as being unattractive, deformed, disfigured, ugly, hideous, or "not right." The face or head is commonly the body area that troubles these individuals, with a focus on skin flaws, defects, blemishes, wrinkles, scars, or supposed acne. Typically, these individuals are preoccupied with their appearance for several hours each day. DSM-5 has changed the initial criterion from preoccupation with an "imagined defect in appearance" to preoccupation with "perceived defects or flaws in physical appearance that are not observable or appear slight to others." This clarifies the criterion's meaning, and eliminating the term *imagined* prevents clinicians from characterizing the disorder as due to psychosis.

Criterion B

All people with body dysmorphic disorder have at some point in their illness performed repetitive, time-consuming behaviors in response to their preoccupations. These behaviors focus on examining, improving, being reassured about, or hiding the perceived defect. These behaviors are often described as "compulsive" in the sense that the urge to perform them is strong and difficult to resist. They are also sometimes referred to as "safety behaviors," meaning that they are performed to prevent a feared catastrophe (e.g., camouflaging "ghostlike" skin with bronzer to prevent feared scrutiny by other people).

Criterion C

This item recognizes that individuals with body dysmorphic disorder experience clinically significant impairment in social, occupational, or other areas of functioning because of their appearance concerns. They also have poor quality of life; about 25% of individuals with body dysmorphic disorder are so distressed that they attempt suicide. However, severity varies, with some individuals appearing to lead relatively normal lives despite the distress and interference they experience.

Criterion D

Body dysmorphic disorder must be distinguished from eating disorders. Body dysmorphic disorder and anorexia nervosa, for example, share disturbed body image and a preoccupation with perceived appearance flaws. Many individuals with anorexia nervosa are preoccupied with aspects of appearance other than weight, such as the size of the stomach or thighs, or even body areas such as the skin or nose. Conversely, some individuals with body dysmorphic disorder are preoccupied with body weight and body shape. Although anorexia nervosa and body dysmorphic disorder have similarities, as well as some overlap, they also appear to have some important differences, including gender distribution (more individuals with anorexia nervosa are female), comorbidity, patterns of familial aggregation of psychiatric disorders, and response to treatment.

Specifiers

In DSM-5, specifiers regarding whether the body dysmorphic disorder focuses on one's body build (muscle dysmorphia, defined as preoccupation with the idea that one's body is too small or not muscular enough) and insight have been added.

Muscle dysmorphia appears to have several important differences from other forms of body dysmorphic disorder (e.g., higher rates of suicidal behavior, comorbid substance use disorders), and the treatment approach may require some modification. Thus, adding this specifier may have clinical utility.

Although the majority of individuals with body dysmorphic disorder also have ideas of reference (thinking that others notice their imagined defect and react to it with dislike or disgust), there appear to be far more similarities than differences between delusional and nondelusional body dysmorphic disorder. The insight specifier reflects the broad range of insight (including delusional thinking) that can characterize body dysmorphic disorder beliefs. These levels of insight are similar to categories in widely used scales for body dysmorphic disorder, and they are the same as those for OCD.

Hoarding Disorder

Hoarding is a persistent difficulty discarding or parting with possessions. The accumulation of possessions makes it hard to use living areas of the home for their intended purposes (Frost et al. 2012; Mataix-Cols et al. 2010). The hoarding causes clinically significant distress or impairment. Hoarding is surprisingly common and potentially disabling. Significant hoarding has been shown to occur in 2%–6% of the general population. Prior to DSM-5, hoarding was mentioned in DSM-IV only in the context of obsessive-compulsive personality disorder (Item 5), but the related text suggests that serious hoarding behavior should be considered a form of OCD. The high prevalence and serious consequences of hoarding disorder, together with research on its distinctiveness from OCD and obsessive-compulsive personality disorder, have led the authors of DSM-5 to classify it as an independent disorder.

Diagnostic Criteria for Hoarding Disorder   300.3 (F42)

A. Persistent difficulty discarding or parting with possessions, regardless of their actual value.
B. This difficulty is due to a perceived need to save the items and to distress associated with discarding them.
C. The difficulty discarding possessions results in the accumulation of possessions that congest and clutter active living areas and substantially compromises their intended use. If living areas are uncluttered, it is only because of the interventions of third parties (e.g., family members, cleaners, authorities).
D. The hoarding causes clinically significant distress or impairment in social, occupational, or other important areas of functioning (including maintaining a safe environment for self and others).
E. The hoarding is not attributable to another medical condition (e.g., brain injury, cerebrovascular disease, Prader-Willi syndrome).
F. The hoarding is not better explained by the symptoms of another mental disorder (e.g., obsessions in obsessive-compulsive disorder, decreased energy in major depressive disorder, delusions in schizophrenia or another psychotic disorder, cognitive deficits in major neurocognitive disorder, restricted interests in autism spectrum disorder).

Specify if:

With excessive acquisition: If difficulty discarding possessions is accompanied by excessive acquisition of items that are not needed or for which there is no available space.

Specify if:

With good or fair insight: The individual recognizes that hoarding-related beliefs and behaviors (pertaining to difficulty discarding items, clutter, or excessive acquisition) are problematic.

With poor insight: The individual is mostly convinced that hoarding-related beliefs and behaviors (pertaining to difficulty discarding items, clutter, or excessive acquisition) are not problematic despite evidence to the contrary.
With absent insight/delusional beliefs: The individual is completely convinced that hoarding-related beliefs and behaviors (pertaining to difficulty discarding items, clutter, or excessive acquisition) are not problematic despite evidence to the contrary.

Criterion A

The desire to retain objects of value, either sentimental or financial, is common. With hoarding disorder, the difficulty with discarding possessions seems driven by fears of losing important things. Criterion A refers to the core characteristic, which is difficulty discarding. The wording "discarding or parting with" is intended to make clear that this difficulty is not confined to throwing things away, but rather to any attempt to let go of a possession, including giving it away, recycling it, or selling it. The second clause, "regardless of their actual value," distinguishes this definition from that used to define hoarding as a symptom of obsessive-compulsive personality disorder in DSM-IV, in which the hoarding was defined as being "unable to discard worn-out or worthless objects." What is considered worthless or worn out varies considerably from person to person. The most frequently hoarded items include clothes, newspapers, and magazines. Many of these items, especially clothes, are frequently new and never worn.

Criterion B

A central feature of hoarding disorder is the need to save possessions. Clutter that results is due to purposeful saving and reluctance to discard items because they have sentimental significance, are potentially useful, or have intrinsic aesthetic value. The nature of emotional attachment is reflected in the person's reaction to getting rid of a possession; the emotion experienced is either anxiety or a feeling of grief at the loss. Associated with this is the tendency to assign humanlike qualities to possessions. Another form of emotional attachment concerns a sense of comfort and security provided by possessions. The thought of getting rid of a possession appears to violate feelings of safety.

Criterion C

The major consequence of hoarding is disorganized clutter, which elicits great concern from family and friends. Clutter makes a space unusable or unsanitary, and finding important items may be nearly impossible. This criterion emphasizes the living areas of the home or workspace rather than locations such as attics, basements, or garages, which are sometimes cluttered in homes of persons without hoarding disorder. In some cases, family members keep the living area from being cluttered, and in such cases, the individual can still receive a diagnosis of hoarding disorder if sufficient distress or other impairment is generated by the behavior.

Criterion D

People who hoard experience distress largely due to the consequences of the behavior, such as conflict with family members over the clutter, and not due to the thoughts or behaviors themselves. Research suggests that functioning is impaired in a variety of domains. People are often unable to use living spaces in the home, and in severe cases appliances are not functional and utilities such as water and electricity are shut off. Hoarding poses a serious public health burden (e.g., fire hazards, infestations) and increases costs to the public in the form of involvement by social service agencies.

Criterion E

Several other medical conditions can lead to clutter and difficulty discarding possessions. For example, hoarding behaviors have occurred in people with lesions in the anterior ventromedial prefrontal and cingulate cortices. Also, many individuals with Prader-Willi syndrome (a rare genetic disorder associated with short stature, hyperphagia, insatiability, and food-seeking behavior) display hoarding behavior, mostly associated with food, but with nonfood items as well.

Criterion F

In some people, hoarding may be related to OCD, generalized anxiety disorder, or major depressive disorder instead of being an independent disorder. These disorders need to be ruled out. Hoarding behavior can also occur in individuals with severe dementia; however, hoarding associated with dementia appears to stem from significant cognitive deterioration rather than from excessive attachment to objects. Hoarding is also described in institutionalized patients with schizophrenia, but the behavior does not appear to be motivated by a true attachment to objects. OCD is the disorder most closely associated with hoarding, and about approximately 20% of individuals with OCD have hoarding symptoms. In some cases where the hoarding behavior appears to be secondary to more classic OCD symptoms, such as contamination, the diagnosis of hoarding disorder would not be appropriate.

Specifiers

DSM-5 includes the specifier "with excessive acquisition." People with hoarding problems tend to buy and carry with them a large number of "just in case" items, and studies have confirmed excessive acquiring in the context of hoarding. Acquisition of free things also tends to be excessive. Stealing is another form of excessive acquisition associated with hoarding. Although only a small percentage of people with hoarding disorder steal, kleptomania is not uncommon (10%). The diagnostic criteria do not include excessive acquisition, because a small percentage (10%–15%) of people who hoard report no excessive acquisition.

Insight specifiers similar to those for OCD are also available. When the disorder is severe, the hoarding may appear to take on delusional proportions. Clinicians generally rate hoarding patients as having poor or limited insight compared with more typical individuals with OCD. Sometimes the term *insight* is confused with *overvalued ideation,* which refers to a belief maintained despite evidence to the contrary. In the context of hoarding, overvalued ideation involves beliefs about the value or useful-ness of possessions. Many individuals with hoarding recognize the problem with their behavior, but their unreasonable ideas about the value of their possessions make it impossible for them to discard. This may appear to an observer as a lack of insight, but in reality these beliefs about the value and usefulness of possessions may repre-sent part of the disorder.

Trichotillomania (Hair-Pulling Disorder)

Trichotillomania involves repetitive hair pulling leading to noticeable hair loss, sub-jective distress, and social or occupational impairment. Research has shown that the prevalence of trichotillomania among adults and adolescents in the United States ranges from 1% to 2%. Trichotillomania was included in the DSM-IV chapter "Im-pulse-Control Disorders Not Elsewhere Classified."

The name has been modified in DSM-5 by including a more descriptive term—*hair-pulling disorder*—parenthetically. Given that research in clinical phenomenology, neurobi-ology, and genetics has suggested an association between trichotillomania and OCD, DSM-5 includes trichotillomania with the obsessive-compulsive and related disorders.

Diagnostic Criteria for Trichotillomania (Hair-Pulling Disorder)   312.39 (F63.3)

A. Recurrent pulling out of one's hair, resulting in hair loss.
B. Repeated attempts to decrease or stop hair pulling.
C. The hair pulling causes clinically significant distress or impairment in social, occu-pational, or other important areas of functioning.
D. The hair pulling or hair loss is not attributable to another medical condition (e.g., a dermatological condition).
E. The hair pulling is not better explained by the symptoms of another mental disorder (e.g., attempts to improve a perceived defect or flaw in appearance in body dys-morphic disorder).

Criterion A

Hair pulling may occur in any body region. The most common sites are the scalp, eye-brows, and eyelids; less common sites are axillary, facial, pubic, and perirectal regions. Hair-pulling sites may vary over time, and hair pulling may occur in brief episodes scat-tered throughout the day or in less frequent but more sustained periods. Criterion A re-quires that hair pulling lead to hair loss, but unlike in DSM-IV, this criterion does not require that the hair loss be "noticeable." In fact, individuals with trichotillomania may pull hair in a widely distributed pattern (i.e., pulling single hairs from all over a site) such that hair loss may not be clearly visible. Alternatively, individuals may attempt to conceal or camouflage hair loss (e.g., with makeup, scarves, or wigs).

Criterion B

This item requires that individuals with trichotillomania attempt unsuccessfully to control their pulling. This criterion reflects the intense drive underlying the behavior. The criterion also more accurately represents what many individuals with the condition report (i.e., that they do not feel tension before pulling or experience relief or gratification after pulling). This item replaces DSM-IV's Criteria B ("sense of tension immediately before pulling") and C ("pleasure, gratification, or relief when pulling out the hair") based on evidence that some individuals with trichotillomania did not have these symptoms and thus their presentations did not qualify for the diagnosis.

Criterion C

Trichotillomania is associated with subjective distress as well as with social and occupational impairment. The disorder causes significant embarrassment. People attempt to avoid pulling in front of others and to avoid situations where the consequences of pulling may be noticed (e.g., swimming, sexual intimacy). Individuals also attempt to camouflage bald spots with wigs or scarfs. In addition, there may be irreversible damage to hair growth and hair quality. Infrequent medical consequences of behavior include digit purpura, musculoskeletal injury (e.g., carpal tunnel syndrome; back, shoulder, and neck pain), blepharitis, and dental damage (e.g., worn or broken teeth due to hair biting). Swallowing of hair (trichophagia) may lead to trichobezoars, with subsequent anemia, abdominal pain, hematemesis, nausea and vomiting, bowel obstruction, and even perforation.

Criterion D

Trichotillomania is not diagnosed when the hair pulling or hair loss is due to another medical condition (e.g., inflammation of the skin or other dermatological conditions). Other causes of scarring alopecia (e.g., alopecia areata, androgenetic alopecia, telogen effluvium) or nonscarring alopecia (e.g., chronic discoid lupus erythematosus, lichen planopilaris, central centrifugal cicatricial alopecia, pseudopelade, folliculitis decalvans, dissecting folliculitis, acne keloidalis) should be considered in individuals with hair loss who deny hair pulling. Skin biopsy or dermoscopy can be used to differentiate individuals with trichotillomania from those with dermatological disorders.

Criterion E

Individuals with body dysmorphic disorder may remove body hair they perceive as ugly or abnormal. People with OCD may pull out hairs as part of their symmetry rituals. Hair pulling may meet the definition of stereotyped behaviors (as in stereotypic movement disorder), but the diagnostic criteria for stereotypic movement disorder exclude symptoms better explained by trichotillomania. Individuals with a psychosis may remove hair in response to delusions or hallucinations. Trichotillomania is not diagnosed in such cases. Although hair-pulling symptoms may be exacerbated by certain substances, such as stimulants, it is not clear that substances can be the primary cause of recurrent hair pulling.

Excoriation (Skin-Picking) Disorder

Excoriation disorder is characterized by the recurrent, compulsive picking of skin, leading to skin lesions. Although long described in the medical literature, excoriation disorder is new to DSM-5, partly in response to the growing body of data emphasizing its prevalence and potentially disabling nature. There are significant clinical similarities between excoriation disorder and trichotillomania, and the criteria for the two disorders are very similar. The criteria for excoriation disorder are supported by a field survey.

Prevalence studies have found that excoriation disorder occurs in 1.4%–5.4% of the general population. Often considered chronic, the disorder fluctuates in intensity and severity. Few people with this disorder seek treatment.

Diagnostic Criteria for Excoriation (Skin-Picking) Disorder
698.4 (L98.1)

A. Recurrent skin picking resulting in skin lesions.
B. Repeated attempts to decrease or stop skin picking.
C. The skin picking causes clinically significant distress or impairment in social, occupational, or other important areas of functioning.
D. The skin picking is not attributable to the physiological effects of a substance (e.g., cocaine) or another medical condition (e.g., scabies).
E. The skin picking is not better explained by symptoms of another mental disorder (e.g., delusions or tactile hallucinations in a psychotic disorder, attempts to improve a perceived defect or flaw in appearance in body dysmorphic disorder, stereotypies in stereotypic movement disorder, or intention to harm oneself in nonsuicidal self-injury).

Criterion A

All individuals at some time pick at their skin, either to smooth out irregularities or to improve blemishes or acne. Criterion A requires that picking be recurrent and result in lesions, thereby reflecting the frequency and intensity of the picking. Although the face is the most commonly reported site of picking, areas such as the hands, fingers, torso, arms, and legs are also common targets. Individuals with excoriation disorder report multiple sites of picking and the use of multiple instruments (e.g., fingernails, knives, tweezers, pins). Picking may result in significant tissue damage and may lead to medical complications such as localized infections and septicemia.

Criterion B

This criterion requires that the person has tried to decrease or stop the picking, reflecting the intense drive underlying the behavior. Neurocognitive data support the idea that individuals with this disorder have difficulty inhibiting motor behaviors once the behaviors have begun.

Criterion C

Individuals with excoriation disorder spend a significant amount of time picking their skin, with many reporting that the behavior takes up several hours each day. Because of the amount of time spent picking, individuals report missing or being late for work, school, or social activities. The picking also leads to problems with self-esteem and difficulties in personal relationships.

Criterion D

Use of stimulant drugs such as cocaine and amphetamines can lead to skin picking and should be ruled out. In addition, many dermatological conditions, including scabies, atopic dermatitis, psoriasis, and blistering skin disorders, can lead to scratching or picking.

Criterion E

Excoriation disorder is often misdiagnosed as either OCD or body dysmorphic disorder. The repetitive motor symptoms of excoriation disorder resemble compulsive rituals, although individuals are less likely to report obsessive thoughts about their skin and may even be unaware of their picking behavior because of its automatic nature. Individuals with body dysmorphic disorder pick at their skin to improve their appearance.

Substance/Medication-Induced Obsessive-Compulsive and Related Disorder

It is important to consider whether any of the symptoms associated with OCD or related disorders are due to the direct effects of a substance, in which case the appropriate diagnosis is substance intoxication, substance withdrawal, or substance/medication-induced obsessive-compulsive and related disorder. A range of obsessive thoughts and compulsive behaviors occur as part of substance intoxication or substance withdrawal. If the obsessive thoughts or compulsive behaviors persist for a substantial period of time after the cessation of acute withdrawal or severe intoxication, and are in excess of what is expected and warrant independent clinical attention, then the diagnosis of substance/medication-induced obsessive-compulsive and related disorder is appropriate.

Diagnostic Criteria for Substance/Medication-Induced Obsessive-Compulsive and Related Disorder

---

A. Obsessions, compulsions, skin picking, hair pulling, other body-focused repetitive behaviors, or other symptoms characteristic of the obsessive-compulsive and related disorders predominate in the clinical picture.

B. There is evidence from the history, physical examination, or laboratory findings of both (1) and (2):

1. The symptoms in Criterion A developed during or soon after substance intoxication or withdrawal or after exposure to a medication.
2. The involved substance/medication is capable of producing the symptoms in Criterion A.

C. The disturbance is not better explained by an obsessive-compulsive and related disorder that is not substance/medication-induced. Such evidence of an independent obsessive-compulsive and related disorder could include the following:

> The symptoms precede the onset of the substance/medication use; the symptoms persist for a substantial period of time (e.g., about 1 month) after the cessation of acute withdrawal or severe intoxication; or there is other evidence suggesting the existence of an independent non-substance/medication-induced obsessive-compulsive and related disorder (e.g., a history of recurrent non-substance/medication-related episodes).

D. The disturbance does not occur exclusively during the course of a delirium.
E. The disturbance causes clinically significant distress or impairment in social, occupational, or other important areas of functioning.

Note: This diagnosis should be made in addition to a diagnosis of substance intoxication or substance withdrawal only when the symptoms in Criterion A predominate in the clinical picture and are sufficiently severe to warrant clinical attention.

Coding note: The ICD-9-CM and ICD-10-CM codes for the [specific substance/medication]-induced obsessive-compulsive and related disorders are indicated in the table below. Note that the ICD-10-CM code depends on whether or not there is a comorbid substance use disorder present for the same class of substance. If a mild substance use disorder is comorbid with the substance-induced obsessive-compulsive and related disorder, the 4th position character is "1," and the clinician should record "mild [substance] use disorder" before the substance-induced obsessive-compulsive and related disorder (e.g., "mild cocaine use disorder with cocaine-induced obsessive-compulsive and related disorder"). If a moderate or severe substance use disorder is comorbid with the substance-induced obsessive-compulsive and related disorder, the 4th position character is "2," and the clinician should record "moderate [substance] use disorder" or "severe [substance] use disorder," depending on the severity of the comorbid substance use disorder. If there is no comorbid substance use disorder (e.g., after a one-time heavy use of the substance), then the 4th position character is "9," and the clinician should record only the substance-induced obsessive-compulsive and related disorder.

		ICD-10-CM		
	ICD-9-CM	With use disorder, mild	With use disorder, moderate or severe	Without use disorder
Amphetamine (or other stimulant)	292.89	F15.188	F15.288	F15.988
Cocaine	292.89	F14.188	F14.288	F14.988
Other (or unknown) substance	292.89	F19.188	F19.288	F19.988

Specify if (see Table 16–1 in the chapter "Substance-Related and Addictive Disorders" for diagnoses associated with substance class):

With onset during intoxication: If the criteria are met for intoxication with the substance and the symptoms develop during intoxication.

With onset during withdrawal: If criteria are met for withdrawal from the substance and the symptoms develop during, or shortly after, withdrawal.

With onset after medication use: Symptoms may appear either at initiation of medication or after a modification or change in use.

Obsessive-Compulsive and Related Disorder Due to Another Medical Condition

The initial evaluation of obsessive-compulsive and related disorders requires that the clinician rule out medical conditions as a cause of the symptoms. If a medical condition is present, and the OCD or related disorder is determined to be the direct pathophysiological consequence of the medical condition, then the person should be diagnosed with obsessive-compulsive and related disorder due to another medical condition. When communicating or recording the diagnosis, the clinician should use the name of the etiological medical condition. That said, although cases have been reported in the literature of various medical conditions inducing obsessive-compulsive behaviors, they are rare.

Diagnostic Criteria for Obsessive-Compulsive and Related Disorder Due to Another Medical Condition   294.8 (F06.8)

A. Obsessions, compulsions, preoccupations with appearance, hoarding, skin picking, hair pulling, other body-focused repetitive behaviors, or other symptoms characteristic of obsessive-compulsive and related disorder predominate in the clinical picture.

B. There is evidence from the history, physical examination, or laboratory findings that the disturbance is the direct pathophysiological consequence of another medical condition.

C. The disturbance is not better explained by another mental disorder.

D. The disturbance does not occur exclusively during the course of a delirium.

E. The disturbance causes clinically significant distress or impairment in social, occupational, or other important areas of functioning.

Specify if:

With obsessive-compulsive disorder–like symptoms: If obsessive-compulsive disorder–like symptoms predominate in the clinical presentation.

With appearance preoccupations: If preoccupation with perceived appearance defects or flaws predominates in the clinical presentation.

With hoarding symptoms: If hoarding predominates in the clinical presentation.

With hair-pulling symptoms: If hair pulling predominates in the clinical presentation.

With skin-picking symptoms: If skin picking predominates in the clinical presentation.

Coding note: Include the name of the other medical condition in the name of the mental disorder (e.g., 294.8 [F06.8] obsessive-compulsive and related disorder due to cerebral infarction). The other medical condition should be coded and listed separately immediately before the obsessive-compulsive and related disorder due to the medical condition (e.g., 438.89 [I69.398] cerebral infarction; 294.8 [F06.8] obsessive-compulsive and related disorder due to cerebral infarction).

Other Specified Obsessive-Compulsive and Related Disorder and Unspecified Obsessive-Compulsive and Related Disorder

These are residual categories to use for individuals with symptoms of an obsessive-compulsive or related disorder who have distress or impairment but whose symptoms do not meet criteria for a more specific disorder in the class. The category other specified obsessive-compulsive and related disorder is used when the clinician chooses to communicate the reason that the presentation does not meet full criteria. The clinician is encouraged to record the specific reason (e.g., body dysmorphic–like disorder with actual flaws).

The category unspecified obsessive-compulsive and related disorder is used when the clinician chooses not to specify the reason the criteria are not met, or there is insufficient information to make a more specific diagnosis.

Other Specified Obsessive-Compulsive and Related Disorder   300.3 (F42)

This category applies to presentations in which symptoms characteristic of an obsessive-compulsive and related disorder that cause clinically significant distress or impairment in social, occupational, or other important areas of functioning predominate but do not meet the full criteria for any of the disorders in the obsessive-compulsive and related disorders diagnostic class. The other specified obsessive-compulsive and related disorder category is used in situations in which the clinician chooses to communicate the specific reason that the presentation does not meet the criteria for any specific obsessive-compulsive and related disorder. This is done by recording "other specified obsessive-compulsive and related disorder" followed by the specific reason (e.g., "body-focused repetitive behavior disorder").

Examples of presentations that can be specified using the "other specified" designation include the following:

1. **Body dysmorphic–like disorder with actual flaws:** This is similar to body dysmorphic disorder except that the defects or flaws in physical appearance are clearly observable by others (i.e., they are more noticeable than "slight"). In such cases, the preoccupation with these flaws is clearly excessive and causes significant impairment or distress.
2. **Body dysmorphic–like disorder without repetitive behaviors:** Presentations that meet body dysmorphic disorder except that the individual has not performed repetitive behaviors or mental acts in response to the appearance concerns.
3. **Body-focused repetitive behavior disorder:** This is characterized by recurrent body-focused repetitive behaviors (e.g., nail biting, lip biting, cheek chewing) and repeated attempts to decrease or stop the behaviors. These symptoms cause clinically significant distress or impairment in social, occupational, or other important areas of functioning and are not better explained by trichotillomania (hair-pulling disorder), excoriation (skin-picking) disorder, stereotypic movement disorder, or nonsuicidal self-injury.
4. **Obsessional jealousy:** This is characterized by nondelusional preoccupation with a partner's perceived infidelity. The preoccupations may lead to repetitive behaviors or mental acts in response to the infidelity concerns; they cause clinically significant distress or impairment in social, occupational, or other important areas of functioning; and they are not better explained by another mental disorder such as delusional disorder, jealous type, or paranoid personality disorder.
5. *Shubo-kyofu:* A variant of *taijin kyofusho* (see "Glossary of Cultural Concepts of Distress" in the Appendix to DSM-5) that is similar to body dysmorphic disorder and is characterized by excessive fear of having a bodily deformity.
6. *Koro:* Related to *dhat syndrome* (see "Glossary of Cultural Concepts of Distress" in the Appendix to DSM-5), an episode of sudden and intense anxiety that the penis (or the vulva and nipples in females) will recede into the body, possibly leading to death.
7. *Jikoshu-kyofu:* A variant of *taijin kyofusho* (see "Glossary of Cultural Concepts of Distress" in the Appendix to DSM-5) characterized by fear of having an offensive body odor (also termed *olfactory reference syndrome*).

Unspecified Obsessive-Compulsive and Related Disorder

300.3 (F42)

This category applies to presentations in which symptoms characteristic of an obsessive-compulsive and related disorder that cause clinically significant distress or impairment in social, occupational, or other important areas of functioning predominate but do not meet the full criteria for any of the disorders in the obsessive-compulsive and related disorders diagnostic class. The unspecified obsessive-compulsive and related disorder category is used in situations in which the clinician chooses *not* to specify the reason that the criteria are not met for a specific obsessive-compulsive and related disorder, and includes presentations in which there is insufficient information to make a more specific diagnosis (e.g., in emergency room settings).

KEY POINTS

- This chapter is new and reflects the scientific understanding that a spectrum of disorders related to obsessive-compulsive disorder (OCD) is sufficiently distinct from anxiety disorders that it should stand alone.

- Hoarding disorder and excoriation (skin-picking) disorder are new, both achieving full disorder status because of data showing their high prevalence, associated functional impairment, and familial relationship to OCD.

- Trichotillomania is now termed "trichotillomania (hair-pulling disorder)" and has been moved from the DSM-IV chapter "Impulse-Control Disorders Not Elsewhere Classified." Body dysmorphic disorder has been moved from the DSM-IV "Somatoform Disorders" chapter. In each case, the Anxiety, Obsessive-Compulsive Spectrum, Posttraumatic, and Dissociative Disorders Work Group recognized the putative etiological relationship with OCD.

- A "muscle dysmorphia" specifier for body dysmorphic disorder has been added in recognition of the growing literature on this distinction.

- The OCD criteria have been revised to emphasize that obsessions are often urges, not impulses, and that they are intrusive and unwanted rather than merely inappropriate. The DSM-IV "with poor insight" specifier has been refined, and an analogous specifier has been added for body dysmorphic disorder.

CHAPTER 8

Trauma- and Stressor-Related Disorders

313.89 (F94.1) Reactive Attachment Disorder
313.89 (F94.2) Disinhibited Social Engagement Disorder
309.81 (F43.10) Posttraumatic Stress Disorder
308.3 (F43.0) Acute Stress Disorder
Adjustment Disorders
309.89 (F43.8) Other Specified Trauma- and Stressor-Related Disorder
309.9 (F43.9) Unspecified Trauma- and Stressor-Related Disorder

Trauma- and stressor-related disorders is a new diagnostic class that brings together conditions previously listed in DSM-IV as anxiety disorders (acute stress disorder, posttraumatic stress disorder [PTSD]); disorders that are usually first diagnosed in infancy, childhood, or adolescence (reactive attachment disorder, the new disinhibited social engagement disorder); and adjustment disorders. All disorders in this class, listed in Table 8–1, result from exposure to traumatic or stressful situations or events explicitly recognized in the diagnostic criteria. In DSM-5, the trauma- and stressor-related disorders are placed directly following the obsessive-compulsive and related disorders and precede the dissociative disorders. The close placement of these disorders is a reflection of the manual's metastructure, whereby the proximity of disorders denotes presumed etiological relationships. Many of the symptoms of these disorders resemble those observed in individuals with obsessive-compulsive disorder (i.e., uncontrolled thoughts and preoccupations), whereas dissociative symptoms may occur in individuals with acute stress disorder, PTSD, or adjustment disorders.

The DSM-5 Anxiety, Obsessive-Compulsive Spectrum, Posttraumatic, and Dissociative Disorders Work Group recommended creating a separate diagnostic class for trauma- and stressor-related disorders because of research showing variations in the clinical expression of psychological distress following exposure to traumatic or stressful events (Andrews et al. 2009). Rather than a fear- or anxiety-based response, which

TABLE 8–1.   DSM-5 trauma- and stressor-related disorders
Reactive attachment disorder
Disinhibited social engagement disorder
Posttraumatic stress disorder
Acute stress disorder
Adjustment disorders
Other specified trauma- and stressor-related disorder
Unspecified trauma- and stressor-related disorder

had been the justification for placing acute stress disorder and PTSD with the anxiety disorders, the most prominent clinical features are anhedonic and dysphoric symptoms, anger and aggressive symptoms, or dissociative symptoms, thus calling for a new and separate diagnostic class. Furthermore, it was thought logical to combine these with the adjustment disorders, which also result from exposure to stressful events and have a variable presentation. The childhood-onset reactive attachment disorder and disinhibited social engagement disorder both result from social neglect, defined as the absence of appropriate caregiving during childhood, and therefore fit well within this new diagnostic class.

Important changes have been made to the DSM-5 criteria for the disorders. With acute stress disorder, the traumatic event is now more explicitly specified as having been experienced directly, witnessed, or experienced indirectly. DSM-IV's Criterion A2, regarding the person's subjective reaction, has been eliminated. Based on evidence that acute posttraumatic reactions vary considerably, and evidence that DSM-IV's emphasis on dissociative symptoms was overly restricting, the menu of symptoms has been expanded to 14 qualifying as intrusion, negative mood, dissociative, avoidance, and/or arousal symptoms.

PTSD is no longer considered narrowly as a fear- and anxiety-based disorder, but has been reconceptualized to include a wide spectrum of negative responses to traumatic experiences, including anhedonia-like and externalizing symptoms. The elimination of the requirement for a subjective negative response *at the time of* the event is one of the changes that led to removing PTSD from the anxiety disorders and placing it in a class with other disorders that arise in response to traumatic or stressful events that precede the emergence of symptoms. DSM-IV's Criterion A2, which related to the person's subjective reaction to the event, has been deleted, as it was for acute stress disorder. In addition, rather than three symptom clusters (reexperiencing, avoidance/numbing, and arousal), there are now four clusters, because the avoidance/numbing cluster has been split into two (described more fully in the section "Posttraumatic Stress Disorder" later in this chapter). A "with dissociative symptoms" subtype is new, having been added to acknowledge the fact that these symptoms are frequent and constitute the presentation of a definable group of individuals with PTSD. Also, a criteria set for PTSD in children 6 years and younger has been developed for use in preschool children, with a lowered diagnostic threshold. For that reason, PTSD is now developmentally sensitive.

In DSM-IV, reactive attachment disorder was a childhood diagnosis characterized by aberrant social behaviors that resulted from what was described as "pathogenic care" involving disregard for the child's emotional and physical needs, in addition to changes of primary caregiver that prevented the development of stable attachments. There were two subtypes: *inhibited,* in which the child showed little responsiveness to others and no discriminated attachments, and *disinhibited,* in which the child showed no reticence with unfamiliar adults and a pattern of social boundary violations. In DSM-5, these two subtypes are now distinct disorders: reactive attachment disorder and disinhibited social engagement disorder.

These two disorders essentially result from social neglect and/or other situations that limit a child's opportunity to form selective attachments. Despite their etiological similarities, they differ in important respects. Reactive attachment disorder resembles internalizing disorders and overlaps modestly with depression, whereas disinhibited social engagement disorder resembles externalizing disorders, particularly attention-deficit/hyperactivity disorder, with which it partially overlaps. Furthermore, the disorders have distinctive relationships with attachment behaviors. Reactive attachment disorder involves the lack of, or incompletely formed preferred attachments to, caregiving adults. On the other hand, disinhibited social engagement disorder occurs in children who lack attachments, children who have established attachments, and even children with secure attachments. The two disorders also differ in their clinical correlates, course, and response to intervention. For these reasons, the work group recommended two separate diagnoses in DSM-5.

Last, the adjustment disorders are relatively unchanged from DSM-IV, apart from their new placement in this chapter (Strain and Friedman 2011).

Reactive Attachment Disorder

Reactive attachment disorder has been refashioned from the broad DSM-IV conceptualization and, as noted in the introduction above, is characterized by absent or underdeveloped attachment between the child and caregivers. Because it is caused by grossly inadequate parenting, the disorder may be associated with signs of severe neglect (e.g., malnutrition, poor hygiene) and may co-occur with developmental delays in language acquisition and cognitive ability. The children show little responsiveness to others and make scant effort to obtain comfort, support, nurturance, or protection from caregivers. In addition, these children have episodes of negative emotions (e.g., irritability, sadness, fearfulness) that are not easily explained. The diagnosis is not appropriate for children developmentally unable to form selective attachments. For this reason, the child must have the cognitive capacity of at least a 9-month-old to receive the diagnosis.

Diagnostic Criteria for Reactive Attachment Disorder   **313.89** (F94.1)

A. A consistent pattern of inhibited, emotionally withdrawn behavior toward adult caregivers, manifested by both of the following:

    1. The child rarely or minimally seeks comfort when distressed.

    2. The child rarely or minimally responds to comfort when distressed.

B. A persistent social and emotional disturbance characterized by at least two of the following:

    1. Minimal social and emotional responsiveness to others.

    2. Limited positive affect.

    3. Episodes of unexplained irritability, sadness, or fearfulness that are evident even during nonthreatening interactions with adult caregivers.

C. The child has experienced a pattern of extremes of insufficient care as evidenced by at least one of the following:

    1. Social neglect or deprivation in the form of persistent lack of having basic emotional needs for comfort, stimulation, and affection met by caregiving adults.

    2. Repeated changes of primary caregivers that limit opportunities to form stable attachments (e.g., frequent changes in foster care).

    3. Rearing in unusual settings that severely limit opportunities to form selective attachments (e.g., institutions with high child-to-caregiver ratios).

D. The care in Criterion C is presumed to be responsible for the disturbed behavior in Criterion A (e.g., the disturbances in Criterion A began following the lack of adequate care in Criterion C).

E. The criteria are not met for autism spectrum disorder.

F. The disturbance is evident before age 5 years.

G. The child has a developmental age of at least 9 months.

Specify if:

    Persistent: The disorder has been present for more than 12 months.

Specify current severity:

    Reactive attachment disorder is specified as **severe** when a child exhibits all symptoms of the disorder, with each symptom manifesting at relatively high levels.

Criterion A

This criterion defines disturbed and inappropriate attachment behaviors observed in the child toward adult caregivers. The child rarely or minimally seeks nurturance from an attachment figure and rarely or minimally responds to comfort when distressed. Although some have suggested that social impairment or social communication is a core of this disorder, it is likely that the absence of a selective attachment necessarily impairs social functioning, and that social behaviors improve markedly once the child is in a more favorable environment, making attachment the core of the disorder.

Criterion B

This criterion indicates that the diagnosis requires a persistent social and emotional disturbance characterized by at least two of three behaviors: minimal social and emotional responsiveness to others, limited positive affect, and episodes of unexplained irritability, sadness, or fearfulness even during nonthreatening interactions with caregivers. Separating these behaviors from Criterion A restricts the diagnosis to those children who have both of these features, which are highlighted in the DSM-5 criteria, and the absence of an attachment figure, implied but not spelled out in DSM-IV (Criterion A).

Criterion C

This criterion requires that "a pattern of extremes of insufficient care" be present, as evidenced by at least one of three caregiver behaviors: disregard for a child's needs for comfort, stimulation, and affection; repeated changes of primary caregivers; and rearing in unusual settings that severely limit opportunities to form selective attachments, such as institutions with a high child:caregiver ratio. From a practical point of view, this criterion poses challenges for the clinician, because insufficient care is not always disclosed and cannot always be clearly identified. Many young children cannot describe their own experiences, and caregivers may be implicated in inadequate care (and therefore have no reason to self-report). Yet, retaining Criterion C precludes making the diagnosis of reactive attachment disorder in children whose maltreatment is unknown to the clinician. On the other hand, there are no case reports of young children exhibiting reactive attachment disorder without at least a reasonable inference of seriously inadequate caregiving. The revisions are intended to describe in more detail what is known about the types of care that appear to predispose children to reactive attachment disorder. The criteria remain less specific than desirable, but this is a challenging area of investigation and data are limited.

Criterion D

This criterion is unchanged from DSM-IV. It is presumed that the pattern of extremes of insufficient care described in Criterion C is responsible for the child's aberrant behavior.

Criterion E

Because of symptom overlap, autism spectrum disorder needs to be ruled out. Aberrant social behaviors manifest in young children with reactive attachment disorder, but they are also features of autism spectrum disorder. The two disorders can be distinguished on the basis of developmental histories of neglect, the presence of restricted interests or ritualized behaviors, specific deficits in social communication, and the presence of selective attachment behaviors. Although the work group acknowledged that autism spectrum disorder and reactive attachment disorder could be comorbid, the lack of data combined with the concern about mistaking the former for the latter led them to recommend that the criterion be included.

Criteria F and G

The symptoms must be evident before age 5 years (Criterion F), as in DSM-IV. New to DSM-5, however, is the requirement that the child has reached a developmental age of 9 months (Criterion G). This criterion has been added to ensure that an attachment disorder is not diagnosed in children who are developmentally incapable of demonstrating a focused attachment. Stranger wariness and separation protest, in addition to selective comfort seeking or behavioral indicators of selective attachment, typically emerge between ages 7 and 9 months.

Specifiers

The specifiers may be used to indicate chronicity (present for more than 12 months) and current severity.

Disinhibited Social Engagement Disorder

Disinhibited social engagement disorder is new in DSM-5, having been split off from the DSM-IV reactive attachment disorder of infancy or early childhood. The essential feature of disinhibited social engagement disorder is a pattern of behavior that involves inappropriate and overly familiar behavior with unfamiliar adults or relative strangers, thus violating the social boundaries of the culture. The child must have the cognitive capacity of at least a 9-month-old. The disorder is uncommon, even among those who were severely neglected and subsequently placed in foster care or raised in group facilities. Disinhibited social engagement disorder has been described from the second year of life through adolescence. At very young ages, children are usually reticent when interacting with strangers. Children with this disorder not only lack such reticence but willingly engage with strangers and will even go off with unfamiliar adults. In preschool children, verbal and social intrusiveness are common, often accompanied by attention-seeking behaviors. When the disorder persists into middle childhood, verbal and physical overfamiliarity manifest, as well as inauthentic expression of emotions, and by adolescence indiscriminate behavior extends to peers. Peer relationships tend to be superficial and characterized by conflict.

Like reactive attachment disorder, disinhibited social engagement disorder is associated with cognitive and language delays, stereotypies, and other signs of severe neglect, including malnutrition and poor hygiene. Signs of the disorder may persist even when the neglect is no longer present. Thus, disinhibited social engagement disorder may be seen in children with a history of neglect who lack attachments or whose attachment to their caregivers ranges from disturbed to secure.

Diagnostic Criteria for Disinhibited Social
Engagement Disorder   313.89 (F94.2)

A. A pattern of behavior in which a child actively approaches and interacts with unfamiliar adults and exhibits at least two of the following:

1. Reduced or absent reticence in approaching and interacting with unfamiliar adults.

2. Overly familiar verbal or physical behavior (that is not consistent with culturally sanctioned and with age-appropriate social boundaries).

3. Diminished or absent checking back with adult caregiver after venturing away, even in unfamiliar settings.
4. Willingness to go off with an unfamiliar adult with minimal or no hesitation.

B. The behaviors in Criterion A are not limited to impulsivity (as in attention-deficit/hyperactivity disorder) but include socially disinhibited behavior.

C. The child has experienced a pattern of extremes of insufficient care as evidenced by at least one of the following:

1. Social neglect or deprivation in the form of persistent lack of having basic emotional needs for comfort, stimulation, and affection met by caregiving adults.
2. Repeated changes of primary caregivers that limit opportunities to form stable attachments (e.g., frequent changes in foster care).
3. Rearing in unusual settings that severely limit opportunities to form selective attachments (e.g., institutions with high child-to-caregiver ratios).

D. The care in Criterion C is presumed to be responsible for the disturbed behavior in Criterion A (e.g., the disturbances in Criterion A began following the pathogenic care in Criterion C).

E. The child has a developmental age of at least 9 months.

Specify if:

Persistent: The disorder has been present for more than 12 months.

Specify current severity:

Disinhibited social engagement disorder is specified as **severe** when the child exhibits all symptoms of the disorder, with each symptom manifesting at relatively high levels.

Criterion A

This criterion focuses the disorder more on aberrant social behavior than on disordered attachment behavior. The diagnosis requires that two or more of four examples of disinhibited behavior be present. These include reduced (or absent) reticence in approaching and interacting with unfamiliar adults, overly familiar verbal or physical behavior, diminished or absent checking back with the caregiver, and willingness to go off with an unfamiliar adult. These behaviors are aberrant in many cultures, where a child would typically become upset in these situations. The items composing the criterion are empirically derived from investigations of the construct.

Criterion B

This criterion is presumed necessary from several lines of evidence suggesting co-occurrence of attention-deficit/hyperactivity disorder (ADHD) signs and the social impulsivity that characterizes the indiscriminately social/disinhibited phenotype. For that reason, it is important that the behavior not be explained as a result of the impulsivity typically seen in children with ADHD. It appears that one may have ADHD with socially indiscriminate behavior and that one may have socially indiscriminate behavior without ADHD, but there are often moderately strong correlations between the two symptom profiles. Thus, rather than make ADHD a rule-out for disinhibited social engagement disorder, it seems more useful to direct attention to the distinctness of the latter from ADHD.

Criterion C

Extremes of insufficient care must be present as evidenced by at least one of three caregiver patterns: disregard for a child's need for comfort, stimulation, and affection; repeated changes of caregivers; and rearing in unusual settings that severely limit opportunities to form selective attachments, such as institutions with a high child:caregiver ratio. Insufficient care is retained in Criterion C (as in DSM-IV for the disinhibited type of reactive attachment disorder) for the important reason that children with adequate caregiving but chromosome 7 deletion demonstrate behavior phenotypically similar to that of individuals with disinhibited social engagement disorder. Insufficient care is described exactly as in reactive attachment disorder because no evidence suggests that certain types of pathogenic care are more or less likely to lead to reactive attachment disorder or to disinhibited social engagement disorder.

Criterion D

This criterion is retained from DSM-IV for the same reason that it was retained in reactive attachment disorder, described in the previous section: the presumption is that the pathogenic care situation described in Criterion C is responsible for the child's disturbed behavior.

Criterion E

The requirement that the child has reached a developmental age of 9 months serves the same purpose as Criterion G for reactive attachment disorder, as noted earlier.

Specifiers

The specifiers may be used to indicate chronicity (present for more than 12 months) and current severity.

Posttraumatic Stress Disorder

PTSD was introduced in DSM-III, but in the past this syndrome was recognized as "shell shock" or "war neurosis" because it was most commonly seen in wartime situations. Many of its symptoms, such as intrusive thoughts and autonomic hyperarousal, were also seen in victims of other traumatic events, including natural disasters. In DSM-I, the disorder was recognized as "gross stress reaction," considered one of several transient situational personality disorders:

> Under conditions of great or unusual stress, a normal personality may utilize established patterns of reaction to deal with overwhelming fear. The patterns of such reactions differ from those of neurosis or psychosis chiefly with respect to clinical history, reversibility of reaction, and its transient character. When promptly and adequately treated, the condition may clear rapidly. It is also possible that the condition may progress to one of the

neurotic reactions....This diagnosis is justified only in situations in which the individual has been exposed to severe physical demands or extreme emotional stress, such as in combat or in civilian catastrophe (fire, earthquake, explosion, etc.). (p. 40)

PTSD is common in the general population and can occur at any age, even in young children. In women the most frequent precipitating event is a physical assault, whereas in men the event often involves a combat experience. PTSD generally begins soon after the event is experienced, but onset can be delayed. For many individuals, PTSD is chronic, but symptoms can fluctuate and may worsen during stressful times.

The major etiological factor leading to PTSD is a traumatic event that involves exposure to actual or threatened death, serious injury, or sexual violence. The event is typically outside the range of normal human experience. Business losses, marital conflicts, and the death of a loved one are *not* stressors that cause PTSD. A person's age, history of psychiatric illness, level of social support, and proximity to the stressor are all factors that affect the likelihood of developing PTSD.

The DSM-5 criteria depart from those in DSM-IV in several important respects (Friedman et al. 2011). The stressor (Criterion A) is more explicitly described, and the subjective reaction (Criterion A2 in DSM-IV) has been eliminated. Whereas DSM-IV had three major symptom clusters corresponding to Criteria B, C, and D (reexperiencing, avoidance/numbing, and arousal, respectively), DSM-5 has four because the avoidance/numbing cluster has been split into two distinct clusters: persistent avoidance and negative alterations in cognitions and mood. The latter includes new or reconceptualized symptoms such as persistent and exaggerated negative expectations about oneself, others, and the world itself; persistent distorted cognitions about the cause or consequences of the event; and persistent negative emotional state. The final cluster, arousal, now includes reckless or self-destructive behavior (Criterion E2), but is otherwise unchanged. Diagnostic thresholds have been lowered for children, and a specific preschool subtype is included.

The work group dropped DSM-IV Criterion A2, which required individuals to have subjectively experienced fear, helplessness, or horror at the time of a traumatic event. In the past, it was believed that PTSD required an intense emotional reaction at the time of an adverse event, but not all people respond to traumatic events in the same way. Clinical and research experience show that Criterion A2 was not useful in predicting who would later exhibit symptoms of PTSD. Furthermore, the criterion tended to exclude people for whom exposure to a traumatic event was an occupational hazard for which they had been extensively trained, and who were just "doing their job," and therefore did not experience a horrific reaction at the time.

The work group has also added a new symptom cluster. The avoidance and numbing symptoms have been separated, with numbing symptoms renamed as a fourth cluster called "negative alterations in cognitions and mood" (Criterion D). The cluster is defined as showing evidence of two or more of seven specified symptoms in persons over age 6. The criteria reflect the anhedonic component of PTSD in which persons with PTSD are unable to experience positive emotions of joy or love, or enjoyment of pleasure, which can be devastating to marriages and relationships.

The subtype for children 6 years and younger was created to lower symptom thresholds and eliminate some symptoms that are difficult to assess in preschool children.

Research had shown that the prevalence of PTSD in children when using the DSM-IV criteria was lower than expected (Scheeringa et al. 2011).

The "with dissociative symptoms" subtype was created because it has long been known that people exposed to traumatic events can experience dissociation (15%–30% of persons with PTSD), mainly depersonalization and derealization (Lanius et al. 2012). These people respond differently to treatment, and neuroimaging studies show that those who dissociate have distinctive patterns of altered neurocircuitry. The body of information justified creating a specific subtype to recognize this specific subset of individuals with PTSD.

Diagnostic Criteria for
Posttraumatic Stress Disorder   **309.81** (F43.10)

Posttraumatic Stress Disorder

Note: The following criteria apply to adults, adolescents, and children older than 6 years. For children 6 years and younger, see corresponding criteria below.

A. Exposure to actual or threatened death, serious injury, or sexual violence in one (or more) of the following ways:

1. Directly experiencing the traumatic event(s).
2. Witnessing, in person, the event(s) as it occurred to others.
3. Learning that the traumatic event(s) occurred to a close family member or close friend. In cases of actual or threatened death of a family member or friend, the event(s) must have been violent or accidental.
4. Experiencing repeated or extreme exposure to aversive details of the traumatic event(s) (e.g., first responders collecting human remains; police officers repeatedly exposed to details of child abuse).

   Note: Criterion A4 does not apply to exposure through electronic media, television, movies, or pictures, unless this exposure is work related.

B. Presence of one (or more) of the following intrusion symptoms associated with the traumatic event(s), beginning after the traumatic event(s) occurred:

1. Recurrent, involuntary, and intrusive distressing memories of the traumatic event(s).

   Note: In children older than 6 years, repetitive play may occur in which themes or aspects of the traumatic event(s) are expressed.
2. Recurrent distressing dreams in which the content and/or affect of the dream are related to the traumatic event(s).

   Note: In children, there may be frightening dreams without recognizable content.
3. Dissociative reactions (e.g., flashbacks) in which the individual feels or acts as if the traumatic event(s) were recurring. (Such reactions may occur on a continuum, with the most extreme expression being a complete loss of awareness of present surroundings.)

   Note: In children, trauma-specific reenactment may occur in play.

4. Intense or prolonged psychological distress at exposure to internal or external cues that symbolize or resemble an aspect of the traumatic event(s).
5. Marked physiological reactions to internal or external cues that symbolize or resemble an aspect of the traumatic event(s).

C. Persistent avoidance of stimuli associated with the traumatic event(s), beginning after the traumatic event(s) occurred, as evidenced by one or both of the following:

1. Avoidance of or efforts to avoid distressing memories, thoughts, or feelings about or closely associated with the traumatic event(s).
2. Avoidance of or efforts to avoid external reminders (people, places, conversations, activities, objects, situations) that arouse distressing memories, thoughts, or feelings about or closely associated with the traumatic event(s).

D. Negative alterations in cognitions and mood associated with the traumatic event(s), beginning or worsening after the traumatic event(s) occurred, as evidenced by two (or more) of the following:

1. Inability to remember an important aspect of the traumatic event(s) (typically due to dissociative amnesia and not to other factors such as head injury, alcohol, or drugs).
2. Persistent and exaggerated negative beliefs or expectations about oneself, others, or the world (e.g., "I am bad," "No one can be trusted," "The world is completely dangerous," "My whole nervous system is permanently ruined").
3. Persistent, distorted cognitions about the cause or consequences of the traumatic event(s) that lead the individual to blame himself/herself or others.
4. Persistent negative emotional state (e.g., fear, horror, anger, guilt, or shame).
5. Markedly diminished interest or participation in significant activities.
6. Feelings of detachment or estrangement from others.
7. Persistent inability to experience positive emotions (e.g., inability to experience happiness, satisfaction, or loving feelings).

E. Marked alterations in arousal and reactivity associated with the traumatic event(s), beginning or worsening after the traumatic event(s) occurred, as evidenced by two (or more) of the following:

1. Irritable behavior and angry outbursts (with little or no provocation) typically expressed as verbal or physical aggression toward people or objects.
2. Reckless or self-destructive behavior.
3. Hypervigilance.
4. Exaggerated startle response.
5. Problems with concentration.
6. Sleep disturbance (e.g., difficulty falling or staying asleep or restless sleep).

F. Duration of the disturbance (Criteria B, C, D, and E) is more than 1 month.
G. The disturbance causes clinically significant distress or impairment in social, occupational, or other important areas of functioning.
H. The disturbance is not attributable to the physiological effects of a substance (e.g., medication, alcohol) or another medical condition.

Specify whether:

With dissociative symptoms: The individual's symptoms meet the criteria for posttraumatic stress disorder, and in addition, in response to the stressor, the individual experiences persistent or recurrent symptoms of either of the following:

1. **Depersonalization:** Persistent or recurrent experiences of feeling detached from, and as if one were an outside observer of, one's mental processes or body (e.g., feeling as though one were in a dream; feeling a sense of unreality of self or body or of time moving slowly).

2. **Derealization:** Persistent or recurrent experiences of unreality of surroundings (e.g., the world around the individual is experienced as unreal, dreamlike, distant, or distorted).

Note: To use this subtype, the dissociative symptoms must not be attributable to the physiological effects of a substance (e.g., blackouts, behavior during alcohol intoxication) or another medical condition (e.g., complex partial seizures).

Specify if:

With delayed expression: If the full diagnostic criteria are not met until at least 6 months after the event (although the onset and expression of some symptoms may be immediate).

Posttraumatic Stress Disorder for Children 6 Years and Younger

A. In children 6 years and younger, exposure to actual or threatened death, serious injury, or sexual violence in one (or more) of the following ways:

1. Directly experiencing the traumatic event(s).
2. Witnessing, in person, the event(s) as it occurred to others, especially primary caregivers.

   Note: Witnessing does not include events that are witnessed only in electronic media, television, movies, or pictures.

3. Learning that the traumatic event(s) occurred to a parent or caregiving figure.

B. Presence of one (or more) of the following intrusion symptoms associated with the traumatic event(s), beginning after the traumatic event(s) occurred:

1. Recurrent, involuntary, and intrusive distressing memories of the traumatic event(s).

   Note: Spontaneous and intrusive memories may not necessarily appear distressing and may be expressed as play reenactment.

2. Recurrent distressing dreams in which the content and/or affect of the dream are related to the traumatic event(s).

   Note: It may not be possible to ascertain that the frightening content is related to the traumatic event.

3. Dissociative reactions (e.g., flashbacks) in which the child feels or acts as if the traumatic event(s) were recurring. (Such reactions may occur on a continuum, with the most extreme expression being a complete loss of awareness of present surroundings.) Such trauma-specific reenactment may occur in play.

4. Intense or prolonged psychological distress at exposure to internal or external cues that symbolize or resemble an aspect of the traumatic event(s).

5. Marked physiological reactions to reminders of the traumatic event(s).

C. One (or more) of the following symptoms, representing either persistent avoidance of stimuli associated with the traumatic event(s) or negative alterations in cognitions and mood associated with the traumatic event(s), must be present, beginning after the event(s) or worsening after the event(s):

Persistent Avoidance of Stimuli

1. Avoidance of or efforts to avoid activities, places, or physical reminders that arouse recollections of the traumatic event(s).
2. Avoidance of or efforts to avoid people, conversations, or interpersonal situations that arouse recollections of the traumatic event(s).

Negative Alterations in Cognitions

3. Substantially increased frequency of negative emotional states (e.g., fear, guilt, sadness, shame, confusion).
4. Markedly diminished interest or participation in significant activities, including constriction of play.
5. Socially withdrawn behavior.
6. Persistent reduction in expression of positive emotions.

D. Alterations in arousal and reactivity associated with the traumatic event(s), beginning or worsening after the traumatic event(s) occurred, as evidenced by two (or more) of the following:

1. Irritable behavior and angry outbursts (with little or no provocation) typically expressed as verbal or physical aggression toward people or objects (including extreme temper tantrums).
2. Hypervigilance.
3. Exaggerated startle response.
4. Problems with concentration.
5. Sleep disturbance (e.g., difficulty falling or staying asleep or restless sleep).

E. The duration of the disturbance is more than 1 month.

F. The disturbance causes clinically significant distress or impairment in relationships with parents, siblings, peers, or other caregivers or with school behavior.

G. The disturbance is not attributable to the physiological effects of a substance (e.g., medication or alcohol) or another medical condition.

Specify whether:

With dissociative symptoms: The individual's symptoms meet the criteria for posttraumatic stress disorder, and the individual experiences persistent or recurrent symptoms of either of the following:

1. **Depersonalization:** Persistent or recurrent experiences of feeling detached from, and as if one were an outside observer of, one's mental processes or body (e.g., feeling as though one were in a dream; feeling a sense of unreality of self or body or of time moving slowly).
2. **Derealization:** Persistent or recurrent experiences of unreality of surroundings (e.g., the world around the individual is experienced as unreal, dreamlike, distant, or distorted).

Note: To use this subtype, the dissociative symptoms must not be attributable to the physiological effects of a substance (e.g., blackouts) or another medical condition (e.g., complex partial seizures).

Specify if:

With delayed expression: If the full diagnostic criteria are not met until at least 6 months after the event (although the onset and expression of some symptoms may be immediate).

Criterion A

This criterion has been edited to remove ambiguities and tighten the definition of a traumatic event. The criteria make clear that exposure involves actual or threatened death, serious injury, or sexual violence (the latter replaced the phrase "threat to the physical integrity of self or others"). The ways in which a person may be exposed are more explicit than in DSM-IV as well, and include directly experiencing or witnessing the event, or learning about an event that a close relative or friend experienced, although in the latter cases the actual or threatened death must have been violent or accidental. Learning that a relative has died from natural causes, for example, is not qualifying exposure. Criterion A4 is new and requires that the experience be repeated or that there be extreme exposure to aversive details for an event (such as that experienced by first responders). Although the DSM-IV language may well have included such exposures, it became clear following the terrorist attacks of September 11, 2001, that those involved in cleanup activities can develop symptoms (even though they may not have witnessed the event). DSM-5 also makes clear, in a note, that media exposure is an insufficient qualifier (e.g., reading about the event, or watching the event on television).

Criteria B, C, D, and E

Instead of three major symptom clusters as in DSM-IV, there are now four: intrusion symptoms (Criterion B), avoidance (Criterion C), negative alterations in cognitions and mood associated with the event (Criterion D), and marked alteration in arousal and reactivity (Criterion E). Reckless or self-destructive behavior (E2) has been added as a possible alteration in arousal and reactivity.

The traumatic event can be reexperienced in various ways. The individual may have recurrent, involuntary, and intrusive recollections of the event (B1). The emphasis is on spontaneous or triggered recurrent memories of the event that usually include sensory, emotional, or physiological behavioral components. A common reexperiencing symptom is distressing dreams during which the event is replayed or represented by related dangers (B2). Distressing dreams may contain themes that are representative of or thematically related to the major threats involved in the traumatic event (e.g., in the case of a motor vehicle accident survivor, the dreams may involve crashing cars). There may be dissociative states during which components of the event are relived and the person behaves as though reexperiencing the event. Dissociative reactions ("flashbacks") are typically brief but may cause great distress (B3).

The individual persistently avoids stimuli associated with the trauma (Criterion C). An individual may refuse to discuss his or her traumatic experience, or may engage in avoidance strategies to minimize awareness of emotional reactions, such as avoiding watching news coverage of traumatic experiences, refusing to return to the place where the trauma occurred, or avoiding interacting with others who shared the same experience (C2).

The individual may have negative alteration in cognitions and mood associated with the traumatic event—for example, being unable to recall important aspects of the event (dissociative amnesia) (D1), or exaggerated negative beliefs about oneself (e.g., I'm a bad person.") (D2). Some may experience a sustained negative emotional state, including fear, horror, or anger (D4), or develop feelings of detachment or estrangement from others (D6), such as *depersonalization,* a detached sense of oneself, or *derealization,* having a distorted view of one's surroundings. Others may report an inability to feel positive emotions such as happiness or joy (D7), symptoms sometimes referred to as emotional or psychic numbing.

The person must have two or more symptoms of arousal, such as an exaggerated startle response or problems with concentration. Some individuals experience irritable behavior and angry outbursts (E1). In response to research findings, this symptom description has been expanded in DSM-5 to indicate that the behavior may occur with little (or no) provocation and may involve verbal or physical aggression toward others or objects. This helps to distinguish PTSD from other causes of aggression, such as antisocial personality disorder.

Criterion F

The duration is more than 1 month. This is unchanged from DSM-IV (Criterion E) and helps separate PTSD from acute stress disorder.

Criterion G

This criterion is unchanged from DSM-IV and requires that symptoms cause significant distress or impairment in important areas of functioning.

Criterion H

The "rule-out" criterion is new to DSM-5 and brings PTSD into conformity with other disorders whereby substances of abuse, medications, and other medical conditions are eliminated as the cause of the disturbance. An important condition to rule out is a postconcussive syndrome, or traumatic brain injury, that is responsible for a variety of symptoms that could be due to PTSD, such as difficulty concentrating, irritability or anger, or sensitivity to light or noises. It is possible for an individual to have both conditions.

Acute Stress Disorder

Acute stress disorder was introduced in DSM-IV to recognize that dissociative symptoms could occur immediately following a traumatic event and that this would predict the development of PTSD. In DSM-5, the symptoms have been collapsed into a list of 14 possible symptoms (Criterion B), of which at least 9 must be present to indicate a diagnosis, none mandatory. Dissociative symptoms are included, but they are not required as they were in DSM-IV. Research has shown that acute stress reactions are variable and that many people with intense and disabling reactions never experience dissociation (Bryant et al. 2011).

The clinical presentation of this disorder typically involves an anxiety response with some form of reexperiencing or reactivity to the traumatic event. In some persons, a dissociative or detached presentation can predominate, although these individuals typically will also display strong emotional or physiological reactivity in response to trauma reminders. In others, there can be a strong anger response in which reactivity is characterized by irritable or even aggressive responses.

Diagnostic Criteria for Acute Stress Disorder   308.3 (F43.0)

A. Exposure to actual or threatened death, serious injury, or sexual violation in one (or more) of the following ways:

1. Directly experiencing the traumatic event(s).
2. Witnessing, in person, the event(s) as it occurred to others.
3. Learning that the event(s) occurred to a close family member or close friend. **Note:** In cases of actual or threatened death of a family member or friend, the event(s) must have been violent or accidental.
4. Experiencing repeated or extreme exposure to aversive details of the traumatic event(s) (e.g., first responders collecting human remains, police officers repeatedly exposed to details of child abuse).

Note: This does not apply to exposure through electronic media, television, movies, or pictures, unless this exposure is work related.

B. Presence of nine (or more) of the following symptoms from any of the five categories of intrusion, negative mood, dissociation, avoidance, and arousal, beginning or worsening after the traumatic event(s) occurred:

Intrusion Symptoms

1. Recurrent, involuntary, and intrusive distressing memories of the traumatic event(s). **Note:** In children, repetitive play may occur in which themes or aspects of the traumatic event(s) are expressed.
2. Recurrent distressing dreams in which the content and/or affect of the dream are related to the event(s). **Note:** In children, there may be frightening dreams without recognizable content.
3. Dissociative reactions (e.g., flashbacks) in which the individual feels or acts as if the traumatic event(s) were recurring. (Such reactions may occur on a continuum, with the most extreme expression being a complete loss of awareness of present surroundings.) **Note:** In children, trauma-specific reenactment may occur in play.
4. Intense or prolonged psychological distress or marked physiological reactions in response to internal or external cues that symbolize or resemble an aspect of the traumatic event(s).

Negative Mood

5. Persistent inability to experience positive emotions (e.g., inability to experience happiness, satisfaction, or loving feelings).

Dissociative Symptoms

6. An altered sense of the reality of one's surroundings or oneself (e.g., seeing oneself from another's perspective, being in a daze, time slowing).
7. Inability to remember an important aspect of the traumatic event(s) (typically

due to dissociative amnesia and not to other factors such as head injury, alcohol, or drugs).

Avoidance Symptoms

8. Efforts to avoid distressing memories, thoughts, or feelings about or closely associated with the traumatic event(s).
9. Efforts to avoid external reminders (people, places, conversations, activities, objects, situations) that arouse distressing memories, thoughts, or feelings about or closely associated with the traumatic event(s).

Arousal Symptoms

10. Sleep disturbance (e.g., difficulty falling or staying asleep, restless sleep).
11. Irritable behavior and angry outbursts (with little or no provocation), typically expressed as verbal or physical aggression toward people or objects.
12. Hypervigilance.
13. Problems with concentration.
14. Exaggerated startle response.

C. Duration of the disturbance (symptoms in Criterion B) is 3 days to 1 month after trauma exposure.

Note: Symptoms typically begin immediately after the trauma, but persistence for at least 3 days and up to a month is needed to meet disorder criteria.

D. The disturbance causes clinically significant distress or impairment in social, occupational, or other important areas of functioning.
E. The disturbance is not attributable to the physiological effects of a substance (e.g., medication or alcohol) or another medical condition (e.g., mild traumatic brain injury) and is not better explained by brief psychotic disorder.

Criterion A

This criterion describes the range of exposure that may lead to the development of symptoms and is identical to Criterion A for PTSD, described above. DSM-IV Criterion A2 was deleted because it required that the person's response involve "intense fear, helplessness, or horror" and the criterion was thought by the work group to have little clinical utility.

Criterion B

Nine or more of 14 items are required for the diagnosis, and they roughly correspond to those described above that occur in PTSD (Criteria B, C, D, and E).

Criterion C

Instead of a minimum duration of 2 days as in DSM-IV (Criterion G), this item requires that the full symptom picture be present for at least 3 days following a traumatic event but no longer than 1 month following the event. The purpose of this criterion is to separate acute stress disorder from PTSD, which lasts more than 1 month.

Criterion D

The symptoms must cause significant distress or impairment. The extreme level of anxiety may interfere with sleep, energy levels, and capacity to attend to tasks. Avoidance in acute stress disorder can result in generalized withdrawal from many situations perceived as potentially threatening, which can result in nonattendance at medical appointments, avoidance of driving, and absenteeism from work.

Criterion E

The symptoms must not be attributable to the physiological effects of a substance or another medical condition. When brain injury occurs in the context of a traumatic event, symptoms of acute stress disorder may appear. It is important to recognize that whatever caused the head trauma may also constitute a psychologically traumatic event and that postconcussive and acute stress disorder symptoms are not mutually exclusive and may co-occur.

Adjustment Disorders

Adjustment disorders are conditions in which people develop symptoms of emotional distress or behavioral symptoms in response to stressful events, or feel overwhelmed by their circumstances, but the symptoms fail to meet criteria for a more specific diagnosis such as acute stress disorder or PTSD. With adjustment disorders, people can experience varied symptoms, ranging from depression, to anxiety, to impaired work ability. These "walking wounded" may have symptoms sufficiently severe to require treatment or care.

Adjustment disorders were accorded a separate class beginning in DSM-III. Earlier DSMs recognized that individuals could develop symptoms in response to "a difficult situation or to newly experienced environmental factors" (DSM-I, p. 41) in the absence of serious personality difficulties, yet adjustment disorders were included in the category "transient situational personality disorders." Because adjustment disorders develop in response to identifiable stressors, the work group thought it appropriate to place them in the diagnostic class trauma- and stressor-related disorders in DSM-5.

It is important to understand that if the individual's symptoms lead to a more specific disorder, such as major depressive disorder or panic disorder, that diagnosis trumps adjustment disorder, even when a stressor appears central to the onset of the disorder.

Diagnostic Criteria for Adjustment Disorders

A. The development of emotional or behavioral symptoms in response to an identifiable stressor(s) occurring within 3 months of the onset of the stressor(s).
B. These symptoms or behaviors are clinically significant, as evidenced by one or both of the following:

1. Marked distress that is out of proportion to the severity or intensity of the stressor, taking into account the external context and the cultural factors that might influence symptom severity and presentation.
2. Significant impairment in social, occupational, or other important areas of functioning.

C. The stress-related disturbance does not meet the criteria for another mental disorder and is not merely an exacerbation of a preexisting mental disorder.
D. The symptoms do not represent normal bereavement.
E. Once the stressor or its consequences have terminated, the symptoms do not persist for more than an additional 6 months.

Specify whether:

309.0 (F43.21) With depressed mood: Low mood, tearfulness, or feelings of hopelessness are predominant.

309.24 (F43.22) With anxiety: Nervousness, worry, jitteriness, or separation anxiety is predominant.

309.28 (F43.23) With mixed anxiety and depressed mood: A combination of depression and anxiety is predominant.

309.3 (F43.24) With disturbance of conduct: Disturbance of conduct is predominant.

309.4 (F43.25) With mixed disturbance of emotions and conduct: Both emotional symptoms (e.g., depression, anxiety) and a disturbance of conduct are predominant.

309.9 (F43.20) Unspecified: For maladaptive reactions that are not classifiable as one of the specific subtypes of adjustment disorder.

Criterion A

There must be an identifiable stressor, and symptoms must begin within 3 months of its onset. Symptoms can be emotional or behavioral (e.g., depression, anxiety, acting out). The operative question in suspected cases of adjustment disorder is, "What is the individual having trouble adjusting to?"

Criterion B

This criterion is important because it describes the significant impairment in functioning or subjective distress that distinguishes adjustment disorder from normal responses that many persons experience in the face of a stressful situation or event. Adjustment disorders now require distress and/or impairment, rather than either distress or impairment as in DSM-IV.

Criteria C and D

The disturbance is not merely an exacerbation of a preexisting condition, such as major depressive disorder, and a more specific mental disorder has been ruled out. For example, if a person experiencing anxiety in response to a stressor has symptoms that otherwise meet criteria for panic disorder, that disorder—and not adjustment disorder—is the appropriate diagnosis.

The symptoms cannot represent normal bereavement, which is not considered a mental disorder. That said, should a bereaved individual develop symptoms consistent with major depressive episode, the correct diagnosis is major depressive disorder because the so-called bereavement exclusion has been removed (see Chapter 5, "Mood Disorders," for a discussion of the bereavement exclusion).

Criterion E

Adjustment disorders are time-limited reactions that occur in response to stressors and that resolve when the stressor or its consequences end; the symptoms do not persist for more than an additional 6 months. If symptoms persist, the person most likely has some other condition, such as generalized anxiety disorder.

Subtypes

Once an adjustment disorder is diagnosed, the clinician can specify a subtype, which will differ depending on the person's presenting symptoms. Adjustment disorders are varied but in most cases involve either depressive or anxiety-related symptoms, or a mixture of depression and anxiety. In some cases, the stressor may lead an individual to act out or misbehave, justifying the subtype "with disturbance of conduct." For example, an adolescent may shoplift or steal, or an adult may engage in an extramarital affair or embezzle funds. Sometimes a person may experience a mixture of emotions and behavior problems, leading to the subtype "with mixed disturbance of emotions and conduct."

Other Specified Trauma- and Stressor-Related Disorder and Unspecified Trauma- and Stressor-Related Disorder

These are residual categories to use for individuals with symptoms of a trauma- or stressor-related disorder who have distress or impairment but whose symptoms do not meet criteria for a more specific disorder in the class. The category other specified trauma- and stressor-related disorder is used when the clinician chooses to communicate the reason that the presentation does not meet the full criteria. The clinician is encouraged to record the specific reason (e.g., *ataque de nervios*).

The category unspecified trauma- and stressor-related disorder is used when the clinician chooses not to specify the reason the criteria are not met, or there is insufficient information to make a more specific diagnosis.

Other Specified Trauma- and Stressor-Related Disorder	309.89 (F43.8)

This category applies to presentations in which symptoms characteristic of a trauma- and stressor-related disorder that cause clinically significant distress or impairment in social, occupational, or other important areas of functioning predominate but do not meet the full criteria for any of the disorders in the trauma- and stressor-related disorders diagnostic class. The other specified trauma- and stressor-related disorder category is used in situations in which the clinician chooses to communicate the specific reason that the presentation does not meet the criteria for any specific trauma- and stressor-related disorder. This is done by recording "other specified trauma- and stressor-related disorder" followed by the specific reason (e.g., "persistent complex bereavement disorder").

Examples of presentations that can be specified using the "other specified" designation include the following:

1. **Adjustment-like disorders with delayed onset of symptoms that occur more than 3 months after the stressor.**
2. **Adjustment-like disorders with prolonged duration of more than 6 months without prolonged duration of stressor.**
3. ***Ataque de nervios:*** See "Glossary of Cultural Concepts of Distress" in the Appendix to DSM-5.
4. **Other cultural syndromes:** See "Glossary of Cultural Concepts of Distress" in the Appendix to DSM-5.
5. **Persistent complex bereavement disorder:** This disorder is characterized by severe and persistent grief and mourning reactions (see Chapter 22, "Conditions for Further Study," this volume).

Unspecified Trauma- and Stressor-Related Disorder   309.9 (F43.9)

This category applies to presentations in which symptoms characteristic of a trauma- and stressor-related disorder that cause clinically significant distress or impairment in social, occupational, or other important areas of functioning predominate but do not meet the full criteria for any of the disorders in the trauma- and stressor-related disorders diagnostic class. The unspecified trauma- and stressor-related disorder category is used in situations in which the clinician chooses *not* to specify the reason that the criteria are not met for a specific trauma- and stressor-related disorder, and includes presentations in which there is insufficient information to make a more specific diagnosis (e.g., in emergency room settings).

KEY POINTS

- This new chapter brings together conditions in which an identifiable traumatic event or stressor or insufficient parenting has induced the disorder.
- DSM-IV reactive attachment disorder has been split to create a reformulated reactive attachment disorder and the new disinhibited social engagement disorder. This change was made to recognize that some children exposed to a pattern of extremes of insufficient care develop emotionally withdrawn behavior, whereas others become indiscriminately social.

- The stressor criterion (A) for acute stress disorder and posttraumatic stress disorder (PTSD) has been revised to be more explicit in describing the types of events that lead to these disorders. Also, PTSD is now defined by the development of symptoms in each of four clusters, rather than three clusters. The avoidance/numbing cluster has been split into an avoidance cluster and a negative alterations in cognitions and mood cluster. A developmentally sensitive criteria set for PTSD has been included for children 6 years and younger.

- Adjustment disorders are mostly unchanged but specifically exclude those experiencing normal bereavement.

CHAPTER 9

Dissociative Disorders

300.14 (F44.81) Dissociative Identity Disorder
300.12 (F44.0) Dissociative Amnesia
300.6 (F48.1) Depersonalization/Derealization Disorder
300.15 (F44.89) Other Specified Dissociative Disorder
300.15 (F44.9) Unspecified Dissociative Disorder

Dissociative disorders retain an important role in DSM-5, whose metastructure recognizes that dissociative symptoms are a feature of disorders in other diagnostic classes in the manual. For that reason, the placement of dissociative disorders between the trauma- and stressor-related disorders and the somatic symptom and related disorders is meant to reflect the close relationship among these categories. Acute stress disorder and posttraumatic stress disorder include dissociative symptoms, such as amnesia, flashbacks, and numbing. The somatic symptom and related disorders also include syndromes involving interference with sensory and motor function that are dissociative in nature, such as pseudoseizures and other pseudoneurological symptoms.

Dissociative states have a long and rich history, their hallmark being a disruption of and/or discontinuity in the normal integration of conscience, memory, identity, emotion, perception, body representation, motor control, and behavior. They were first formally recognized in DSM-I as "dissociative reaction." DSM-II included the diagnosis "hysterical neurosis, dissociative type" as one of two neuroses (the other was "hysterical neurosis, conversion type"). According to DSM-II, "In the dissociative type, alterations may occur in the patient's state of consciousness or in his identity, to produce such symptoms as amnesia, somnambulism, fugue, and multiple personality" (p. 40).

Dissociative disorders were accorded a separate class in DSM-III, which included diagnostic criteria for the many forms of dissociation and depersonalization that had been described, including multiple personality disorder (renamed "dissociative identity disorder" in DSM-IV).

Some believe that dissociative disorders are rare, but research suggests they are relatively common, particularly in hospital and clinic settings (Foote et al. 2006; Sar et al. 2007). Subclinical forms of dissociation are frequent in the general population and are not inherently maladaptive (e.g., daydreaming). Experiences of pathological possession and other forms of identity disruption may be even more common in non-Western cultures. They are frequently found in the aftermath of trauma, and many of the symptoms are hidden or confusing to individuals, making careful diagnostic evaluation important.

Dissociative disorders cause substantial distress and disability and can disrupt every important area of psychological function. Symptoms can be experienced as unwanted intrusions into awareness and behavior with accompanying loss of continuity in subjective experience, or as an inability to access information or control mental functions that are normally readily amenable to access or control.

There are several important changes in the dissociative disorders in DSM-5 (Spiegel et al. 2011). First, *derealization*—the feeling of estrangement or detachment from one's environment—has been merged with depersonalization in depersonalization/derealization disorder. This replaces DSM-IV's depersonalization disorder. The change is an acknowledgment of the importance of these symptoms and recognizes that they often co-occur. Research evidence shows that people with prominent derealization alone do not differ in any important respect from those with depersonalization accompanied by derealization.

Next, dissociative fugue is now a specifier for dissociative amnesia rather than an independent disorder, as in DSM-IV. The criteria for dissociative identity disorder have been changed to indicate that disruption of identity and conscience may be reported by the individual as well as observed by others, and that the accompanying amnesia can be for everyday events and for important personal information, not just for traumatic events.

The dissociative disorders are mutually exclusive and are presented hierarchically. When present, dissociative identity disorder takes precedence over dissociative amnesia and depersonalization/derealization disorder. The categories other specified dissociative disorder and unspecified dissociative disorder can be used for dissociative symptoms that do not meet more specific criteria. Table 9–1 lists the DSM-5 dissociative disorders.

TABLE 9–1.   DSM-5 dissociative disorders

Dissociative identity disorder

Dissociative amnesia

Depersonalization/derealization disorder

Other specified dissociative disorder

Unspecified dissociative disorder

Dissociative Identity Disorder

Described for centuries and first recognized in DSM-III as "multiple personality disorder," dissociative identity disorder is defined in DSM-5 as requiring two or more fully distinct personality states, which in some cultures may be described as an experience of possession. The disorder is reported to begin in childhood and has been attributed to adaptation to overwhelming circumstances, such as physical or sexual abuse.

Individuals with dissociative identity disorder may first present with symptoms of emotional and behavioral turmoil. Some may notice memory gaps and incidents of out-of-character behavior. These symptoms result from different "alters," or alternate identities, controlling an individual's behavior for varying lengths of time. Switches have been observed with stressful situations, disputes among alters, and other psychological conflicts.

Diagnostic Criteria for Dissociative Identity Disorder   300.14 (F44.81)

A. Disruption of identity characterized by two or more distinct personality states, which may be described in some cultures as an experience of possession. The disruption in identity involves marked discontinuity in sense of self and sense of agency, accompanied by related alterations in affect, behavior, consciousness, memory, perception, cognition, and/or sensory-motor functioning. These signs and symptoms may be observed by others or reported by the individual.
B. Recurrent gaps in the recall of everyday events, important personal information, and/or traumatic events that are inconsistent with ordinary forgetting.
C. The symptoms cause clinically significant distress or impairment in social, occupational, or other important areas of functioning.
D. The disturbance is not a normal part of a broadly accepted cultural or religious practice.
   Note: In children, the symptoms are not better explained by imaginary playmates or other fantasy play.
E. The symptoms are not attributable to the physiological effects of a substance (e.g., blackouts or chaotic behavior during alcohol intoxication) or another medical condition (e.g., complex partial seizures).

Criterion A

This criterion has been revised to be more specific with regard to how the disorder disturbs the person's functioning. The language was changed to acknowledge a marked discontinuity in the sense of self and sense of agency. DSM-IV required two or more distinct "identities or personality states," but the distinction between "identities" and "personality states" was never clear, nor was it clear that switches had to represent a break with the person's usual thinking and behavior. These changes may be observed by others or reported by the individual (in DSM-IV this was unstated). The concept of *possession* appears as well (it wasn't specified in DSM-IV).

Criterion B

In DSM-IV Criterion C, memory gaps were described as involving "important personal information." More guidance is given to clinicians in DSM-5 with regard to memory lapses, in that they are described as affecting recall of "everyday events, important personal information, and/or traumatic events." Clearly, with dissociative identity disorder, memory gaps tend to occur when one or more of the alters take control of the person's executive function, and the individual reports "losing time." The quality and extent of the memory loss are not consistent with ordinary forgetting. For example, the person may report that he or she is unable to recall the past 2 days despite having excellent recall of events immediately preceding and following the period of amnesia.

Criterion C

This criterion, new to DSM-5, recognizes that dissociative identity disorder causes clinically significant distress or impairment in functioning in important life domains. Symptoms are consciously experienced and are often quite disturbing to the person, reflecting an alter's intrusion into the person's conscious functioning. When this occurs, the person's sense of self is disrupted. The person's sense of directing his or her speech and actions may be lost, and voices may intrude into the conscious mind; strong emotions and impulses may emerge suddenly. People may become depersonalized observers of their actions, which they may feel powerless to stop. The person's body may suddenly feel very different—for example, like that of a small child or an individual of the opposite gender—and all of these alterations in sense of self and this loss of personal agency may be accompanied by feelings that the person recognizes are "not mine." These changes can be highly distressing, and for many people these symptoms will adversely affect relationships, marriages, parenting function, and one's occupational and professional life.

Criterion D

This criterion recognizes that cultural and religious practices that include or even celebrate dissociation must be excluded as explanations for the disorder. Some indigenous societies believe in the concept of *spirit possession*. These beliefs are not uncommon in the developing world and non-Western societies, but they may also be found in certain religious groups in the United States and elsewhere. In these situations, alters may present as spirits, demons, animals, or mythical figures.

Criterion E

This criterion recognizes that substances of abuse or a medical condition could be associated with dissociation and therefore must be ruled out. For example, hallucinogens and phencyclidine (PCP) can induce dissociative-like experiences. Brain tumors or seizure disorders (e.g., complex partial seizures) have been known to cause dissociative states. These conditions must be ruled out as part of a medical evaluation.

Dissociative Amnesia

Dissociative amnesia is characterized by the inability to recall important autobiographical information, usually of a traumatic or stressful nature, that is considered too extensive to be explained by ordinary forgetfulness. With dissociative amnesia, the person is typically confused and perplexed and may not recall significant personal information or even his or her own name. The amnesia typically develops suddenly and can last from minutes to days, or even longer. Most cases last less than 1 week. In DSM-5, two primary forms are listed: 1) *localized* or *selective* amnesia for specific event(s) and 2) *generalized* amnesia for identity and life history. Although some individuals with amnesia notice that they have "lost time" or that they have a gap in their memory, most people with dissociative disorders are initially unaware of their amnesias.

A major change in DSM-5 is that dissociative fugue is now a specifier for dissociative amnesia, not a separate diagnosis as in DSM-IV. This change was prompted by the fact that the disorder is uncommon, is rarely diagnosed, and typically occurs in the context of an amnesic episode. The fugue usually involves sudden, unexpected travel away from home or one's workplace, and the associated amnesia is characterized by inability to recall one's past and the assumption of a new identity that may be partial or complete. Fugues can last for months and lead to a complicated pattern of travel and identity formation.

Diagnostic Criteria for Dissociative Amnesia 300.12 (F44.0)

A. An inability to recall important autobiographical information, usually of a traumatic or stressful nature, that is inconsistent with ordinary forgetting.
   Note: Dissociative amnesia most often consists of localized or selective amnesia for a specific event or events; or generalized amnesia for identity and life history.
B. The symptoms cause clinically significant distress or impairment in social, occupational, or other important areas of functioning.
C. The disturbance is not attributable to the physiological effects of a substance (e.g., alcohol or other drug of abuse, a medication) or a neurological or other medical condition (e.g., partial complex seizures, transient global amnesia, sequelae of a closed head injury/traumatic brain injury, other neurological condition).
D. The disturbance is not better explained by dissociative identity disorder, posttraumatic stress disorder, acute stress disorder, somatic symptom disorder, or major or mild neurocognitive disorder.

Coding note: The code for dissociative amnesia without dissociative fugue is **300.12 (F44.0)**. The code for dissociative amnesia with dissociative fugue is **300.13 (F44.1)**.

Specify if:
   300.13 (F44.1) With dissociative fugue: Apparently purposeful travel or bewildered wandering that is associated with amnesia for identity or for other important autobiographical information.

Criterion A

Dissociative amnesia primarily affects the ability to recall personal information about oneself, and it may be selective for specific events or more global. Unlike in DSM-IV, the criterion now specifies two types of amnesia: localized or selective, and generalized.

Criterion B

The diagnosis requires clinically significant distress or impairment in functioning. With this disorder, the person may feel that he or she is "going crazy" or may have concerns about self-identity.

Criteria C and D

Amnesia must be distinguished from the effect of a substance or a neurological or other medical condition that can induce amnesia. For example, individuals may experience blackouts during periods of heavy alcohol use, and people who experience seizures may be amnesic for varying periods of time prior to or following a seizure. Major neurocognitive disorders can cause amnesia, but in these disorders the amnestic symptoms generally do not occur in isolation, and other symptoms typical of a dementia, such as behavioral disturbance, will be present.

Dissociative amnesia must be distinguished from other mental disorders. This is important because amnesia may be seen in other disorders, such as somatic symptom disorder and posttraumatic stress disorder. For example, a person with dissociative identity disorder may experience amnesia when an alter takes control.

Specifier

The specifier "with dissociative fugue" is used when the person unexpectedly travels away from home or the workplace, or wanders bewilderedly, during an episode of dissociative amnesia.

Depersonalization/Derealization Disorder

Depersonalization/derealization disorder is characterized by clinically significant persistent or recurrent experiences of depersonalization and/or derealization. Transient depersonalization and derealization symptoms are very common. Research shows that these symptoms comprise four or five factors: numbing, unreality of self, unreality of others, temporal disintegration, and perceptual alterations. There is no evidence of any distinction between individuals with predominantly depersonalization or derealization symptoms. The disorder rarely begins after age 40 years and can become chronic, resulting in significant distress and disability.

Diagnostic Criteria for Depersonalization/Derealization Disorder
300.6 (F48.1)

A. The presence of persistent or recurrent experiences of depersonalization, derealization, or both:

1. **Depersonalization:** Experiences of unreality, detachment, or being an outside observer with respect to one's thoughts, feelings, sensations, body, or actions (e.g., perceptual alterations, distorted sense of time, unreal or absent self, emotional and/or physical numbing).

2. **Derealization:** Experiences of unreality or detachment with respect to surroundings (e.g., individuals or objects are experienced as unreal, dreamlike, foggy, lifeless, or visually distorted).

B. During the depersonalization or derealization experiences, reality testing remains intact.

C. The symptoms cause clinically significant distress or impairment in social, occupational, or other important areas of functioning.

D. The disturbance is not attributable to the physiological effects of a substance (e.g., a drug of abuse, medication) or another medical condition (e.g., seizures).

E. The disturbance is not better explained by another mental disorder, such as schizophrenia, panic disorder, major depressive disorder, acute stress disorder, posttraumatic stress disorder, or another dissociative disorder.

Criteria A, B, and C

Criterion A requires the presence of persistent or recurrent experiences of depersonalization and/or derealization. *Depersonalization* involves feeling detached from oneself or one's surroundings, as though one were an outside observer (e.g., a "dreamlike" state). A person may feel cut off from his or her thoughts, emotions, or identity. Another may feel like a robot or automaton. *Derealization* produces a sense of unreality or detachment with respect to one's surroundings.

Criterion B recognizes that despite the strange thoughts and sensations the person is experiencing, he or she is not psychotic or out of touch with reality. Intact reality testing excludes the possibility of a psychotic disorder.

The diagnosis requires the presence of distress or impairment in functioning (Criterion C). The symptoms may be highly distressing; the affectively flattened and robotic demeanor seen in some individuals may be incongruent with the extreme emotional pain they report. Impairment is often experienced in both interpersonal and occupational domains, largely due to the sense of hypoemotionality. Others may experience subjective difficulty in focusing and retaining information, and feel a general sense of disconnectedness from life.

Criteria D and E

Depersonalization and derealization can result from the use of substances (e.g., marijuana, hallucinogens) or from a medical condition (Criterion D). Presentation after age 40 years should suggest the possibility of an underlying medical condition, such as a seizure disorder, brain tumor, or stroke. Complex partial seizures are known to induce depersonalization and derealization, but they are uncommon.

Depersonalization/derealization disorder needs to be distinguished from other mental disorders associated with these symptoms (Criterion E). Individuals with schizophrenia may experience depersonalization and derealization symptoms, but these occur in the context of hallucinations and delusions. Some persons with major depressive disorder experience feelings of numbness or feel emotionally dead inside, but these feelings occur only during a mood episode. People with panic disorder can experience these symptoms, but the symptoms occur during panic attacks and are not chronic. Depersonalization/derealization symptoms may occur in other dissociative disorders, but in that case the diagnosis of depersonalization/derealization disorder is preempted.

Other Specified Dissociative Disorder and Unspecified Dissociative Disorder

The other specified and unspecified dissociative disorder diagnoses replace DSM-IV's category dissociative disorder not otherwise specified but serve a similar function as a residual category for dissociative symptoms that do not fit within a more specific category.

Other specified dissociative disorder is used when symptoms characteristic of a dissociative disorder are present and cause distress or impairment but do not meet the full criteria for a more specific disorder in the class. The category is used when the clinician chooses to communicate the reason that the presentation does not meet full criteria. The clinician is encouraged to record the specific reason (e.g., chronic or recurrent syndromes of mixed dissociative symptoms).

The category unspecified dissociative disorder is used when the individual's symptoms do not meet full criteria for a more specific disorder that causes distress or impairment, and the clinician chooses not to specify the reason the criteria are not met, or there is insufficient information to make a more specific diagnosis.

Other Specified Dissociative Disorder   300.15 (F44.89)

This category applies to presentations in which symptoms characteristic of a dissociative disorder that cause clinically significant distress or impairment in social, occupational, or other important areas of functioning predominate but do not meet the full criteria for any of the disorders in the dissociative disorders diagnostic class. The other specified dissociative disorder category is used in situations in which the clinician chooses to communicate the specific reason that the presentation does not meet the criteria for any specific dissociative disorder. This is done by recording "other specified dissociative disorder" followed by the specific reason (e.g., "dissociative trance").

Examples of presentations that can be specified using the "other specified" designation include the following:

1. **Chronic and recurrent syndromes of mixed dissociative symptoms:** This category includes identity disturbance associated with less-than-marked discontinuities in sense of self and agency, or alterations of identity or episodes of possession in an individual who reports no dissociative amnesia.

2. **Identity disturbance due to prolonged and intense coercive persuasion:** Individuals who have been subjected to intense coercive persuasion (e.g., brainwashing, thought reform, indoctrination while captive, torture, long-term political imprisonment, recruitment by sects/cults or by terror organizations) may present with prolonged changes in, or conscious questioning of, their identity.

3. **Acute dissociative reactions to stressful events:** This category is for acute, transient conditions that typically last less than 1 month, and sometimes only a few hours or days. These conditions are characterized by constriction of consciousness; depersonalization; derealization; perceptual disturbances (e.g., time slowing, macropsia); micro-amnesias; transient stupor; and/or alterations in sensory-motor functioning (e.g., analgesia, paralysis).

4. **Dissociative trance:** This condition is characterized by an acute narrowing or complete loss of awareness of immediate surroundings that manifests as profound unresponsiveness or insensitivity to environmental stimuli. The unresponsiveness may be accompanied by minor stereotyped behaviors (e.g., finger movements) of which the individual is unaware and/or that he or she cannot control, as well as transient paralysis or loss of consciousness. The dissociative trance is not a normal part of a broadly accepted collective cultural or religious practice.

Unspecified Dissociative Disorder   300.15 (F44.9)

This category applies to presentations in which symptoms characteristic of a dissociative disorder that cause clinically significant distress or impairment in social, occupational, or other important areas of functioning predominate but do not meet the full criteria for any of the disorders in the dissociative disorders diagnostic class. The unspecified dissociative disorder category is used in situations in which the clinician chooses *not* to specify the reason that the criteria are not met for a specific dissociative disorder, and includes presentations for which there is insufficient information to make a more specific diagnosis (e.g., in emergency room settings).

KEY POINTS

- The criteria for dissociative identity disorder have been changed to indicate that disruption of identity and conscience may be reported by the individual as well as observed, and that the accompanying amnesia can involve everyday events and important personal information, as well as traumatic events.

- Dissociative fugue is now a specifier for dissociative amnesia, rather than an independent disorder as in DSM-IV.

- Depersonalization/derealization disorder is new to DSM-5 and, by merging derealization with depersonalization, acknowledges that these symptoms often co-occur.

CHAPTER 10

Somatic Symptom and Related Disorders

300.82 (F45.1) Somatic Symptom Disorder
300.7 (F45.21) Illness Anxiety Disorder
300.11 (F44._) Conversion Disorder (Functional Neurological Symptom Disorder)
316 (F54) Psychological Factors Affecting Other Medical Conditions
300.19 (F68.10) Factitious Disorder (Imposed on Self and Imposed on Another)
300.89 (F45.8) Other Specified Somatic Symptom and Related Disorder
300.82 (F45.9) Unspecified Somatic Symptom and Related Disorder

The somatic symptom and related disorders are unified by the presence of physical symptoms and/or excessive concern regarding medical illnesses or symptoms. The new diagnostic class name was recommended by the DSM-5 Somatic Symptoms Disorders Work Group because it better reflects the content of the category and creates less confusion regarding its member disorders than did the former term *somatoform disorders*.

The concept of unexplained physical complaints was recognized in early editions of DSM. A broad category of psychoneurotic disorders in DSM-I included "conversion reaction," in which it was said that the "impulse causing anxiety is 'converted' into functional symptoms in organs or parts of the body..." (American Psychiatric Association 1952, p. 32). DSM-II introduced the new category "hysterical neurosis," characterized as an "involuntary psychogenic loss of disorder of function...symbolic of underlying conflicts" (American Psychiatric Association 1968, p. 39). Two subcategories were specified: "hysterical neurosis, conversion type" and "hysterical neurosis, dissociative type." The former represented continuity with DSM-I's conversion reaction and the latter with DSM-I's dissociative reaction. DSM-III introduced the new class of *somatoform disorders,* which included somatization disorder, a syndrome of unexplained physical complaints, patterned after Briquet's syndrome (Feighner et al. 1972) and named after a 19th-century French psychiatrist. Other conditions included conversion disorder, psychogenic pain disorder (renamed *somatoform pain disorder* in DSM-III-R and *simplified to pain disorder* in DSM-IV), hypochondriasis, and atypical somatoform disorder. Body dysmorphic disorder (dysmorphophobia), undifferentiated somatoform disorder, and the residual category somatoform disorder not otherwise specified were added to the class in DSM-III-R. The class was mostly unchanged in DSM-IV except that criteria for somatization disorder were simplified.

The chapter has been reformulated for DSM-5 and brings together disorders that were spread among several DSM-IV chapters. Many were listed in DSM-IV in the "Somatoform Disorders" chapter. In addition, factitious disorder was moved to this chapter from its own chapter, and psychological factors affecting other medical conditions was moved from "Other Conditions That May Be a Focus of Clinical Attention." On the other hand, body dysmorphic disorder was moved from "Somatoform Disorders" to the new chapter "Obsessive-Compulsive and Related Disorders" (see Chapter 7). The somatic symptom and related disorders are listed in Table 10–1.

TABLE 10–1. DSM-5 somatic symptom disorders

Somatic symptom disorder

Illness anxiety disorder

Conversion disorder (functional neurological symptom disorder)

Psychological factors affecting other medical conditions

Factitious disorder (imposed on self and imposed on another)

Other specified somatic symptom and related disorder

Unspecified somatic symptom and related disorder

Although disorders characterized by the presence of somatic symptoms or concerns are common, nonpsychiatric physicians found the earlier DSM diagnoses confusing and difficult to understand. DSM-IV's somatoform disorder diagnoses overlapped, and clinicians had trouble distinguishing one from another. For these reasons, the diagnoses were rarely used and were often ignored. As a case in point, the diagnosis of somatization disorder was thought by many to be difficult to use because of the requirement for what seemed like arbitrary and lengthy symptom counts that changed with each new DSM edition. The DSM-5 classification minimizes the overlap by reducing the total number of disorders and their subcategories. Clinicians should find the reformulated chapter and the revised criteria more user friendly (Dimsdale and Creed 2009).

There are several important changes from the DSM-IV somatoform disorders. First, somatic symptom disorder is a new diagnosis that replaces somatization disorder, hypochondriasis, pain disorder, and undifferentiated somatoform disorder. Because these disorders all shared the presence of somatic symptoms and similar cognitive distortions, the work group decided there was little reason for separate diagnoses that were rarely used. In reconceptualizing these disorders, the work group aimed to make them more useful.

A major criterion for several of these disorders was that symptoms were medically unexplained. Because of the general unreliability of a clinician's determination of whether a symptom is medically based or not, and the fact that such a determination only encourages "mind-body dualism," medically unexplained symptoms are no longer emphasized as core features. Furthermore, unexplained somatic symptoms sometimes accompany other psychiatric disorders (e.g., major depressive disorder, schizophrenia) and some medical conditions, and therefore are often a poor basis for distinguishing "functional" from genuine physical disorders.

Although many clinicians have had difficulty with the concept of somatoform disorders in general, and patients have found the diagnoses unhelpful and stigmatizing, these disorders remain important because they can cause considerable subjective distress and impair functioning. Many individuals with these disorders have repeated surgeries, develop drug or alcohol use disorders, experience marital instability, and attempt suicide. Co-occurring mood and anxiety disorders are common. The disorders tend to be chronic, with fluctuations in frequency and severity of symptoms.

In DSM-5, instead of an emphasis on the absence of a medical explanation serving as an organizing principle for the disorders, the focus is on distressing somatic symptoms and abnormal thoughts, feelings, and behaviors. Basing a diagnosis on the *absence* of a medical explanation for the symptoms was as unsatisfying to clinicians as it was to patients. The work group concluded that incorporating affective, cognitive, and behavioral components into the criteria improves the validity and clinical utility of the criteria. Individuals formerly diagnosed with hypochondriasis will now be split between somatic symptom disorder—for those with somatic symptoms—and illness anxiety disorder—a new diagnosis for those whose main problem is illness anxiety that occurs primarily in the absence of somatic symptoms. Pain disorder has been eliminated as a diagnosis because it was rarely used and was not useful. It was easily misinterpreted as implying that the person's pain was psychologically motivated and "in the patient's head." In most cases, individuals had medical disorders that explained the pain, but it was clear that psychological factors contributed to the pain.

Conversion disorder has been renamed conversion disorder (functional neurological symptom disorder) to acknowledge that neurological symptoms are the focus of concern. The criteria emphasize the importance of the neurological examination and recognize that relevant psychological factors may not be demonstrable at the time of the diagnosis. Although the chapter has de-emphasized medically unexplained symptoms, they remain key features of conversion disorder and pseudocyesis (listed as an example of an other specified somatic symptom and related disorder). In each case, medical evaluation can demonstrate that these disorders are inconsistent with known mechanisms of pathophysiology.

Somatic Symptom Disorder

Somatic symptom disorder is a new omnibus category that replaces DSM-IV's somatization disorder, hypochondriasis, pain disorder, and undifferentiated somatoform disorder. These diagnoses were rarely used and created confusion for both clinicians and patients. The new diagnosis de-emphasizes medically unexplained symptoms, which had a central organizing role for many of the somatoform disorders. Instead, the category is defined on the basis of distressing somatic symptoms, and the excessive thoughts, feelings, and behaviors that arise in response to these symptoms. The work group felt that the DSM-IV criteria for somatization disorder were overly restrictive and that those for undifferentiated somatoform disorder and somatoform disorder not otherwise specified had such low thresholds that either diagnosis could apply to a large proportion of individuals seen in primary care. The new diagnosis is expected to overcome these problems and will be more user friendly.

This new diagnosis follows in the long tradition of recognizing psychiatric disorders whose primary manifestations are somatic symptoms or concerns. Somatic symptom disorder will likely be used for individuals formerly diagnosed with somatization disorder, hypochondriasis, or pain disorder. To diagnose DSM-IV's somatization disorder, the clinician followed a complicated algorithm that required the presence of at least eight medically unexplained symptoms, including four pain, two gastrointestinal, one sexual, and one pseudoneurological. The ensuing distress or impairment had to be greater than would be expected from the history, physical examination, or laboratory findings. Many additional patients with fewer unexplained symptoms were relegated to receiving a diagnosis of undifferentiated somatoform disorder or somatoform disorder not otherwise specified.

Diagnostic Criteria for Somatic Symptom Disorder   300.82 (F45.1)

A. One or more somatic symptoms that are distressing or result in significant disruption of daily life.

B. Excessive thoughts, feelings, or behaviors related to the somatic symptoms or associated health concerns as manifested by at least one of the following:

   1. Disproportionate and persistent thoughts about the seriousness of one's symptoms.

   2. Persistently high level of anxiety about health or symptoms.

   3. Excessive time and energy devoted to these symptoms or health concerns.

C. Although any one somatic symptom may not be continuously present, the state of being symptomatic is persistent (typically more than 6 months).

Specify if:

With predominant pain (previously pain disorder): This specifier is for individuals whose somatic symptoms predominantly involve pain.

Specify if:

Persistent: A persistent course is characterized by severe symptoms, marked impairment, and long duration (more than 6 months).

Specify current severity:

Mild: Only one of the symptoms specified in Criterion B is fulfilled.

Moderate: Two or more of the symptoms specified in Criterion B are fulfilled.

Severe: Two or more of the symptoms specified in Criterion B are fulfilled, plus there are multiple somatic complaints (or one very severe somatic symptom).

Criterion A

This item requires the presence of one or more somatic symptoms that are distressing or result in significant disruption of daily life. The high bar set by DSM-IV with the requirement for eight medically unexplained symptoms was confusing. This simplified requirement should encompass the presentation of most of the individuals whose symptoms formerly met criteria for somatization disorder, pain disorder, and hypochondriasis.

Persons with somatic symptom disorder are excessively worried about their health, see their bodily symptoms as unduly threatening, and fear the medical seriousness of their symptoms. Health concerns often become an organizing principle for the individual's life, dominating all other concerns. Quality of life may be markedly impaired, and the disorder can lead to a high level of medical care utilization.

Criterion B

Rather than focusing on the medically unexplained nature of symptoms (the emphasis since DSM-III), this criterion now requires the presence of excessive thoughts, feelings, and behaviors related to these somatic symptoms or associated health concerns. This criterion requires at least one of the following: disproportionate and persistent thoughts about the seriousness of one's symptoms, persistently high level of anxiety about health or symptoms, or excessive time and energy devoted to these symptoms or health concerns.

Criterion C

This criterion requires the person to have been persistently symptomatic (typically for more than 6 months), but not necessarily with any one symptom. Symptom migration, in which an individual previously preoccupied with a particular symptom focuses on a new symptom, is not uncommon. For many individuals, preoccupation with somatic concerns begins early in life and lasts years or decades.

Specifiers

The specifiers allow the clinician to identify individuals whose predominant symptom is pain, as well as to rate the current severity of the condition as mild, moderate, or severe. Typically, the disorder is more severe when multiple somatic symptoms are present. The clinician can also specify whether the disorder's course is persistent.

Illness Anxiety Disorder

Research suggests that about one-quarter of persons with hypochondriasis had few somatic symptoms but were highly anxious and suspicious about the presence of a serious but undiagnosed medical illness. Most of these patients' presentations now fit the new diagnosis illness anxiety disorder. Unlike hypochondriasis, wherein failure to respond to reassurance is an explicit criterion, illness anxiety disorder has as its primary focus preoccupation with having or acquiring a serious (and undiagnosed) medical illness.

Although the individual's concern may be derived from a nonpathological physical sign or sensation, the distress tends not to come from the physical complaint itself, but rather from his or her anxiety about its meaning, significance, or cause. If the physical sign or symptom is present, it is often a normal physiological sensation, a benign and self-limited dysfunction, or a bodily discomfort not generally considered indicative of disease. If a diagnosable medical condition is present, the person's anxiety and preoccupation are clearly excessive and disproportionate to the severity of the condition. Individuals with this condition are easily alarmed about ill health and do not respond to appropriate medical reassurance, negative diagnostic tests, or a benign course. The clinician's attempt to reassure the patient is frequently not helpful. Incessant worry becomes frustrating to family members and may lead to considerable strain within marriages and families.

Diagnostic Criteria for Illness Anxiety Disorder   300.7 (F45.21)

A. Preoccupation with having or acquiring a serious illness.
B. Somatic symptoms are not present or, if present, are only mild in intensity. If another medical condition is present or there is a high risk for developing a medical condition (e.g., strong family history is present), the preoccupation is clearly excessive or disproportionate.
C. There is a high level of anxiety about health, and the individual is easily alarmed about personal health status.
D. The individual performs excessive health-related behaviors (e.g., repeatedly checks his or her body for signs of illness) or exhibits maladaptive avoidance (e.g., avoids doctor appointments and hospitals).
E. Illness preoccupation has been present for at least 6 months, but the specific illness that is feared may change over that period of time.
F. The illness-related preoccupation is not better explained by another mental disorder, such as somatic symptom disorder, panic disorder, generalized anxiety disorder, body dysmorphic disorder, obsessive-compulsive disorder, or delusional disorder, somatic type.

Specify whether:
   Care-seeking type: Medical care, including physician visits or undergoing tests and procedures, is frequently used.
   Care-avoidant type: Medical care is rarely used.

Criterion A

This criterion implies that somatic symptoms, if present, are relatively mild. This is important because the essence of this disorder is not the presence of symptoms, but rather the presence of health-related anxieties and preoccupations.

Criterion B

This criterion is similar to DSM-IV's Criterion A for hypochondriasis because both focus on the concern that one might have a serious illness. The operative word is *preoccupation* that is clearly excessive or disproportionate.

Criterion C

Although some people rarely think about health concerns, the person whose anxiety and alarm satisfy this criterion is hypervigilant about his or her health. Such people tend to monitor their bodies, enlarging the importance of each ache, pain, discoloration, bowel change, or noise.

Criterion D

Like the person with obsessive-compulsive disorder, the person who fears for his or her health engages in checking behaviors (e.g., to make sure there are no tumors or swellings) or copes with these feelings through avoidance behaviors.

Criterion E

Preoccupation with the illness must last 6 months or longer, but the specific illness feared may change over that period of time. In most cases, the clinician will note that the preoccupation has been chronic for months or years.

Criterion F

Because some psychiatric disorders can be associated with excessive health concerns, these other mental disorders and medical conditions must be ruled out as a cause of the disturbance. Individuals with obsessive-compulsive disorder will have other symptoms (e.g., washing, counting, hoarding). Although individuals with panic disorder may have concerns about having a heart attack, this concern occurs in the context of a panic attack.

Subtypes

The subtypes will enable the clinician to identify whether the individual is care seeking or care avoidant.

Conversion Disorder (Functional Neurological Symptom Disorder)

Conversion disorders have a long history in psychiatry. Individuals with this disorder have symptoms that simulate or mimic neurological illness. Typical symptoms include paralysis, abnormal movements, inability to speak (aphonia), blindness, and deafness. Pseudoseizures are also common and may occur in individuals with genuine epileptic seizures. Individuals with conversion disorders are commonly seen on neurology wards and on psychiatry consultation-liaison services at general hospitals.

Conversion disorders were described in the nineteenth century by Charcot and Freud and were considered a form of hysteria. Conversion reaction was included as a diagnosis in DSM-I. The disorder was renamed hysterical neurosis, conversion type, in DSM-II, which described it as "an involuntary psychogenic loss or disorder of function," with such symptoms as "blindness, deafness, anosmia, anesthesias, paresthesias, paralyses, ataxias, akinesias, and dyskinesias" (American Psychiatric Association 1968, pp. 39–40). Criteria were enumerated in DSM-III, with minor wording changes in subsequent editions.

For DSM-5, the name has been changed to include a parenthetical "functional neurological symptom disorder" because the disorder is often seen by neurologists. In addition, this term is more acceptable to patients. Importantly, DSM-IV Criterion B— "Psychological factors are judged to be associated with the symptom or deficit because the initiation or exacerbation of the symptom or deficit is preceded by conflicts or other stressors" (American Psychiatric Association 2000, p. 457)—has been deleted. This criterion was always problematic because it was difficult to reliably assess and required considerable subjective judgment on the part of the clinician. The work group proposed that the criterion be eliminated and that any discussion about a proposed etiological factor be placed in the text. Additional concerns were that this DSM-IV criterion was inconsistent with data showing that observed psychological factors are often nonspecific—that is, they occur in individuals with other conditions, often with a similar frequency. Furthermore, in many cases psychological factors cannot be convincingly demonstrated.

Another change is the deletion of DSM-IV Criterion C: "The symptom or deficit is not intentionally produced or feigned (as in Factitious Disorder or Malingering)" (American Psychiatric Association 2000, p. 457). This criterion was always difficult for clinicians to use because it is nearly impossible to know with any degree of confidence whether or not a person is feigning. Also, there is little evidence that feigning is more common in individuals with conversion disorder than in persons with other mental disorders.

Diagnostic Criteria for Conversion Disorder (Functional Neurological Symptom Disorder)

A. One or more symptoms of altered voluntary motor or sensory function.
B. Clinical findings provide evidence of incompatibility between the symptom and recognized neurological or medical conditions.
C. The symptom or deficit is not better explained by another medical or mental disorder.
D. The symptom or deficit causes clinically significant distress or impairment in social, occupational, or other important areas of functioning or warrants medical evaluation.

Coding note: The ICD-9-CM code for conversion disorder is **300.11,** which is assigned regardless of the symptom type. The ICD-10-CM code depends on the symptom type (see below).

Specify symptom type:
   (F44.4) With weakness or paralysis
   (F44.4) With abnormal movement (e.g., tremor, dystonic movement, myoclonus, gait disorder)
   (F44.4) With swallowing symptoms
   (F44.4) With speech symptom (e.g., dysphonia, slurred speech)
   (F44.5) With attacks or seizures
   (F44.6) With anesthesia or sensory loss
   (F44.6) With special sensory symptom (e.g., visual, olfactory, or hearing disturbance)
   (F44.7) With mixed symptoms
Specify if:
   Acute episode: Symptoms present for less than 6 months.
   Persistent: Symptoms occurring for 6 months or more.
Specify if:
   With psychological stressor *(specify stressor)*
   Without psychological stressor

Criterion A

The essential feature of conversion disorder is the presence of symptoms or subjective deficits affecting motor or sensory functioning, or apparent impairment in level of consciousness. Motor symptoms include weakness or paralysis of a body part; abnormal movements, such as tremor, jerky movements, and other hyper- or hypokinetic movement abnormalities; gait abnormalities; and abnormal limb posturing. Sensory symptoms include altered, reduced, or absent skin sensation, vision, or hearing. Episodes of abnormal generalized limb shaking with apparent impaired or loss of consciousness may resemble epileptic seizures (pseudoseizures). The person may collapse and be motionless and unresponsive in an episode resembling syncope or coma. Other symptoms include reduced or absent speech volume, a sensation of a lump in the throat, and diplopia.

Criterion B

Neurological disease must be excluded as a cause of the symptoms, and there must be positive evidence of functional neurological symptoms. Positive evidence depends on the demonstration of either internal inconsistency or incompatibility with disease. Internal inconsistency means physical evidence of a symptom, such as weakness, that can be demonstrated to be inconsistently present. For example, in Hoover's sign, weakness of hip extension returns to normal strength with contralateral hip flexion against resistance.

Criterion C

Other recognized medical conditions and mental disorders must be ruled out. Research shows that some individuals who receive a diagnosis of conversion disorder are later found to have medical or neurological illnesses that, in retrospect, accounted for their symptoms. Clinicians need to keep this information in mind and to have a healthy degree of skepticism. Conversion symptoms sometimes occur in individuals with depressive or bipolar disorders, anxiety disorders, and even schizophrenia. In these situations, the symptoms are likely attributable to the primary disorder. The possibility of feigning, as part of either factitious disorder or malingering, should be considered in the differential diagnosis.

Criterion D

People with functional neurological symptoms may have substantial physical and mental disability. The severity can be similar to that experienced by individuals with comparable neurological disease. For example, the disability of individuals with functional weakness is similar to that of individuals with multiple sclerosis of similar duration, and the effect of pseudoseizures on social and occupational functioning is similar to that experienced by people with epilepsy.

Specifiers

The clinician can choose to specify the patient's predominant symptoms (e.g., "with weakness or paralysis"), as well as course (acute episode or persistent), and whether a psychological stressor is present or not.

Psychological Factors Affecting Other Medical Conditions

The category currently called *psychological factors affecting other medical conditions* has a long history. DSM-I had detailed sections describing 10 *psychophysiologic autonomic and visceral disorders* (a term used in preference to *psychosomatic disorders*), each involving a different organ system (e.g., skin, musculoskeletal, respiratory), in which emotional factors were presumed to play a causative role. DSM-I stated, "These reactions represent the visceral expression of affect which may be thereby largely prevented from being conscious. These symptoms are due to a chronic and exaggerated state of the normal physiological expression of emotion, with the feeling, or subjective part, repressed. Such long continued visceral states may eventually lead to structural changes" (p. 29).

The category continued in DSM-II mostly unchanged other than shortening the term to *psychophysiologic disorder*. DSM-III revamped the concept to create a single category called psychological factors affecting physical condition. The authors of DSM-III noted that the diagnosis was rarely used and perpetuated the notion—since discredited—that physical symptoms were caused by emotional factors. Also, the term *psychophysiological* was discarded because the decision about whether the condition was psychophysiological or organic was arbitrary. The term was believed to decrease collaboration between specialists and was thought to perpetuate simplistic ideas about disease causation.

In DSM-III, psychological contributions to medical illness were integrated into the new multiaxial system. The approach taken was that psychological factors may be associated with the initiation or exacerbation of a physical disorder, which could be recorded on Axis III. However, "psychological factors affecting physical condition" was considered a category, not a specific diagnosis. With DSM-IV, the authors chose to move the category to the chapter "Other Conditions That May Be a Focus of Clinical Attention," and it was no longer considered a mental disorder. To make the category more useful, DSM-IV contained a subcategorization format that allowed clinicians to specify the ways in which the psychological or behavioral factors could affect medical conditions. For instance, the clinician could choose "personality traits or coping style affecting…" and then specify the general medical condition involved. (For example, a person could experience an exacerbation of his coronary artery disease because his denial leads him to ignore warnings to minimize physical exertion.)

In DSM-5, this category has been moved to this chapter on somatic symptom and related disorders to acknowledge the fact that somatic concerns are the main focus. The criteria have had only minor wording changes. In DSM-IV, psychological factors affecting medical condition had six subtypes. The subtypes were rarely used, however, and have been eliminated.

Psychological factors affecting other medical conditions may be confused with other DSM-5 categories that involve both psychological factors and medical symptoms. During differential diagnosis, the clinician should distinguish psychological factors affecting other medical conditions from the somatic symptom disorders; for example, with conversion disorder an individual may present with symptoms that suggest a neurological condition and are related to psychological factors. Unlike individuals with psychological factors affecting other medical conditions, those with somatic symptom disorders have no medical condition that adequately explains the physical symptoms.

The essential feature of psychological factors affecting other medical conditions is the presence of one or more clinically significant psychological or behavioral factors that adversely affect a medical condition by increasing the risk for suffering, death, or disability. These factors can adversely affect the medical condition by influencing its course or treatment, by constituting an additional health risk factor, or by exacerbating the physiology related to the medical condition. Psychological or behavioral factors include psychological distress, patterns of interpersonal interaction, coping styles, and maladaptive help behaviors, such as denial of symptoms or poor adherence to medical recommendations. Common examples are the person with anxiety exacerbating his or her asthma, denial of the need for treatment of acute chest pain, and manipulation of insulin by a person with diabetes wishing to lose weight. Current severity can be indicated using a specifier.

Diagnostic Criteria for Psychological Factors Affecting Other Medical Conditions   316 (F54)

A. A medical symptom or condition (other than a mental disorder) is present.
B. Psychological or behavioral factors adversely affect the medical condition in one of the following ways:

1. The factors have influenced the course of the medical condition as shown by a close temporal association between the psychological factors and the development or exacerbation of, or delayed recovery from, the medical condition.
2. The factors interfere with the treatment of the medical condition (e.g., poor adherence).
3. The factors constitute additional well-established health risks for the individual.
4. The factors influence the underlying pathophysiology, precipitating or exacerbating symptoms or necessitating medical attention.

C. The psychological and behavioral factors in Criterion B are not better explained by another mental disorder (e.g., panic disorder, major depressive disorder, posttraumatic stress disorder).

Specify current severity:
   Mild: Increases medical risk (e.g., inconsistent adherence with antihypertension treatment).
   Moderate: Aggravates underlying medical condition (e.g., anxiety aggravating asthma).
   Severe: Results in medical hospitalization or emergency room visit.
   Extreme: Results in severe, life-threatening risk (e.g., ignoring heart attack symptoms).

Criterion A

A medical symptom or condition other than a mental disorder must be present. As in the past, this could involve a disorder from any organ system.

Criteria B and C

Criterion B has been edited but is otherwise unchanged. It lists the ways in which the "psychological or behavioral factors" adversely affect the medical condition: this includes a clear-cut temporal relationship between these factors and the development and exacerbation of, or recovery from, the medical condition. It is important to establish that the factors interfere with treatment, constitute a well-established health risk, or influence the underlying physiology and pathophysiology to such an extent that they precipitate or exacerbate symptoms or necessitate medical attention. Other mental disorders need to be ruled out as a cause of the disturbance (Criterion C).

Specifiers

The clinician can indicate current severity indicators (mild, moderate, severe, or extreme) that track to indicators of medical risk.

Factitious Disorder

Factitious disorder involves the intentional falsification of physical or psychological signs or symptoms of illness, which in some cases leads the person to make hospitalization a way of life. The term *Munchausen syndrome* also has been used to describe patients who move from hospital to hospital simulating various illnesses. Cases of *Munchausen syndrome by proxy* have also been observed. In this instance, a parent induces (or simulates) illness in his or her child so that the child is repeatedly hospitalized. No reliable prevalence data are available, but factitious disorder is not uncommon.

Individuals are known to use various strategies to simulate illness. Some report symptoms suggesting an illness without having them. Others produce false evidence of an illness, such as a factitious fever produced by applying friction to a thermometer, or intentionally produce symptoms of illness, such as by injecting feces to produce infection. Factitious disorder is chronic and begins in early adulthood. Research evidence suggests that many persons with factitious disorder worked in health care occupations, and many have severely maladaptive personality traits. The disorder can severely impair social and occupational functioning.

The Somatic Symptoms Disorders Work Group recommended that factitious disorder be placed in the somatic symptom disorders chapter because physical symptoms are the main focus of concern. This placement should facilitate differential diagnosis for individuals who present with persistent problems related to illness perception, frequently including unexpected and/or unexplained psychological and/or physical symptoms. This move may also facilitate research on the broad spectrum of symptom-reporting phenomena, including the feigning of symptoms. The criteria recognize factitious disorder imposed on self and factitious disorder imposed on another (i.e., by proxy). The clinician can specify whether the disorder is a single episode or is recurrent.

Diagnostic Criteria for Factitious Disorder   300.19 (F68.10)

Factitious Disorder Imposed on Self

A. Falsification of physical or psychological signs or symptoms, or induction of injury or disease, associated with identified deception.
B. The individual presents himself or herself to others as ill, impaired, or injured.
C. The deceptive behavior is evident even in the absence of obvious external rewards.
D. The behavior is not better explained by another mental disorder, such as delusional disorder or another psychotic disorder.

Specify:
   Single episode
   Recurrent episodes (two or more events of falsification of illness and/or induction of injury)

Factitious Disorder Imposed on Another
(Previously Factitious Disorder by Proxy)

A. Falsification of physical or psychological signs or symptoms, or induction of injury or disease, in another, associated with identified deception.

B. The individual presents another individual (victim) to others as ill, impaired, or injured.

C. The deceptive behavior is evident even in the absence of obvious external rewards.

D. The behavior is not better explained by another mental disorder, such as delusional disorder or another psychotic disorder.

Note: The perpetrator, not the victim, receives this diagnosis.

Specify:

Single episode

Recurrent episodes (two or more events of falsification of illness and/or induction of injury)

Other Specified Somatic Symptom and Related Disorder and Unspecified Somatic Symptom and Related Disorder

Individuals whose somatic symptoms do not fit more specific diagnoses are diagnosed with other specified or unspecified somatic symptom and related disorder, both of which replace DSM-IV's somatoform disorder not otherwise specified.

The category other specified somatic symptom and related disorder is used when the clinician chooses to communicate the reason that the presentation does not meet full criteria. The clinician is encouraged to record the specific reason (e.g., brief somatic symptom disorder).

The category unspecified somatic symptom and related disorder is used when the individual does not meet full criteria for a more specific disorder that causes distress or impairment and the clinician chooses not to specify the reason the criteria are not met, or there is insufficient information to make a more specific diagnosis.

Other Specified Somatic Symptom and Related Disorder
300.89 (F45.8)

This category applies to presentations in which symptoms characteristic of a somatic symptom and related disorder that cause clinically significant distress or impairment in social, occupational, or other important areas of functioning predominate but do not meet the full criteria for any of the disorders in the somatic symptom and related disorders diagnostic class.

Examples of presentations that can be specified using the "other specified" designation include the following:

1. **Brief somatic symptom disorder:** Duration of symptoms is less than 6 months.
2. **Brief illness anxiety disorder:** Duration of symptoms is less than 6 months.
3. **Illness anxiety disorder without excessive health-related behaviors:** Criterion D for illness anxiety disorder is not met.

4. **Pseudocyesis:** A false belief of being pregnant that is associated with objective signs and reported symptoms of pregnancy.

Unspecified Somatic Symptom and Related Disorder

300.82 (F45.9)

This category applies to presentations in which symptoms characteristic of a somatic symptom and related disorder that cause clinically significant distress or impairment in social, occupational, or other important areas of functioning predominate but do not meet the full criteria for any of the disorders in the somatic symptom and related disorders diagnostic class. The unspecified somatic symptom and related disorder category should not be used unless there are decidedly unusual situations where there is insufficient information to make a more specific diagnosis.

KEY POINTS

- Somatic symptom and related disorders is a reformulated diagnostic class that replaces the somatoform disorders. The key element is that all disorders focus on physical symptoms and/or excessive health-related concerns. The class emphasizes affective, cognitive, and behavioral features of the disorders rather than focusing on physical symptoms.

- Somatic symptom disorder is a new diagnosis that replaces DSM-IV's somatization disorder, hypochondriasis, pain disorder, and undifferentiated somatoform disorder. The DSM-IV diagnoses were not well used, were considered pejorative, and did not foster positive doctor-patient interactions.

- Illness anxiety disorder is new to DSM-5 and is used to describe a preoccupation with having or acquiring a serious illness.

- Body dysmorphic disorder has been moved to a new chapter, "Obsessive-Compulsive and Related Disorders," based on research evidence showing its relatedness to obsessive-compulsive disorder.

- Factitious disorder and psychological factors affecting other medical conditions have been moved to this diagnostic class because of their central focus on physical symptoms.

CHAPTER 11

Feeding and Eating Disorders

307.52 (F__._) Pica
307.53 (F98.21) Rumination Disorder
307.59 (F50.8) Avoidant/Restrictive Food Intake Disorder
307.1 (F50.0_) Anorexia Nervosa
307.51 (F50.2) Bulimia Nervosa
307.51 (F50.8) Binge-Eating Disorder
307.59 (F50.8) Other Specified Feeding or Eating Disorder
307.50 (F50.9) Unspecified Feeding or Eating Disorder

The chapter on feeding and eating disorders has combined the feeding disorders (pica, rumination disorder) from the DSM-IV chapter "Disorders Usually First Diagnosed in Infancy, Childhood, or Adolescence" with the eating disorders (anorexia nervosa, bulimia nervosa) to better reflect their shared phenomenology and pathophysiology. The diagnosis avoidant/restrictive food intake disorder replaces and extends the DSM-IV diagnosis feeding disorder of infancy or early childhood. In addition, binge-eating disorder, previously included in DSM-IV's Appendix B, has now achieved full disorder status. Feeding and eating disorders reflect dysfunctional appetitive drive and behavior and can span the entire age range. Table 11–1 lists the disorders included in this chapter.

Disordered eating and eating-related behaviors have been recognized for centuries. Richard Morton (1636–1698) is credited with making the first clinical description of anorexia nervosa in 1689, but it was Sir William Gull (1816–1890) who coined the term in the late nineteenth century. Gull's patients were mostly emaciated young women with amenorrhea, constipation, and an abnormally slow pulse who were nonetheless remarkably overactive. His account of the disorder remains noteworthy for its attention to detail.

Despite Gull's and other descriptions, eating and feeding disorders were not listed in DSM until DSM-III, when they were included in the chapter "Disorders Usually First

TABLE 11–1. DSM-5 feeding and eating disorders
Pica
Rumination disorder
Avoidant/restrictive food intake disorder
Anorexia nervosa
Bulimia nervosa
Binge-eating disorder
Other specified feeding or eating disorder
Unspecified feeding or eating disorder

Diagnosed in Infancy, Childhood, or Adolescence." Eating disorders were given their own chapter in DSM-IV because it was clear that they could occur across the age range. In revisiting the issue, the DSM-5 Eating Disorders Work Group recommended that feeding disorders also be included in the same chapter with eating disorders because they, too, can occur across the age range.

Pica

The essential feature of pica is the eating of nonnutritive nonfood substances on a persistent basis for a period of at least 1 month. Medical accounts that resemble the modern-day definition of pica date back many centuries. Historically, pica has been considered either as an accompaniment to conditions such as pregnancy or developmental disabilities or as a symptom of medical disorders such as iron deficiency. Children up to age 24 months frequently mouth or even eat nonnutritive items, but this behavior does not suggest that the child has pica. Although frequently associated with children with developmental delays, pica is not confined to children or to individuals with intellectual developmental disorders.

Pica has been regarded as an independent disorder since its inclusion in DSM-III. The criteria were revised for DSM-5 to ensure that they can be used with individuals of any age.

Diagnostic Criteria for Pica

A. Persistent eating of nonnutritive, nonfood substances over a period of at least 1 month.

B. The eating of nonnutritive, nonfood substances is inappropriate to the developmental level of the individual.

C. The eating behavior is not part of a culturally supported or socially normative practice.

D. If the eating behavior occurs in the context of another mental disorder (e.g., intellectual disability [intellectual developmental disorder], autism spectrum disorder, schizophrenia) or medical condition (including pregnancy), it is sufficiently severe to warrant additional clinical attention.

Coding note: The ICD-9-CM code for pica is **307.52** and is used for children or adults. The ICD-10-CM codes for pica are **(F98.3)** in children and **(F50.8)** in adults.

Specify if:

In remission: After full criteria for pica were previously met, the criteria have not been met for a sustained period of time.

Criterion A

A single ingestion of a nonnutritive, nonfood substance is not sufficient to merit the diagnosis of pica. The eating must be persistent over a 1-month period. Changes to DSM-5 include the addition of the term *nonfood*; the wording "nonnutritive substances" was potentially problematic because, with nonfood not specified, the term could include foodstuffs with no nutritional value, such as diet soda.

Criterion B

Mouthing of objects, including nonnutritive, nonfood substances, is developmentally normal in young infants. A minimum age of 2 years is recommended because pica is not an appropriate diagnosis for young children.

Criterion C

People around the world eat clay or dirt (called *geophagy*) for a variety of reasons. Commonly, geophagy is a traditional cultural activity that takes place during pregnancy, for religious ceremonies, or as a remedy for disease, particularly in Central Africa and the Southern United States. The indigenous Pomo of Northern California also include dirt in their diet. Although it is a cultural practice, it may also fill a physiological need (or perceived need) for nutrients.

Criterion D

Pica frequently occurs in individuals with developmental delays and sometimes in pregnant women. Individuals with schizophrenia may have delusional beliefs about the need to ingest nonfood substances. If the eating behavior is severe enough to warrant independent clinical attention, then the additional diagnosis of pica is appropriate. DSM-5 has changed the wording from "during the course of" to "in the context of" to retain consistency with parallel criteria for rumination disorder and avoidant/restrictive food intake disorder, and because the example given (intellectual developmental disorder) does not run a course.

Rumination Disorder

Rumination disorder is characterized by the repeated regurgitation of food. Included in some form in the medical literature from the seventeenth century onward, rumination disorder occurs across the age range and in both genders. Individuals with this disorder repeatedly regurgitate swallowed or partially digested food, which may then be rechewed and either reswallowed or expelled. Adolescents and adults may be less likely to rechew regurgitated material. There is no involuntary retching, nausea, heartburn, odors, or abdominal pains associated with the regurgitation, as there is with typical vomiting. Although the disorder occurs more commonly in infants, young children, and individuals with developmental disabilities, it also occurs in otherwise healthy adolescents and adults. Unlike in typical vomiting, the regurgitation is typically described as effortless and unforced.

DSM-III included rumination disorder of infancy as an independent disorder. The criteria have been modified for DSM-5 to ensure that they are appropriate for individuals of any age.

Diagnostic Criteria for Rumination Disorder   307.53 (F98.21)

A. Repeated regurgitation of food over a period of at least 1 month. Regurgitated food may be re-chewed, re-swallowed, or spit out.
B. The repeated regurgitation is not attributable to an associated gastrointestinal or other medical condition (e.g., gastroesophageal reflux, pyloric stenosis).
C. The eating disturbance does not occur exclusively during the course of anorexia nervosa, bulimia nervosa, binge-eating disorder, or avoidant/restrictive food intake disorder.
D. If the symptoms occur in the context of another mental disorder (e.g., intellectual disability [intellectual developmental disorder] or another neurodevelopmental disorder), they are sufficiently severe to warrant additional clinical attention.

Specify if:
   In remission: After full criteria for rumination disorder were previously met, the criteria have not been met for a sustained period of time.

Criterion A

This criterion requires repeated regurgitation of food for at least 1 month. Not all individuals with rumination disorder, particularly older individuals and those with normal intelligence, rechew the regurgitated food. Therefore, DSM-5 has deleted the rechewing requirement and instead states, "Regurgitated food may be re-chewed, re-swallowed, or spit out." In addition, the DSM-IV requirement that the behavior follow "a period of normal functioning" has been deleted because this may be difficult to determine.

Criterion B

Individuals with rumination disorder may have a history of reflux, and it may be difficult clinically to reliably parse out the medical and psychological components of the behavior. In recognition of this clinical difficulty, DSM-5 requires ruling out an associated gastrointestinal or other medical condition.

Criterion C

Rumination behavior is well documented to occur in persons with conventional eating disorders. This criterion requires that the rumination be more than a symptom of one of the eating disorders. If it occurs apart from the eating disorder, then it can be independently diagnosed.

Criterion D

Rumination disorder commonly occurs in the context of developmental delays, often as a means of self-stimulation. In these cases, this behavior is more appropriately considered a symptom of these other disorders or conditions. If the rumination behavior is severe enough to warrant independent clinical attention, then the additional diagnosis of rumination disorder is appropriate. DSM-5 has changed the wording from "during the course of" to "in the context of" to maintain consistency with parallel criteria for pica and avoidant/restrictive food intake disorder and because the example given (intellectual disability [intellectual developmental disorder]) does not, strictly speaking, run a course.

Avoidant/Restrictive Food Intake Disorder

Avoidant/restrictive food intake disorder replaces and extends feeding disorder of infancy or early childhood from DSM-IV. This disorder is a disturbance of eating or feeding behavior that takes the form of avoiding or restricting food intake. The change in the formal name of the disorder reflects the fact that there are a number of types of presentation that occur across the age range rather than being restricted to infancy and early childhood. Three main subtypes have been identified in the existing literature: individuals who do not eat enough or show little interest in feeding or eating; individuals who accept only a limited diet in relation to sensory features; and individuals whose food refusal is related to aversive experience.

Avoidance or restriction associated with insufficient intake or lack of interest in food usually develops in infancy or early childhood, although it can begin in adolescence; onset in adulthood is rare. This disorder does not include developmentally normal food avoidance, which is characterized by picky eating in childhood or reduced food intake associated with advanced age. Pregnant women may restrict intake or avoid certain foods because of altered sensory sensitivities, but this is a self-limited behavior and the diagnosis of avoidant/restrictive food intake disorder is not warranted unless the eating disturbance is extreme and full criteria are met.

Avoidant/restrictive food intake disorder appears equally common in males and females in infancy and childhood. Various functional consequences are associated with this disorder: impairments in physical development, relationship and social difficulties, caregiver stress, and problems in family functioning.

This diagnosis has been renamed from feeding disorder of infancy or early childhood in DSM-IV, a diagnosis that was rarely used. In revamping this category, the authors of DSM-5 expect that the new category will be more useful. The category should potentially fill a clinical need because a substantial number of individuals—not exclusively children and adolescents—restrict their food intake and develop significant physiological and/or psychosocial problems, but their presentations fail to meet criteria for an eating disorder. Avoidance/restrictive food intake disorder is a broad category intended to capture this range of presentations.

Diagnostic Criteria for Avoidant/Restrictive Food Intake Disorder   307.59 (F50.8)

A. An eating or feeding disturbance (e.g., apparent lack of interest in eating or food; avoidance based on the sensory characteristics of food; concern about aversive consequences of eating) as manifested by persistent failure to meet appropriate nutritional and/or energy needs associated with one (or more) of the following:

1. Significant weight loss (or failure to achieve expected weight gain or faltering growth in children).
2. Significant nutritional deficiency.
3. Dependence on enteral feeding or oral nutritional supplements.
4. Marked interference with psychosocial functioning.

B. The disturbance is not better explained by lack of available food or by an associated culturally sanctioned practice.

C. The eating disturbance does not occur exclusively during the course of anorexia nervosa or bulimia nervosa, and there is no evidence of a disturbance in the way in which one's body weight or shape is experienced.

D. The eating disturbance is not attributable to a concurrent medical condition or not better explained by another mental disorder. When the eating disturbance occurs in the context of another condition or disorder, the severity of the eating disturbance exceeds that routinely associated with the condition or disorder and warrants additional clinical attention.

Specify if:

In remission: After full criteria for avoidant/restrictive food intake disorder were previously met, the criteria have not been met for a sustained period of time.

Criterion A

Many young children with avoidant/restrictive food intake difficulties had symptoms that failed to meet DSM-IV criteria for feeding disorder because of the primary focus in those criteria on failure to gain weight or weight loss, as well as the fact that certain features of presentation are also commonly seen in older individuals. "Feeding disturbance" has been replaced by "an eating or feeding disturbance" to account for the wider age range of people who have this disorder. Consequences resulting from food avoidance or restriction may persist, and this criterion has been expanded beyond weight loss or inability to gain weight. Faltering growth, nutritional deficiency, or dependency on enteral feeding or oral nutritional supplements, and marked interference with psychosocial functioning have been added because these are common clinically significant consequences of such eating or feeding disturbances.

Criterion B

Because extreme poverty and cultural practices, such as religious fasting, can also result in significant weight loss, this criterion includes the phrase "not better explained by lack of available food" and the requirement that there be no evidence that a "culturally sanctioned" practice alone, such as particular religious or cultural observations, might account for the disorder.

Criterion C

Restriction of energy intake relative to requirements resulting in weight loss is a core feature of anorexia nervosa and may be a compensatory behavior in bulimia nervosa. For older children or young adolescents, these disorders share a number of features, such as low weight and food avoidance. Anorexia nervosa, however, is associated with fear of gaining weight and perceptual disturbances regarding one's body weight or shape. In the case of bulimia nervosa, the restriction or fasting is a compensatory behavior for the recurrent episodes of binge eating. It is necessary to make a distinction between restricted food intake in the context of eating disorders, in which there are weight or shape concerns, and restricted food intake in which such concerns are not present.

Criterion D

Gastrointestinal (e.g., gastroesophageal reflux), endocrinological (e.g., diabetes), and neurological (e.g., those related to oral/esophageal/pharyngeal structural or functional problems) conditions can cause feeding disturbances and need to be distinguished from avoidant/restrictive food intake disorder.

Anorexia Nervosa

Anorexia nervosa is characterized by persistent energy intake restriction, an intense fear of gaining weight, and a distorted body self-perception. Anorexia nervosa was the first eating disorder described and appears to have been present at different points in history and to be present throughout different cultures. The disorder is associated with distorted self-image and other cognitive distortions regarding food and eating. Individuals with anorexia nervosa sometimes engage in repeated weighing, measuring, and assessing of their body in the mirror. The key clinical feature is defined as a refusal to maintain body weight at or above a minimally normal level for age, sex, developmental trajectory, and physical health. Anorexia nervosa is associated with high rates of morbidity (e.g., cardiac arrhythmias, growth retardation, osteoporosis) and mortality.

Anorexia nervosa typically has an onset in adolescence and is more prevalent among females. The disorder can affect men and women of any age, race or ethnicity, and socioeconomic background. The disorder has an estimated prevalence of 0.3%–1% in women and 0.1% in men.

Anorexia nervosa was listed in DSM-I as an example of psychophysiological gastrointestinal reaction and in DSM-II as a feeding disturbance within the special symptoms category. It finally achieved full disorder status in DSM-III. The core diagnostic criteria for anorexia nervosa are conceptually unchanged from DSM-IV, with one exception: *the requirement for amenorrhea has been eliminated* (DSM-IV's Criterion D). Some individuals with anorexia nervosa may exhibit all other symptoms and signs of the disorder and report at least some menstrual activity. In addition, this criterion could not be applied to premenarcheal girls, women taking oral contraceptives, postmenopausal women, or males. Because some data indicate that women who endorse amenorrhea have poorer bone health than do women who fail to meet this criterion, the information is clinically important even if not required for the diagnosis. In addition, the clinical characteristics and course for women with presentations that meet all the DSM-IV criteria for anorexia nervosa except amenorrhea closely resemble the characteristics of women with presentations that meet all of the criteria.

Diagnostic Criteria for Anorexia Nervosa

A. Restriction of energy intake relative to requirements, leading to a significantly low body weight in the context of age, sex, developmental trajectory, and physical health. *Significantly low weight* is defined as a weight that is less than minimally normal or, for children and adolescents, less than that minimally expected.

B. Intense fear of gaining weight or of becoming fat, or persistent behavior that interferes with weight gain, even though at a significantly low weight.

C. Disturbance in the way in which one's body weight or shape is experienced, undue influence of body weight or shape on self-evaluation, or persistent lack of recognition of the seriousness of the current low body weight.

Coding note: The ICD-9-CM code for anorexia nervosa is **307.1,** which is assigned regardless of the subtype. The ICD-10-CM code depends on the subtype (see below).

Specify whether:

(F50.01) Restricting type: During the last 3 months, the individual has not engaged in recurrent episodes of binge eating or purging behavior (i.e., self-induced vomiting or the misuse of laxatives, diuretics, or enemas). This subtype describes presentations in which weight loss is accomplished primarily through dieting, fasting, and/or excessive exercise.

(F50.02) Binge-eating/purging type: During the last 3 months, the individual has engaged in recurrent episodes of binge eating or purging behavior (i.e., self-induced vomiting or the misuse of laxatives, diuretics, or enemas).

Specify if:

In partial remission: After full criteria for anorexia nervosa were previously met, Criterion A (low body weight) has not been met for a sustained period, but either Criterion B (intense fear of gaining weight or becoming fat or behavior that interferes with weight gain) or Criterion C (disturbances in self-perception of weight and shape) is still met.

In full remission: After full criteria for anorexia nervosa were previously met, none of the criteria have been met for a sustained period of time.

Specify current severity:
The minimum level of severity is based, for adults, on current body mass index (BMI) (see below) or, for children and adolescents, on BMI percentile. The ranges below are derived from World Health Organization categories for thinness in adults; for children and adolescents, corresponding BMI percentiles should be used. The level of severity may be increased to reflect clinical symptoms, the degree of functional disability, and the need for supervision.

Mild: BMI $\geq$ 17 kg/m^2
Moderate: BMI 16–16.99 kg/m^2
Severe: BMI 15–15.99 kg/m^2
Extreme: BMI < 15 kg/m^2

Criterion A

The DSM-IV wording "Refusal to maintain body weight at or above a minimally normal weight for age and height" has been changed to emphasize the importance of energy homeostasis for maintenance of a minimally normal weight. This change allows for applicability of the diagnosis to individuals who employ increased activity as a means of reducing weight.

Criterion B

DSM-IV required "fear of weight gain." A significant minority of individuals with anorexia nervosa, however, explicitly deny experiencing such fear. Therefore, DSM-5 has added a clause to focus on behavior, "persistent behavior that interferes with weight gain, even though at a significantly low weight."

Criterion C

The wording of this item has changed from "denial of the seriousness of the current low body weight" in DSM-IV to "persistent lack of recognition of the seriousness of the current low body weight." The word *denial* was removed because of the lack of empirical evidence supporting its use and the concern that it conveyed a paternalistic and pejorative attitude.

Subtypes and Specifiers

In DSM-5, the subtypes restricting and binge-eating/purging are specified for the last 3 months. Although data suggest that subtyping is useful clinically and for research purposes, there is significant crossover between subtypes, and clinicians had difficulty specifying the subtype for the "current episode" of illness (the DSM-IV standard).

Clinicians can also specify whether the person's disorder is in full remission or in partial remission. The distinction is that with partial remission, in which low body weight (Criterion A) is no longer an issue, the person still has an intense fear of gaining weight or of being fat, or has a disturbed body image.

Current severity can be indicated by specifying whether the disorder is mild, moderate, severe, or extreme, based on body mass index.

Bulimia Nervosa

Bulimia nervosa is characterized by episodes of bingeing on food (i.e., consuming a large amount of food in a short amount of time), followed by attempts to purge the body of the food via vomiting, laxatives, or excessive exercise. The behavior is performed in the context of overconcern with weight and shape. Russell (1979) observed that both anorexia nervosa and bulimia nervosa are developmental disorders that share the characteristics fear of fatness and body image distortion. As with anorexia nervosa, there are medical consequences of bulimia nervosa, including loss of electrolytes, erosion of tooth enamel (due to repeated exposure to acidic gastric contents), cavities, stomach ulcers, stomach or esophagus ruptures, constipation, irregular heartbeat, and an increased tendency toward suicidal behavior. Bulimia nervosa also exhibits marked differences from anorexia nervosa. Individuals with bulimia nervosa tend to develop eating disorder symptoms later in life, generally lose less weight, and have a tendency to be more extroverted and impulsive than persons with anorexia nervosa.

This disorder, simply called "bulimia," was included in DSM-III. The name was changed to bulimia nervosa in DSM-III-R. Approximately 90% of people diagnosed with bulimia nervosa are women, and its prevalence is estimated at 1.0%–1.5% in young women.

The only change in the criteria is a reduction in the required minimum average frequency of binge eating and inappropriate compensatory behavior (Criterion C). Clinicians can now rate severity levels that range from mild to extreme depending on the number of episodes of inappropriate compensatory behaviors per week.

Although DSM-IV required that subtype (purging or nonpurging) be specified, a literature review indicated that individuals with the nonpurging subtype closely resembled individuals with binge-eating disorder. In addition, precisely how to define nonpurging inappropriate behaviors (e.g., fasting or excessive exercise) was unclear. For these reasons, DSM-5 has eliminated the purging and nonpurging subtypes for bulimia nervosa. Instead, clinicians can specify whether the disorder is in partial or full remission and the current severity (mild, moderate, severe, extreme).

Diagnostic Criteria for Bulimia Nervosa   307.51 (F50.2)

A. Recurrent episodes of binge eating. An episode of binge eating is characterized by both of the following:

  1. Eating, in a discrete period of time (e.g., within any 2-hour period), an amount of food that is definitely larger than what most individuals would eat in a similar period of time under similar circumstances.

  2. A sense of lack of control over eating during the episode (e.g., a feeling that one cannot stop eating or control what or how much one is eating).

B. Recurrent inappropriate compensatory behaviors in order to prevent weight gain, such as self-induced vomiting; misuse of laxatives, diuretics, or other medications; fasting; or excessive exercise.

C. The binge eating and inappropriate compensatory behaviors both occur, on average, at least once a week for 3 months.

D. Self-evaluation is unduly influenced by body shape and weight.

E. The disturbance does not occur exclusively during episodes of anorexia nervosa.

Specify if:

In partial remission: After full criteria for bulimia nervosa were previously met, some, but not all, of the criteria have been met for a sustained period of time.

In full remission: After full criteria for bulimia nervosa were previously met, none of the criteria have been met for a sustained period of time.

Specify current severity:

The minimum level of severity is based on the frequency of inappropriate compensatory behaviors (see below). The level of severity may be increased to reflect other symptoms and the degree of functional disability.

Mild: An average of 1–3 episodes of inappropriate compensatory behaviors per week.

Moderate: An average of 4–7 episodes of inappropriate compensatory behaviors per week.

Severe: An average of 8–13 episodes of inappropriate compensatory behaviors per week.

Extreme: An average of 14 or more episodes of inappropriate compensatory behaviors per week.

Criterion A

Many people may experience an isolated episode of overeating, such as at a party with unlimited free food. Bulimia nervosa is an appropriate diagnosis in cases in which there are recurrent episodes of binge eating that occur during a discrete period of time and involve the consumption of a large amount of food, and the person reports feeling a lack of control.

Criterion B

The bulimia nervosa diagnosis requires that the binge eating be accompanied by recurrent inappropriate compensatory behaviors intended to counteract the effects of the binge episode and prevent weight gain (e.g., vomiting, laxative abuse, diuretic abuse, excessive exercise).

Criterion C

Although DSM-IV required that episodes of binge eating and inappropriate compensatory behaviors both occur, on average, twice per week over a 3-month period, research found that the clinical characteristics of individuals reporting bingeing and purging once per week were similar to those of individuals whose behavior met the

DSM-IV twice-per-week criterion. DSM-5 therefore requires that the binge eating and inappropriate compensatory behaviors occur at least once a week for 3 months.

Criterion D

Individuals with bulimia nervosa are preoccupied with body shape and weight. They may report low self-esteem due to body image issues.

Criterion E

Individuals with anorexia nervosa may have a presentation that falls under the subtype referred to as *binge-eating/purging type,* which must be differentiated from bulimia nervosa. The diagnosis of anorexia nervosa requires a refusal to maintain normal body weight. When that requirement is met, the appropriate diagnosis is anorexia nervosa.

Binge-Eating Disorder

Binge-eating disorder is characterized by recurrent episodes of binge eating without the recurrent use of compensatory behaviors. It was listed in Appendix B ("Criteria Sets and Axes Provided for Further Study") in DSM-IV, and the DSM-5 Eating Disorders Work Group recommended that it achieve full disorder status. Binge-eating disorder is the most frequent eating disorder in the United States (1.6% of women, 0.8% of men) and is more prevalent among those seeking weight loss treatment than in the general population.

The distinction between binge-eating disorder and bulimia nervosa is sometimes unclear, and the two categories may represent different stages of the same underlying disorder. Compared with individuals with bulimia nervosa, people with binge-eating disorder are generally older, are more likely to be male, and have a later age at onset of the disorder.

Approximately two-thirds of individuals with binge-eating disorder have a history of using inappropriate compensatory behaviors, suggesting a past diagnosis of bulimia nervosa. Although weight and shape concerns are not required for the diagnosis, they are commonly part of the presentation.

Clinicians can rate current severity based on number of binge-eating episodes per week (although the level of severity may be increased to reflect other symptoms and the degree of functional disability). Clinicians can also specify whether the disorder is in partial or full remission.

Diagnostic Criteria for Binge-Eating Disorder   307.51 (F50.8)

A. Recurrent episodes of binge eating. An episode of binge eating is characterized by both of the following:

   1. Eating, in a discrete period of time (e.g., within any 2-hour period), an amount

of food that is definitely larger than what most people would eat in a similar period of time under similar circumstances.

2. A sense of lack of control over eating during the episode (e.g., a feeling that one cannot stop eating or control what or how much one is eating).

B. The binge-eating episodes are associated with three (or more) of the following:

1. Eating much more rapidly than normal.
2. Eating until feeling uncomfortably full.
3. Eating large amounts of food when not feeling physically hungry.
4. Eating alone because of feeling embarrassed by how much one is eating.
5. Feeling disgusted with oneself, depressed, or very guilty afterward.

C. Marked distress regarding binge eating is present.

D. The binge eating occurs, on average, at least once a week for 3 months.

E. The binge eating is not associated with the recurrent use of inappropriate compensatory behavior as in bulimia nervosa and does not occur exclusively during the course of bulimia nervosa or anorexia nervosa.

Specify if:

In partial remission: After full criteria for binge-eating disorder were previously met, binge eating occurs at an average frequency of less than one episode per week for a sustained period of time.

In full remission: After full criteria for binge-eating disorder were previously met, none of the criteria have been met for a sustained period of time.

Specify current severity:

The minimum level of severity is based on the frequency of episodes of binge eating (see below). The level of severity may be increased to reflect other symptoms and the degree of functional disability.

Mild: 1–3 binge-eating episodes per week.

Moderate: 4–7 binge-eating episodes per week.

Severe: 8–13 binge-eating episodes per week.

Extreme: 14 or more binge-eating episodes per week.

Criterion A

The requirement of binge eating mirrors that for bulimia nervosa. The criterion requires "recurrent episodes" to differentiate this disorder from context-specific instances where an individual may binge on food, such as at a wedding or banquet.

Criterion B

Criterion B requires at least three of five indicators of impaired control: eating much more rapidly than usual; eating until feeling uncomfortably full; eating large amounts of food when not hungry; eating alone because of embarrassment; and feeling disgust, depression, or guilt after the episode. The best overall indicators for correctly identifying binge eating are "eating large amounts of food when not feeling physically hungry" and "eating alone because of feeling embarrassed." Among men the most common feature of binge eating is eating more rapidly than usual, whereas among women the most common feature is feeling disgusted, depressed, or very guilty afterward. Research indicates that the requirement for three or more symptoms yields the most accurate prediction of binge eating while minimizing the false positives.

Criterion C

This criterion speaks to the specificity of distress associated with the binge eating. Distress related to co-occurring disorders would not meet this criterion.

Criterion D

Analyses based on once-weekly and twice-weekly classifications were remarkably similar. In DSM-IV Appendix B, it was suggested that the frequency of binge days, as opposed to binge episodes, be assessed, and that a minimum average frequency of twice per week over 6 months be required. Research indicates that criteria identical to those for bulimia nervosa would not change caseness significantly. Therefore, Criterion D was changed to be similar to Criterion C for bulimia nervosa, requiring at least once a week for 3 months.

Criterion E

Binge-eating disorder is characterized by the absence of recurrent use of inappropriate compensatory mechanisms after eating large amounts of food.

Other Specified Feeding or Eating Disorder and Unspecified Feeding or Eating Disorder

Other specified and unspecified feeding or eating disorder should be considered as diagnoses when the individual has symptoms of a feeding and eating disorder that are distressing and cause impairment but do not meet the full criteria for a more specific disorder in the class.

The categories replace DSM-IV's eating disorder not otherwise specified. The category other specified feeding or eating disorder is used when the clinician chooses to communicate the reason that the presentation does not meet full criteria. The clinician is encouraged to record the specific reason (e.g., atypical anorexia nervosa).

The category unspecified feeding or eating disorder is used when the clinician chooses not to specify the reason the criteria are not met, or there is insufficient information to make a more specific diagnosis.

Other Specified Feeding or Eating Disorder

307.59 (F50.8)

This category applies to presentations in which symptoms characteristic of a feeding and eating disorder that cause clinically significant distress or impairment in social, occupational, or other important areas of functioning predominate but do not meet the full criteria for any of the disorders in the feeding and eating disorders diagnostic class. The other specified feeding or eating disorder category is used in situations in which the clinician chooses to communicate the specific reason that the presentation does not meet the criteria for any specific feeding and eating disorder. This is done by recording "other specified feeding or eating disorder" followed by the specific reason (e.g., "bulimia nervosa of low frequency").

Examples of presentations that can be specified using the "other specified" designation include the following:

1. **Atypical anorexia nervosa:** All of the criteria for anorexia nervosa are met, except that despite significant weight loss, the individual's weight is within or above the normal range.
2. **Bulimia nervosa (of low frequency and/or limited duration):** All of the criteria for bulimia nervosa are met, except that the binge eating and inappropriate compensatory behaviors occur, on average, less than once a week and/or for less than 3 months.
3. **Binge-eating disorder (of low frequency and/or limited duration):** All of the criteria for binge-eating disorder are met, except that the binge eating occurs, on average, less than once a week and/or for less than 3 months.
4. **Purging disorder:** Recurrent purging behavior to influence weight or shape (e.g., self-induced vomiting; misuse of laxatives, diuretics, or other medications) in the absence of binge eating.
5. **Night eating syndrome:** Recurrent episodes of night eating, as manifested by eating after awakening from sleep or by excessive food consumption after the evening meal. There is awareness and recall of the eating. The night eating is not better explained by external influences such as changes in the individual's sleep-wake cycle or by local social norms. The night eating causes significant distress and/or impairment in functioning. The disordered pattern of eating is not better explained by binge-eating disorder or another mental disorder, including substance use, and is not attributable to another medical disorder or to an effect of medication.

Unspecified Feeding or Eating Disorder   307.50 (F50.9)

This category applies to presentations in which symptoms characteristic of a feeding and eating disorder that cause clinically significant distress or impairment in social, occupational, or other important areas of functioning predominate but do not meet the full criteria for any of the disorders in the feeding and eating disorders diagnostic class. The unspecified feeding or eating disorder category is used in situations in which the clinician chooses *not* to specify the reason that the criteria are not met for a specific feeding and eating disorder, and includes presentations in which there is insufficient information to make a more specific diagnosis (e.g., in emergency room settings).

KEY POINTS

- This chapter combines the feeding disorders, formerly placed in the DSM-IV chapter "Disorders Usually First Diagnosed in Infancy, Childhood, or Adolescence," with the eating disorders. Both groups of disorders are characterized by disturbed consummatory behaviors.

- The criteria for pica and rumination disorder have been revised to ensure that the disorders can be diagnosed in persons of all ages. Similarly, avoidant/restrictive food intake disorder no longer has an age restriction.

- The requirement that anorexia nervosa be accompanied by amenorrhea has been dropped because research showed little difference between those with or without the symptom.

- With bulimia nervosa, the only change in the criteria is a reduction in the required minimum average frequency of binge eating and inappropriate compensatory behavior to one episode per week (Criterion C), because research did not support the requirement in DSM-IV for two episodes per week.

- Binge-eating disorder has been elevated to full disorder status in DSM-5.

CHAPTER 12

Elimination Disorders

307.6 (F98.0) Enuresis
307.7 (F98.1) Encopresis
Other Specified Elimination Disorder
Unspecified Elimination Disorder

This chapter describes conditions in which the predominant disturbance is related to bowel or bladder problems. Elimination disorders are usually first diagnosed in childhood and include enuresis and encopresis (Table 12–1). Placed in the chapter "Disorders Usually First Diagnosed in Infancy, Childhood, or Adolescence" in DSM-III and DSM-IV, elimination disorders are now contained in a stand-alone chapter, which reflects a change in categorization recommended by the Childhood and Adolescent Disorders Work Group.

TABLE 12–1. DSM-5 elimination disorders

Enuresis

Encopresis

Other specified elimination disorder

Unspecified elimination disorder

Elimination disorders are common, with approximately 1% of children age 5 years having encopresis and 5%–10% of 5-year-olds having nocturnal enuresis. These disorders can continue into adolescence, with approximately 1% of adolescents experiencing nocturnal enuresis.

At least among older children, these disorders can be very embarrassing and have a negative impact on self-esteem. Impairment is often a reflection of how the disorders contribute to social ostracism and social withdrawal by the individuals, and to anger and rejection by caregivers.

Most elimination disorders have a functional cause and are not a neurological or medical condition. Children with these disorders are usually first evaluated by pediatricians and not mental health clinicians. This may reflect not only the obvious physical nature of the symptoms but also the ongoing controversy regarding when and to what extent these disorders are manifestations of underlying emotional problems.

Enuresis

Enuresis is characterized by repeated urination into clothing or the bed. The behavior is most often involuntary but it is sometimes intentional. Enuresis commonly occurs during nighttime sleep (nocturnal subtype) but it may also occur while the person is awake (diurnal subtype). Clinical judgment is necessary to assess the frequency of the behavior, the age beyond which it is appropriate, and the degree of distress or impairment associated with enuresis. The DSM-5 criteria reflect no substantive proposed changes to the DSM-IV criteria for enuresis.

Diagnostic Criteria for Enuresis   307.6 (F98.0)

A. Repeated voiding of urine into bed or clothes, whether involuntary or intentional.
B. The behavior is clinically significant as manifested by either a frequency of at least twice a week for at least 3 consecutive months or the presence of clinically significant distress or impairment in social, academic (occupational), or other important areas of functioning.
C. Chronological age is at least 5 years (or equivalent developmental level).
D. The behavior is not attributable to the physiological effects of a substance (e.g., a diuretic, an antipsychotic medication) or another medical condition (e.g., diabetes, spina bifida, a seizure disorder).

Specify whether:
   Nocturnal only: Passage of urine only during nighttime sleep.
   Diurnal only: Passage of urine during waking hours.
   Nocturnal and diurnal: A combination of the two subtypes above.

Criterion A

This criterion clarifies that enuresis can be either involuntary or intentional. (DSM-III required involuntary voiding.) The inclusion of intentional voiding allows the diagnosis to be made in children who are too embarrassed to ask to use the bathroom.

Criterion B

Given that short-term episodes of bed-wetting are common, the criterion requires a frequency and duration of at least twice weekly for at least 3 consecutive months, or the presence of clinically significant distress or impairment, in order to make the diagnosis. In contrast, the World Health Organization defines enuresis as wetting twice per month (under age 7 years) or once per month (age 7 years and older) in the past 3 months.

Criterion C

The minimal age criterion has been set at 5 years, but medical guidelines vary on when a child is old enough to stay dry. The majority of children are toilet trained for daytime by age 5 years, and nighttime toilet training usually happens several months later than daytime toilet training. Therefore, although it has been common practice to define enuresis as abnormal from age 5 years, many only consider treatment for children when they are at least 7 years old.

Criterion D

Medical conditions must be excluded as a cause of the bed-wetting. These include neurological disorders (e.g., seizures, spina bifida), other medical conditions (e.g., urinary tract infections, sickle cell anemia, diabetes, sleep apnea), and structural causes (e.g., urinary tract obstruction, congenital defect of the posterior valve of the urethra). As with any clinical problem, the clinician must exercise judgment and rule out alternative explanations for the condition.

Subtypes

Nocturnal only is the most common subtype, and bed-wetting typically occurs during the first one-third of the evening. The *diurnal only* subtype is more common in girls. Debate has focused on whether these subtypes are clinically useful or whether expanded subtyping would be more appropriate. For example, "urge incontinence" and "voiding postponement" are proposed subtypes of daytime enuresis that have been associated with distinct behavioral problems and psychiatric comorbidity. The International Children's Continence Society has suggested four subtypes of nocturnal enuresis based on whether the enuresis is primary (no dry period for longer than 6 months) or secondary (relapse after at least a 6-month dry spell) and whether it is monosymptomatic (no daytime bladder dysfunction) or nonmonosymptomatic (bladder symptoms such as urgency or voiding postponement can occur during the day).

Encopresis

Encopresis refers to the repeated involuntary or occasionally intentional passage of feces into inappropriate places after the mental age of 4 years without any underlying organic cause. Encopresis is most often caused by underlying functional constipation, impaction, and retention with subsequent overflow. Encopresis can occur without constipation, an event(s) often referred to as "nonretentive fecal soiling," although this type is less common. Encopresis is more common in boys. Children with soiling problems tend to have more psychological and behavioral problems than those without (Joinson et al. 2006). No changes have been made in the criteria for DSM-5.

Diagnostic Criteria for Encopresis　　　　　　　　307.7 (F98.1)

A. Repeated passage of feces into inappropriate places (e.g., clothing, floor), whether involuntary or intentional.
B. At least one such event occurs each month for at least 3 months.
C. Chronological age is at least 4 years (or equivalent developmental level).
D. The behavior is not attributable to the physiological effects of a substance (e.g., laxatives) or another medical condition except through a mechanism involving constipation.

Specify whether:
　　With constipation and overflow incontinence: There is evidence of constipation on physical examination or by history.
　　Without constipation and overflow incontinence: There is no evidence of constipation on physical examination or by history.

Criteria A and B

A diagnosis of encopresis requires defecating into inappropriate places at least once a month for at least 3 months. This requirement is in keeping with the Rome Diagnostic Criteria, a classification system created by pediatric gastroenterologists who set criteria for functional gastrointestinal disorders in childhood (Drossman and Dumitrascu 2006). These criteria have provided clinicians with a method for standardizing their definition of clinical disorders and have allowed researchers from various fields to study the pathophysiology and treatment of the same disorders from different points of view. The passage of feces may be either involuntary or intentional. When involuntary, the passage of feces is often related to constipation, impaction, and retention with subsequent overflow.

Criterion C

Toilet training is usually completed by age 3 years, and the age requirement of 4 years allows for some variability in normal toilet training. (In the case of children with developmental delays, the mental age must be at least 4 years.)

Criterion D

Medical explanations for the disturbance must be excluded before the diagnosis of encopresis is made. Possible medical causes include use of laxatives, anorectal malformations such as anal stenosis, spinal disorders (e.g., meningomyelocele, spinal tumor), Hirschsprung's disease, cerebral palsy, endocrine disorders (e.g., hypothyroidism, lead intoxication), and neuromuscular disorders.

Subtypes

Encopresis "with constipation and overflow incontinence" may result in feces that are poorly formed and leakage occurring mostly during the day. The incontinence usually resolves after treatment of the constipation. Encopresis "without constipation and overflow incontinence" usually results in feces of normal form and consistency and is more likely to be associated with oppositional defiant disorder or conduct disorder. Although studies of children based on subtyping have found no significant differences in behaviors or in social competence, subtyping of encopresis has treatment implications. Disimpaction and laxatives may be needed if constipation is present, whereas laxatives may worsen encopresis without constipation. Although DSM-5 does not define *constipation*, the Rome Diagnostic Criteria require two of the following symptoms: two or fewer defecations in the toilet per week; at least one episode of fecal incontinence per week; history of retentive posturing or excessive volitional stool retention; history of painful or hard bowel movements; presence of a large fecal mass in the rectum; and history of large-diameter stools that may obstruct the toilet.

Other Specified Elimination Disorder and Unspecified Elimination Disorder

Other specified elimination disorder refers to symptoms of an elimination disorder that cause significant distress or impairment in functioning but fail to meet full diagnostic criteria for any elimination disorder (e.g., passage of feces in inappropriate places for only 2 months). The clinician can use this disorder category and communicate the reason the symptoms or behavior did not meet full criteria for an elimination disorder. The clinician is encouraged to record the specific reason (e.g., "low-frequency enuresis").

Unspecified elimination disorder should be used when an individual presents with symptoms that are characteristic of an elimination disorder, with distress and functional impairment, but that do not meet full diagnostic criteria and the clinician chooses not to specify the reason the full criteria were not met, or there was insufficient information to do so.

Other Specified Elimination Disorder

This category applies to presentations in which symptoms characteristic of an elimination disorder that cause clinically significant distress or impairment in social, occupational, or other important areas of functioning predominate but do not meet the full criteria for any of the disorders in the elimination disorders diagnostic class. The other specified elimination disorder category is used in situations in which the clinician chooses to communicate the specific reason that the presentation does not meet the criteria for any specific elimination disorder. This is done by recording "other specified elimination disorder" followed by the specific reason (e.g., "low-frequency enuresis").

Coding note: Code **788.39 (N39.498)** for other specified elimination disorder with urinary symptoms; **787.60 (R15.9)** for other specified elimination disorder with fecal symptoms.

Unspecified Elimination Disorder

This category applies to presentations in which symptoms characteristic of an elimination disorder that cause clinically significant distress or impairment in social, occupational, or other important areas of functioning predominate but do not meet the full criteria for any of the disorders in the elimination disorders diagnostic class. The unspecified elimination disorder category is used in situations in which the clinician chooses *not* to specify the reason that the criteria are not met for a specific elimination disorder, and includes presentations in which there is insufficient information to make a more specific diagnosis (e.g., in emergency room settings).

Coding note: Code **788.30 (R32)** for unspecified elimination disorder with urinary symptoms; **787.60 (R15.9)** for unspecified elimination disorder with fecal symptoms.

KEY POINTS

- Now a separate diagnostic class, elimination disorders have been moved from the chapter "Disorders Usually First Diagnosed in Infancy, Childhood, or Adolescence."
- DSM-5 recognizes that enuresis may be intentional or involuntary.

CHAPTER 13

Sleep-Wake Disorders

307.42 (F51.01)   Insomnia Disorder
307.44 (F51.11)   Hypersomnolence Disorder
Narcolepsy

Breathing-Related Sleep Disorders
327.23 (G47.33)   Obstructive Sleep Apnea Hypopnea
Central Sleep Apnea
327.2_ (G47.3_)   Sleep-Related Hypoventilation

Circadian Rhythm Sleep-Wake Disorders
307.45 (G47.21)   Delayed Sleep Phase Type
307.45 (G47.22)   Advanced Sleep Phase Type
307.45 (G47.23)   Irregular Sleep-Wake Type
307.45 (G47.24)   Non-24-Hour Sleep-Wake Type
307.45 (G47.26)   Shift Work Type
307.45 (G47.20)   Unspecified Type

Parasomnias
Non–Rapid Eye Movement Sleep Arousal Disorders
307.46 (F51.3)   Sleepwalking Type
307.46 (F51.4)   Sleep Terror Type
307.47 (F51.5)   Nightmare Disorder
327.42 (G47.52)   Rapid Eye Movement Sleep Behavior Disorder
333.94 (G25.81)   Restless Legs Syndrome
Substance/Medication-Induced Sleep Disorder
780.52 (G47.09)   Other Specified Insomnia Disorder
708.52 (G47.00)   Unspecified Insomnia Disorder
780.54 (G47.19)   Other Specified Hypersomnolence Disorder
708.54 (G47.10)   Unspecified Hypersomnolence Disorder
780.59 (G47.8)   Other Specified Sleep-Wake Disorder
780.59 (G47.9)   Unspecified Sleep-Wake Disorder

Dysfunction in sleep or waking is among the most common reasons people seek health care.

The maintenance of a normal cycle of sleep and wakefulness is an important component of successful adaptation across the life cycle because robust circadian rhythms help regulate mood and enhance cognitive performance. Problems with sleep, sleep quality, and daytime alertness have enormous impact on quality of life and level of functioning.

The four stages of sleep include rapid eye movement (REM) sleep and three stages of non–rapid eye movement (NREM) sleep. Stage 1 NREM sleep is characterized by the disappearance of alpha waves and the appearance of theta waves on the electroencephalogram (EEG). Hypnic jerks are common in this stage. In stage 2 NREM sleep, sleep spindles and K-complexes are found on the EEG. Previously separated into two stages, stage 3 NREM sleep is *slow-wave sleep*, or deep sleep. Delta waves are seen on the EEG. Dreaming is more common in this stage than in other stages of NREM sleep but not as common as in REM sleep. REM sleep is characterized by rapid eye movement, low muscle tone, and rapid, low-voltage electroencephalographic activity. REM sleep alternates with periods of NREM sleep approximately every 90 minutes; in adults, REM sleep typically occupies 20%–25% of total sleep. During a normal night's sleep, most adults experience four to five periods of REM sleep. The REM episodes increase in duration during the night. The relative amount of REM sleep varies with age, with older age associated with less efficient sleep and less time spent in REM sleep.

Dysfunction in any of these sleep stages may result in a sleep-wake disorder. DSM has long recognized sleep disorders in some fashion. Somnambulism, or sleepwalking disorder, was the first sleep-wake disorder included in DSM-I. The disorder name was changed to disorder of sleep in DSM-II. DSM-III included both sleepwalking disorder and sleep terror disorder, but they were placed with the "Disorders Usually First Diagnosed in Infancy, Childhood, or Adolescence." A stand-alone chapter was developed for DSM-III-R and included the variety of disorders that are now recognized as sleep disorders. Several disorders were added to DSM-IV, such as narcolepsy and breathing-related sleep disorder.

DSM-5 recognizes 12 specific sleep-wake disorders as well as several other specified and unspecified disorders (Table 13–1). The chapter revision has been influenced by the second edition of the *International Classification of Sleep Disorders* (ICSD-2), published by the American Academy of Sleep Medicine (2005). The ICSD-2 contains over 70 specific sleep-wake diagnoses grouped into eight categories: insomnia, breathing-related sleep disorders, hypersomnias of central origin, circadian rhythm sleep disorders, parasomnias, sleep-related movement disorders, isolated symptoms and normal variants, and other sleep disorders. Although DSM-5 has not incorporated as many diagnoses as are contained in the ICSD-2, the current diagnoses are compatible with them.

The revisions in DSM-5 present a clinically useful approach to diagnosis. In DSM-IV, sleep disorders required the clinician to determine if the sleeping problem was a primary issue or a consequence of another problem. In DSM-5, use of the term *primary* has been dropped in favor of simply listing insomnia disorder if diagnostic criteria are met. Coexisting mental and physical disorders are listed, but without the use of terms

---

TABLE 13–1. DSM-5 sleep-wake disorders

Insomnia disorder

Hypersomnolence disorder

Narcolepsy

Breathing-related sleep disorders

   Obstructive sleep apnea hypopnea

   Central sleep apnea

   Sleep-related hypoventilation

Circadian rhythm sleep-wake disorders

   Delayed sleep phase type

   Advanced sleep phase type

   Irregular sleep-wake type

   Non-24-hour sleep-wake type

   Shift work type

Parasomnias

   Non–rapid eye movement sleep arousal disorders

     Sleepwalking type

     Sleep terror type

   Nightmare disorder

   Rapid eye movement sleep behavior disorder

   Restless legs syndrome

Substance/medication-induced sleep disorder

Other specified insomnia disorder

Unspecified insomnia disorder

Other specified hypersomnolence disorder

Unspecified hypersomnolence disorder

Other specified sleep-wake disorder

Unspecified sleep-wake disorder

---

such as *related to* or *due to,* which were used in DSM-IV. Such terms imply a causal relationship, which often cannot be established. By avoiding etiological assumptions, the classification system reminds clinicians that insomnia disorder usually requires independent clinical attention in addition to management of coexisting mental and physical disorders. The changes also recognize the bidirectional and interactive effects between sleep disorders and coexisting medical and mental disorders.

    The clinician confronted with complaints of sleep disturbance must define the nature of the complaint, whether primarily insomnia, excessive daytime sleepiness, disturbed mentation or behavior during sleep, or difficulties in the circadian placement of sleep. The first step in diagnosis should be to consider the individual's general medical condition, to determine whether the complaint represents a sleep disorder attributable to another medical condition. Furthermore, if the individual is taking a medication or using a substance, the clinician will need to consider the possibility of a substance/medication-induced sleep disorder.

If the main complaint is persistent insomnia and/or difficulty initiating or maintaining sleep, a diagnosis of insomnia disorder may be appropriate. If the primary complaint is excessive sleepiness, the clinician should consider the differential diagnosis of a hypersomnolence disorder, narcolepsy, or one of the breathing-related sleep disorders. If the individual frequently travels or is involved in shift work, or has a problem of sleep timing, a circadian rhythm sleep-wake disorder should be considered. If the individual's symptoms consist of predominantly behavioral or mental events during sleep (e.g., abrupt awakening, frightening dreams, or walking about while sleeping), the clinician should consider a diagnosis of an NREM sleep arousal disorder.

Insomnia Disorder

Insomnia, which is Latin for "no sleep," involves the predominant complaint of an inability to fall asleep or remain asleep. The word is also used to describe the condition of waking up not feeling restored or refreshed. Insomnia is the most common sleep complaint in the general population. It can be either acute (i.e., lasting one to several nights) or chronic (i.e., persisting for 1 month or longer). According to the National Center on Sleep Disorders Research at the National Institutes of Health, about 30%–40% of adults say they have symptoms of insomnia within a given year, and about 10%–15% of adults report chronic insomnia (National Institutes of Health 2005). Among individuals reporting chronic insomnia, most have chronic or intermittent symptoms, meaning that they experience difficulty sleeping for a few nights, followed by a few nights of adequate sleep before the problem returns.

Among those who report insomnia, sleep maintenance insomnia is the most frequent problem, followed by difficulty falling asleep and then early morning awakening. Complaints of poor sleep or insomnia increase with age, paralleling age-related changes in sleep-stage physiology. Young people with insomnia more frequently report difficulty falling asleep, whereas older individuals report middle and terminal insomnia. Furthermore, women of all ages report more sleep problems than men. Despite the large number of people with insomnia complaints, relatively few seek medical attention.

Insomnia can be a disorder in its own right or a symptom of another condition. Stress and worry are frequently blamed for insomnia. Insomnia can also occur with jet lag, shift work, and other major schedule changes. Research has consistently found a robust association between insomnia and psychiatric disorders—particularly depression and anxiety—across the life cycle. Persistent sleep disturbance was identified in the Epidemiologic Catchment Area study as a highly significant risk factor for the *subsequent* development of major depressive disorder (Ford and Kamerow 1989). Hence, early intervention to treat sleep disturbance might protect against depression.

Many changes have been made in the criteria for DSM-5 sleep-wake disorders. Three DSM-IV disorders—primary insomnia, insomnia related to another mental disorder, and sleep disorder due to a general medical condition, insomnia type—have been merged into the single DSM-5 diagnostic entity of insomnia disorder. The change moves away from the need to make causal attributions between co-occurring disorders, and acknowledges the interactive effects between sleep disorders and co-occurring medical or psychiatric conditions. Data show that in the majority of insomnia cases, the individual presents with another psychiatric or medical disorder, as opposed to the insomnia being a disorder on its own (i.e., primary insomnia in DSM-IV). Furthermore, the diagnostic reliability of insomnia, particularly primary insomnia, was relatively poor. Distinguishing between primary insomnia and insomnia due to a mental disorder or a medical condition was often difficult (or impossible), and the construct of secondary insomnia often led to undertreatment. In eliminating the distinction between primary and secondary insomnia, DSM-5 emphasizes that sleep disorders warrant independent clinical attention.

Diagnostic Criteria for Insomnia Disorder   307.42 (F51.01)

A. A predominant complaint of dissatisfaction with sleep quantity or quality, associated with one (or more) of the following symptoms:

1. Difficulty initiating sleep. (In children, this may manifest as difficulty initiating sleep without caregiver intervention.)
2. Difficulty maintaining sleep, characterized by frequent awakenings or problems returning to sleep after awakenings. (In children, this may manifest as difficulty returning to sleep without caregiver intervention.)
3. Early-morning awakening with inability to return to sleep.

B. The sleep disturbance causes clinically significant distress or impairment in social, occupational, educational, academic, behavioral, or other important areas of functioning.
C. The sleep difficulty occurs at least 3 nights per week.
D. The sleep difficulty is present for at least 3 months.
E. The sleep difficulty occurs despite adequate opportunity for sleep.
F. The insomnia is not better explained by and does not occur exclusively during the course of another sleep-wake disorder (e.g., narcolepsy, a breathing-related sleep disorder, a circadian rhythm sleep-wake disorder, a parasomnia).
G. The insomnia is not attributable to the physiological effects of a substance (e.g., a drug of abuse, a medication).
H. Coexisting mental disorders and medical conditions do not adequately explain the predominant complaint of insomnia.

Specify if:
  With non–sleep disorder mental comorbidity, including substance use disorders
  With other medical comorbidity
  With other sleep disorder

  Coding note: The code 780.52 (G47.00) applies to all three specifiers. Code also the relevant associated mental disorder, medical condition, or other sleep disorder immediately after the code for insomnia disorder in order to indicate the association.

Specify if:
> **Episodic:** Symptoms last at least 1 month but less than 3 months.
> **Persistent:** Symptoms last 3 months or longer.
> **Recurrent:** Two (or more) episodes within the space of 1 year.

Note: Acute and short-term insomnia (i.e., symptoms lasting less than 3 months but otherwise meeting all criteria with regard to frequency, intensity, distress, and/or impairment) should be coded as an other specified insomnia disorder.

Criterion A

DSM-5 has integrated the construct of sleep dissatisfaction into the definition of insomnia. Evidence suggests that the presence of sleep dissatisfaction in addition to insomnia symptoms increases considerably the proportion of individuals with daytime impairments relative to those with insomnia symptoms alone. Hence, adding sleep dissatisfaction to the definition of insomnia is likely to improve diagnostic specificity. This change could also improve detection of clinically significant insomnia among subgroups of individuals (e.g., older adults) who typically report little impairment or distress associated with insomnia symptoms but who are otherwise dissatisfied with their sleep. Criterion A requires dissatisfaction with quantity or quality regarding initiating sleep, maintaining sleep, or early morning awakenings. In addition, the criterion specifically highlights how these requirements may differ in children—that children may manifest difficulties initiating or maintaining sleep without caregiver intervention.

Criterion B

This criterion lists specific examples of the distress or impairments in daytime functioning resulting from insomnia. Many individuals with persistent insomnia (e.g., older adults) tend to minimize or underestimate the impact of insomnia on their daytime functioning, partly due to the lack of clear indicators of such impairments. This is likely to lead to underdiagnosis and absence of treatment. The addition of specific examples of impairments may enhance assessment and boost recognition of the impact of insomnia on daytime functioning.

Criteria C and D

Criterion C requires that the sleep disturbance be present for at least 3 nights each week (an addition in DSM-5). The minimum frequency criterion of 3 nights per week will differentiate individuals with occasional (subthreshold) insomnia from those with more clinically meaningful insomnia. Sensitivity and specificity indices are maximized (i.e., correct identification of true insomnia cases and correct exclusion of false positives), with a frequency of occurrence of insomnia falling between 3 and 4 nights per week. Also, this frequency criterion is consistent with that used in ICD-10 and with current research practices in the field. Evidence suggests that the frequency of occurrence of insomnia symptoms is an important determinant of morbidity and impairment.

The minimum duration of 3 months (Criterion D) reflects a change from the previous requirement of 1 month, which was a very short period to define insomnia as a chronic condition. By comparison, few psychiatric or medical conditions are considered chronic before they exceed 6- or 12-month durations. Insomnia lasting only 1 month might be better conceptualized as an *episode* rather than a disorder. Morbidity may also increase with insomnia persisting longer than 3 months.

Criterion E

This criterion requires that the sleep disturbance occur despite adequate opportunity for sleep. This criterion was added to help distinguish clinical insomnia from volitional sleep deprivation.

Criteria F, G, and H

These criteria are for ruling out other mental disorders and medical conditions. They indicate that the insomnia is not better explained by another sleep disorder, such as narcolepsy (or does not occur exclusively during the course of another sleep disorder); is not due to the effects of a substance (e.g., caffeine); and is not better explained by a coexisting medical condition or mental disorder.

Specifiers

Co-occurring mental health, substance use, and sleep disorders can be specified. In addition, there are three specifiers for the course of insomnia disorder: *episodic* (symptoms last at least 1 month but less than 3 months), *persistent* (symptoms last 3 months or longer), and *recurrent* (two or more episodes occur within the space of 1 year). Persistent insomnia is also associated with long-term consequences, including increased risks of major depressive disorder, hypertension, and myocardial infarction; increased absenteeism and reduced productivity at work; reduced quality of life; and increased economic burden.

Hypersomnolence Disorder

Excessive sleepiness poses a great challenge to the nearly one-third of adult Americans who report this problem (Ohayon et al. 2012). Although most healthy people require approximately 7 hours of sleep during the main sleep episode to feel refreshed and alert, many individuals curtail their sleep to meet social, vocational, or other demands. This exacts a high price, and many of these people struggle with excessive daytime sleepiness when they should be fully awake.

Excessive sleepiness can be associated with many sleep disorders, such as obstructive sleep apnea hypopnea, circadian rhythm sleep-wake disorders, and restless legs syndrome. It can also be induced by insomnia disorder, insufficient sleep, or poor sleep hygiene. When excessive sleepiness is associated with other symptoms, it qualifies for the diagnosis hypersomnolence disorder.

Dement et al. (1966) proposed that individuals with excessive daytime sleepiness, but without cataplexy, sleep paralysis, or sleep-onset REM periods, not be considered as having narcolepsy. Roth et al. (1972) later described a type of hypersomnia with sleep drunkenness that consists of difficulty coming to complete wakefulness, confusion, disorientation, poor motor coordination, and slowness, accompanied by deep and prolonged sleep. Abrupt sleep attacks seen in classic narcolepsy are not present in hypersomnolence disorder.

DSM-5 hypersomnolence disorder should be distinguished from excessive sleepiness related to insufficient sleep and from fatigue (tiredness not necessarily relieved by increased sleep and unrelated to sleep quantity or quality). Excessive sleepiness and fatigue are difficult to differentiate from hypersomnolence disorder and may overlap considerably. Individuals with this disorder have no difficulty falling asleep and have a sleep efficiency generally higher than 90%. They may experience confusional arousal upon awakening in the morning but also upon awakening from a daytime nap. During that period, the person appears awake but his or her behavior may be very inappropriate, with memory deficits, disorientation in time and space, and slow mentation and speech. The reduced vigilance and impaired cognitive response return to normal within 30–60 minutes (and sometimes longer). For some individuals with hypersomnolence disorder, the duration of the major sleep episode (nocturnal sleep for most individuals) is 9 hours or more. However, approximately 80% of individuals with a hypersomnolence disorder report their sleep as being nonrestorative, and just as many have difficulties awakening in the morning. Individuals with a hypersomnolence disorder may have daytime naps nearly every day regardless of the nocturnal sleep duration.

Several changes have been made from DSM-IV. DSM-5 has replaced the term *hypersomnia* with *hypersomnolence*. The disorder is characterized by a complaint of excessive sleepiness, which can be expressed in two main categories of symptoms: 1) excessive quantity of sleep, referring to extended nocturnal sleep or involuntary daytime sleep, and 2) deteriorated quality of wakefulness, referring to sleep propensity during wakefulness as shown by difficulty awakening or inability to remain awake when required. With DSM-IV, in many cases, severe excessive sleepiness symptoms remained undiagnosed because the excessive sleepiness was related to the quality of wakefulness, not the *quantity* of sleep. The term *hypersomnia* describes an excessive amount of sleep, whereas *hypersomnolence* refers to the main symptom of excessive sleepiness. Research shows that many individuals have excessive sleepiness that is not explained by another sleep disorder, but with normal amounts of sleep.

Epidemiological and clinical data indicate that individuals with hypersomnolence disorder often present with other psychiatric or medical conditions. DSM-5 has replaced three disorders—primary hypersomnia, hypersomnia related to another mental disorder, and sleep disorder due to a general medical condition, hypersomnia type—with a single diagnostic entity with specification of clinically comorbid conditions. The change in the terminology removes the need to make causal attributions between coexisting disorders and acknowledges the interactive effects of sleep disorders and coexisting medical and/or psychiatric disorders.

Diagnostic Criteria for Hypersomnolence Disorder 307.44 (F51.11)

A. Self-reported excessive sleepiness (hypersomnolence) despite a main sleep period lasting at least 7 hours, with at least one of the following symptoms:

1. Recurrent periods of sleep or lapses into sleep within the same day.
2. A prolonged main sleep episode of more than 9 hours per day that is nonrestorative (i.e., unrefreshing).
3. Difficulty being fully awake after abrupt awakening.

B. The hypersomnolence occurs at least three times per week, for at least 3 months.
C. The hypersomnolence is accompanied by significant distress or impairment in cognitive, social, occupational, or other important areas of functioning.
D. The hypersomnolence is not better explained by and does not occur exclusively during the course of another sleep disorder (e.g., narcolepsy, breathing-related sleep disorder, circadian rhythm sleep-wake disorder, or a parasomnia).
E. The hypersomnolence is not attributable to the physiological effects of a substance (e.g., a drug of abuse, a medication).
F. Coexisting mental and medical disorders do not adequately explain the predominant complaint of hypersomnolence.

Specify if:
   With mental disorder, including substance use disorders
   With medical condition
   With another sleep disorder
   Coding note: The code 780.54 (G47.10) applies to all three specifiers. Code also the relevant associated mental disorder, medical condition, or other sleep disorder immediately after the code for hypersomnolence disorder in order to indicate the association.

Specify if:
   Acute: Duration of less than 1 month.
   Subacute: Duration of 1–3 months.
   Persistent: Duration of more than 3 months.

Specify current severity:
Specify severity based on degree of difficulty maintaining daytime alertness as manifested by the occurrence of multiple attacks of irresistible sleepiness within any given day occurring, for example, while sedentary, driving, visiting with friends, or working.
   Mild: Difficulty maintaining daytime alertness 1–2 days/week.
   Moderate: Difficulty maintaining daytime alertness 3–4 days/week.
   Severe: Difficulty maintaining daytime alertness 5–7 days/week.

Criterion A

The clinical description of excessive sleepiness symptoms in DSM-IV was vague (i.e., complaint of excessive sleepiness "as evidenced by either prolonged sleep episodes or daytime sleep episodes that occur almost daily"). In many cases, severe excessive sleepiness symptoms remained undiagnosed because the excessive sleepiness was related to the *quality* of wakefulness, not the *quantity* of sleep. Additionally, in DSM-IV, no cut point was given to delineate what constituted a prolonged sleep episode. The threshold of 9 hours as indicative of a prolonged main sleep episode will help identify individuals with excessive amount of sleep. The choice of 9 hours was based on clinical evidence that individuals with hypersomnolence disorder (with or without long sleep time) sleep on average 8–8.5 hours on weekdays, and it represents the upper fifth percentile of the normal sleep distribution in the general population.

The DSM-IV symptom "daytime sleep episodes" has been refined: "Recurrent periods of sleep or lapses into sleep within the same day." This change allows for the inclusion of individuals who have a main sleep period of normal duration, defined as at least 7 hours of sleep, and have recurrent sleepiness episodes within the same day (at least two episodes). The duration of 7 hours was adopted because it is the average sleep duration of healthy adults, and it should reduce the possibility of including individuals whose excessive sleepiness might be due to insufficient sleep.

DSM-5 has added "difficulty being fully awake after abrupt awakening" as a core feature of excessive sleepiness. Difficulty in awakening from sleep is present in the majority of individuals (up to 78%) with hypersomnolence characterized by a long sleep time. Sleep inertia (sleep drunkenness) has been reported in 21%–72% of individuals with a hypersomnolence disorder. The addition of this symptom will increase precision in the identification of hypersomnolent individuals.

Criterion B

DSM-5 has added a minimum frequency criterion (i.e., three times per week) with excessive sleepiness. The frequency criterion (at least three times per week) was selected based on population data indicating that it was the best cutoff for sleepiness in terms of identifying individuals reporting impairment or distress associated with excessive sleepiness. The DSM-5 criterion replaces the "almost daily" requirement in DSM-IV and will help distinguish individuals with occasional sleepiness from those with more severe symptoms of excessive sleepiness.

DSM-5 also requires that the excessive sleepiness last at least 3 months. DSM-IV required a duration of 1 month, but that was perceived as too short a period to define excessive sleepiness as a chronic condition. Given that hypersomnolence disorder is generally a chronic condition, typically beginning in early adulthood, a time frame that reflects longer-term chronicity was chosen.

Criterion C

Irritability and cognitive dysfunction are frequent concerns of hypersomnolent individuals. Other symptoms may include anxiety, decreased energy, restlessness, slow speech, loss of appetite, and memory difficulties. Some individuals lose the ability to function in family, social, occupational, or other settings. Motor vehicle accidents are among the most serious of consequences stemming from excessive sleepiness. The National Sleep Foundation's (2005) Sleep in America poll indicated that 60% of behind-the-wheel adults have driven a motor vehicle while drowsy, and 13% have actually fallen asleep while driving at least once per month.

Criteria D, E, and F

Individuals with breathing-related sleep disorders may have patterns of excessive sleepiness, and circadian rhythm sleep-wake disorders are also often characterized by daytime sleepiness. Complaints of daytime sleepiness may occur with medical conditions (e.g., a major neurocognitive disorder), medications (e.g., antipsychotics), or mental disorders (e.g., during a major depressive episode or the depressed phase of bipolar disorder). A diagnosis of hypersomnolence disorder can be made in the presence of another current or past mental disorder as long as the other disorder does not completely explain the hypersomnolence.

Specifiers

The clinician may specify the presence of comorbid conditions: another mental disorder, including substance use disorders; another medical condition; and another sleep disorder. In each case, the specifier helps clarify the individual's condition.

In addition to the specifiers regarding co-occurring conditions, there are three specifiers available to describe course: *acute* (duration of less than 1 month), *subacute* (duration of 1–3 months), and *persistent* (duration of more than 3 months). Severity specifiers, based on difficulty maintaining daytime alertness, are included as well.

Narcolepsy

Narcolepsy is a disorder that leads to instability in the sleep-wake cycle. It causes excessive daytime sleepiness and leads to sudden onsets of REM sleep. Narcolepsy can put severe limitations on individuals' lives because of their inability to stay awake for long periods of time and because of the risk that accompanies sudden bouts of sleeping. It is a chronic condition that is treatable but not curable. Symptoms usually begin either between ages 15 and 25 years or between ages 30 and 35 years, but they can begin at any age. They include episodes of extreme drowsiness every 3–4 hours, dreamlike hallucinations, sleep paralysis, cataplexy (i.e., loss of all muscle tone in the body), and "sleep attacks" (i.e., short attacks triggered by varying conditions such as eating large meals, moments of high stress or tension, or being awake for more than 4 hours). Cataplexy can cause a person's head to drop or knees to buckle, or might cause the person to collapse in his or her seat or onto the floor, potentially leading to dangerous consequences.

The term *narcolepsy* was first used in 1880 by the French neurologist Gélineau, who used the term to describe a syndrome of recurrent, irresistible daytime sleep episodes, sometimes accompanied by sudden falls (Morin and Edinger 2009). The disorder was first included in DSM-IV and continues to be recognized in DSM-5. In the ICSD-2, both narcolepsy with catalepsy and narcolepsy without catalepsy are recognized as distinctive subtypes.

Evidence shows that narcolepsy is associated with a lowered amount of a protein called *hypocretin* in the brain. In the 1990s, hypocretin-2 gene deletions were found to be the disease mechanism in canine narcolepsy. In human studies, low levels of hypocretin-1 are found in the cerebrospinal fluid of narcolepsy patients, and losses of over 80% of hypocretin (orexin)–producing neurons in the dorsolateral hypothalamus have been reported in autopsy studies. One explanation might be that hypocretin-producing cells are destroyed by an autoimmune process.

Diagnostic Criteria for Narcolepsy

A. Recurrent periods of an irrepressible need to sleep, lapsing into sleep, or napping occurring within the same day. These must have been occurring at least three times per week over the past 3 months.

B. The presence of at least one of the following:

1. Episodes of cataplexy, defined as either (a) or (b), occurring at least a few times per month:

   a. In individuals with long-standing disease, brief (seconds to minutes) episodes of sudden bilateral loss of muscle tone with maintained consciousness that are precipitated by laughter or joking.

   b. In children or in individuals within 6 months of onset, spontaneous grimaces or jaw-opening episodes with tongue thrusting or a global hypotonia, without any obvious emotional triggers.

2. Hypocretin deficiency, as measured using cerebrospinal fluid (CSF) hypocretin-1 immunoreactivity values (less than or equal to one-third of values obtained in healthy subjects tested using the same assay, or less than or equal to 110 pg/mL). Low CSF levels of hypocretin-1 must not be observed in the context of acute brain injury, inflammation, or infection.

3. Nocturnal sleep polysomnography showing rapid eye movement (REM) sleep latency less than or equal to 15 minutes, or a multiple sleep latency test showing a mean sleep latency less than or equal to 8 minutes and two or more sleep-onset REM periods.

Specify whether:

347.00 (G47.419) Narcolepsy without cataplexy but with hypocretin deficiency: Criterion B requirements of low CSF hypocretin-1 levels and positive polysomnography/multiple sleep latency test are met, but no cataplexy is present (Criterion B1 not met).

347.01 (G47.411) Narcolepsy with cataplexy but without hypocretin deficiency: In this rare subtype (less than 5% of narcolepsy cases), Criterion B requirements of cataplexy and positive polysomnography/multiple sleep latency test are met, but CSF hypocretin-1 levels are normal (Criterion B2 not met).

347.00 (G47.419) Autosomal dominant cerebellar ataxia, deafness, and narcolepsy: This subtype is caused by exon 21 DNA (cytosine-5)-methyltransferase-1 mutations and is characterized by late-onset (age 30–40 years) narcolepsy (with low or intermediate CSF hypocretin-1 levels), deafness, cerebellar ataxia, and eventually dementia.

347.00 (G47.419) Autosomal dominant narcolepsy, obesity, and type 2 diabetes: Narcolepsy, obesity, and type 2 diabetes and low CSF hypocretin-1 levels have been described in rare cases and are associated with a mutation in the myelin oligodendrocyte glycoprotein gene.

347.10 (G47.429) Narcolepsy secondary to another medical condition: This subtype is for narcolepsy that develops secondary to medical conditions that cause infectious (e.g., Whipple's disease, sarcoidosis), traumatic, or tumoral destruction of hypocretin neurons.

Coding note (for ICD-9-CM code 347.10 only): Code first the underlying medical condition (e.g., 040.2 Whipple's disease; 347.10 narcolepsy secondary to Whipple's disease).

Specify current severity:

Mild: Infrequent cataplexy (less than once per week), need for naps only once or twice per day, and less disturbed nocturnal sleep.

Moderate: Cataplexy once daily or every few days, disturbed nocturnal sleep, and need for multiple naps daily.

Severe: Drug-resistant cataplexy with multiple attacks daily, nearly constant sleepiness, and disturbed nocturnal sleep (i.e., movements, insomnia, and vivid dreaming).

Criterion A

The wording of Criterion A has been changed from "Irresistible attacks of refreshing sleep that occur daily over at least 3 months" to focus on recurrent periods of an irrepressible need to sleep, lapses into sleep, or naps, occurring at least three times per week over the previous 3 months (when the individual is untreated).

Criterion B

In DSM-IV, only one of two criteria had to be met. In this revision, at least one of three criteria has to be met. Narcolepsy was originally described with the presence of cataplexy. Cataplexy is usually triggered by strong emotions, but studies have shown the type of emotions is more important than the intensity. Interestingly, joking is the most specific trigger that distinguishes true cataplexy in individuals with narcolepsy from other experiences reported by individuals without narcolepsy. Laughter is also commonly involved, although it may be more culturally dependent because mirth is the true trigger. In addition, cataplexy is almost always brief, and fewer than 15% of patients report that their attacks last longer than 2 minutes. From 5% to 10% of persons report having one attack per year (or fewer), and less than 20% report having attacks at least monthly (Dauvilliers et al. 2007). For this reason, several attacks per month is considered a reasonable frequency. For young children, the disorder may have a rapid onset that can occur over a few weeks. In these cases, cataplexy manifests differently, by semiconstant, tic-like partial hypotonia of the jaw with tongue protrusion or even a generalized weakness without a clear trigger. These rare cases evolve into the more classic form (with usual trigger) within 6 months to 1 year.

The finding of low cerebrospinal fluid (CSF) hypocretin-1 levels in individuals with narcolepsy has been replicated by investigators around the world. The particular threshold of less than or equal to one-third of mean control values, or ≤ 110 pg/mL, has been established by quantitative ROC (receiver operating characteristic) curves comparing samples drawn from individuals with narcolepsy with samples from healthy controls, patients with other sleep disorders (including narcolepsy without cataplexy, hypersomnia, insomnia), and patients with various acute or chronic neurological conditions (Burgess and Scammell 2012). Additionally, normal subjects essentially never have low CSF hypocretin levels, but some patients with severe acute neurological disorders (e.g., acute meningitis, severe head trauma) can have decreased CSF hypocretin, a finding that is reversible when or if the condition improves. Narcolepsy with cataplexy is almost always caused by hypocretin deficiency. Almost all patients with cataplexy have low or undetectable levels of hypocretin-1 in the CSF. In contrast, only 5%–30% of cases without cataplexy have low CSF hypocretin-1 levels.

In the late 1950s, it was discovered that individuals with narcolepsy also have a short REM sleep latency, a finding that led to using the multiple sleep latency test (MSLT) as a diagnostic test for narcolepsy (nocturnal sleep polysomnography showing mean sleep latency ≤15 minutes or, more recently, MSLT showing mean sleep latency ≤8 minutes with ≥2 sleep-onset REM periods in 4–5 naps as a positive test). The MSLT for narcolepsy-cataplexy has shown about 95% sensitivity and specificity, both when cataplexy is used as a gold standard and when CSF hypocretin has been measured. Research shows that the observation of a short REM latency during a nocturnal sleep study is more specific (~99%) but less sensitive (~50%) than a positive MSLT result (Andlauer et al. 2013). Sleep test criteria consistent with narcolepsy can be either a sleep-onset REM period at night (i.e., REM sleep latency ≤15 minutes) or a positive MSLT finding.

Subtypes and Specifiers

The subtypes allow the clinician to be more specific about causation by pinpointing the relationship of narcolepsy to hypocretin deficiency, chromosome 21 mutations, type 2 diabetes mellitus, neurological disorders, or an infectious cause. Current severity (mild, moderate, severe) may also be specified.

BREATHING-RELATED SLEEP DISORDERS

Rather than having a single set of criteria for breathing-related sleep disorder, as provided in DSM-IV, DSM-5 provides specific diagnostic criteria for a spectrum of breathing-related sleep disorders: obstructive sleep apnea hypopnea, central sleep apnea, and sleep-related hypoventilation. Although these disorders may share common underlying physiological risk factors (respiratory control instability), physiological and anatomical studies indicate differences in the pathogenesis of these disorders, with central sleep apnea less dependent on structural airway abnormalities as compared with obstructive sleep apnea, which is more dependent on increased upper airway resistance, and sleep-related hypoventilation, which is often comorbid with other disorders that depress ventilation. DSM-5 provides an overview of these interrelated disorders and specific definitions for each of these entities.

Obstructive Sleep Apnea Hypopnea

Obstructive sleep apnea hypopnea is the most common category of breathing-related sleep disorders. It is a potentially serious disorder in which breathing repeatedly stops and starts during sleep. A pause in breathing (and therefore total absence of airflow) is called an *apnea* episode. A decrease in airflow during breathing is called a *hypopnea* episode. Almost everyone has brief apnea episodes during sleep. The person with obstructive sleep apnea hypopnea is rarely aware of having difficulty breathing, even upon awakening. When the muscles relax, a person's airway narrows or closes as he or she breathes in, and breathing may be inadequate for 10–20 seconds. This period of inadequate breathing may lower the level of oxygen in the blood. The brain senses this impaired breathing and briefly rouses the person from sleep.

The most noticeable sign of obstructive sleep apnea hypopnea is *snoring.* This is recognized as a problem by others witnessing the individual during sleep episodes or is suspected because of its effects on the body. Because the muscle tone of the body ordinarily relaxes during sleep, and the airway at the throat is composed of walls of soft tissue, which can collapse, it is not surprising that breathing can be obstructed during sleep. Although a very minor degree of obstructive sleep apnea hypopnea is considered to be within the bounds of normal sleep, and many individuals experience episodes of obstructive sleep apnea at some point in life, only a small percentage of people are afflicted with chronic, severe obstructive sleep apnea hypopnea.

Obstructive sleep apnea hypopnea most commonly affects middle-age and older adults and people who are overweight. Signs and symptoms of obstructive sleep apnea hypopnea include excessive daytime sleepiness (hypersomnia), loud snoring, observed episodes of breathing cessation during sleep, abrupt awakenings accompanied by shortness of breath, awakening with a dry mouth or sore throat, morning headache, difficulty staying asleep (insomnia), and difficult-to-control high blood pressure. The breathing disruptions impair the ability to reach the desired deep, restful phases of sleep, resulting in sleepiness during waking hours. Diagnosis is based on polysomnographic findings and on symptoms.

Diagnostic Criteria for Obstructive Sleep Apnea Hypopnea   327.23 (G47.33)

A. Either (1) or (2):

  1. Evidence by polysomnography of at least five obstructive apneas or hypopneas per hour of sleep and either of the following sleep symptoms:

    a. Nocturnal breathing disturbances: snoring, snorting/gasping, or breathing pauses during sleep.

    b. Daytime sleepiness, fatigue, or unrefreshing sleep despite sufficient opportunities to sleep that is not better explained by another mental disorder (including a sleep disorder) and is not attributable to another medical condition.

  2. Evidence by polysomnography of 15 or more obstructive apneas and/or hypopneas per hour of sleep regardless of accompanying symptoms.

Specify current severity:

  Mild: Apnea hypopnea index is less than 15.

  Moderate: Apnea hypopnea index is 15–30.

  Severe: Apnea hypopnea index is greater than 30.

Criterion A

DSM-5 includes symptoms of nocturnal breathing disturbances in the diagnostic criteria for obstructive sleep apnea hypopnea. Nocturnal symptoms reflect the occurrence of breathing disorders during the sleep period. Objective measurements of snoring intensity correlate with apnea hypopnea index. Snoring and gasping contribute significantly to sleep apnea prediction and in some studies are the most significant symptoms associated with sleep apnea. DSM-5 also includes polysomnographic criteria in the diagnostic criteria. Symptom reports are not sufficiently sensitive or specific to diagnose breathing-related sleep disorders, although they can be used as screening tools.

Specifiers

The severity of obstructive sleep apnea hypopnea is delineated based on an apnea hypopnea index (i.e., the number of apneas plus hypopneas per hour of sleep, as determined by polysomnography or other overnight monitoring). The disorder is mild if the index is less than 15, moderate if the index is between 15 and 30, and severe if the index is greater than 30. Regardless of the apnea hypopnea index, the disorder is considered to be more severe when apneas and hypopneas are accompanied by significant oxygen hemoglobin desaturation or when sleep is severely fragmented as shown by an elevated arousal index (arousal index greater than 30) or reduced stages in deep sleep.

Central Sleep Apnea

Central sleep apnea is a disorder in which breathing repeatedly stops and starts during sleep. It occurs because the brain fails to send proper signals to the muscles that control breathing. In contrast, in obstructive sleep apnea hypopnea, a person cannot breathe normally because of upper airway obstruction. Central sleep apnea is less common, accounting for fewer than 5% of sleep apnea cases.

Common signs and symptoms of central sleep apnea include observed episodes of stopped breathing or abnormal breathing patterns during sleep, abrupt awakenings accompanied by shortness of breath, shortness of breath relieved by sitting up, difficulty staying asleep (insomnia), excessive daytime sleepiness (hypersomnia), difficulty concentrating, morning headaches, and snoring. Although snoring indicates some degree of increased obstruction of airflow, snoring may also be heard in the presence of central sleep apnea; however, snoring may not be as prominent with central sleep apnea as it is with obstructive sleep apnea hypopnea. Central sleep apnea is associated with several conditions, including heart failure and chronic opioid use.

In DSM-IV, central sleep apnea was included in the breathing-related sleep disorder diagnosis and did not have separate criteria. Specific diagnostic criteria for central sleep apnea have been developed for DSM-5.

Diagnostic Criteria for Central Sleep Apnea

A. Evidence by polysomnography of five or more central apneas per hour of sleep.

B. The disorder is not better explained by another current sleep disorder.

Specify whether:

327.21 (G47.31) Idiopathic central sleep apnea: Characterized by repeated episodes of apneas and hypopneas during sleep caused by variability in respiratory effort but without evidence of airway obstruction.

786.04 (R06.3) Cheyne-Stokes breathing: A pattern of periodic crescendo-decrescendo variation in tidal volume that results in central apneas and hypopneas at a frequency of at least five events per hour, accompanied by frequent arousal.

780.57 (G47.37) Central sleep apnea comorbid with opioid use: The pathogenesis of this subtype is attributed to the effects of opioids on the respiratory rhythm generators in the medulla as well as the differential effects on hypoxic versus hypercapnic respiratory drive.

Coding note (for 780.57 [G47.37] code only): When an opioid use disorder is present, first code the opioid use disorder: 305.50 (F11.10) mild opioid use disorder or 304.00 (F11.20) moderate or severe opioid use disorder; then code 780.57 (G47.37) central sleep apnea comorbid with opioid use. When an opioid use disorder is not present (e.g., after a one-time heavy use of the substance), code only 780.57 (G47.37) central sleep apnea comorbid with opioid use.

Note: See the section "Diagnostic Features" in DSM-5 text.

Specify current severity:

Severity of central sleep apnea is graded according to the frequency of the breathing disturbances as well as the extent of associated oxygen desaturation and sleep fragmentation that occur as a consequence of repetitive respiratory disturbances.

Criteria A and B

Apnea episodes require polysomnographic data indicating five or more central apneas per hour of sleep. Clinical symptoms are not sufficiently sensitive or specific to diagnose central sleep apnea, although they can be used as a screening tool. Other sleep disorders need to be ruled out as a cause of the disturbance.

Subtypes and Specifiers

Clinicians may indicate if 1) the disorder is idiopathic and unrelated to airway obstruction, 2) a Cheyne-Stokes breathing pattern is present (characterized by a pattern of periodic crescendo-decrescendo variation in tidal volume that results in central apneas and hypopneas occurring at a frequency of at least five events per hour that are accompanied by frequent arousals), or 3) the disorder appears to be comorbid with opioid use. Current severity may also be recorded.

Sleep-Related Hypoventilation

Sleep-related hypoventilation is the result of decreased respiration associated with elevated carbon dioxide levels during sleep. Sleep-related hypoventilation is characterized by frequent episodes of shallow breathing lasting longer than 10 seconds during sleep. It is frequently associated with lung disease or neuromuscular or chest wall disorders, or medication use.

DSM-5 provides specific diagnostic criteria for sleep-related hypoventilation rather than, as in DSM-IV, incorporating the condition within the single criteria set for breathing-related sleep disorder. Although breathing-related sleep disorders may share common underlying physiological risk factors (respiratory control instability), physiological and anatomical studies indicate differences in the pathogenesis of these disorders, with sleep-related hypoventilation often comorbid with other disorders that depress ventilation.

Diagnostic Criteria for Sleep-Related Hypoventilation

A. Polysomnograpy demonstrates episodes of decreased respiration associated with elevated CO_2 levels. (**Note:** In the absence of objective measurement of CO_2, persistent low levels of hemoglobin oxygen saturation unassociated with apneic/hypopneic events may indicate hypoventilation.)

B. The disturbance is not better explained by another current sleep disorder.

Specify whether:

327.24 (G47.34) Idiopathic hypoventilation: This subtype is not attributable to any readily identified condition.

327.25 (G47.35) Congenital central alveolar hypoventilation: This subtype is a rare congenital disorder in which the individual typically presents in the perinatal period with shallow breathing, or cyanosis and apnea during sleep.

327.26 (G47.36) Comorbid sleep-related hypoventilation: This subtype occurs as a consequence of a medical condition, such as a pulmonary disorder (e.g., interstitial lung disease, chronic obstructive pulmonary disease) or a neuromuscular or chest wall disorder (e.g., muscular dystrophies, postpolio syndrome, cervical spinal cord injury, kyphoscoliosis), or medications (e.g., benzodiazepines, opiates). It also occurs with obesity (obesity hypoventilation disorder), where it reflects a combination of increased work of breathing due to reduced chest wall compliance and ventilation-perfusion mismatch and variably reduced ventilatory drive. Such individuals usually are characterized by body mass index of greater than 30 and hypercapnia during wakefulness (with a pCO_2 of greater than 45), without other evidence of hypoventilation.

Specify current severity:

Severity is graded according to the degree of hypoxemia and hypercarbia present during sleep and evidence of end organ impairment due to these abnormalities (e.g., right-sided heart failure). The presence of blood gas abnormalities during wakefulness is an indicator of greater severity.

Criteria A and B

As is the case for the other sleep disorders, specific polysomnographic findings are required for the diagnosis. Other sleep disorders need to be ruled out before making this diagnosis.

Subtypes and Specifiers

The clinician can record whether the hypoventilation is idiopathic, attributable to the rare congenital central alveolar hypoventilation syndrome (which presents in the perinatal period with shallow breathing, or cyanosis and apnea during sleep), or attributable to a comorbid disorder such as a pulmonary disease. Current severity may be indicated as well.

CIRCADIAN RHYTHM SLEEP-WAKE DISORDERS

Circadian Rhythm Sleep-Wake Disorders

Human beings have biological rhythms known as *circadian rhythms* that are controlled by a biological clock and that work on a daily time scale. The rhythms affect body temperature, alertness, appetite, and hormone secretion, as well as sleep timing. Because of a person's circadian clock, sleepiness does not continuously increase as time passes. A person's desire and ability to fall asleep are influenced both by the length of time since the person woke from an adequate sleep and by internal circadian rhythms. Thus, the body is ready for sleep and for wakefulness at different times of the day.

A circadian rhythm sleep-wake disorder is a persistent or recurring pattern of sleep disruption resulting either from an altered sleep-wake schedule or from an inequality between a person's natural sleep-wake cycle and the sleep-related demands placed on him or her. The term *circadian rhythm* refers to a person's internal sleep- and wake-related rhythms that occur throughout a 24-hour period. The sleep disruption leads to insomnia or excessive sleepiness during the day, resulting in impaired functioning. People with circadian rhythm sleep-wake disorders are unable to sleep and wake at the times required for normal work, school, and social needs; however, they are generally able to get enough sleep if allowed to sleep and wake at the times dictated by their body clocks. Unless they also have another sleep disorder, their sleep is of normal quality.

DSM-5 circadian rhythm sleep-wake disorder criteria differ from DSM-IV in two notable areas. First, the name has changed from "circadian rhythm sleep disorders." Although it is well appreciated that individuals with circadian rhythm sleep-wake disorders have difficulty initiating and/or maintaining sleep, they also prominently suffer from impairment of wakefulness and often seek treatment for excessive sleepiness. Thus, the term *sleep-wake* captures the daytime and nighttime impairments in function that are characteristic of circadian dysfunction. Second, specifiers have been revised, as described later in this section.

Diagnostic Criteria for Circadian Rhythm Sleep-Wake Disorders

A. A persistent or recurrent pattern of sleep disruption that is primarily due to an alteration of the circadian system or to a misalignment between the endogenous circadian rhythm and the sleep–wake schedule required by an individual's physical environment or social or professional schedule.

B. The sleep disruption leads to excessive sleepiness or insomnia, or both.

C. The sleep disturbance causes clinically significant distress or impairment in social, occupational, and other important areas of functioning.

Coding note: For ICD-9-CM, code **307.45** for all subtypes. For ICD-10-CM, code is based on subtype.

Specify whether:

307.45 (G47.21) Delayed sleep phase type: A pattern of delayed sleep onset and awakening times, with an inability to fall asleep and awaken at a desired or conventionally acceptable earlier time.

> *Specify* if:
> **Familial:** A family history of delayed sleep phase is present.

> *Specify* if:
> **Overlapping with non-24-hour sleep-wake type:** Delayed sleep phase type may overlap with another circadian rhythm sleep-wake disorder, non-24-hour sleep-wake type.

307.45 (G47.22) Advanced sleep phase type: A pattern of advanced sleep onset and awakening times, with an inability to remain awake or asleep until the desired or conventionally acceptable later sleep or wake times.

> *Specify* if:
> **Familial:** A family history of advanced sleep phase is present.

307.45 (G47.23) Irregular sleep-wake type: A temporally disorganized sleep-wake pattern, such that the timing of sleep and wake periods is variable throughout the 24-hour period.

307.45 (G47.24) Non-24-hour sleep-wake type: A pattern of sleep-wake cycles that is not synchronized to the 24-hour environment, with a consistent daily drift (usually to later and later times) of sleep onset and wake times.

307.45 (G47.26) Shift work type: Insomnia during the major sleep period and/or excessive sleepiness (including inadvertent sleep) during the major awake period associated with a shift work schedule (i.e., requiring unconventional work hours).

307.45 (G47.20) Unspecified type

Specify if:

Episodic: Symptoms last at least 1 month but less than 3 months.

Persistent: Symptoms last 3 months or longer.

Recurrent: Two or more episodes occur within the space of 1 year.

Criteria A, B, and C

The sleep disruption is primarily due to a circadian system alteration or a mismatch between the demands of the person's environment or work/social schedule and the person's internal circadian sleep-wake cycle. This mismatch leads to sleep disturbances, which in turn result in excessive sleepiness or insomnia, or both, as well as distress or functional impairment.

Subtypes and Specifiers

Subtypes include delayed sleep phase type, advanced sleep phase type, irregular sleep-wake type, non-24-hour sleep-wake type, and shift work type, as well as an unspecified type. The delayed sleep phase type may be further specified as familial or overlapping with non-24-hour sleep-wake type.

Delayed sleep phase type is based on a delay in the timing of the major sleep period (usually more than 2 hours) in relation to the desired sleep and wake times, resulting in difficulties waking in the morning and excessive sleepiness at work and impaired sleep at home.

The diagnosis of advanced sleep phase type is based primarily on a history of an advance in the timing of the major sleep period (usually more than 2 hours) in relation to the desired sleep and wake times, which results in symptoms of early morning insomnia and excessive daytime sleepiness. The rationale for inclusion of advanced sleep phase type was based on strong empirical evidence of earlier timing of circadian biomarkers, including melatonin and core body temperature rhythms, occurring 2–4 hours earlier than normal.

The diagnosis of irregular sleep-wake type is based primarily on a history of symptoms of insomnia at night (during the usual sleep period) and excessive sleepiness (napping) during the day. This type is characterized by a lack of discernible sleep-wake circadian rhythm. The individual has no major sleep period, and sleep is fragmented into at least three periods during the 24-hour day. In otherwise healthy subjects, the condition may be a result of very poor sleep hygiene; however, the irregular sleep-wake type is commonly associated with neurological impairment, such as developmental disability in children and dementia in older adults.

The diagnosis of non-24-hour sleep-wake type is based primarily on a history of symptoms of insomnia and/or excessive sleepiness due to lack of a stable entrainment or synchronization between the timing of the endogenous circadian rhythm and the 24-hour light-dark cycle. Individuals will typically present with periods of insomnia, excessive sleepiness, or both, alternating with asymptomatic periods. Starting with the asymptomatic period when the individual's sleep phase is aligned to the external environment, sleep latency will gradually increase and the individual will complain of sleep-onset insomnia. As the sleep phase continues to drift so that clock-drive for sleep is now in the daytime, individuals will have trouble staying awake during the day and complain of sleepiness, with subsequent negative impact on affect, cognition, and function. Because the circadian period is not aligned to the external 24-hour environment, symptoms will depend on when an individual tries to sleep in relation to the circadian rhythm of sleep propensity. The diagnosis of shift work type is based on a history of regularly scheduled work outside the daytime window of 8:00 A.M. to 6:00 P.M. This results in excessive sleepiness at work and impaired sleep at home.

The DSM-IV jet lag subtype has been dropped. The jet lag subtype was removed because travel across time zones typically involves transient or short-term impairments, and the sleep-wake dysfunction may represent normal physiology rather than a pathological response.

PARASOMNIAS

Parasomnias are disorders characterized by abnormal behavioral, experiential, or physiological events occurring in association with sleep, specific sleep stages, or sleep-wake transitions.

Non–Rapid Eye Movement Sleep Arousal Disorders

The conditions making up the NREM sleep arousal disorders—sleepwalking and sleep terrors—represent variations of the simultaneous admixture of elements of both wakefulness and NREM sleep, a combination that results in the appearance of complex motor behavior without conscious awareness (sometimes called "state dissociation"). The overlap of these conditions in people and in animals is well established. The fact that human sleep can be characterized by the simultaneous coexistence of wake-like and sleeplike electroencephalographic patterns in different cortical areas supports the state-dissociation concept of NREM sleep arousal disorders.

Diagnostic Criteria for Non–Rapid Eye Movement Sleep Arousal Disorders

---

A. Recurrent episodes of incomplete awakening from sleep, usually occurring during the first third of the major sleep episode, accompanied by either one of the following:

1. **Sleepwalking:** Repeated episodes of rising from bed during sleep and walking about. While sleepwalking, the individual has a blank, staring face; is relatively unresponsive to the efforts of others to communicate with him or her; and can be awakened only with great difficulty.
2. **Sleep terrors:** Recurrent episodes of abrupt terror arousals from sleep, usually beginning with a panicky scream. There is intense fear and signs of autonomic arousal, such as mydriasis, tachycardia, rapid breathing, and sweating, during each episode. There is relative unresponsiveness to efforts of others to comfort the individual during the episodes.

B. No or little (e.g., only a single visual scene) dream imagery is recalled.
C. Amnesia for the episodes is present.
D. The episodes cause clinically significant distress or impairment in social, occupational, or other important areas of functioning.

E. The disturbance is not attributable to the physiological effects of a substance (e.g., a drug of abuse, a medication).

F. Coexisting mental and medical disorders do not explain the episodes of sleep-walking or sleep terrors.

Coding note: For ICD-9-CM, code **307.46** for all subtypes. For ICD-10-CM, code is based on subtype.

Specify whether:

307.46 (F51.3) Sleepwalking type

Specify if:

With sleep-related eating

With sleep-related sexual behavior (sexsomnia)

307.46 (F51.4) Sleep terror type

Criteria A, B, and C

NREM sleep arousal disorders are characterized by repeated episodes of incomplete arousals from sleep, usually beginning during the first third of the major sleep episode. The individual may *sleepwalk* (defined as repeated episodes of complex motor behavior initiated during sleep, including rising from bed and walking about) or experience *sleep terrors* (repeated occurrence of precipitous awakenings from sleep in abrupt terror, usually beginning with a panicky scream). If the individual awakens after these arousals, little or none of the dream or only fragmentary, single images are recalled and the person has amnesia for the episode.

Criteria D, E, and F

Consistent with other DSM-5 disorders, NREM sleep arousal disorders must be associated with clinically significant distress or impairment. The physiological effects of a substance (e.g., a drug of abuse, a medication) must be ruled out as a cause, as must coexisting other mental disorders and medical conditions.

Nightmare Disorder

Nightmare disorder is characterized by recurrent dreams that feel threatening or frightening or cause dysphoria. The person becomes fully oriented when awakened and can usually remember the dream. Because nightmares are relatively common in the general population, nightmare disorder should be considered only in cases where the nightmares are recurrent and result in significant distress or impairment.

Diagnostic Criteria for Nightmare Disorder · 307.47 (F51.5)

A. Repeated occurrences of extended, extremely dysphoric, and well-remembered dreams that usually involve efforts to avoid threats to survival, security, or physical integrity and that generally occur during the second half of the major sleep episode.

B. On awakening from the dysphoric dreams, the individual rapidly becomes oriented and alert.

C. The sleep disturbance causes clinically significant distress or impairment in social, occupational, or other important areas of functioning.

D. The nightmare symptoms are not attributable to the physiological effects of a substance (e.g., a drug of abuse, a medication).

E. Coexisting mental and medical disorders do not adequately explain the predominant complaint of dysphoric dreams.

Specify if:

During sleep onset

Specify if:

With associated non–sleep disorder, including substance use disorders
With associated other medical condition
With associated other sleep disorder

Coding note: The code 307.47 (F51.5) applies to all three specifiers. Code also the relevant associated mental disorder, medical condition, or other sleep disorder immediately after the code for nightmare disorder in order to indicate the association.

Specify if:

Acute: Duration of period of nightmares is 1 month or less.
Subacute: Duration of period of nightmares is greater than 1 month but less than 6 months.
Persistent: Duration of period of nightmares is 6 months or greater.

Specify current severity:

Severity can be rated by the frequency with which the nightmares occur:

Mild: Less than one episode per week on average.
Moderate: One or more episodes per week but less than nightly.
Severe: Episodes nightly.

Criteria A and B

DSM-5 has replaced "repeated awakenings" with "repeated occurrences." The change removes the requirement that nightmares awaken the individual and thereby removes the distinction made by some between nightmares (which cause awakenings) and bad dreams (which do not). The distress due to nightmares extends beyond the disruptions of nocturnal sleep that awakenings produce. First, up to 36% of chronic and 56% of acute nightmare patients report not suffering from awakenings from sleep, whereas as few as 11% claim that their nightmares always awaken them. Second, 69% of patients with nightmare disorder report having had at least one (nonawakening) bad dream whose emotional intensity is of equal or greater magnitude than that reported for their nightmares. For 22% of individuals, mean intensity ratings for their bad dreams equal or exceed mean intensity ratings for their nightmares (Hasler and Germain 2009). Third, even the most unpleasant dreams do not necessarily awaken the sleeper; clinicians have described many individuals who dream of dying violently in their dreams without waking up. These findings together point to the existence of a substantial group of individuals who have extremely intense, disturbing dreams that do not awaken them. When nightmares terminate upon awakening, the person exhibits a rapid return to full alertness. Dysphoria may persist into wakefulness and contribute to difficulty returning to sleep and lasting daytime distress.

DSM-5 has also changed "extended and extremely frightening dreams, usually involving threats to survival, security, or self-esteem" to "extended, extremely dysphoric, and well-remembered dreams that usually involve efforts to avoid threats to survival, security, or physical integrity." Fear may be the most common emotion characterizing nightmares, but it is by no means the only one. Studies indicate that a variety of dysphoric emotions occur in nightmares, including anger, sadness, frustration, disgust, confusion, and guilt. In fact, 30% of nightmares and 51% of bad dreams contain primary emotions other than fear (Nielsen and Zadra 2010)

Criterion C

Nightmares cause more significant subjective distress than demonstrable social or occupational impairment. If nightmares result in frequent awakenings or sleep avoidance, however, individuals may experience excessive daytime sleepiness, poor concentration, depression, anxiety, or irritability. Some individuals with nightmare disorder minimize or underestimate the impact of nightmares on their functioning, partly due to the lack of clear indicators of such impairments. This could lead to underdiagnosis and undertreatment.

Criteria D and E

The nightmare symptoms are not attributable to the physiological effects of a substance. The term *attributable to* more accurately reflects the fact that the precise causality of the nightmares is not known. Other mental disorders (e.g., panic disorder) and medical conditions (e.g., nocturnal seizures) need to be ruled out as possible causes of the dysphoric dreams. Bereavement may also be a cause of the dreams.

Rapid Eye Movement Sleep Behavior Disorder

REM sleep behavior disorder in both human beings and animals is well established and has the potential to cause dramatic and potentially violent or injurious behavior arising from REM sleep. Seen in animal experiments in the 1960s, REM sleep behavior disorder was first described in humans in 1986. Since then, it has been identified as one of the major types of parasomnias, likely second only in prevalence to the NREM sleep arousal disorders. The clinical features, polysomnographic findings (present in nearly every case), and response to medication have been well characterized. REM sleep behavior disorder is one of the most important causes of sleep-related injurious or violent behavior.

The extraordinary relationship between REM sleep behavior disorder and neurodegenerative disorders (particularly Parkinson's disease, dementia with Lewy bodies, and multiple system atrophy) has been clearly established. At least 50% of individuals with REM sleep behavior disorder presenting in sleep clinics will eventually (often with a delay of over 10 years) develop one of these conditions. REM sleep behavior disorder may be more prevalent in psychiatric populations. In addition, iatrogenic REM sleep behavior disorder induced by medications commonly prescribed by psychiatrists, including tricyclic antidepressants, selective serotonin reuptake inhibitors, or serotonin-norepinephrine reuptake inhibitors, is becoming increasingly recognized.

Diagnostic Criteria for Rapid Eye Movement Sleep Behavior Disorder   327.42 (G47.52)

A. Repeated episodes of arousal during sleep associated with vocalization and/or complex motor behaviors.

B. These behaviors arise during rapid eye movement (REM) sleep and therefore usually occur more than 90 minutes after sleep onset, are more frequent during the later portions of the sleep period, and uncommonly occur during daytime naps.

C. Upon awakening from these episodes, the individual is completely awake, alert, and not confused or disoriented.

D. Either of the following:
1. REM sleep without atonia on polysomnographic recording.
2. A history suggestive of REM sleep behavior disorder and an established synucleinopathy diagnosis (e.g., Parkinson's disease, multiple system atrophy).

E. The behaviors cause clinically significant distress or impairment in social, occupational, or other important areas of functioning (which may include injury to self or the bed partner).

F. The disturbance is not attributable to the physiological effects of a substance (e.g., a drug of abuse, a medication) or another medical condition.

G. Coexisting mental and medical disorders do not explain the episodes.

Criteria A, B, C, and D

REM sleep behavior disorder is characterized by repeated episodes of arousal, often associated with vocalizations and/or complex motor behaviors, during REM sleep. These behaviors often reflect motor responses to the content of action-filled or violent dreams and have been referred to as "dream-enacting behaviors." These behaviors may be very bothersome to the individual and the bed partner and can result in significant injury (e.g., falling, jumping out of bed, punching, or kicking). These behaviors occur only during REM sleep. Upon awakening, the individual is immediately alert and oriented and can usually recall the dream content. Further, either 1) REM sleep without atonia on polysomnographic recording or 2) a history suggestive of REM sleep behavior disorder and an established synucleinopathy diagnosis (e.g., Parkinson's disease) is present.

Criteria E, F, and G

The diagnosis of REM sleep behavior disorder requires clinically significant distress or impairment. The physiological effects of a substance (e.g., a drug of abuse, a medication) or another medical condition must be ruled out as causing the disturbance, and coexisting mental or medical disorders must have also been ruled out as a cause.

Restless Legs Syndrome

Restless legs syndrome is a sensorimotor, neurological sleep disorder characterized by a desire to move the legs (or arms), usually associated with uncomfortable sensations typically described as creeping, crawling, tingling, burning, or itching. Symptoms are worse when the individual is at rest, and frequent movements of the legs occur in an effort to relieve the uncomfortable sensations. Symptoms are worse in the evening or night and in some individuals occur only in the evening or night. In DSM-5, restless legs syndrome has been elevated to disorder status. DSM-IV included a brief summary of restless legs syndrome within the broader category of dyssomnia not otherwise specified.

Restless legs syndrome is common, with prevalence rates from 2.7% to 7.2% (the lower rates reflecting the added requirement of at least moderate distress). Women are 1.5–2 times more likely than men to have restless legs syndrome (Allen et al. 2005).

Restless legs syndrome is associated with significant clinical and functional impairment. The disorder is well documented to be associated with reduced sleep time, sleep fragmentation, and reports of more sleep disturbance. Objective studies demonstrate significant, objective sleep abnormalities for individuals with restless legs syndrome, with increased latency to sleep and higher arousal index as the most consistent findings.

Diagnostic Criteria for Restless Legs Syndrome   333.94 (G25.81)

A. An urge to move the legs, usually accompanied by or in response to uncomfortable and unpleasant sensations in the legs, characterized by all of the following:

 1. The urge to move the legs begins or worsens during periods of rest or inactivity.
 2. The urge to move the legs is partially or totally relieved by movement.
 3. The urge to move the legs is worse in the evening or at night than during the day, or occurs only in the evening or at night.

B. The symptoms in Criterion A occur at least three times per week and have persisted for at least 3 months.

C. The symptoms in Criterion A are accompanied by significant distress or impairment in social, occupational, educational, academic, behavioral, or other important areas of functioning.

D. The symptoms in Criterion A are not attributable to another mental disorder or medical condition (e.g., arthritis, leg edema, peripheral ischemia, leg cramps) and are not better explained by a behavioral condition (e.g., positional discomfort, habitual foot tapping).

E. The symptoms are not attributable to the physiological effects of a drug of abuse or medication (e.g., akathisia).

Criteria A and B

Criteria A and B are in line with the essential diagnostic features as defined in DSM-IV and are compatible with descriptions in the literature. Urges to move the legs must occur at least three times per week over a 3-month period to qualify for the diagnosis. This helps ensure that the disorder is not simply a transient disturbance.

Criterion C

Restless legs syndrome must significantly affect functioning or cause distress. Although the impact of milder symptoms is not well characterized, people may complain of disruption in at least one activity of daily living, with half reporting a negative impact on mood and nearly half reporting lack of energy. The most common consequences of restless legs syndrome are sleep disturbances, including reduced sleep time and sleep fragmentation.

Criteria D and E

Symptoms of restless legs syndrome cannot be solely accounted for by another mental disorder or medical or behavioral condition or by medication effects. The differentiation of restless legs syndrome from other conditions is important because many people report some urge or need to move the legs while at rest and do not have the disorder. The most important mimics of restless legs syndrome are leg cramps, positional discomfort, arthralgias or arthritis, myalgias, positional ischemia (numbness), leg edema, peripheral neuropathy, radiculopathy, and habitual foot tapping. Muscle "knots" or cramps, relief with a single postural shift, limitation in joints, soreness on palpation, and other abnormalities on physical examination are not characteristic of the syndrome. Worsening at night and periodic limb movements are more common in restless legs syndrome than in medication-induced akathisia or peripheral neuropathy.

Substance/Medication-Induced Sleep Disorder

In DSM-5, substance- and medication-induced sleep disturbances are combined in a single category. The essential feature of substance/medication-induced sleep disorder is a prominent sleep disturbance judged to be primarily associated with the known effects of a substance of abuse or a medication. These disturbances are relatively common in clinical settings but are not always straightforward to diagnose, and they depend on several factors, including the type of substance (or medication), the individual's response to the agent, and the substance's pharmacology. For example, caffeine is one of the most common causes of disrupted sleep and needs to be ruled out as a cause in any investigation of insomnia. Depending on the substance, one of four subtypes of sleep disturbance may be reported: insomnia type, daytime sleepiness type, parasomnia type, and a mixed type for cases in which more than one type of sleep disturbance is present and none predominates.

DSM-5 has included tobacco-induced sleep disorder in the list of diagnoses. Empirical evidence indicates that nicotine may be a sleep-disturbing substance.

Diagnostic Criteria for Substance/Medication-Induced Sleep Disorder

A. A prominent and severe disturbance in sleep.

B. There is evidence from the history, physical examination, or laboratory findings of both (1) and (2):

1. The symptoms in Criterion A developed during or soon after substance intoxication or after withdrawal from or exposure to a medication.

2. The involved substance/medication is capable of producing the symptoms in Criterion A.

C. The disturbance is not better explained by a sleep disorder that is not substance/medication-induced. Such evidence of an independent sleep disorder could include the following:

The symptoms precede the onset of the substance/medication use; the symptoms persist for a substantial period of time (e.g., about 1 month) after the cessation of acute withdrawal or severe intoxication; or there is other evidence suggesting the existence of an independent non-substance/medication-induced sleep disorder (e.g., a history of recurrent non-substance/medication-related episodes).

D. The disturbance does not occur exclusively during the course of a delirium.

E. The disturbance causes clinically significant distress or impairment in social, occupational, or other important areas of functioning.

Note: This diagnosis should be made instead of a diagnosis of substance intoxication or substance withdrawal only when the symptoms in Criterion A predominate in the clinical picture and when they are sufficiently severe to warrant clinical attention.

Coding note: The ICD-9-CM and ICD-10-CM codes for the [specific substance/medication]-induced sleep disorders are indicated in the table below. Note that the ICD-10-CM code depends on whether or not there is a comorbid substance use disorder present for the same class of substance. If a mild substance use disorder is comorbid with the substance-induced sleep disorder, the 4th position character is "1," and the clinician should record "mild [substance] use disorder" before the substance-induced sleep disorder (e.g., "mild cocaine use disorder with cocaine-induced sleep disorder"). If a moderate or severe substance use disorder is comorbid with the substance-induced sleep disorder, the 4th position character is "2," and the clinician should record "moderate [substance] use disorder" or "severe [substance] use disorder," depending on the severity of the comorbid substance use disorder. If there is no comorbid substance use disorder (e.g., after a one-time heavy use of the substance), then the 4th position character is "9," and the clinician should record only the substance-induced sleep disorder. A moderate or severe tobacco use disorder is required in order to code a tobacco-induced sleep disorder; it is not permissible to code a comorbid mild tobacco use disorder or no tobacco use disorder with a tobacco-induced sleep disorder.

		ICD-10-CM		
	ICD-9-CM	With use disorder, mild	With use disorder, moderate or severe	Without use disorder
Alcohol	291.82	F10.182	F10.282	F10.982
Caffeine	292.85	F15.182	F15.282	F15.982
Cannabis	292.85	F12.188	F12.288	F12.988
Opioid	292.85	F11.182	F11.282	F11.982
Sedative, hypnotic, or anxiolytic	292.85	F13.182	F13.282	F13.982
Amphetamine (or other stimulant)	292.85	F15.182	F15.282	F15.982
Cocaine	292.85	F14.182	F14.282	F14.982
Tobacco	292.85	NA	F17.208	NA
Other (or unknown) substance	292.85	F19.182	F19.282	F19.982

Specify whether:
Insomnia type: Characterized by difficulty falling asleep or maintaining sleep, frequent nocturnal awakenings, or nonrestorative sleep.
Daytime sleepiness type: Characterized by predominant complaint of excessive sleepiness/fatigue during waking hours or, less commonly, a long sleep period.
Parasomnia type: Characterized by abnormal behavioral events during sleep.
Mixed type: Characterized by a substance/medication-induced sleep problem characterized by multiple types of sleep symptoms, but no symptom clearly predominates.
Specify if (see Table 16–1 in the chapter "Substance-Related and Addictive Disorders" for diagnoses associated with substance class):
With onset during intoxication: This specifier should be used if criteria are met for intoxication with the substance/medication and symptoms developed during the intoxication period.
With onset during discontinuation/withdrawal: This specifier should be used if criteria are met for discontinuation/withdrawal from the substance/medication and symptoms developed during, or shortly after, discontinuation of the substance/medication.

Criteria A and B

The criteria require that the sleep disturbance be severe. This limits the diagnosis to sleep problems that merit independent clinical attention. The criteria further require that one can attribute the sleep disturbance to the pharmacological effects of the substance.

Criterion C

Criterion C requires that the disturbance not be better accounted for by a sleep disorder that is not induced by a substance or medication. Evidence could include the following: 1) symptoms precede onset of the substance or medication use; 2) symptoms persist for a substantial period of time (e.g., about 1 month) after the cessation of acute withdrawal or severe intoxication; or 3) there is other evidence suggesting the existence of an independent non-substance/medication-induced sleep disorder (e.g., a history of recurrent non-substance/medication-related episodes).

Criterion D

If the sleep disturbance occurs only during the course of a delirium, it should not warrant a separate diagnosis.

Criterion E

The sleep disturbance from the substance needs to result in clinically significant distress or impairment. Increased risk for relapse is one unique functional consequence of this disorder.

Other Specified Insomnia Disorder and Unspecified Insomnia Disorder

These are residual categories to use for symptoms of an insomnia disorder that cause clinically significant distress or impairment but do not meet criteria for a more specific disorder in the class. The category other specified insomnia disorder is used when the clinician chooses to communicate the reason that the presentation does not meet full criteria. The clinician is encouraged to record the specific reason (e.g., brief insomnia disorder).

The category unspecified insomnia disorder is used when the clinician chooses *not* to specify the reason the criteria are not met, or there is insufficient information to make a more specific diagnosis.

Other Specified Insomnia Disorder   780.52 (G47.09)

This category applies to presentations in which symptoms characteristic of insomnia disorder that cause clinically significant distress or impairment in social, occupational, or other important areas of functioning predominate but do not meet the full criteria for insomnia disorder or any of the disorders in the sleep-wake disorders diagnostic class. The other specified insomnia disorder category is used in situations in which the clinician chooses to communicate the specific reason that the presentation does not meet the criteria for insomnia disorder or any specific sleep-wake disorder. This is done by recording "other specified insomnia disorder" followed by the specific reason (e.g., "brief insomnia disorder").

Examples of presentations that can be specified using the "other specified" designation include the following:

1. **Brief insomnia disorder:** Duration is less than 3 months.
2. **Restricted to nonrestorative sleep:** Predominant complaint is nonrestorative sleep unaccompanied by other sleep symptoms such as difficulty falling asleep or remaining asleep.

Unspecified Insomnia Disorder   780.52 (G47.00)

This category applies to presentations in which symptoms characteristic of insomnia disorder that cause clinically significant distress or impairment in social, occupational, or other important areas of functioning predominate but do not meet the full criteria for insomnia disorder or any of the disorders in the sleep-wake disorders diagnostic class. The unspecified insomnia disorder category is used in situations in which the clinician chooses *not* to specify the reason that the criteria are not met for insomnia disorder or a specific sleep-wake disorder, and includes presentations in which there is insufficient information to make a more specific diagnosis.

Other Specified Hypersomnolence Disorder and Unspecified Hypersomnolence Disorder

These are residual categories to use for symptoms of a hypersomnolence disorder that cause clinically significant distress or impairment but do not meet criteria for a more specific disorder in the class. The category other specified hypersomnolence disorder is used when the clinician chooses to communicate the reason that the presentation does not meet full criteria. The clinician is encouraged to record the specific reason (e.g., brief-duration hypersomnolence).

The category unspecified hypersomnolence disorder is used when the clinician chooses *not* to specify the reason the criteria are not met, or there is insufficient information to make a more specific diagnosis.

Other Specified Hypersomnolence Disorder   780.54 (G47.19)

This category applies to presentations in which symptoms characteristic of hypersomnolence disorder that cause clinically significant distress or impairment in social, occupational, or other important areas of functioning predominate but do not meet the full criteria for hypersomnolence disorder or any of the disorders in the sleep-wake disorders diagnostic class. The other specified hypersomnolence disorder category is used in situations in which the clinician chooses to communicate the specific reason that the presentation does not meet the criteria for hypersomnolence disorder or any specific sleep-wake disorder. This is done by recording "other specified hypersomnolence disorder" followed by the specific reason (e.g., "brief-duration hypersomnolence," as in Kleine-Levin syndrome).

Unspecified Hypersomnolence Disorder   780.54 (G47.10)

This category applies to presentations in which symptoms characteristic of hypersomnolence disorder that cause clinically significant distress or impairment in social, occupational, or other important areas of functioning predominate but do not meet the full criteria for hypersomnolence disorder or any of the disorders in the sleep-wake disorders diagnostic class. The unspecified hypersomnolence disorder category is used in situations in which the clinician chooses *not* to specify the reason that the criteria are not met for hypersomnolence disorder or a specific sleep-wake disorder, and includes presentations in which there is insufficient information to make a more specific diagnosis.

Other Specified Sleep-Wake Disorder and Unspecified Sleep-Wake Disorder

The other specified sleep-wake disorder category applies in situations in which symptoms characteristic of a sleep-wake disorder that cause clinically significant distress or functional impairment predominate but do not meet full criteria for any of the disorders in the sleep-wake disorders diagnostic class, and do not qualify for a diagnosis of other specified insomnia disorder or other specified hypersomnolence disorder.

The unspecified sleep-wake disorder category applies in situations in which the clinician chooses not to specify the reason that the criteria are not met for a specific sleep-wake disorder, or there is insufficient information to make a more specific diagnosis.

Other Specified Sleep-Wake Disorder   780.59 (G47.8)

This category applies to presentations in which symptoms characteristic of a sleep-wake disorder that cause clinically significant distress or impairment in social, occupational, or other important areas of functioning predominate but do not meet the full criteria for any of the disorders in the sleep-wake disorders diagnostic class and do not qualify for a diagnosis of other specified insomnia disorder or other specified hypersomnolence disorder. The other specified sleep-wake disorder category is used in situations in which the clinician chooses to communicate the specific reason that the presentation does not meet the criteria for any specific sleep-wake disorder. This is done by recording "other specified sleep-wake disorder" followed by the specific reason (e.g., "repeated arousals during rapid eye movement sleep without polysomnography or history of Parkinson's disease or other synucleinopathy").

Unspecified Sleep-Wake Disorder   780.59 (G47.9)

This category applies to presentations in which symptoms characteristic of a sleep-wake disorder that cause clinically significant distress or impairment in social, occupational, or other important areas of functioning predominate but do not meet the full criteria for any of the disorders in the sleep-wake disorders diagnostic class and do not qualify for a diagnosis of unspecified insomnia disorder or unspecified hypersomnolence disorder. The unspecified sleep-wake disorder category is used in situations in which the clinician chooses *not* to specify the reason that the criteria are not met for a specific sleep-wake disorder, and includes presentations in which there is insufficient information to make a more specific diagnosis.

KEY POINTS

- The revision of the sleep disorders chapter for DSM-5 has been influenced by the second edition of the *International Classification of Sleep Disorders,* published by the American Academy of Sleep Medicine.

- The diagnosis primary insomnia has been renamed *insomnia disorder* to avoid the differentiation between primary and secondary insomnia. Narcolepsy—now known to be associated with hypocretin—is distinguished from other forms of hypersomnolence (hypersomnolence disorder).

- Breathing-related sleep disorders are divided into three distinct disorders: obstructive sleep apnea hypopnea, central sleep apnea, and sleep-related hypoventilation.

- The subtypes of circadian rhythm sleep disorders (now called *circadian rhythm sleep-wake disorders*) have been expanded to include advanced sleep phase type and irregular sleep-wake type, and the jet lag type has been omitted.

- Rapid eye movement sleep behavior disorder and restless legs syndrome have achieved independent disorder status. Both were included in DSM-IV as examples of a "not otherwise specified" diagnosis.

CHAPTER 14

Sexual Dysfunctions, Gender Dysphoria, and Paraphilic Disorders

Sexual Dysfunctions

302.74 (F52.32) Delayed Ejaculation
302.72 (F52.21) Erectile Disorder
302.73 (F52.31) Female Orgasmic Disorder
302.72 (F52.22) Female Sexual Interest/Arousal Disorder
302.76 (F52.6) Genito-Pelvic Pain/Penetration Disorder
302.71 (F52.0) Male Hypoactive Sexual Desire Disorder
302.75 (F52.4) Premature (Early) Ejaculation
Substance/Medication-Induced Sexual Dysfunction
302.79 (F52.8) Other Specified Sexual Dysfunction
302.70 (F52.9) Unspecified Sexual Dysfunction

Gender Dysphoria

302.6 (F64.2) Gender Dysphoria in Children
302.85 (F64.1) Gender Dysphoria in Adolescents and Adults
302.6 (F64.8) Other Specified Gender Dysphoria
302.6 (F64.9) Unspecified Gender Dysphoria

Paraphilic Disorders

302.82 (F65.3) Voyeuristic Disorder
302.4 (F65.2) Exhibitionistic Disorder
302.89 (F65.81) Frotteuristic Disorder
302.83 (F65.51) Sexual Masochism Disorder
302.84 (F65.52) Sexual Sadism Disorder
302.2 (F65.4) Pedophilic Disorder
302.81 (F65.0) Fetishistic Disorder
302.3 (F65.1) Transvestic Disorder
302.89 (F65.89) Other Specified Paraphilic Disorder
302.9 (F65.9) Unspecified Paraphilic Disorder

DSM-5 includes separate chapters for sexual dysfunctions, gender dysphoria, and paraphilic disorders. *Sexual dysfunctions* are disorders characterized by a disturbance in a person's ability to respond sexually or to experience sexual pleasure. *Gender dysphoria* refers to a person's affective/cognitive discontent with the assigned gender. *Paraphilic disorders* involve sexual preferences other than genital stimulation or preparatory fondling. DSM classification of these disorders has varied over the years, reflecting the growing knowledge about the disorders as well as the greater concern that individuals, clinicians, and researchers have about them.

Sexual dysfunctions were first recognized in DSM-II within the diagnosis "psycho-physiologic genito-urinary disorder," which included problems such as "disturbances of menstruation and micturition, dyspareunia, and impotence in which emotional factors play a causative role" (p. 47). Their attribution to "emotional factors" reflected the thinking at the time, which minimized the role of a physical etiology for these disorders. In DSM-III, sexual dysfunctions came into their own and were placed in the umbrella chapter "Psychosexual Disorders," which also included gender identity disorders and paraphilias.

Whereas the gender identity disorders were first recognized in DSM-III, paraphilias were first listed in DSM-I under "sexual deviation," a subcategory of sociopathic personality disturbance. DSM-I stated the following: "This diagnosis is reserved for deviant sexuality which is not symptomatic of more extensive syndromes, such as schizophrenic and obsessional reactions. The term includes most of the cases formerly classified as 'psychopathic personality with pathologic sexuality.' The diagnosis will specify the type of the pathologic behavior, such as homosexuality, transvestism, pedophilia, fetishism and sexual sadism (including rape, sexual assault, mutilation)" (pp. 38–39).

In DSM-II, the paraphilias continued to be grouped within the category of personality disorders and certain other nonpsychotic mental disorders, but a more complete listing of sexual deviations was created that resembles the current classification, with the exception of homosexuality, which was deleted from DSM in 1973 by vote of the American Psychiatric Association (APA) Board of Trustees. DSM-III introduced operational diagnostic criteria for the paraphilias and included ego-dystonic homosexuality under the subcategory of other psychosexual disorders. It was finally deleted from DSM-III-R, although "persistent and marked distress" about one's sexual orientation continued in DSM-III-R, DSM-IV, and DSM-IV-TR as an example of a sexual disorder not otherwise specified. This concern is no longer acknowledged in DSM-5, reflecting the evolving views of the psychiatric field and society at large.

During DSM-5 deliberations, there was some controversy about the possibility of including hypersexual disorder, which is characterized by sexual behavior that is excessive or poorly controlled (commonly referred to as either "sex addiction" or "compulsive sexual behavior"), and paraphilic coercive disorder, which consists of a sexual preference for coerced sexual activity (i.e., rape). After considerable discussion and input from fellow APA members, the decision was made not to include these disorders in DSM-5.

Sexual dysfunctions, gender dysphoria, and paraphilic disorders will be discussed in turn, beginning with the sexual dysfunctions.

SEXUAL DYSFUNCTIONS

Sexual dysfunction involves either a disturbance in the processes that characterize the sexual response cycle or pain or discomfort associated with sexual intercourse (see list of disorders in Table 14–1). Epidemiological data suggest that sexual dysfunctions are frequent and occur in 10%–30% of adults. Especially common are premature (early) ejaculation, female orgasmic disorder, and erectile disorder. The sexual response cycle has four phases—sexual excitement, plateau, orgasm, and resolution.

TABLE 14–1. DSM-5 sexual dysfunctions

Delayed ejaculation

Erectile disorder

Female orgasmic disorder

Female sexual interest/arousal disorder

Genito-pelvic pain/penetration disorder

Male hypoactive sexual desire disorder

Premature (early) ejaculation

Substance/medication-induced sexual dysfunction

Other specified sexual dysfunction

Unspecified sexual dysfunction

The first phase, *sexual excitement,* consists of muscle tension, changes in breathing and heart rate, swelling of the genitals, and vaginal lubrication. This phase may last from a few minutes to a few hours. The second phase, the *plateau* phase, intensifies the feelings of the first phase and extends to the point of orgasm. The physiological responses during the plateau phase become more intense. Several DSM-5 disorders correspond to these first two phases. These include male hypoactive sexual desire disorder, female sexual interest/arousal disorder, and erectile disorder. Several changes have been made for DSM-5. First, the DSM-IV categories hypoactive sexual desire disorder (as it relates to females) and female sexual arousal disorder have been merged into a single category: female sexual interest/arousal disorder. Second, in DSM-5, hypoactive sexual desire disorder is now specifically focused on men and has been renamed male hypoactive sexual desire disorder. Third, sexual aversion disorder has been eliminated.

Orgasm, the third phase of the sexual response cycle, is the shortest phase and may last only a few seconds or minutes. This phase consists of a release of sexual tension, ejaculation of semen, and vaginal contractions. DSM-5 disorders corresponding to this phase include female orgasmic disorder, delayed ejaculation, and premature (early) ejaculation. The DSM-IV disorders male orgasmic disorder and premature ejaculation have been replaced by delayed ejaculation and premature (early) ejaculation, respectively.

During *resolution,* the final stage of the sexual response cycle, the body slowly returns to normal, with swelling and erection resolving, and a sense of well-being occurring. No DSM-5 disorders correspond to this phase.

In addition to disorders associated with the sexual response cycle, DSM-5 includes genito-pelvic pain/penetration disorder, which involves experiencing physical pain or discomfort during sexual intercourse. Having a single disorder referring to pain or discomfort reflects a change from DSM-IV, in which two specific pain disorders—dyspareunia and vaginismus—were included. DSM-5 has also expanded the previous category of substance-induced sexual dysfunction to include medication (substance/medication-induced sexual dysfunction).

DSM-5 criteria for the sexual dysfunctions have several elements in common. Criterion A describes the disorder, Criteria B–D are the same for all disorders (except substance/medication-induced sexual dysfunction, which has an additional criterion), and the subtypes and specifiers are identical for most disorders (with some variation for genito-pelvic pain/penetration disorder and for substance/medication-induced sexual dysfunction). In addition, the sexual dysfunction category includes an other specified and an unspecified disorder to account for symptoms that do not meet the full criteria for any of the disorders in the diagnostic class. These replace the DSM-IV "not otherwise specified" categories.

To avoid redundancy, the criteria for delayed ejaculation are presented as an example, and readers are referred to DSM-5 for the specific criteria for the other sexual dysfunctions. Because occasional sexual dysfunction is an inherent part of human sexuality and not indicative of a disorder, only symptoms that persist are considered for purposes of a diagnosis.

Sexual Dysfunction

Diagnostic Criteria for Delayed Ejaculation   302.74 (F52.32)

A. Either of the following symptoms must be experienced on almost all or all occasions (approximately 75%–100%) of partnered sexual activity (in identified situational contexts or, if generalized, in all contexts), and without the individual desiring delay:

  1. Marked delay in ejaculation.
  2. Marked infrequency or absence of ejaculation.

B. The symptoms in Criterion A have persisted for a minimum duration of approximately 6 months.

C. The symptoms in Criterion A cause clinically significant distress in the individual.

D. The sexual dysfunction is not better explained by a nonsexual mental disorder or as a consequence of severe relationship distress or other significant stressors and is not attributable to the effects of a substance/medication or another medical condition.

Specify whether:

Lifelong: The disturbance has been present since the individual became sexually active.

Acquired: The disturbance began after a period of relatively normal sexual function.

Specify whether:
 Generalized: Not limited to certain types of stimulation, situations, or partners.
 Situational: Only occurs with certain types of stimulation, situations, or partners.
Specify current severity:
 Mild: Evidence of mild distress over the symptoms in Criterion A.
 Moderate: Evidence of moderate distress over the symptoms in Criterion A.
 Severe: Evidence of severe or extreme distress over the symptoms in Criterion A.

Criterion A

This item describes the symptoms of sexual dysfunction and establishes the frequency for the symptoms. In most cases, the symptoms must be experienced on approximately 75%–100% of all occasions of sexual activity. This reflects a change from DSM-IV, which stated that the sexual dysfunction had to be "persistent and recurrent," providing the clinician with little guidance to evaluating symptom frequency. This criterion also prevents the overdiagnosis of a sexual dysfunction.

Criterion B

This item establishes the minimum duration of symptoms required for diagnosis with the sexual dysfunction. In most cases, the symptoms need to be present for a minimum duration of approximately 6 months.

Criterion C

This item states that the symptoms of sexual dysfunction "cause clinically significant distress." This criterion, like the first two, differentiates sexual dysfunctions from temporary difficulties with sexual functioning that are part of everyday life. The clinically significant distress may take the form of social isolation, depression, and poor self-esteem. Impairment from sexual dysfunction may include unstable relationships, lack of dating, and abuse of substances to help cope. Criterion C reflects a change from DSM-IV's Criterion B, which stated, "the disturbance causes marked distress or interpersonal difficulty." The phrases "marked distress" and "interpersonal difficulty" have been variously interpreted by clinicians and researchers, and the new language provides greater clarity.

Criterion D

Other disorders or behaviors that could possibly exhibit themselves as a sexual dysfunction must be excluded. In DSM-IV, only substances and general medical conditions were excluded. In DSM-5, the exclusions have been expanded to include distress from a relationship and other stressors. For example, when a man is experiencing a contentious divorce and reports low sexual desire only during the time of the extended proceedings, the diagnosis of male hypoactive sexual desire disorder would not be appropriate.

Subtypes and Specifiers

DSM-5 provides subtypes and specifiers for each of the sexual dysfunctions. Although the subtypes are carried over from DSM-IV, the specifiers have been expanded to more accurately reflect the variety of factors that can impact sexual functioning.

The lifelong and acquired subtypes apply to the onset of the sexual dysfunction. *Lifelong* refers to the failure to develop normal sexual functioning from first sexual experiences, whereas *acquired* refers to situations in which the person develops sexual disorders after a period of relatively normal functioning.

The generalized and situational subtypes have also been carried over. *Generalized* refers to sexual difficulties that are not limited to certain situations, partners, or types of stimulation. *Situational* refers to sexual difficulties that only occur with particular partners, in certain situations, or with certain types of stimulation.

Current severity specifiers are provided to rate each disorder as mild (evidence of mild distress over the symptoms in Criterion A), moderate (evidence of moderate distress over the symptoms in Criterion A), or severe (evidence of severe or extreme distress over the symptoms in Criterion A).

Delayed Ejaculation

Delayed ejaculation applies when a man has a marked delay in or marked infrequency or absence of orgasm. For some men, only certain types of stimulation lead to orgasm. Others may experience an orgasm but only after prolonged and intense sexual activity or stimulation.

Delayed ejaculation is the new name for DSM-IV male orgasmic disorder. The name change reflects current terminology in the field. Given that men's experiences of sexual excitement are not uniform, the phrase "following a normal sexual excitement phase" was eliminated from the diagnostic criteria.

Erectile Disorder

Erectile disorder applies to situations when a man is unable to attain or maintain an adequate erection (Segraves 2010). This can happen at the outset of or during a sexual encounter. Erectile disorder can interfere with fertility and produce low self-esteem.

In addition to the general changes for the overall category of sexual dysfunctions, the diagnosis of erectile disorder underwent several changes in DSM-5. Whereas DSM-IV stated that the disorder was defined as an "inability to attain, or to maintain until completion of the sexual activity, an adequate erection," DSM-5 requires one of three possible symptoms: marked difficulty in obtaining an erection during sexual activity, marked difficulty in maintaining an erection until completion of sexual activity, or marked decrease in erectile rigidity.

Female Orgasmic Disorder

Female orgasmic disorder involves recurrent delay in, marked infrequency of, or absence of orgasm, or markedly reduced intensity of orgasmic sensations. Women demonstrate wide variability in the type and intensity of stimulation needed for orgasm. For this reason, the diagnosis requires that the symptoms are experienced on almost all occasions of sexual activity.

DSM-5 includes three important changes to female orgasmic disorder. "Marked infrequency" of orgasms and "reduced intensity of orgasmic sensations" have been added as symptoms, either of which can fulfill the diagnosis. The addition of "markedly reduced intensity of orgasmic sensations" reflects the fact that orgasm is not an "all or nothing" phenomenon and that diminished intensity of orgasm may be a problem for some women. In addition, in DSM-5, the phrase "following a normal sexual excitement phase" has been deleted because a woman's experience of sexual excitement is not uniform, there is good evidence of substantial variability, and none of the prevalence studies have assessed what constitutes a "normal sexual excitement phase."

Female Sexual Interest/Arousal Disorder

In DSM-5, aspects of both hypoactive sexual desire disorder and female sexual arousal disorder have been combined to create female sexual interest/arousal disorder. The diagnosis applies when a woman has either a lack of interest in sexual activity or an inability to attain or maintain arousal.

The name change reflects the common experience that desire and (at least subjective) arousal highly overlap. In some women, desire precedes arousal; in other women, desire follows arousal. There are inconsistencies in how desire is defined, with some definitions focusing on sexual behavior as an indicator of desire, others focusing on spontaneous sexual thoughts and fantasies, and still others emphasizing the responsive nature of women's desire. The word *desire* in DSM-IV hypoactive sexual desire disorder has been changed to *interest* because *desire* connotes a deficiency and often implies a biological urge. The phrase "an adequate lubrication-swelling response of sexual excitement" in DSM-IV female sexual arousal disorder has been eliminated because evidence suggests that increases in vaginal blood flow during exposure to sexual stimuli may be a relatively "automatic response," and one that women may or may not be aware of. Furthermore, there is little evidence that women with a sexual arousal disorder have impaired genital response; lubrication may or may not co-occur with subjective arousal. Finally, there is evidence that women report a wide range of nongenital and genital changes, and it is unclear how common the "lubrication-swelling response" is.

Genito-Pelvic Pain/Penetration Disorder

Genito-pelvic pain/penetration disorder applies when a person has pain or discomfort, muscular tightening, or fear or anxiety about pain when having sexual intercourse. This disorder reflects a change from DSM-IV, in which two distinct disorders—dyspareunia and vaginismus—were used to diagnose sexual pain disorders, both now subsumed within this new category. Dyspareunia and vaginismus were unreliable diagnoses, and it was difficult for clinicians to distinguish between them. The new category will correct that situation, yet allow for the diagnosis of pain and penetration disorders. This will also provide a framework to facilitate clinician evaluation, diagnosis, and referral.

Male Hypoactive Sexual Desire Disorder

Male hypoactive sexual desire disorder applies when a man has diminished desire for sexual activity and few if any sexual thoughts or fantasies (Brotto 2010). Because DSM-5 has a new diagnosis for low sexual desire and arousal problems in women (i.e., female sexual interest/arousal disorder), male hypoactive sexual desire disorder was created to enable a clinician to diagnose a man's diminished sexual desire. Other than the general changes to the category of sexual dysfunction in DSM-5, as stated earlier in this chapter, the criteria for male hypoactive sexual desire disorder are essentially unchanged from DSM-IV.

Premature (Early) Ejaculation

Early ejaculation is a condition in which a man ejaculates "during partnered sexual activity within approximately 1 minute following vaginal penetration and before the individual wishes it." Early ejaculation is more common in novel sexual situations and in men who have had a substantial interval since last orgasm.

The definition of early ejaculation has been operationalized by the use of "approximately 1 minute" as the amount of time after initiation of sexual activity that ejaculation occurs.

DSM-5 notes that premature (early) ejaculation can occur during nonvaginal sexual activities, but that specific duration criteria have not been established and thus are not included.

Substance/Medication-Induced Sexual Dysfunction

Substance/medication-induced sexual dysfunction applies when a clinically significant sexual dysfunction develops during or soon after substance intoxication or withdrawal or exposure to a medication, and the substance/medication is capable of producing the symptoms. Acute intoxication with or chronic abuse of various substances (e.g., alcohol, nicotine, opiates, sedatives) may result in sexual dysfunction. In addition, many medications (e.g., antihypertensives, antidepressants, antipsychotics) may cause a decrease in sexual interest and result in sexual performance difficulties.

Diagnostic Criteria for Substance/Medication-Induced Sexual Dysfunction

A. A clinically significant disturbance in sexual function is predominant in the clinical picture.

B. There is evidence from the history, physical examination, or laboratory findings of both (1) and (2):

   1. The symptoms in Criterion A developed during or soon after substance intoxication or withdrawal or after exposure to a medication.
   2. The involved substance/medication is capable of producing the symptoms in Criterion A.

C. The disturbance is not better explained by a sexual dysfunction that is not substance/medication-induced. Such evidence of an independent sexual dysfunction could include the following:

   The symptoms precede the onset of the substance/medication use; the symptoms persist for a substantial period of time (e.g., about 1 month) after the cessation of acute withdrawal or severe intoxication; or there is other evidence suggesting the existence of an independent non-substance/medication-induced sexual dysfunction (e.g., a history of recurrent non-substance/medication-related episodes).

D. The disturbance does not occur exclusively during the course of a delirium.

E. The disturbance causes clinically significant distress in the individual.

Note: This diagnosis should be made instead of a diagnosis of substance intoxication or substance withdrawal only when the symptoms in Criterion A predominate in the clinical picture and are sufficiently severe to warrant clinical attention.

Coding note: The ICD-9-CM and ICD-10-CM codes for the [specific substance/medication]-induced sexual dysfunctions are indicated in the table below. Note that the ICD-10-CM code depends on whether or not there is a comorbid substance use disorder present for the same class of substance. If a mild substance use disorder is comorbid with the substance-induced sexual dysfunction, the 4th position character is "1," and the clinician should record "mild [substance] use disorder" before the substance-induced sexual dysfunction (e.g., "mild cocaine use disorder with cocaine-induced sexual dysfunction"). If a moderate or severe substance use disorder is comorbid with the substance-induced sexual dysfunction, the 4th position character is "2," and the clinician should record "moderate [substance] use disorder" or "severe [substance] use disorder," depending on the severity of the comorbid substance use disorder. If there is no comorbid substance use disorder (e.g., after a one-time heavy use of the substance), then the 4th position character is "9," and the clinician should record only the substance-induced sexual dysfunction.

		ICD-10-CM		
	ICD-9-CM	With use disorder, mild	With use disorder, moderate or severe	Without use disorder
Alcohol	291.89	F10.181	F10.281	F10.981
Opioid	292.89	F11.181	F11.281	F11.981
Sedative, hypnotic, or anxiolytic	292.89	F13.181	F13.281	F13.981
Amphetamine (or other stimulant)	292.89	F15.181	F15.281	F15.981
Cocaine	292.89	F14.181	F14.281	F14.981
Other (or unknown) substance	292.89	F19.181	F19.281	F19.981

Specify if (see Table 16–1 in the chapter "Substance-Related and Addictive Disorders" for diagnoses associated with substance class):

With onset during intoxication: If the criteria are met for intoxication with the substance and the symptoms develop during intoxication.

With onset during withdrawal: If criteria are met for withdrawal from the substance and the symptoms develop during, or shortly after, withdrawal.

With onset after medication use: Symptoms may appear either at initiation of medication or after a modification or change in use.

Specify current severity:

Mild: Occurs on 25%–50% of occasions of sexual activity.

Moderate: Occurs on 50%–75% of occasions of sexual activity.

Severe: Occurs on 75% or more of occasions of sexual activity.

The DSM-5 criteria state that the dysfunction has to have started during or soon after substance intoxication or withdrawal or after exposure to a medication. These criteria reflect a change from DSM-IV, which failed to account for changes in dosage increase and discontinuation being potential causes of the sexual dysfunction.

Other Specified Sexual Dysfunction and Unspecified Sexual Dysfunction

Sexual dysfunctions that do not meet criteria for any specific sexual dysfunction are classified as other specified or unspecified sexual dysfunction. The "other specified" diagnosis is appropriate when the clinician has concluded that a sexual dysfunction is present but does not meet the full criteria for any of the disorders. In this instance the clinician chooses to communicate the specific reason the presentation does not meet the criteria (e.g., by specifying "sexual aversion"). The category unspecified sexual dysfunction applies when symptoms of sexual dysfunction are present but the clinician chooses not to specify why the criteria are not met for a specific disorder. It may also be used when there is insufficient information to make a more specific diagnosis of a sexual dysfunction.

GENDER DYSPHORIA

Gender dysphoria refers to the distress that may accompany the mismatch between one's assigned gender and how a person perceives their true gender. The DSM classifications of this disorder reflect the tension within the field as to how best to conceptualize the disorder. In DSM-III, transsexualism and gender identity disorder of childhood were introduced, both placed in the chapter titled "Psychosexual Disorders." In DSM-III-R, both disorders were moved to the chapter titled "Disorders First Evident in Infancy, Childhood, or Adolescence." Also included was the diagnosis gender identity disorder of adolescence or adulthood, nontranssexual type, for cross-gender-identified individuals who did not pursue sex reassignment. DSM-IV and DSM-IV-TR included only one specific diagnosis, gender identity disorder, along with gender identity disorder not otherwise specified, in the chapter titled "Sexual and Gender Identity Disorders." Although the DSM terminology and categorization of gender identity disorders have varied over time, the fundamental nature of the disorder—distress about one's assigned gender—remains a consistent and unifying feature. Table 14–2 lists the DSM-5 gender dysphoria diagnoses.

TABLE 14–2. DSM-5 gender dysphoria

Gender dysphoria in children

Gender dysphoria in adolescents and adults

Other specified gender dysphoria

Unspecified gender dysphoria

Gender Dysphoria in Children

Gender dysphoria is characterized by marked incongruence between the person's assigned gender and their expressed gender.

In response to criticisms that the term *gender identity disorder* was stigmatizing, it has been renamed *gender dysphoria* in DSM-5. In addition, subtypes pertaining to sexual attraction were eliminated, and a new subtype categorization that recognizes individuals with a medical disorder of sex development was introduced.

Diagnostic Criteria for Gender Dysphoria in Children   302.6 (F64.2)

A. A marked incongruence between one's experienced/expressed gender and assigned gender, of at least 6 months' duration, as manifested by at least six of the following (one of which must be Criterion A1):

   1. A strong desire to be of the other gender or an insistence that one is the other gender (or some alternative gender different from one's assigned gender).

2. In boys (assigned gender), a strong preference for cross-dressing or simulating female attire; or in girls (assigned gender), a strong preference for wearing only typical masculine clothing and a strong resistance to the wearing of typical feminine clothing.
3. A strong preference for cross-gender roles in make-believe play or fantasy play.
4. A strong preference for the toys, games, or activities stereotypically used or engaged in by the other gender.
5. A strong preference for playmates of the other gender.
6. In boys (assigned gender), a strong rejection of typically masculine toys, games, and activities and a strong avoidance of rough-and-tumble play; or in girls (assigned gender), a strong rejection of typically feminine toys, games, and activities.
7. A strong dislike of one's sexual anatomy.
8. A strong desire for the primary and/or secondary sex characteristics that match one's experienced gender.

B. The condition is associated with clinically significant distress or impairment in social, school, or other important areas of functioning.

Specify if:

With a disorder of sex development (e.g., a congenital adrenogenital disorder such as 255.2 [E25.0] congenital adrenal hyperplasia or 259.50 [E34.50] androgen insensitivity syndrome).

Coding note: Code the disorder of sex development as well as gender dysphoria.

Criterion A

Because some degree of cross-gender identification is not pathological, DSM-5 has eliminated the DSM-IV wording "strong and persistent" and instead introduced a minimum duration requirement of 6 months and raised the threshold from four to six indicators of "marked incongruence between one's experienced/expressed gender and assigned gender." These changes reflect the intensity and duration of cross-gender identification and help avoid the problem of overdiagnosis.

Criterion B

The condition causes clinically significant distress or impairment. In children, this may include problems in school performance, refusal to attend school (where they may be exposed to taunts and bullying), social isolation, and depression. They may feel that no one understands them and that they do not fit in with other children.

Specifiers

The specifiers have replaced DSM-IV Criterion C, which stated, "The disturbance is not concurrent with a physical intersex condition." A specifier has been added: "with a disorder of sex development" (e.g., a congenital adrenogenital disorder such as congenital adrenal hyperplasia or androgen insensitivity syndrome). Gender dysphoria is common in individuals with and without intersex conditions, now referred to as *disorders of sex development*.

Gender Dysphoria in Adolescents and Adults

The diagnosis of gender dysphoria requires discomfort with one's own assigned gender and clinically significant distress or impairment. In adolescents and adults, the disturbance is manifested by symptoms such as stated desire to be of the other gender, frequent passing as the other gender, desire to live as the other gender, and the conviction that the person has the typical feelings and reactions of the other gender.

Diagnostic Criteria for Gender Dysphoria in Adolescents and Adults   302.85 (F64.1)

A. A marked incongruence between one's experienced/expressed gender and assigned gender, of at least 6 months' duration, as manifested by at least two of the following:

1. A marked incongruence between one's experienced/expressed gender and primary and/or secondary sex characteristics (or in young adolescents, the anticipated secondary sex characteristics).
2. A strong desire to be rid of one's primary and/or secondary sex characteristics because of a marked incongruence with one's experienced/expressed gender (or in young adolescents, a desire to prevent the development of the anticipated secondary sex characteristics).
3. A strong desire for the primary and/or secondary sex characteristics of the other gender.
4. A strong desire to be of the other gender (or some alternative gender different from one's assigned gender).
5. A strong desire to be treated as the other gender (or some alternative gender different from one's assigned gender).
6. A strong conviction that one has the typical feelings and reactions of the other gender (or some alternative gender different from one's assigned gender).

B. The condition is associated with clinically significant distress or impairment in social, occupational, or other important areas of functioning.

Specify if:

With a disorder of sex development (e.g., a congenital adrenogenital disorder such as 255.2 [E25.0] congenital adrenal hyperplasia or 259.50 [E34.50] androgen insensitivity syndrome).

Coding note: Code the disorder of sex development as well as gender dysphoria.

Specify if:

Posttransition: The individual has transitioned to full-time living in the desired gender (with or without legalization of gender change) and has undergone (or is preparing to have) at least one cross-sex medical procedure or treatment regimen—namely, regular cross-sex hormone treatment or gender reassignment surgery confirming the desired gender (e.g., penectomy, vaginoplasty in a natal male; mastectomy or phalloplasty in a natal female).

Criterion A

The focus is on the discrepancy between experienced or expressed gender (which can be either male, female, in between, or otherwise) and assigned gender (in most societies male or female) rather than cross-gender identification and same-gender aversion. For the adult criteria, DSM-5 requires at least two of six indicators of the condition.

Criterion B

The condition causes clinically significant distress or impairment. Adolescents and adults with gender dysphoria may become socially isolated, abuse alcohol or other drugs to cope, and have difficulties with work or interpersonal relationships.

Specifiers

Two specifiers have replaced the DSM-IV criterion "The disturbance is not concurrent with a physical intersex condition." First, the specifier "with a disorder of sex development" (e.g., a congenital adrenogenital disorder such as congenital adrenal hyperplasia or androgen insensitivity syndrome) has been added to further describe the gender dysphoria. Gender dysphoria is common in individuals with and without intersex conditions, now referred to as *disorders of sex development.* Second, "posttransition" has been added as the other specifier. This addition was prompted by the observation that for many individuals, after transition, no criteria for gender dysphoria are met, but they continue to undergo chronic hormone treatment, further gender-confirming surgery, or intermittent psychotherapy or counseling to facilitate adaptation to life in the desired gender and the social consequences of the transition. The concept of posttransition is modeled on the concept "in partial or full remission," which is used for mood disorders.

Other Specified Gender Dysphoria and Unspecified Gender Dysphoria

These diagnostic categories apply to presentations in which symptoms characteristic of gender dysphoria that cause significant distress or functional impairment predominate but do not meet the full criteria for gender dysphoria. The other specified category is used when the clinician chooses to communicate the specific reason that the presentation does not meet the criteria for gender dysphoria. The unspecified category is used when the clinician chooses not to specify the reason that the criteria are not met for gender dysphoria, and includes presentations in which there is insufficient information to make a more specific diagnosis.

PARAPHILIC DISORDERS

Paraphilic disorders are characterized by intense and persistent sexual interest other than sexual interest in genital stimulation or preparatory fondling with mature consenting humans.

The paraphilias have been recognized for centuries. In terms of formal classification, paraphilias were recognized in DSM-I and DSM-II as a form of personality disturbance, but in DSM-III they were placed in the chapter "Psychosexual Disorders" and diagnostic criteria were developed. The paraphilias continued relatively unchanged through subsequent editions, included in chapters containing the sexual dysfunctions (and gender identity disorder in DSM-IV). In DSM-5, paraphilic disorders have their own chapter.

Because not all paraphilias are considered mental disorders, DSM-5 makes a distinction between paraphilias and paraphilic disorders. A paraphilic disorder diagnosis requires that a paraphilia cause distress or impairment to the individual, or entail personal harm, or risk of harm, to others. A paraphilia is a necessary but not a sufficient condition for having a paraphilic disorder. Having a paraphilia does not in and of itself automatically justify or require clinical intervention.

In the diagnostic criteria set for each of the listed paraphilic disorders, Criterion A specifies the qualitative nature of the paraphilia (e.g., cross-dressing) and Criterion B specifies the negative consequences of the paraphilia (significant distress or impairment in important areas of functioning).

Course specifiers have been added for each of the paraphilic disorders, allowing for the documentation of changes in an individual's status. "In a controlled environment" is included because the propensity of an individual to act on paraphilic urges may be more difficult to assess objectively when the individual has no opportunity to act on such urges. "In full remission" indicates that the individual has not acted on the urges with a nonconsenting person and/or has had no distress or impairment in functioning for at least 5 years while in an uncontrolled environment.

DSM-5 includes 10 paraphilic disorders, as listed in Table 14–3. Each is discussed in turn, and changes from DSM-IV are highlighted.

TABLE 14–3. DSM-5 paraphilic disorders

Voyeuristic disorder

Exhibitionistic disorder

Frotteuristic disorder

Sexual masochism disorder

Sexual sadism disorder

Pedophilic disorder

Fetishistic disorder

Transvestic disorder

Other specified paraphilic disorder

Unspecified paraphilic disorder

Voyeuristic Disorder

Voyeuristic disorder is defined by the act of observing an unsuspecting person(s) who is naked, in the process of disrobing, or engaged in sexual activity. The individual has acted on these sexual urges with a nonconsenting person, or the sexual urges or fantasies have resulted in clinically significant distress or functional impairment.

Diagnostic Criteria for Voyeuristic Disorder   302.82 (F65.3)

A. Over a period of at least 6 months, recurrent and intense sexual arousal from observing an unsuspecting person who is naked, in the process of disrobing, or engaging in sexual activity, as manifested by fantasies, urges, or behaviors.
B. The individual has acted on these sexual urges with a nonconsenting person, or the sexual urges or fantasies cause clinically significant distress or impairment in social, occupational, or other important areas of functioning.
C. The individual experiencing the arousal and/or acting on the urges is at least 18 years of age.

Specify if:
  In a controlled environment: This specifier is primarily applicable to individuals living in institutional or other settings where opportunities to engage in voyeuristic behavior are restricted.
  In full remission: The individual has not acted on the urges with a nonconsenting person, and there has been no distress or impairment in social, occupational, or other areas of functioning, for at least 5 years while in an uncontrolled environment.

Exhibitionistic Disorder

Exhibitionistic disorder is defined by the exposure of one's genitalia to an unsuspecting individual, with the additional requirement that the person has acted on these sexual urges with a nonconsenting person or the sexual urges or fantasies have resulted in clinically significant distress or functional impairment.

In addition to the overall changes to the paraphilic disorders in DSM-5, specifiers have been added for exhibitionistic disorder regarding the age of the unsuspecting individuals.

Diagnostic Criteria for Exhibitionistic Disorder   302.4 (F65.2)

A. Over a period of at least 6 months, recurrent and intense sexual arousal from the exposure of one's genitals to an unsuspecting person, as manifested by fantasies, urges, or behaviors.
B. The individual has acted on these sexual urges with a nonconsenting person, or the sexual urges or fantasies cause clinically significant distress or impairment in social, occupational, or other important areas of functioning.

Specify whether:
  Sexually aroused by exposing genitals to prepubertal children
  Sexually aroused by exposing genitals to physically mature individuals

Sexually aroused by exposing genitals to prepubertal children and to physically mature individuals

Specify if:

In a controlled environment: This specifier is primarily applicable to individuals living in institutional or other settings where opportunities to expose one's genitals are restricted.

In full remission: The individual has not acted on the urges with a nonconsenting person, and there has been no distress or impairment in social, occupational, or other areas of functioning, for at least 5 years while in an uncontrolled environment.

Frotteuristic Disorder

Frotteuristic disorder involves sexual arousal from touching or rubbing against a nonconsenting person. The individual has acted on these sexual urges with a nonconsenting person, or the individual's sexual urges or fantasies cause clinically significant distress or functional impairment.

Diagnostic Criteria for Frotteuristic Disorder   302.89 (F65.81)

A. Over a period of at least 6 months, recurrent and intense sexual arousal from touching or rubbing against a nonconsenting person, as manifested by fantasies, urges, or behaviors.

B. The individual has acted on these sexual urges with a nonconsenting person, or the sexual urges or fantasies cause clinically significant distress or impairment in social, occupational, or other important areas of functioning.

Specify if:

In a controlled environment: This specifier is primarily applicable to individuals living in institutional or other settings where opportunities to touch or rub against a nonconsenting person are restricted.

In full remission: The individual has not acted on the urges with a nonconsenting person, and there has been no distress or impairment in social, occupational, or other areas of functioning, for at least 5 years while in an uncontrolled environment.

Sexual Masochism Disorder

Sexual masochism disorder involves the act of being humiliated, beaten, bound, or otherwise made to suffer. The fantasies, urges, or behaviors need to also result in clinically significant distress or functional impairment.

In DSM-5, the unique specifier regarding asphyxiophilia has been added because of the high rates of mortality associated with the behavior.

Diagnostic Criteria for Sexual Masochism Disorder 302.83 (F65.51)

A. Over a period of at least 6 months, recurrent and intense sexual arousal from the act of being humiliated, beaten, bound, or otherwise made to suffer, as manifested by fantasies, urges, or behaviors.
B. The fantasies, sexual urges, or behaviors cause clinically significant distress or impairment in social, occupational, or other important areas of functioning.

Specify if:
   With asphyxiophilia: If the individual engages in the practice of achieving sexual arousal related to restriction of breathing.

Specify if:
   In a controlled environment: This specifier is primarily applicable to individuals living in institutional or other settings where opportunities to engage in masochistic sexual behaviors are restricted.
   In full remission: There has been no distress or impairment in social, occupational, or other areas of functioning for at least 5 years while in an uncontrolled environment.

Sexual Sadism Disorder

Sexual sadism disorder involves acts in which the person recurrently derives intense sexual arousal from the physical or psychological suffering of another person. For the behavior to merit a disorder, however, the individual has to have acted on these sexual urges with a nonconsenting person, or the sexual urges or fantasies must cause clinically significant distress or functional impairment.

Diagnostic Criteria for Sexual Sadism Disorder   302.84 (F65.52)

A. Over a period of at least 6 months, recurrent and intense sexual arousal from the physical or psychological suffering of another person, as manifested by fantasies, urges, or behaviors.
B. The individual has acted on these sexual urges with a nonconsenting person, or the sexual urges or fantasies cause clinically significant distress or impairment in social, occupational, or other important areas of functioning.

Specify if:
   In a controlled environment: This specifier is primarily applicable to individuals living in institutional or other settings where opportunities to engage in sadistic sexual behaviors are restricted.
   In full remission: The individual has not acted on the urges with a nonconsenting person, and there has been no distress or impairment in social, occupational, or other areas of functioning, for at least 5 years while in an uncontrolled environment.

Pedophilic Disorder

Pedophilic disorder is defined by sexually arousing fantasies, urges, or behaviors involving sexual activities with a prepubescent child (generally age 13 years or younger). Some individuals with this disorder are only attracted to children, whereas others are also attracted to adults. For the criteria for pedophilic disorder to be met, however, the individual has to have acted on these sexual urges, or the sexual urges or fantasies must cause marked distress or interpersonal difficulty. The individual must be at least 16 years old and at least 5 years older than the child to whom the fantasies or behavior is directed.

DSM-5 has included unique specifiers to designate whether the individual is also attracted to adults, which gender the individual is attracted to, and whether the attraction is only to family members (incest).

Diagnostic Criteria for Pedophilic Disorder   302.2 (F65.4)

A. Over a period of at least 6 months, recurrent, intense sexually arousing fantasies, sexual urges, or behaviors involving sexual activity with a prepubescent child or children (generally age 13 years or younger).
B. The individual has acted on these sexual urges, or the sexual urges or fantasies cause marked distress or interpersonal difficulty.
C. The individual is at least age 16 years and at least 5 years older than the child or children in Criterion A.
   Note: Do not include an individual in late adolescence involved in an ongoing sexual relationship with a 12- or 13-year-old.
Specify whether:
   Exclusive type (attracted only to children)
   Nonexclusive type
Specify if:
   Sexually attracted to males
   Sexually attracted to females
   Sexually attracted to both
Specify if:
   Limited to incest

Fetishistic Disorder

Fetishistic disorder involves the use of nonliving objects, such as underwear or shoes, or a highly specific focus on a nongenital body part(s) for sexual arousal. For the behavior to merit a diagnosis, however, the fantasies, urges, or behaviors need to result in clinically significant distress or functional impairment.

Criterion C reflects the need to distinguish fetishistic disorder from transvestic disorder. In DSM-5, a unique specifier has been added that details the object of the fetish (e.g., body part[s]).

Diagnostic Criteria for Fetishistic Disorder   302.81 (F65.0)

A. Over a period of at least 6 months, recurrent and intense sexual arousal from either the use of nonliving objects or a highly specific focus on nongenital body part(s), as manifested by fantasies, urges, or behaviors.
B. The fantasies, sexual urges, or behaviors cause clinically significant distress or impairment in social, occupational, or other important areas of functioning.
C. The fetish objects are not limited to articles of clothing used in cross-dressing (as in transvestic disorder) or devices specifically designed for the purpose of tactile genital stimulation (e.g., vibrator).

Specify:
Body part(s)
Nonliving object(s)
Other

Specify if:
In a controlled environment: This specifier is primarily applicable to individuals living in institutional or other settings where opportunities to engage in fetishistic behaviors are restricted.
In full remission: There has been no distress or impairment in social, occupational, or other areas of functioning for at least 5 years while in an uncontrolled environment.

Transvestic Disorder

Transvestic disorder is characterized by recurrent and intense sexual arousal from cross-dressing. In addition, the urges, fantasies, or behavior causes the person clinically significant distress or functional impairment.

The name has changed from transvestic fetishism to transvestic disorder. DSM-5 does not include Criterion C from the DSM-IV criteria, which stated that the cross-dressing could not occur exclusively during the course of gender identity disorder. In addition, DSM-5 has removed the requirement that the disorder only be diagnosed in heterosexual males. Unique specifiers have been added to the DSM-5 criteria regarding whether the objects are the main driving force or whether the individual imagines himself as the female.

Diagnostic Criteria for Transvestic Disorder   302.3 (F65.1)

A. Over a period of at least 6 months, recurrent and intense sexual arousal from cross-dressing, as manifested by fantasies, urges, or behaviors.
B. The fantasies, sexual urges, or behaviors cause clinically significant distress or impairment in social, occupational, or other important areas of functioning.

Specify if:
　With fetishism: If sexually aroused by fabrics, materials, or garments.
　With autogynephilia: If sexually aroused by thoughts or images of self as female.

Specify if:
　In a controlled environment: This specifier is primarily applicable to individuals living in institutional or other settings where opportunities to cross-dress are restricted.
　In full remission: There has been no distress or impairment in social, occupational, or other areas of functioning for at least 5 years while in an uncontrolled environment.

Other Specified Paraphilic Disorder and Unspecified Paraphilic Disorder

Other specified and unspecified paraphilic disorders are residual categories that replace DSM-IV's paraphilia not otherwise specified. The former is a category for paraphilic disorders that cause distress or impairment but do not meet the full criteria for any of the specific paraphilic disorders. It is used in situations in which the clinician chooses to communicate the reason (e.g., zoophilia). The category unspecified paraphilic disorder is used when the paraphilic disorder causes distress or impairment but does not meet the full criteria for any of the specific paraphilic disorders and the clinician chooses not to specify the reason that the criteria are not met, and includes presentations in which there is insufficient information to make a more specific diagnosis.

Other Specified Paraphilic Disorder　　302.89 (F65.89)

This category applies to presentations in which symptoms characteristic of a paraphilic disorder that cause clinically significant distress or impairment in social, occupational, or other important areas of functioning predominate but do not meet the full criteria for any of the disorders in the paraphilic disorders diagnostic class. The other specified paraphilic disorder category is used in situations in which the clinician chooses to communicate the specific reason that the presentation does not meet the criteria for any specific paraphilic disorder. This is done by recording "other specified paraphilic disorder" followed by the specific reason (e.g., "zoophilia").

Examples of presentations that can be specified using the "other specified" designation include, but are not limited to, recurrent and intense sexual arousal involving *telephone scatologia* (obscene phone calls), *necrophilia* (corpses), *zoophilia* (animals), *coprophilia* (feces), *klismaphilia* (enemas), or *urophilia* (urine) that has been present for at least 6 months and causes marked distress or impairment in social, occupational, or other important areas of functioning. Other specified paraphilic disorder can be specified as in remission and/or as occurring in a controlled environment.

Unspecified Paraphilic Disorder   302.9 (F65.9)

This category applies to presentations in which symptoms characteristic of a paraphilic disorder that cause clinically significant distress or impairment in social, occupational, or other important areas of functioning predominate but do not meet the full criteria for any of the disorders in the paraphilic disorders diagnostic class. The unspecified paraphilic disorder category is used in situations in which the clinician chooses *not* to specify the reason that the criteria are not met for a specific paraphilic disorder, and includes presentations in which there is insufficient information to make a more specific diagnosis.

KEY POINTS

- Each of the three classes of disorders discussed in this chapter—sexual dysfunctions, gender dysphoria, and paraphilic disorders—has its own chapter in DSM-5, rather than all being grouped together as in DSM-IV.

- The DSM-IV categories hypoactive sexual desire disorder (as it relates to females) and female sexual arousal disorder are now combined into a single disorder: female sexual interest/arousal disorder. Hypoactive sexual desire disorder as it relates to men is now called male hypoactive sexual desire disorder. Sexual aversion disorder has been eliminated.

- Gender identity disorder has been renamed *gender dysphoria* to help avoid stigma associated with the word *disorder.*

- Paraphilias have been renamed *paraphilic disorders* to help distinguish the disorders from nonpathological sexual preference (paraphilia).

CHAPTER 15

Disruptive, Impulse-Control, and Conduct Disorders

313.81 (F91.3) Oppositional Defiant Disorder
312.34 (F63.81) Intermittent Explosive Disorder
Conduct Disorder
301.7 (F60.2) Antisocial Personality Disorder
312.33 (F63.1) Pyromania
312.32 (F63.3) Kleptomania
312.89 (F91.8) Other Specified Disruptive, Impulse-Control, and Conduct Disorder
312.9 (F91.9) Unspecified Disruptive, Impulse-Control, and Conduct Disorder

This new chapter on disruptive, impulse-control, and conduct disorders brings together disorders that appeared in the DSM-IV chapters "Disorders Usually First Diagnosed in Infancy, Childhood, or Adolescence" (oppositional defiant disorder, conduct disorder), "Personality Disorders" (antisocial personality disorder—see Chapter 18 for diagnostic criteria and a detailed description), and "Impulse-Control Disorders Not Elsewhere Classified" (intermittent explosive disorder, pyromania, kleptomania). The chapter represents a departure from DSM-IV, but reflects the approach taken by the DSM-5 Task Force to group related disorders based on clinical and biological evidence. The disorders are listed in Table 15–1.

These disorders are unified by the presence of impaired self-regulation that results in difficult, disruptive, aggressive, or antisocial behavior. These behaviors are usually multidetermined and associated with physical or verbal injury to self, others, or objects, or with violating the rights of others. They appear in several forms and may be defensive, premeditated, or impulsive. Whereas defensive aggression is normative, premeditated and impulsive forms of aggression are viewed as pathological. Additionally, some disruptive behavior may be normative during adolescent development, but repeated disruptive behavior may represent a maladaptive behavioral trait that begins early in life and continues into adulthood.

TABLE 15–1. DSM-5 disruptive, impulse-control, and conduct disorders

---

Oppositional defiant disorder

Intermittent explosive disorder

Conduct disorder

Antisocial personality disorder

Pyromania

Kleptomania

Other specified disruptive, impulse-control, and conduct disorder

Unspecified disruptive, impulse-control, and conduct disorder

---

Throughout the history of DSM, anger, rage, and aggression have characterized a number of personality and problematic behavior disorders. In DSM-I, aggression was specifically identified as occurring in persons with passive-aggressive personality, aggressive type. In DSM-II, explosive personality (epileptoid personality disorder) was added and was described as follows: "This behavior pattern is characterized by gross outbursts of rage or of verbal or physical aggressiveness. These outbursts are strikingly different from the patient's usual behavior, and he may be regretful and repentant for them" (American Psychiatric Association 1968, p. 42).

Several additional disorders occurring in adults have specifically featured aggression as a symptom. Intermittent explosive disorder was introduced in DSM-III to describe persons with episodes of aggression grossly out of proportion to precipitating stressors, and was considered a rough equivalent to explosive personality. The disorder continued mostly unchanged through DSM-IV. Isolated explosive disorder, also introduced in DSM-III, was used to describe persons with a single, discrete episode of uncharacteristic aggression. This disorder was dropped from subsequent editions because of its limited utility. Aggressive behavior was listed as a criterion for antisocial personality disorder in DSM-III (Criterion C5) and DSM-IV (Criterion A4).

Among youth, several diagnoses have featured aggressive or oppositional behavior. Most prominent is oppositional defiant disorder, which describes a persistent pattern of negativistic, hostile, defiant, and disobedient behaviors toward others. Another is conduct disorder, which is a persistent pattern of behavior that involves significant violations of the rights of others and/or major societal norms.

The history of disruptive, impulse-control, and conduct disorders dates to DSM-II and the category "Behavior Disorders of Childhood and Adolescence," which was limited to a small number of diagnoses described as arising from divergent environmental factors: runaway reaction, unsocialized aggressive reaction, and group delinquent reaction. (Interestingly, although the word *reaction* was discarded for DSM-II adult diagnoses, the word was retained for use in child and adolescent diagnoses.) The runaway reaction diagnosis described individuals who fled threatening situations at home and engaged in covert acts of stealing as a means of self-preservation. The unsocialized aggressive reaction diagnosis described loners with a pattern of hostile disobedience, aggressiveness, stealing, and lying, whose behaviors arose primarily as a reaction to inconsistent discipline and parental rejection. The group delinquent reaction diagnosis included individuals who committed predominately nonaggressive acts as part of a delinquent peer group, and their behavior problems were purportedly a consequence of being poorly monitored in an impoverished neighborhood.

In DSM-III, this category was renamed "Disorders Usually First Diagnosed in Infancy, Childhood, or Adolescence" and was expanded to include a large number of diagnoses of varying degrees of severity and stability. Oppositional disorder and conduct disorder were among the new diagnoses. The former was renamed oppositional defiant disorder in DSM-III-R. Conduct disorder was considered the childhood precursor to antisocial personality disorder, which was not to be diagnosed unless the individual was at least age 18 years. This condition was distinct from oppositional disorder, which primarily involved disobedient opposition to authority figures, but not overt aggression. The presence of conduct disorder excluded the diagnosis of oppositional disorder because it was believed that oppositional behavior was a feature of most individuals with conduct disorder.

In DSM-5, oppositional defiant disorder and conduct disorder are now grouped with antisocial personality disorder and intermittent explosive disorder, thereby reflecting emerging evidence supporting their clinical and biological commonality along a developmental spectrum. Antisocial personality disorder involves violations of the rights of others. Intermittent explosive disorder is characterized by impulsive aggressive and assaultive behaviors that are out of proportion to stressors.

Oppositional Defiant Disorder

Irritability, anger, defiance, and temper are specific descriptors of oppositional defiant disorder (Burke et al. 2002). In DSM-III, this disorder was introduced as oppositional disorder and was characterized by a negative and disobedient opposition to authority. The authors of DSM-5 consider oppositional defiant disorder to be a developmental antecedent for some youth with conduct disorder, thereby suggesting that the disorders may reflect different stages of a spectrum of disruptive behavior. In fact, DSM-5 organizes oppositional defiant disorder, conduct disorder, and antisocial personality disorder hierarchically and developmentally to reflect age-dependent expressions of the same underlying diathesis. Transient oppositional behavior is very common in childhood and adolescence, but oppositional defiant disorder occurs in 1%–11% of youth. The disorder is more prevalent in boys before puberty and has an equal gender prevalence for young people after puberty. Clinicians can specify whether the disorder is mild, moderate, or severe.

Diagnostic Criteria for Oppositional Defiant Disorder 313.81 (F91.3)

A. A pattern of angry/irritable mood, argumentative/defiant behavior, or vindictiveness lasting at least 6 months as evidenced by at least four symptoms from any of the following categories, and exhibited during interaction with at least one individual who is not a sibling.

Angry/Irritable Mood

1. Often loses temper.
2. Is often touchy or easily annoyed.
3. Is often angry and resentful.

Argumentative/Defiant Behavior

4. Often argues with authority figures or, for children and adolescents, with adults.
5. Often actively defies or refuses to comply with requests from authority figures or with rules.
6. Often deliberately annoys others.
7. Often blames others for his or her mistakes or misbehavior.

Vindictiveness

8. Has been spiteful or vindictive at least twice within the past 6 months.

Note: The persistence and frequency of these behaviors should be used to distinguish a behavior that is within normal limits from a behavior that is symptomatic. For children younger than 5 years, the behavior should occur on most days for a period of at least 6 months unless otherwise noted (Criterion A8). For individuals 5 years or older, the behavior should occur at least once per week for at least 6 months, unless otherwise noted (Criterion A8). While these frequency criteria provide guidance on a minimal level of frequency to define symptoms, other factors should also be considered, such as whether the frequency and intensity of the behaviors are outside a range that is normative for the individual's developmental level, gender, and culture.

B. The disturbance in behavior is associated with distress in the individual or others in his or her immediate social context (e.g., family, peer group, work colleagues), or it impacts negatively on social, educational, occupational, or other important areas of functioning.
C. The behaviors do not occur exclusively during the course of a psychotic, substance use, depressive, or bipolar disorder. Also, the criteria are not met for disruptive mood dysregulation disorder.

Specify current severity:

Mild: Symptoms are confined to only one setting (e.g., at home, at school, at work, with peers).
Moderate: Some symptoms are present in at least two settings.
Severe: Some symptoms are present in three or more settings.

Criterion A

Even well-adjusted children can display behaviors consistent with one or more of the symptoms of oppositional defiant disorder. Symptoms of oppositional defiant disorder, however, must be part of a pattern of behavior that is frequent and not typical for the child's developmental level. Over a 6-month period, the child must demonstrate at least four of eight behavioral symptoms, which have been grouped into three logical categories: angry/irritable mood, argumentative/defiant behavior, and vindictiveness. Although in DSM-IV the criterion stated that the behaviors are exhibited "often," little guidance was provided about how to objectively define *often*. DSM-5 provides clarification as to the necessary frequency of behavior and distinguishes it by age: "For children younger than 5 years, the behavior should occur on most days for a period of at least 6 months unless otherwise noted (Criterion A8)." For individuals 5 years or older, the behavior should occur at least once per week for at least 6 months, unless otherwise noted (Criterion A8)."

The essential behaviors have not changed from those in DSM-IV except that vindictive behavior has been refined to require at least two episodes during the past 6 months. Another change requires that these behaviors not have been exhibited only in relation to a sibling.

In DSM-5, the behaviors are grouped depending on whether they are emotional or behavioral in nature. Research suggests that the symptoms of oppositional defiant disorder are highly intercorrelated and that all contribute to the prediction of disruptive behavior disorder outcomes. However, the emotional symptoms independently predict mood and anxiety disorders.

Criterion B

The disorder is associated with distress in the individual or in others in his or her immediate social context, or impacts negatively on social, educational, vocational, or other important areas of functioning. This criterion helps distinguish occasional disruptive behavior in an otherwise well-adjusted child or adolescent from disruptive behavior of someone with a diagnosis of oppositional defiant disorder. In a study of youth with DSM-IV oppositional defiant disorder (Burke et al 2002), nearly all subjects reported trouble at home (96%) and in school (85%), and fewer had trouble with peers (67%).

Criterion C

DSM-5 does not include the exclusionary criterion of DSM-IV that allowed for the diagnosis of oppositional defiant disorder only if the criteria for conduct disorder were not met. *The two diagnoses may now be comorbid.* This change was based on research which suggested that presence or absence of comorbid oppositional defiant disorder helped predict outcome in conduct disorder.

Intermittent Explosive Disorder

Intermittent explosive disorder was introduced in DSM-III, but precursors included the DSM-I passive-aggressive personality, aggressive type, characterized as "persistent reaction to frustration with irritability, temper tantrums, and destructive behavior," and the DSM-II explosive personality. Individuals with the latter were aggressive individuals with intermittently violent behavior. In DSM-III, this behavior pattern was codified as intermittent explosive disorder and assigned to Axis I of the new multiaxial system, rather than as a personality disorder on Axis II.

Aggressive outbursts in this disorder are characterized by rapid onset and short duration; there is usually little or no prodrome. Episodes involve verbal assault, destructive and nondestructive property assault, or injurious or noninjurious physical assault. Aggressive outbursts most commonly occur in response to a minor provocation by a close intimate or associate, and subjects with intermittent explosive disorder often have less severe episodes of verbal and nondestructive property assault between the more severe destructive-assaultive episodes. Episodes lead to substantial subjective distress, impairment in social functioning, occupational difficulty, or legal or financial problems. Research evidence suggests that "recurrent, problematic, impulsive aggression" has a prevalence of 5%–7% in the general adult population and perhaps a higher percentage in psychiatric hospitals and clinics (Coccaro 2012).

Diagnostic Criteria for Intermittent Explosive Disorder
312.34 (F63.81)

A. Recurrent behavioral outbursts representing a failure to control aggressive impulses as manifested by either of the following:

  1. Verbal aggression (e.g., temper tantrums, tirades, verbal arguments or fights) or physical aggression toward property, animals, or other individuals, occurring twice weekly, on average, for a period of 3 months. The physical aggression does not result in damage or destruction of property and does not result in physical injury to animals or other individuals.
  2. Three behavioral outbursts involving damage or destruction of property and/or physical assault involving physical injury against animals or other individuals occurring within a 12-month period.

B. The magnitude of aggressiveness expressed during the recurrent outbursts is grossly out of proportion to the provocation or to any precipitating psychosocial stressors.

C. The recurrent aggressive outbursts are not premeditated (i.e., they are impulsive and/or anger-based) and are not committed to achieve some tangible objective (e.g., money, power, intimidation).

D. The recurrent aggressive outbursts cause either marked distress in the individual or impairment in occupational or interpersonal functioning, or are associated with financial or legal consequences.

E. Chronological age is at least 6 years (or equivalent developmental level).

F. The recurrent aggressive outbursts are not better explained by another mental disorder (e.g., major depressive disorder, bipolar disorder, disruptive mood dysregulation disorder, a psychotic disorder, antisocial personality disorder, borderline personality disorder) and are not attributable to another medical condition (e.g., head trauma, Alzheimer's disease) or to the physiological effects of a substance (e.g., a drug of abuse, a medication). For children ages 6–18 years, aggressive behavior that occurs as part of an adjustment disorder should not be considered for this diagnosis.

Note: This diagnosis can be made in addition to the diagnosis of attention-deficit/hyperactivity disorder, conduct disorder, oppositional defiant disorder, or autism spectrum disorder when recurrent impulsive aggressive outbursts are in excess of those usually seen in these disorders and warrant independent clinical attention.

Criterion A

The DSM-5 criteria operationalize the scope, frequency, and time frame for aggressive behavior required, allowing intermittent explosive disorder to be diagnosed in the presence of aggressive outbursts of high frequency and low intensity (Criterion A1) or of low frequency and high intensity (Criterion A2). The A1 threshold was set at an average of two outbursts per week for at least 3 months because this level of low-intensity aggression responds well to treatment. The threshold for Criterion A2 was set at three severe outbursts per year because this level of high-intensity aggression distinguishes individuals who are significantly more aggressive from those with a lower frequency of severe aggressive outbursts.

Criterion B

The essence of the disorder is that the outburst is grossly out of proportion to what might occur in most persons faced with a stressful situation. Clearly, aggressive behavior occurs for many reasons in people with and without mental illnesses. This criterion helps to define what is (or is not) attributable to a mental illness, by establishing that the behavioral response is out of bounds.

Criterion C

This new criterion requires that the aggressive behavior be impulsive in nature, an important distinction because empirical data clearly separate impulsive from premeditated aggression. This distinction helps to separate aggressive behavior that is planned from that which occurs spontaneously and without reflection. The criterion also helps to separate the outbursts in intermittent explosive disorder from aggressive outbursts calculated to achieve an objective, such as frightening or intimidating others, as might occur in a person with antisocial personality disorder.

Criterion D

In keeping with other disorders, intermittent explosive disorder in DSM-5 includes the requirement that marked subjective distress or social or occupational dysfunction be linked to the aggressive behavior. The disorder may cause considerable subjective distress as the individual copes with the consequences of his or her behavior. For most, the behavior is ego-dystonic and leads to feelings of embarrassment and remorse (unlike in antisocial personality disorder, in which the individual may not experience either emotion). Because the outburst is disproportionate, it may disrupt relationships, lead to occupational problems (e.g., being fired), or contribute to legal problems if victims suffer personal injuries or must deal with property damage. Although not stated, the intent of the diagnosis is not to provide legal cover for those whose aggressive acts have selfish, financial, or political motives.

Criterion E

Intermittent explosive disorder appears as early as prepubertal childhood and peaks in mid-adolescence, with a mean onset age ranging from about 13 to 21 years. Data also suggest that the disorder is persistent and follows a chronic course of at least 12 years. By establishing a minimum age (or equivalent developmental level) of 6 years, DSM-5 authors are encouraging clinicians to use other diagnoses for children with recurrent temper outbursts (i.e., disruptive mood dysregulation disorder), because the course of such outbursts in a young child is of unclear significance.

Criterion F

Exclusions have changed. DSM-5 allows individuals with autism spectrum disorder, other disruptive behavior disorders (conduct disorder, oppositional defiant disorder), or attention-deficit/hyperactivity disorder (ADHD) to be diagnosed with intermittent explosive disorder. Although individuals with these disorders are sometimes aggressive, the pattern of aggressive acts in these conditions tends to differ from that seen in intermittent explosive disorder. For that reason, the DSM-5 ADHD and Disruptive Behavior Disorders Work Group recommended that these exclusions be dropped. Importantly, other exclusions remain, including antisocial and borderline personality disorders. Also, aggressive behavior occurring in children ages 6–18 years who have an adjustment disorder is not counted toward a diagnosis of intermittent explosive disorder.

Conduct Disorder

The essential feature of conduct disorder is a repetitive and persistent pattern of behavior in which the basic rights of others or major age-appropriate social norms or rules are violated (Burke et al. 2002). The behaviors may entail aggressive conduct that causes or threatens harm to others or animals, nonaggressive behavior resulting in property damage, deceitfulness or theft, or serious violations of rules. General population surveys report prevalence rates ranging from 2% to more than 10%, and the rates are higher in boys than in girls.

Conduct disorder was introduced in DSM-III. Four primary subtypes were proposed on the basis of whether the individual exhibited aggressive (e.g., assault, rape) or nonaggressive (e.g., lying, stealing) conduct problems and whether the individual was socialized (e.g., has lasting friendships, feels guilt/remorse) or unsocialized (e.g., has no close friendships, lacks guilt/remorse). These subtypes were based largely on subtypes of delinquency originally described in DSM-II, and symptoms and diagnostic thresholds were specified for each subgroup. The criteria were simplified in DSM-III-R to include a single set of symptoms (e.g., being physically cruel to people, destroying property, stealing, being truant) rather than having four subtypes. Each symptom had to be present for at least 6 months to reach diagnostic threshold. DSM-IV field trials supported adding bullying, threatening, or intimidating others to the diagnostic criteria, as well as often staying out after dark without permission beginning before age 13 years.

The criteria are essentially unchanged from DSM-IV. In addition to maintaining the age-at-onset subtypes (childhood-onset type, adolescence-onset type), the work group added the specifier "with limited prosocial emotions" to describe the childhood equivalent of the adult with psychopathy. *Psychopathy* is a distinct syndrome that falls within the antisocial spectrum and is characterized by lack of empathy and concern for the feelings, wishes, and well-being of others. These traits are found in a minority of youth with conduct disorder. Research suggests that individuals with conduct disorder who exhibit callous and unemotional traits have a worse outcome and poorer response to treatment than do those without these traits.

Diagnostic Criteria for Conduct Disorder

A. A repetitive and persistent pattern of behavior in which the basic rights of others or major age-appropriate societal norms or rules are violated, as manifested by the presence of at least three of the following 15 criteria in the past 12 months from any of the categories below, with at least one criterion present in the past 6 months:

Aggression to People and Animals

1. Often bullies, threatens, or intimidates others.
2. Often initiates physical fights.
3. Has used a weapon that can cause serious physical harm to others (e.g., a bat, brick, broken bottle, knife, gun).
4. Has been physically cruel to people.
5. Has been physically cruel to animals.
6. Has stolen while confronting a victim (e.g., mugging, purse snatching, extortion, armed robbery).
7. Has forced someone into sexual activity.

Destruction of Property

8. Has deliberately engaged in fire setting with the intention of causing serious damage.
9. Has deliberately destroyed others' property (other than by fire setting).

Deceitfulness or Theft

10. Has broken into someone else's house, building, or car.
11. Often lies to obtain goods or favors or to avoid obligations (i.e., "cons" others).
12. Has stolen items of nontrivial value without confronting a victim (e.g., shoplifting, but without breaking and entering; forgery).

Serious Violations of Rules

13. Often stays out at night despite parental prohibitions, beginning before age 13 years.
14. Has run away from home overnight at least twice while living in the parental or parental surrogate home, or once without returning for a lengthy period.
15. Is often truant from school, beginning before age 13 years.

B. The disturbance in behavior causes clinically significant impairment in social, academic, or occupational functioning.

C. If the individual is age 18 years or older, criteria are not met for antisocial personality disorder.

Specify whether:

312.81 (F91.1) Childhood-onset type: Individuals show at least one symptom characteristic of conduct disorder prior to age 10 years.

312.82 (F91.2) Adolescent-onset type: Individuals show no symptom characteristic of conduct disorder prior to age 10 years.

312.89 (F91.9) Unspecified onset: Criteria for a diagnosis of conduct disorder are met, but there is not enough information available to determine whether the onset of the first symptom was before or after age 10 years.

Specify if:

With limited prosocial emotions: To qualify for this specifier, an individual must have displayed at least two of the following characteristics persistently over at least 12 months and in multiple relationships and settings. These characteristics reflect the individual's typical pattern of interpersonal and emotional functioning over this period and not just occasional occurrences in some situations. Thus, to assess the criteria for the specifier, multiple information sources are necessary. In addition to the individual's self-report, it is necessary to consider reports by others who have known the individual for extended periods of time (e.g., parents, teachers, co-workers, extended family members, peers).

Lack of remorse or guilt: Does not feel bad or guilty when he or she does something wrong (exclude remorse when expressed only when caught and/or facing punishment). The individual shows a general lack of concern about the negative consequences of his or her actions. For example, the individual is not remorseful after hurting someone or does not care about the consequences of breaking rules.

Callous—lack of empathy: Disregards and is unconcerned about the feelings of others. The individual is described as cold and uncaring. The person appears more concerned about the effects of his or her actions on himself or herself, rather than their effects on others, even when they result in substantial harm to others.

Unconcerned about performance: Does not show concern about poor/problematic performance at school, at work, or in other important activities. The individual does not put forth the effort necessary to perform well, even when expectations are clear, and typically blames others for his or her poor performance.

Shallow or deficient affect: Does not express feelings or show emotions to others, except in ways that seem shallow, insincere, or superficial (e.g., actions contradict the emotion displayed; can turn emotions "on" or "off" quickly) or when emotional expressions are used for gain (e.g., emotions displayed to manipulate or intimidate others).

Specify current severity:

Mild: Few if any conduct problems in excess of those required to make the diagnosis are present, and conduct problems cause relatively minor harm to others (e.g., lying, truancy, staying out after dark without permission, other rule breaking).

Moderate: The number of conduct problems and the effect on others are intermediate between those specified in "mild" and those in "severe" (e.g., stealing without confronting a victim, vandalism).

Severe: Many conduct problems in excess of those required to make the diagnosis are present, or conduct problems cause considerable harm to others (e.g., forced sex, physical cruelty, use of a weapon, stealing while confronting a victim, breaking and entering).

Criterion A

The list of 15 problem areas is unchanged from DSM-IV, as are the requirements that three or more be present in the past 12 months and that the pattern of behavior be repetitive and persistent. Most children with conduct disorder have far more than three symptoms. Although occasional problematic behaviors are normal (and even expected) to some extent in children, the severity and variety of these behaviors characterize the person with conduct disorder.

Criterion B

Conduct disorder causes clinically significant impairment and distress to the child, family, school, and community because of the inevitable conflicts that occur with parents, teachers, and peers. Financial and legal repercussions, as well as physical injuries from accidents or fights, are common. Poor frustration tolerance, irritability, temper outbursts, and recklessness are frequently associated symptoms. Conduct disorder behaviors may lead to school suspension or expulsion, problems in work adjustment, sexually transmitted diseases, and unwanted pregnancy. These problems may preclude attendance in ordinary schools or living in the parental home.

Criterion C

Conduct disorder and antisocial personality disorder lie along a continuum. Although conduct disorder technically can be diagnosed at any age, the intention is that it describes a childhood behavioral syndrome that is the precursor to antisocial personality disorder. Approximately 40% of young people with conduct disorder will manifest antisocial personality disorder later in life.

Subtypes and Specifiers

Age-at-onset subtypes are unchanged from DSM-IV. The age at onset should be obtained from both the youth and the caregiver. These subtypes have clinical and treatment ramifications, because an individual with the childhood-onset subtype is more likely to have co-occurring ADHD, to display physical aggression toward others, and to develop antisocial personality disorder.

DSM-5 includes the new descriptive feature specifier "with limited prosocial emotions." These traits were suggested in the DSM-III "undersocialized type." However, this subtype was not continued in subsequent DSM editions because the term *undersocialized* was thought to be overly focused on social attachment. On the other hand, research shows that the presence of limited prosocial emotions can delineate a subtype with a particularly severe and recalcitrant form of antisocial behavior; distinct neurological, cognitive, emotional, and social characteristics (e.g., deficits in processing signs of fear and distress in others, less sensitivity to punishment, more fearless or thrill-seeking behavior); and poorer treatment outcomes. In addition, limited prosocial emotions are relatively stable from childhood to early adolescence and early adulthood, and may be genetically influenced.

Antisocial Personality Disorder

Antisocial personality disorder is characterized by a pervasive pattern of poor social conformity, deceitfulness, impulsivity, criminality, and lack of remorse. Because the disorder is closely connected with the spectrum of externalizing disorders discussed in this class, it is dually coded here and in the chapter on personality disorders. For a complete description of antisocial personality disorder and the DSM-5 criteria, see Chapter 18, "Personality Disorders."

Pyromania

Pyromania is characterized by an impulse to set fires. The disorder was first formally recognized in DSM-III in the new category "Disorders of Impulse-Control Not Elsewhere Classified." Similar to the earlier idea of monomania, the definition focused on the recurrent failure to resist impulses to set fire in persons who were not psychotic, cognitively impaired, or antisocial. In DSM-III-R, these exclusions were removed and an item was added to recognize that persons with pyromania tend to be fascinated with or curious about fires. In DSM-IV, exclusions for mania and antisocial personality disorder were restored. Other than minor editing, the DSM-5 criteria are unchanged.

The essential features of pyromania are the presence of multiple episodes of deliberate and purposeful fire setting and the failure to resist an impulse to set fires. Persons with pyromania like watching fire. They may be recognized as regular "watchers" at fires in their communities and enjoy setting off false fire alarms. Their fascination leads some to seek employment or to volunteer as firefighters. They may be indifferent to the consequences of the fire and its effect on life and property, and they may get satisfaction from the resulting destruction. The behavior may lead to property damage, legal consequences, or injury or loss of life to the fire setter or to others.

Diagnostic Criteria for Pyromania   312.33 (F63.1)

A. Deliberate and purposeful fire setting on more than one occasion.
B. Tension or affective arousal before the act.
C. Fascination with, interest in, curiosity about, or attraction to fire and its situational contexts (e.g., paraphernalia, uses, consequences).
D. Pleasure, gratification, or relief when setting fires or when witnessing or participating in their aftermath.
E. The fire setting is not done for monetary gain, as an expression of sociopolitical ideology, to conceal criminal activity, to express anger or vengeance, to improve

one's living circumstances, in response to a delusion or hallucination, or as a result of impaired judgment (e.g., in major neurocognitive disorder, intellectual disability [intellectual developmental disorder], substance intoxication).

F. The fire setting is not better explained by conduct disorder, a manic episode, or antisocial personality disorder.

Criterion A

This criterion requires that fire setting occur on more than one occasion. This sets the bar at a minimum of two lifetime episodes. In truth, most persons with pyromania will have committed far more episodes of fire setting, with some individuals setting fires on a regular basis.

Criteria B, C, and D

These criteria get at the essence of the disorder. The sense of excitation is captured by the individual's sense of tension or affective arousal before the act, as well as pleasure, gratification, or relief during or after the act. Most persons with pyromania have a fascination with fire that may be reflected by their interest in watching fires. They spend considerable time planning, setting, and watching fires.

Criteria E and F

These criteria exclude those individuals who set fires for political or other reasons (such as arson for monetary gain) and those who set fires during a manic episode or as part of a pattern of antisocial personality disorder.

Kleptomania

Although kleptomania has long been recognized, it was not officially designated a psychiatric disorder until DSM-III, when it was placed in the category "Disorders of Impulse-Control Not Elsewhere Classified." In DSM-5, the criteria are essentially unchanged.

The prevalence of kleptomania has been estimated at 0.3%–0.6% in the general population. Among individuals hospitalized for mental health reasons, however, research has demonstrated that nearly 8% endorse symptoms consistent with the current diagnosis of kleptomania and 9% endorse a lifetime diagnosis (Grant et al. 2005). The literature suggests that the majority of people with kleptomania are women, although the gender disparity may be due to the fact that women are more likely to present for treatment. The disorder typically has an onset by late adolescence (but may begin in adulthood) and is often comorbid with mood, anxiety, and substance use disorders.

People with kleptomania experience significant impairment in social and occupational functioning. Their intrusive thoughts and urges related to stealing can interfere with their ability to concentrate at home and at work. Others report missing work, often in the afternoon, in order to steal. Inability to control their behavior leads to subjective feelings of shame and guilt. The disorder also leads to high levels of stress that worsen as the stealing behavior intensifies. Additionally, many people with kleptomania face legal difficulties and experience public humiliation from arrests.

Diagnostic Criteria for Kleptomania   312.32 (F63.2)

A. Recurrent failure to resist impulses to steal objects that are not needed for personal use or for their monetary value.
B. Increasing sense of tension immediately before committing the theft.
C. Pleasure, gratification, or relief at the time of committing the theft.
D. The stealing is not committed to express anger or vengeance and is not in response to a delusion or a hallucination.
E. The stealing is not better explained by conduct disorder, a manic episode, or antisocial personality disorder.

Criterion A

This item focuses on the stealing that is performed in response to senseless urges for unneeded items. This has often been considered the criterion that distinguishes individuals with kleptomania from ordinary shoplifters. Interpretation of this criterion is controversial. The stereotype of the middle-aged female kleptomania patient who steals particular items may not adequately account for all people with kleptomania. Individuals with kleptomania may in fact desire the items they steal and be able to use them, but they do not need them. This may be particularly the case with individuals with kleptomania who also hoard items. These individuals may steal multiple versions of the same item; although the item itself may be desired, it is not needed.

Criteria B and C

Many individuals will report a sense of tension immediately before committing the theft, as well as pleasure or gratification afterward. These criteria have sometimes been problematic because occasional individuals will deny feelings of tension or arousal prior to the act and may deny feelings of pleasure or relief following the thefts, yet they clearly have a problem with stealing of unneeded objects.

Criterion D

This item helps to separate people with a motivation to steal ("to express anger or vengeance") from the ordinary person with kleptomania who simply fails to resist an impulse. Furthermore, the stealing is not motivated by psychotic thinking.

Criterion E

These exclusions are needed because during manic episodes, individuals may take objects in response to their abnormal thinking and behavior. A youth with a conduct disorder and an adult with antisocial personality disorder may steal because they want the items; this is stealing in the ordinary sense. Their stealing is done without concern for the consequences of their behavior or the people they may hurt in the process.

Other Specified Disruptive, Impulse-Control, and Conduct Disorder and Unspecified Disruptive, Impulse-Control, and Conduct Disorder

These two residual categories are available to clinicians for use in diagnosing presentations characteristic of disruptive, impulse-control, and conduct disorder that cause distress or impairment but do not meet the full criteria for any of the disorders in the class. The category other specified disruptive, impulse-control, and conduct disorder is also used in situations in which the clinician chooses to communicate the specific reason that the presentation does not meet full criteria (e.g., "recurrent behavioral outbursts of insufficient frequency").

Other Specified Disruptive, Impulse-Control, and Conduct Disorder 312.89 (F91.8)

This category applies to presentations in which symptoms characteristic of a disruptive, impulse-control, and conduct disorder that cause clinically significant distress or impairment in social, occupational, or other important areas of functioning predominate but do not meet the full criteria for any of the disorders in the disruptive, impulse-control, and conduct disorders diagnostic class. The other specified disruptive, impulse-control, and conduct disorder category is used in situations in which the clinician chooses to communicate the specific reason that the presentation does not meet the criteria for any specific disruptive, impulse-control, and conduct disorder. This is done by recording "other specified disruptive, impulse-control, and conduct disorder" followed by the specific reason (e.g., "recurrent behavioral outbursts of insufficient frequency").

The category unspecified disruptive, impulse-control, and conduct disorder is used in situations in which the clinician chooses not to specify the reason that the criteria for a specific disorder are not met, or there is insufficient information to make a more specific diagnosis.

Unspecified Disruptive, Impulse-Control, and Conduct Disorder 312.9 (F91.9)

This category applies to presentations in which symptoms characteristic of a disruptive, impulse-control, and conduct disorder that cause clinically significant distress or impairment in social, occupational, or other important areas of functioning predominate but do not meet the full criteria for any of the disorders in the disruptive, impulse-control, and conduct disorders diagnostic class. The unspecified disruptive, impulse-control, and conduct disorder category is used in situations in which the clinician chooses *not* to specify the reason that the criteria are not met for a specific disruptive, impulse-control, and conduct disorder, and includes presentations in which there is insufficient information to make a more specific diagnosis (e.g., in emergency room settings).

KEY POINTS

- This new chapter brings together disorders unified by the presence of difficult, disruptive, aggressive, or antisocial behavior. The disorders include oppositional defiant disorder, conduct disorder, intermittent explosive disorder, antisocial personality disorder, pyromania, and kleptomania.

- DSM-5 has removed the exclusionary criterion of DSM-IV that allowed for the diagnosis of oppositional defiant disorder only if the criteria for conduct disorder were not met. The two diagnoses may now be comorbid.

- Intermittent explosive disorder requires outbursts to be either high frequency and low intensity (at least two outbursts per week for 3 months) or low frequency and high intensity (three or more severe outbursts a year).

- Conduct disorder now has a "with limited prosocial emotions" specifier that allows clinicians to denote youth with the childhood equivalent of psychopathic traits such as lack of remorse or guilt, or callousness. These youth typically have a worse prognosis and response to treatment.

- While antisocial personality disorder is listed with this class, the criteria and text remain in the chapter on personality disorders.

CHAPTER 16

Substance-Related and Addictive Disorders

Alcohol-Related Disorders
Alcohol Use Disorder
303.00 (F10.___) Alcohol Intoxication
291.8 (F10.23_) Alcohol Withdrawal
Other Alcohol-Induced Disorders
291.9 (F10.99) Unspecified Alcohol-Related Disorder

Caffeine-Related Disorders
305.90 (F15.929) Caffeine Intoxication
292.0 (F15.93) Caffeine Withdrawal
Other Caffeine-Induced Disorders
292.9 (F15.99) Unspecified Caffeine-Related Disorder

Cannabis-Related Disorders
Cannabis Use Disorder
292.89 (F12.___) Cannabis Intoxication
292.0 (F12.288) Cannabis Withdrawal
Other Cannabis-Induced Disorders
292.9 (F12.99) Unspecified Cannabis-Related Disorder

Hallucinogen-Related Disorders
Phencyclidine Use Disorder
Other Hallucinogen Use Disorder
292.89 (F16.___) Phencyclidine Intoxication
292.89 (F16.___) Other Hallucinogen Intoxication
292.89 (F16.983) Hallucinogen Persisting Perception Disorder
Other Phencyclidine-Induced Disorders
Other Hallucinogen-Induced Disorders
292.9 (F16.99) Unspecified Phencyclidine-Related Disorder
292.9 (F16.99) Unspecified Hallucinogen-Related Disorder

Inhalant-Related Disorders
Inhalant Use Disorder

292.89 (F18.___)   Inhalant Intoxication
                        Other Inhalant-Induced Disorders
292.9 (F18.99)   Unspecified Inhalant-Related Disorder

Opioid-Related Disorders
                        Opioid Use Disorder
292.89 (F11.___)   Opioid Intoxication
292.0 (F11.23)   Opioid Withdrawal
                        Other Opioid-Induced Disorders
292.9 (F11.99)   Unspecified Opioid-Related Disorder

Sedative-, Hypnotic-, or Anxiolytic-Related Disorders
                        Sedative, Hypnotic, or Anxiolytic Use Disorder
292.89 (F13.___)   Sedative, Hypnotic, or Anxiolytic Intoxication
292.0 (F13.23_)   Sedative, Hypnotic, or Anxiolytic Withdrawal
                        Other Sedative-, Hypnotic-, or Anxiolytic-Induced Disorders
292.9 (F13.99)   Unspecified Sedative-, Hypnotic-, or Anxiolytic-Related Disorder

Stimulant-Related Disorders
                        Stimulant Use Disorder
                        Stimulant Intoxication
                        Stimulant Withdrawal
                        Other Stimulant-Induced Disorders
                        Unspecified Stimulant-Related Disorder

Tobacco-Related Disorders
                        Tobacco Use Disorder
292.0 (F17.203)   Tobacco Withdrawal
                        Other Tobacco-Induced Disorders
292.9 (F17.209)   Unspecified Tobacco-Related Disorder

Other (or Unknown) Substance–Related Disorders
                        Other (or Unknown) Substance Use Disorder
292.89 (F19.___)   Other (or Unknown) Substance Intoxication
292.0 (F19.239)   Other (or Unknown) Substance Withdrawal
                        Other (or Unknown) Substance–Induced Disorders
292.9 (F19.99)   Unspecified Other (or Unknown) Substance–Related Disorder

Non-Substance-Related Disorders
312.31 (F63.0)   Gambling Disorder

The substance-related disorders are divided according to 10 classes

of substances: alcohol; caffeine; cannabis; hallucinogens; inhalants; opioids; sedatives, hypnotics, or anxiolytics; stimulants; tobacco; and other (or unknown) substances. These are presented in separate sections, but they are not fully distinct because all drugs taken in excess activate the brain's reward circuitry, and their co-occurring use is common. Instead of achieving reward system activation through adaptive behaviors, drugs of abuse short-circuit the normal processes that directly activate these structures. Each class produces a range of behavioral effects, including the "high" that fuels their use. The hallucinogens are an exception in that curiosity rather than euphoria is a major motivation for taking them.

Many substances described in this chapter, along with some prescribed and over-the-counter drugs, can also cause substance-induced disorders that resemble independent mood or anxiety disorders, psychotic disorders, or other disorders, except that the substance-induced disorders are usually temporary. These categories of disorder are discussed in the relevant chapters on the basis of symptoms (e.g., anxiety disorders, depressive disorders).

An important departure from DSM-IV is that the current chapter now includes gambling disorder, formerly listed as pathological gambling in the chapter "Impulse-Control Disorders Not Elsewhere Classified." The disorder has been moved because of evidence showing that gambling activates the same brain reward system, with effects similar to those produced by drugs of abuse (Potenza 2006). Other behaviors (the so-called *behavioral addictions*, such as Internet use and compulsive shopping) appear to have a similar effect on reward systems, but the Substance-Related Disorders Work Group concluded that the research on these behaviors was insufficient for their inclusion. Nonetheless, Internet gaming disorder has been placed in the chapter "Conditions for Further Study" in Section III to encourage research.

The substance use disorders have been recognized in all DSM editions. In DSM-I, the *addictions* (alcoholism, drug addiction) were placed within the umbrella category "sociopathic personality disturbance," reflecting the thinking at the time that individuals with these problems were ill in terms of "society and of conformity with the prevailing cultural milieu" (p. 38). In DSM-II, *alcoholism* and the renamed *drug dependence* were placed within the class "personality disorders and certain other non-psychotic mental disorders." Alcoholism was further divided into *episodic excessive drinking, habitual excessive drinking,* and *alcohol addiction.* The latter diagnosis was reserved for individuals considered dependent on alcohol. Ten subcategories were created for various drug dependencies (e.g., "opium, opium alkaloids, and their derivatives"). In DSM-III, the substance use disorders were finally given their own chapter, and the class was greatly expanded to recognize the many drugs that were commonly misused. Criteria, as well as the major divisions of abuse and dependence, were developed for DSM-III, with refinement of the diagnostic class continuing in DSM-5.

The chapter is organized such that disorders (i.e., use disorders, intoxication, and withdrawal) are placed according to substance. The broad diagnostic categories associated with each specific group of substances are shown in Table 16–1. Stimulant-related disorder diagnoses have replaced the categories for amphetamine and cocaine use disorders. Cannabis use disorder and cannabis withdrawal are new. Caffeine withdrawal has been elevated to the status of an independent disorder from DSM-IV's Appendix B, "Criteria Sets and Axes Provided for Further Study." Nicotine use disorders are now called tobacco-related disorders.

Perhaps the most important change is that a distinction is no longer made between "abuse" of and "dependence" on alcohol or other drugs, and the two diagnoses have been merged. In fact, the term *dependence* is not used in this chapter in DSM-5 to avoid overlap with the use of the term to describe pharmacological tolerance and withdrawal. Also, rather than having generic "substance abuse" and "substance de-

TABLE 16–1. Diagnoses associated with substance class

	Psychotic disorders	Bipolar disorders	Depressive disorders	Anxiety disorders	Obsessive-compulsive and related disorders	Sleep disorders	Sexual dysfunctions	Delirium	Neurocognitive disorders	Substance use disorders	Substance intoxication	Substance withdrawal
Alcohol	I/W	I/W	I/W	I/W		I/W	I/W	I/W	I/W/P	X	X	X
Caffeine				I		I/W		I			X	X
Cannabis	I			I		I/W		I		X	X	X
Hallucinogens												
Phencyclidine	I	I	I	I				I		X	X	
Other hallucinogens	I*	I	I	I				I		X	X	
Inhalants	I		I	I				I	I/P	X	X	
Opioids			I/W	W		I/W	I/W	I/W		X	X	X
Sedatives, hypnotics, or anxiolytics	I/W	I/W	I/W	W		I/W	I/W	I/W	I/W/P	X	X	X
Stimulants**	I	I/W	I/W	I/W	I/W	I/W	I	I		X	X	X
Tobacco						W				X		X
Other (or unknown)	I/W	I/W	I/W	I/W	I/W	I/W	I/W	I/W	I/W/P	X	X	X

Note. X = The category is recognized in DSM-5.
I = The specifier "with onset during intoxication" may be noted for the category.
W = The specifier "with onset during withdrawal" may be noted for the category.
I/W = Either "with onset during intoxication" or "with onset during withdrawal" may be noted for the category.
P = The disorder is persisting.
*Also hallucinogen persisting perception disorder (flashbacks).
**Includes amphetamine-type substances, cocaine, and other or unspecified stimulants.

pendence" criteria sets, each class of drug has its own criteria set for a "use disorder." The historic distinction had been based on the belief that a dependence syndrome was a psychobiological process leading to impaired control resulting from persistent, heavy drinking or drug use. A dependence syndrome was thought to have a different cause from that of excessive alcohol or drug use that resulted only in social or personal problems, giving rise to a "biaxial" concept of substance misuse, with dependence on one axis and consequences (i.e., abuse) on the other. These concepts were incorporated into the substance use disorders chapters in DSM-III, DSM-III-R, and DSM-IV. Furthermore, in DSM-III-R and DSM-IV, dependence took precedence hierarchically over abuse. DSM-IV required that three of seven criteria be met for dependence and one of four for abuse.

There were several reasons to combine abuse and dependence. First, clinicians had trouble distinguishing the syndromes. Whereas studies showed that test-retest reliability of DSM-IV dependence was uniformly very good to excellent, the reliability of DSM-IV abuse was lower and more variable. Many assumed that abuse was often a prodromal phase of dependence, but several prospective studies showed that this was not the case. Second, epidemiological studies showed that the most common way for DSM-IV alcohol abuse to be diagnosed was with a single criterion (Criterion A2)— that is, hazardous use (generally driving after drinking). Although this behavior is certainly unwise and risky, basing a psychiatric diagnosis on a single symptom is questionable. Third, the division between abuse and dependence led to "diagnostic orphans," whereby a person could meet two criteria for dependence but none for abuse. Such individuals, who could have substance use problems of the same severity as others with a diagnosis, were left undiagnosed. Subsequent analyses on the structure of abuse and dependence in clinical and epidemiological samples suggested that DSM-IV abuse and dependence criteria could be considered to form a unidimensional structure, with abuse and dependence criteria interspersed across the severity spectrum. Considering this evidence, the work group recommended that abuse and dependence be combined into a single disorder of graded clinical severity, with two criteria required for the diagnosis (Helzer et al. 2006). An additional recommendation was to eliminate the legal problems criterion for addictive disorders (Criterion A3 for DSM-IV substance abuse). Data from the National Epidemiologic Survey on Alcohol and Related Conditions and other studies had shown that the item had a low prevalence relative to other criteria and that its deletion would have little effect on the prevalence of substance use disorders, while adding little information to the diagnoses in the aggregate. For that reason, the criterion has been deleted from the criteria sets for all addictive disorders.

Intoxication is a separate disorder for each substance. *Intoxication* is considered a reversible substance-specific syndrome resulting from the recent use of a substance. The *disorder* of intoxication requires that this syndrome result in clinically significant impairment or problematic behavioral or psychological changes. Likewise, *withdrawal* is listed for most of the substances as a distinct disorder. The drug withdrawal syndrome consists of a cluster of symptoms that 1) are valid and reliably observed and 2) have a clear time course that includes onset closely following cessation of the drug and a return to baseline levels. Furthermore, the syndrome must be pharmacologically specific to deprivation of the drug or one of its components and associated with clinically important consequences (e.g., contributes to relapse, causes significant physical or psychological problems).

Finally, *craving* is defined as a strong desire for a substance, usually a specific substance. It is a common symptom and tends to be present toward the severe end of the severity spectrum. It has been variously defined as a trait with a time component (present or recent past) or as a lifetime component (ever experienced in one's life). As a time-limited state, craving has often been frequently used as an outcome measure, and brain imaging studies have demonstrated subjective craving precipitated by drug-related cues and correlated with increased activity and dopamine release in specific parts of the brain reward system. On the basis of these data, craving has been added as a symptom for substance use disorders.

Each of the substance use disorders, as well as gambling disorder, has specifiers for "early remission" and "sustained remission." "In early remission" indicates that for at least 3 months but for less than 12 months, none of the items in Criterion A have been met except the criterion relating to craving. "In sustained remission" indicates none of the items in Criterion A have been met for 12 months or longer, except the criterion relating to craving. Gambling disorder has the same definitions for early and sustained remission but does not include the craving exception because that is not a criterion for gambling disorder. In the case of opioid and tobacco use disorders, the specifier "on maintenance therapy" may also be used. This additional specifier is used if the individual is taking a prescribed agonist medication, such as methadone or buprenorphine, or nicotine replacement medication, and none of the criteria for opioid or tobacco use disorder have been met for that class of medication (except tolerance to, or withdrawal from, the agonist or replacement medication).

The additional specifier "in a controlled environment" indicates that the person has been in an environment where access to alcohol and drugs is restricted, such as jails, therapeutic communities, and locked hospital units. The "controlled environment" specifier does not apply to gambling disorder. Finally, each use disorder has a severity specifier (mild, moderate, severe) based on the number of criteria met for that disorder. Unlike the substance use disorders, gambling disorder has the additional specifier for whether the disorder is episodic (i.e., meeting diagnostic criteria at more than one time point, with symptoms subsiding between periods of gambling disorder for at least several months) or persistent (i.e., continuous symptoms meeting diagnostic criteria for multiple years) (Table 16–2).

ALCOHOL-RELATED DISORDERS

Alcohol is a commonly abused substance throughout the world and is associated with significant morbidity and mortality. At some point in their lives, at least 80% of adults in the United States have had some experience with alcohol, and a substantial percentage have had one or more alcohol-related adverse events.

This section contains discussion specific to the alcohol-related disorders to convey their unique features. Alcohol-induced disorders are also described in DSM-5 sections on disorders with which they share symptoms.

TABLE 16–2. **Substance-related and addictive disorders**

Alcohol-related disorders
    Alcohol use disorder
    Alcohol intoxication
    Alcohol withdrawal
    Other alcohol-induced disorders
    Unspecified alcohol-related disorder
Caffeine-related disorders
    Caffeine intoxication
    Caffeine withdrawal
    Other caffeine-induced disorders
    Unspecified caffeine-related disorder
Cannabis-related disorders
    Cannabis use disorder
    Cannabis intoxication
    Cannabis withdrawal
    Other cannabis-induced disorders
    Unspecified cannabis-related disorder
Hallucinogen-related disorders
    Phencyclidine use disorder
    Other hallucinogen use disorder
    Phencyclidine intoxication
    Other hallucinogen intoxication
    Hallucinogen persisting perception disorder
    Other phencyclidine-induced disorders
    Other hallucinogen-induced disorders
    Unspecified phencyclidine-related disorder
    Unspecified hallucinogen-related disorder
Inhalant-related disorders
    Inhalant use disorder
    Inhalant intoxication
    Other inhalant-induced disorders
    Unspecified inhalant-related disorder
Opioid-related disorders
    Opioid use disorder
    Opioid intoxication
    Opioid withdrawal
    Other opioid-induced disorders
    Unspecified opioid-related disorder

TABLE 16–2. **Substance-related and addictive disorders** *(continued)*

Sedative-, hypnotic-, or anxiolytic-related disorders

    Sedative, hypnotic, or anxiolytic use disorder

    Sedative, hypnotic, or anxiolytic intoxication

    Sedative, hypnotic, or anxiolytic withdrawal

    Other sedative-, hypnotic-, or anxiolytic-induced disorders

Unspecified sedative-, hypnotic-, or anxiolytic-related disorder

Stimulant-related disorders

    Stimulant use disorder

    Stimulant intoxication

    Stimulant withdrawal

    Other stimulant-induced disorders

    Unspecified stimulant-related disorder

Tobacco-related disorders

    Tobacco use disorder

    Tobacco withdrawal

    Other tobacco-induced disorders

    Unspecified tobacco-related disorder

Other (or unknown) substance–related disorders

    Other (or unknown) substance use disorder

    Other (or unknown) substance intoxication

    Other (or unknown) substance withdrawal

    Other (or unknown) substance–induced disorders

    Unspecified other (or unknown) substance–related disorder

Non-substance-related disorders

    Gambling disorder

Alcohol Use Disorder

Alcohol use disorder describes a problematic pattern of alcohol use leading to clinically significant impairment or distress. Two or more of 11 problematic behaviors must occur within a 12-month period for the diagnosis to be made. This diagnosis replaces the clinician's choice in DSM-IV for a diagnosis of alcohol "abuse" or "dependence," and the 11 DSM-5 symptoms represent a merging of those listed for each DSM-IV disorder. The diagnosis of abuse required one of four symptoms, whereas dependence required three of seven symptoms.

    Although the criteria are not differentially weighted, clinicians historically have often paid special attention to tolerance and withdrawal (particularly the latter) as indications of a physiological component. Alcohol withdrawal is characterized by withdrawal symptoms that develop 4–12 hours after the reduction of intake following prolonged, heavy ingestion. Because withdrawal can be unpleasant and intense, individuals who experience this condition may continue to consume alcohol despite its adverse consequences. Some withdrawal symptoms, such as sleep problems, can persist at a lower intensity for months and are felt to contribute to relapse. A minority of individuals with an alcohol use disorder never experience clinically relevant levels of alcohol withdrawal, and less than 10% ever experience severe complications, such as delirium or seizures.

Craving is indicated by a strong desire to drink that makes it difficult to think of much else. School and job performance may suffer either from the effects of drinking or from actual intoxication on the job or at school. Child care or household responsibilities may be neglected. Alcohol-related absences may occur as well. The individual may use alcohol in physically hazardous circumstances. Finally, individuals with alcohol use disorder may continue to consume alcohol despite the knowledge that continued consumption poses significant social or interpersonal problems for them.

Diagnostic Criteria for Alcohol Use Disorder

A. A problematic pattern of alcohol use leading to clinically significant impairment or distress, as manifested by at least two of the following, occurring within a 12-month period:

1. Alcohol is often taken in larger amounts or over a longer period than was intended.
2. There is a persistent desire or unsuccessful efforts to cut down or control alcohol use.
3. A great deal of time is spent in activities necessary to obtain alcohol, use alcohol, or recover from its effects.
4. Craving, or a strong desire or urge to use alcohol.
5. Recurrent alcohol use resulting in a failure to fulfill major role obligations at work, school, or home.
6. Continued alcohol use despite having persistent or recurrent social or interpersonal problems caused or exacerbated by the effects of alcohol.
7. Important social, occupational, or recreational activities are given up or reduced because of alcohol use.
8. Recurrent alcohol use in situations in which it is physically hazardous.
9. Alcohol use is continued despite knowledge of having a persistent or recurrent physical or psychological problem that is likely to have been caused or exacerbated by alcohol.
10. Tolerance, as defined by either of the following:
    a. A need for markedly increased amounts of alcohol to achieve intoxication or desired effect.
    b. A markedly diminished effect with continued use of the same amount of alcohol.

11. Withdrawal, as manifested by either of the following:

    a. The characteristic withdrawal syndrome for alcohol (refer to Criteria A and B of the criteria set for alcohol withdrawal).

    b. Alcohol (or a closely related substance, such as a benzodiazepine) is taken to relieve or avoid withdrawal symptoms.

Specify if:

In early remission: After full criteria for alcohol use disorder were previously met, none of the criteria for alcohol use disorder have been met for at least 3 months but for less than 12 months (with the exception that Criterion A4, "Craving, or a strong desire or urge to use alcohol," may be met).

In sustained remission: After full criteria for alcohol use disorder were previously met, none of the criteria for alcohol use disorder have been met at any time during a period of 12 months or longer (with the exception that Criterion A4, "Craving, or a strong desire or urge to use alcohol," may be met).

Specify if:

In a controlled environment: This additional specifier is used if the individual is in an environment where access to alcohol is restricted.

Code based on current severity: Note for ICD-10-CM codes: If an alcohol intoxication, alcohol withdrawal, or another alcohol-induced mental disorder is also present, do not use the codes below for alcohol use disorder. Instead, the comorbid alcohol use disorder is indicated in the 4th character of the alcohol-induced disorder code (see the coding note for alcohol intoxication, alcohol withdrawal, or a specific alcohol-induced mental disorder). For example, if there is comorbid alcohol intoxication and alcohol use disorder, only the alcohol intoxication code is given, with the 4th character indicating whether the comorbid alcohol use disorder is mild, moderate, or severe: F10.129 for mild alcohol use disorder with alcohol intoxication or F10.229 for a moderate or severe alcohol use disorder with alcohol intoxication.

Specify current severity:

305.00 (F10.10) Mild: Presence of 2–3 symptoms.

303.90 (F10.20) Moderate: Presence of 4–5 symptoms.

303.90 (F10.20) Severe: Presence of 6 or more symptoms.

Alcohol Intoxication

The essential feature of alcohol intoxication is the presence of clinically significant problematic behavioral or psychological changes that develop in the context of the ingestion of alcohol. These changes are accompanied by evidence of impaired functioning and judgment and, if intoxication is intense, can result in a life-threatening situation. The symptoms must not be better explained by another medical condition, are not a reflection of conditions such as delirium, and are not related to intoxication with other depressant drugs such as sedatives and hypnotics. The levels of incoordination can interfere with driving abilities and with performing usual activities to the point of causing accidents.

Alcohol intoxication is sometimes associated with amnesia for the events that occurred during the course of the intoxication ("blackouts"). This phenomenon may be related to the presence of high blood alcohol levels and, perhaps, to the rapidity with which this level is reached. Even during mild alcohol intoxication, different symptoms are likely to be observed at different time points. Evidence of mild intoxication can be seen in most people after approximately two drinks. Early in the drinking period, with blood alcohol levels rising, symptoms often include talkativeness, a sense of well-being, and a bright, expansive mood. Later, particularly when levels are falling, the individuals likely become progressively more depressed, withdrawn, and cognitively impaired. At very high levels, a nontolerant person is likely to fall asleep and enter a first stage of anesthesia. Higher blood alcohol levels can cause inhibition of respiration and pulse and even death.

Diagnostic Criteria for Alcohol Intoxication

A. Recent ingestion of alcohol.

B. Clinically significant problematic behavioral or psychological changes (e.g., inappropriate sexual or aggressive behavior, mood lability, impaired judgment) that developed during, or shortly after, alcohol ingestion.

C. One (or more) of the following signs or symptoms developing during, or shortly after, alcohol use:

1. Slurred speech.
2. Incoordination.
3. Unsteady gait.
4. Nystagmus.
5. Impairment in attention or memory.
6. Stupor or coma.

D. The signs or symptoms are not attributable to another medical condition and are not better explained by another mental disorder, including intoxication with another substance.

Coding note: The ICD-9-CM code is **303.00.** The ICD-10-CM code depends on whether there is a comorbid alcohol use disorder. If a mild alcohol use disorder is comorbid, the ICD-10-CM code is **F10.129,** and if a moderate or severe alcohol use disorder is comorbid, the ICD-10-CM code is **F10.229.** If there is no comorbid alcohol use disorder, then the ICD-10-CM code is **F10.929.**

Alcohol Withdrawal

The essential feature of alcohol withdrawal is the presence of a characteristic syndrome that develops after the cessation of or reduction in heavy and prolonged alcohol use. The withdrawal syndrome includes two or more of the symptoms listed in Criterion B. The symptoms cause clinically significant distress or functional impairment. The symptoms must not be due to another medical condition or mental or substance-related disorder. Symptoms can be relieved by the use of alcohol or the administration of benzodiazepines. The withdrawal symptoms typically begin when blood concentrations of alcohol decline sharply, generally within 4–12 hours after alcohol use has stopped or been reduced. Because of the relatively fast metabolism of alcohol, the intensity of symptoms usually peaks during the second day of abstinence and the symptoms generally improve after 4–5 days from the last alcohol use. Symptoms of anxiety, insomnia, and autonomic dysfunction may persist for up to 6 months at lower levels of intensity.

Diagnostic Criteria for Alcohol Withdrawal

A. Cessation of (or reduction in) alcohol use that has been heavy and prolonged.
B. Two (or more) of the following, developing within several hours to a few days after the cessation of (or reduction in) alcohol use described in Criterion A:

1. Autonomic hyperactivity (e.g., sweating or pulse rate greater than 100 bpm).
2. Increased hand tremor.
3. Insomnia.
4. Nausea or vomiting.
5. Transient visual, tactile, or auditory hallucinations or illusions.
6. Psychomotor agitation.
7. Anxiety.
8. Generalized tonic-clonic seizures.

C. The signs or symptoms in Criterion B cause clinically significant distress or impairment in social, occupational, or other important areas of functioning.
D. The signs or symptoms are not attributable to another medical condition and are not better explained by another mental disorder, including intoxication or withdrawal from another substance.

Specify if:

With perceptual disturbances: This specifier applies in the rare instance when hallucinations (usually visual or tactile) occur with intact reality testing, or auditory, visual, or tactile illusions occur in the absence of a delirium.

Coding note: The ICD-9-CM code is **291.81.** The ICD-10-CM code for alcohol withdrawal without perceptual disturbances is **F10.239,** and the ICD-10-CM code for alcohol withdrawal with perceptual disturbances is **F10.232.** Note that the ICD-10-CM code indicates the comorbid presence of a moderate or severe alcohol use disorder, reflecting the fact that alcohol withdrawal can only occur in the presence of a moderate or severe alcohol use disorder. It is not permissible to code a comorbid mild alcohol use disorder with alcohol withdrawal.

Other Alcohol-Induced Disorders and Unspecified Alcohol-Related Disorder

Individuals are diagnosed with other alcohol-induced disorders, such as alcohol-induced anxiety disorder or alcohol-induced sleep disorder, when the symptoms are sufficiently severe to warrant independent clinical attention from intoxication or withdrawal.

Unspecified alcohol-related disorder can be diagnosed when symptoms that cause clinically significant distress or functional impairment do not meet full criteria for other disorders in this diagnostic class.

CAFFEINE-RELATED DISORDERS

Caffeine is one of the most commonly used psychoactive substances in the world. Coffee is one of the most potent sources of caffeine, although certain "energy" drinks may have more caffeine per ounce than coffee. Tea, soft drinks, and chocolate have less caffeine. Caffeine is also found in nonprescription products such as those for headaches.

Available scientific evidence supports the diagnoses of both caffeine intoxication and caffeine withdrawal. Some caffeine users, however, appear to display symptoms consistent with problematic use. Because data are not available at this time to determine the clinical significance of or scientific foundation for a caffeine use disorder, proposed criteria for caffeine use disorder are included in DSM-5 Section III to facilitate research (see Chapter 22, "Conditions for Further Study").

Caffeine Intoxication

Essential features of caffeine intoxication are recent consumption of caffeine and five or more symptoms that develop during or shortly after caffeine use. Symptoms that can appear following the ingestion of as little as 200 mg of caffeine (i.e., 1–2 cups of coffee) per day include restlessness, nervousness, excitement, insomnia, flushed face, diuresis, and gastrointestinal complaints. More severe symptoms, such as muscle twitching, rambling flow of thought or speech, tachycardia, periods of inexhaustibility, and psychomotor agitation, generally appear at levels of more than 1 g/day. Caffeine intoxication may not occur despite a high caffeine intake, however, because of the development of tolerance in some persons. For this diagnosis, the symptoms must cause clinically significant distress or impairment in social, occupational, or other important areas of functioning.

Prevalence of the disorder is unclear, but research suggests that about 7% of individuals in the general population experience five or more symptoms along with functional impairment consistent with the diagnosis of caffeine intoxication. Symptoms usually remit within the first day or so and do not have any known long-lasting consequences.

Diagnostic Criteria for Caffeine Intoxication   305.90 (F15.929)

A. Recent consumption of caffeine (typically a high dose well in excess of 250 mg).
B. Five (or more) of the following signs or symptoms developing during, or shortly after, caffeine use:
   1. Restlessness.

2. Nervousness.
3. Excitement.
4. Insomnia.
5. Flushed face.
6. Diuresis.
7. Gastrointestinal disturbance.
8. Muscle twitching.
9. Rambling flow of thought and speech.
10. Tachycardia or cardiac arrhythmia.
11. Periods of inexhaustibility.
12. Psychomotor agitation.

C. The signs or symptoms in Criterion B cause clinically significant distress or impairment in social, occupational, or other important areas of functioning.
D. The signs or symptoms are not attributable to another medical condition and are not better explained by another mental disorder, including intoxication with another substance.

Caffeine Withdrawal

Caffeine withdrawal is new to DSM-5. The diagnosis was included in DSM-IV's Appendix B, "Criteria Sets and Axes Provided for Further Study," to encourage further research. The major reason it was not previously included as a full-fledged disorder is that the syndrome was not considered severe enough to warrant clinical attention. Research has since accumulated to show that caffeine withdrawal can produce distress and impairment. The severity of symptoms can vary from mild to extreme. Overall, rates of functional impairment vary from about 10% to as high as 55%. Several lines of evidence indicate that repeated caffeine use can produce a physical dependence state that impairs the user's ability to control caffeine use.

Because caffeine is often integrated into social customs and daily rituals, caffeine consumers may be unaware of their physical dependence on caffeine. Thus, withdrawal symptoms can be unexpected and misattributed to other causes. Furthermore, withdrawal symptoms may occur when individuals are required to abstain from foods and beverages prior to medical procedures, or when a caffeine dose is missed because of a change in routine. The probability and severity of withdrawal symptoms are generally related to usual daily caffeine dose, but there is a large variability among (and within) individuals in the incidence, severity, and time course of withdrawal.

Diagnostic Criteria for Caffeine Withdrawal   292.0 (F15.93)

A. Prolonged daily use of caffeine.
B. Abrupt cessation of or reduction in caffeine use, followed within 24 hours by three (or more) of the following signs or symptoms:

1. Headache.
2. Marked fatigue or drowsiness.
3. Dysphoric mood, depressed mood, or irritability.
4. Difficulty concentrating.
5. Flu-like symptoms (nausea, vomiting, or muscle pain/stiffness).

C. The signs or symptoms in Criterion B cause clinically significant distress or impairment in social, occupational, or other important areas of functioning.

D. The signs or symptoms are not associated with the physiological effects of another medical condition (e.g., migraine, viral illness) and are not better explained by another mental disorder, including intoxication or withdrawal from another substance.

Other Caffeine-Induced Disorders and Unspecified Caffeine-Related Disorder

Individuals are diagnosed with other caffeine-induced disorders, such as caffeine-induced anxiety disorder and caffeine-induced sleep disorder, instead of caffeine intoxication or caffeine withdrawal only when the symptoms are sufficiently severe to warrant independent clinical attention. Individuals are diagnosed with unspecified caffeine-related disorder if they have symptoms characteristic of a caffeine-related disorder that are not classifiable as caffeine intoxication, caffeine withdrawal, or a caffeine-induced disorder.

CANNABIS-RELATED DISORDERS

Cannabis-related disorders may result from use of *Cannabis sativa*, commonly referred to as marijuana, weed, pot, herb, grass, reefer, and so on. The concentration extract from cannabis (hashish) is also commonly used. *Cannabis* is a generic term and also refers to other forms, including synthetic cannabinoid compounds. Synthetic oral formulations are available by prescription for medical indications in some areas. The primary psychoactive ingredient in cannabis is delta-9-tetrahydrocannabinol (delta-9-THC). Cannabis has diverse effects on the brain, prominent among which are actions on CB1 and CB2 cannabinoid receptors found throughout the central nervous system. Cannabis that is generally available varies greatly in potency. Although cannabis is more commonly smoked, it is sometimes ingested orally after being mixed into food. Also, devices have been developed in which cannabis is "vaporized." A new disorder listed in DSM-5 is cannabis withdrawal.

Cannabis Use Disorder

People who regularly use cannabis can develop all the general diagnostic features of a substance use disorder. Cannabis use disorder may occur by itself, but it frequently occurs along with use of other substances, such as alcohol, cocaine, and opioids. People who abuse multiple types of substances may minimize the impact of symptoms related to cannabis. Pharmacological and behavioral tolerance to most of the effects of cannabis have been reported in people who use the drug chronically. Tolerance is lost when cannabis use is discontinued for a significant period of time. Abrupt cessation of daily or near-daily use can result in withdrawal symptoms such as irritability, anger, anxiety, depressed mood, restlessness, and sleep difficulty.

People with a cannabis use disorder may use cannabis throughout the day for periods of months or years and may spend many hours per day under its influence. Others may use less frequently but still experience recurrent use-related problems. Use of cannabis at home may lead to arguments with spouses or parents, and its use in the presence of children can adversely impact family functioning. Use of cannabis on the job or while working at a job that requires drug testing can be a sign of a cannabis use disorder. Those who continue using despite knowledge of physical or psychological problems show evidence of a disorder.

Diagnostic Criteria for Cannabis Use Disorder

A. A problematic pattern of cannabis use leading to clinically significant impairment or distress, as manifested by at least two of the following, occurring within a 12-month period:

  1. Cannabis is often taken in larger amounts or over a longer period than was intended.
  2. There is a persistent desire or unsuccessful efforts to cut down or control cannabis use.
  3. A great deal of time is spent in activities necessary to obtain cannabis, use cannabis, or recover from its effects.
  4. Craving, or a strong desire or urge to use cannabis.
  5. Recurrent cannabis use resulting in a failure to fulfill major role obligations at work, school, or home.
  6. Continued cannabis use despite having persistent or recurrent social or interpersonal problems caused or exacerbated by the effects of cannabis.
  7. Important social, occupational, or recreational activities are given up or reduced because of cannabis use.
  8. Recurrent cannabis use in situations in which it is physically hazardous.
  9. Cannabis use is continued despite knowledge of having a persistent or recurrent physical or psychological problem that is likely to have been caused or exacerbated by cannabis.
  10. Tolerance, as defined by either of the following:
      a. A need for markedly increased amounts of cannabis to achieve intoxication or desired effect.
      b. Markedly diminished effect with continued use of the same amount of cannabis.
  11. Withdrawal, as manifested by either of the following:
      a. The characteristic withdrawal syndrome for cannabis (refer to Criteria A and B of the criteria set for cannabis withdrawal).
      b. Cannabis (or a closely related substance) is taken to relieve or avoid withdrawal symptoms.

Specify if:

In early remission: After full criteria for cannabis use disorder were previously met, none of the criteria for cannabis use disorder have been met for at least 3 months but for less than 12 months (with the exception that Criterion A4, "Craving, or a strong desire or urge to use cannabis," may be met).

In sustained remission: After full criteria for cannabis use disorder were previously met, none of the criteria for cannabis use disorder have been met at any time during a period of 12 months or longer (with the exception that Criterion A4, "Craving, or a strong desire or urge to use cannabis," may be present).

Specify if:

In a controlled environment: This additional specifier is used if the individual is in an environment where access to cannabis is restricted.

Code based on current severity: Note for ICD-10-CM codes: If a cannabis intoxication, cannabis withdrawal, or another cannabis-induced mental disorder is also present, do not use the codes below for cannabis use disorder. Instead, the comorbid cannabis use disorder is indicated in the 4th character of the cannabis-induced disorder code (see the coding note for cannabis intoxication, cannabis withdrawal, or a specific cannabis-induced mental disorder). For example, if there is comorbid cannabis-induced anxiety disorder and cannabis use disorder, only the cannabis-induced anxiety disorder code is given, with the 4th character indicating whether the comorbid cannabis use disorder is mild, moderate, or severe: F12.180 for mild cannabis use disorder with cannabis-induced anxiety disorder or F12.280 for a moderate or severe cannabis use disorder with cannabis-induced anxiety disorder.

Specify current severity:

305.20 (F12.10) Mild: Presence of 2–3 symptoms.

304.30 (F12.20) Moderate: Presence of 4–5 symptoms.

304.30 (F12.20) Severe: Presence of 6 or more symptoms.

Cannabis Intoxication

The essential feature of cannabis intoxication is the presence of clinically significant problematic behavioral or psychological changes that develop during or shortly after cannabis use. Intoxication usually begins with a "high," followed by symptoms that include euphoria with inappropriate laughter and grandiosity, sedation, lethargy, impairment in short-term memory, difficulty carrying out complex mental processes, and impaired judgment. Occasionally, anxiety, dysphoria, or social withdrawal may occur. These effects are accompanied by two or more of the following physical signs, developing within 2 hours of cannabis use: conjunctival injection, increased appetite, dry mouth, and tachycardia.

Intoxication develops within minutes if cannabis is smoked but may take a few hours to develop if orally ingested. The effects usually last 3–4 hours, the duration being somewhat longer when the substance is ingested orally.

Diagnostic Criteria for Cannabis Intoxication

A. Recent use of cannabis.

B. Clinically significant problematic behavioral or psychological changes (e.g., impaired motor coordination, euphoria, anxiety, sensation of slowed time, impaired judgment, social withdrawal) that developed during, or shortly after, cannabis use.

C. Two (or more) of the following signs or symptoms developing within 2 hours of cannabis use:

   1. Conjunctival injection.
   2. Increased appetite.
   3. Dry mouth.
   4. Tachycardia.

D. The signs or symptoms are not attributable to another medical condition and are not better explained by another mental disorder, including intoxication with another substance.

Specify if:

   With perceptual disturbances: Hallucinations with intact reality testing or auditory, visual, or tactile illusions occur in the absence of a delirium.

Coding note: The ICD-9-CM code is **292.89.** The ICD-10-CM code depends on whether or not there is a comorbid cannabis use disorder and whether or not there are perceptual disturbances.

   For cannabis intoxication, without perceptual disturbances: If a mild cannabis use disorder is comorbid, the ICD-10-CM code is **F12.129,** and if a moderate or severe cannabis use disorder is comorbid, the ICD-10-CM code is **F12.229.** If there is no comorbid cannabis use disorder, then the ICD-10-CM code is **F12.929.**

   For cannabis intoxication, with perceptual disturbances: If a mild cannabis use disorder is comorbid, the ICD-10-CM code is **F12.122,** and if a moderate or severe cannabis use disorder is comorbid, the ICD-10-CM code is **F12.222.** If there is no comorbid cannabis use disorder, then the ICD-10-CM code is **F12.922.**

Cannabis Withdrawal

Research on cannabis withdrawal conducted since the publication of DSM-IV clearly supports its inclusion in DSM-5. Studies have shown that the syndrome can be reliably identified and that it has a time course typical of other substance withdrawal syndromes. Nonhuman and human laboratory studies provide clear evidence of the pharmacological specificity of the withdrawal syndrome. Furthermore, research suggests that the syndrome is not rare.

Evidence also shows that the syndrome is clinically important. Cannabis users report using cannabis to relieve withdrawal symptoms, suggesting that withdrawal might contribute to ongoing abuse. A substantial proportion of adults and adolescents in treatment for cannabis use admit to moderate to severe withdrawal symptoms, and report that these symptoms make cessation more difficult. People living with cannabis users observe significant withdrawal effects, suggesting that such symptoms are disruptive to daily living.

Diagnostic Criteria for Cannabis Withdrawal 292.0 (F12.288)

A. Cessation of cannabis use that has been heavy and prolonged (i.e., usually daily or almost daily use over a period of at least a few months).

B. Three (or more) of the following signs and symptoms develop within approximately 1 week after Criterion A:

1. Irritability, anger, or aggression.
2. Nervousness or anxiety.
3. Sleep difficulty (e.g., insomnia, disturbing dreams).
4. Decreased appetite or weight loss.
5. Restlessness.
6. Depressed mood.
7. At least one of the following physical symptoms causing significant discomfort: abdominal pain, shakiness/tremors, sweating, fever, chills, or headache.

C. The signs or symptoms in Criterion B cause clinically significant distress or impairment in social, occupational, or other important areas of functioning.

D. The signs or symptoms are not attributable to another medical condition and are not better explained by another mental disorder, including intoxication or withdrawal from another substance.

Coding note: The ICD-9-CM code is 292.0. The ICD-10-CM code for cannabis withdrawal is F12.288. Note that the ICD-10-CM code indicates the comorbid presence of a moderate or severe cannabis use disorder, reflecting the fact that cannabis withdrawal can only occur in the presence of a moderate or severe cannabis use disorder. It is not permissible to code a comorbid mild cannabis use disorder with cannabis withdrawal.

Other Cannabis-Induced Disorders and Unspecified Cannabis-Related Disorder

Individuals are diagnosed with other cannabis-induced disorders, such as cannabis-induced psychotic disorder, cannabis-induced anxiety disorder, cannabis-induced sleep disorder, or cannabis intoxication delirium, instead of cannabis intoxication or cannabis withdrawal when the symptoms are sufficiently severe to warrant independent clinical attention. Individuals are diagnosed with unspecified cannabis-related disorder if they have symptoms characteristic of a cannabis-related disorder that are not classifiable as cannabis use disorder, cannabis intoxication, cannabis withdrawal, or a cannabis-induced disorder.

HALLUCINOGEN-RELATED DISORDERS

Phencyclidine and Other Hallucinogen Use Disorders

Hallucinogens have been used for thousands of years and in multiple cultures. They include LSD (lysergic acid diethylamide), mescaline, MDMA (3,4-methylenedioxymethamphetamine), and psilocybin. DSM-IV contained separate sections for phencyclidine and for hallucinogenic drugs. From both clinical and pharmacological perspectives, however, phencyclidine is a drug of abuse with hallucinogenic properties. For that reason, DSM-5 has included phencyclidine in the clinically similar but pharmacologically heterogeneous category of hallucinogens. All drugs in this category produce hallucinations, but by different mechanisms.

Diagnostic Criteria for Phencyclidine Use Disorder

A. A pattern of phencyclidine (or a pharmacologically similar substance) use leading to clinically significant impairment or distress, as manifested by at least two of the following, occurring within a 12-month period:

1. Phencyclidine is often taken in larger amounts or over a longer period than was intended.
2. There is a persistent desire or unsuccessful efforts to cut down or control phencyclidine use.
3. A great deal of time is spent in activities necessary to obtain phencyclidine, use the phencyclidine, or recover from its effects.
4. Craving, or a strong desire or urge to use phencyclidine.
5. Recurrent phencyclidine use resulting in a failure to fulfill major role obligations at work, school, or home (e.g., repeated absences from work or poor work performance related to phencyclidine use; phencyclidine-related absences, suspensions, or expulsions from school; neglect of children or household).
6. Continued phencyclidine use despite having persistent or recurrent social or interpersonal problems caused or exacerbated by the effects of the phencyclidine (e.g., arguments with a spouse about consequences of intoxication; physical fights).
7. Important social, occupational, or recreational activities are given up or reduced because of phencyclidine use.
8. Recurrent phencyclidine use in situations in which it is physically hazardous (e.g., driving an automobile or operating a machine when impaired by a phencyclidine).
9. Phencyclidine use is continued despite knowledge of having a persistent or recurrent physical or psychological problem that is likely to have been caused or exacerbated by the phencyclidine.

10. Tolerance, as defined by either of the following:
    a. A need for markedly increased amounts of the phencyclidine to achieve intoxication or desired effect.
    b. A markedly diminished effect with continued use of the same amount of the phencyclidine.

Note: Withdrawal symptoms and signs are not established for phencyclidines, and so this criterion does not apply. (Withdrawal from phencyclidines has been reported in animals but not documented in human users.)

Specify if:
In early remission: After full criteria for phencyclidine use disorder were previously met, none of the criteria for phencyclidine use disorder have been met for at least 3 months but for less than 12 months (with the exception that Criterion A4, "Craving, or a strong desire or urge to use the phencyclidine," may be met).

In sustained remission: After full criteria for phencyclidine use disorder were previously met, none of the criteria for phencyclidine use disorder have been met at any time during a period of 12 months or longer (with the exception that Criterion A4, "Craving, or a strong desire or urge to use the phencyclidine," may be met).

Specify if:
In a controlled environment: This additional specifier is used if the individual is in an environment where access to phencyclidines is restricted.

Coding based on current severity: Note for ICD-10-CM codes: If a phencyclidine intoxication or another phencyclidine-induced mental disorder is also present, do not use the codes below for phencyclidine use disorder. Instead, the comorbid phencyclidine use disorder is indicated in the 4th character of the phencyclidine-induced disorder code (see the coding note for phencyclidine intoxication or a specific phencyclidine-induced mental disorder). For example, if there is comorbid phencyclidine-induced psychotic disorder, only the phencyclidine-induced psychotic disorder code is given, with the 4th character indicating whether the comorbid phencyclidine use disorder is mild, moderate, or severe: F16.159 for mild phencyclidine use disorder with phencyclidine-induced psychotic disorder or F16.259 for a moderate or severe phencyclidine use disorder with phencyclidine-induced psychotic disorder.

Specify current severity:
305.90 (F16.10) Mild: Presence of 2–3 symptoms.
304.60 (F16.20) Moderate: Presence of 4–5 symptoms.
304.60 (F16.20) Severe: Presence of 6 or more symptoms.

Diagnostic Criteria for Other Hallucinogen Use Disorder

A. A problematic pattern of hallucinogen (other than phencyclidine) use leading to clinically significant impairment or distress, as manifested by at least two of the following, occurring within a 12-month period:

1. The hallucinogen is often taken in larger amounts or over a longer period than was intended.
2. There is a persistent desire or unsuccessful efforts to cut down or control hallucinogen use.

3. A great deal of time is spent in activities necessary to obtain the hallucinogen, use the hallucinogen, or recover from its effects.

4. Craving, or a strong desire or urge to use the hallucinogen.

5. Recurrent hallucinogen use resulting in a failure to fulfill major role obligations at work, school, or home (e.g., repeated absences from work or poor work performance related to hallucinogen use; hallucinogen-related absences, suspensions, or expulsions from school; neglect of children or household).

6. Continued hallucinogen use despite having persistent or recurrent social or interpersonal problems caused or exacerbated by the effects of the hallucinogen (e.g., arguments with a spouse about consequences of intoxication; physical fights).

7. Important social, occupational, or recreational activities are given up or reduced because of hallucinogen use.

8. Recurrent hallucinogen use in situations in which it is physically hazardous (e.g., driving an automobile or operating a machine when impaired by the hallucinogen).

9. Hallucinogen use is continued despite knowledge of having a persistent or recurrent physical or psychological problem that is likely to have been caused or exacerbated by the hallucinogen.

10. Tolerance, as defined by either of the following:

    a. A need for markedly increased amounts of the hallucinogen to achieve intoxication or desired effect.

    b. A markedly diminished effect with continued use of the same amount of the hallucinogen.

Note: Withdrawal symptoms and signs are not established for hallucinogens, and so this criterion does not apply.

Specify **the particular hallucinogen.**

Specify if:

In early remission: After full criteria for other hallucinogen use disorder were previously met, none of the criteria for other hallucinogen use disorder have been met for at least 3 months but for less than 12 months (with the exception that Criterion A4, "Craving, or a strong desire or urge to use the hallucinogen," may be met).

In sustained remission: After full criteria for other hallucinogen use disorder were previously met, none of the criteria for other hallucinogen use disorder have been met at any time during a period of 12 months or longer (with the exception that Criterion A4, "Craving, or a strong desire or urge to use the hallucinogen," may be met).

Specify if:

In a controlled environment: This additional specifier is used if the individual is in an environment where access to hallucinogens is restricted.

Coding based on current severity: Note for ICD-10-CM codes: If a hallucinogen intoxication or another hallucinogen-induced mental disorder is also present, do not use the codes below for hallucinogen use disorder. Instead, the comorbid hallucinogen use disorder is indicated in the 4th character of the hallucinogen-induced disorder code (see the coding note for hallucinogen intoxication or specific hallucinogen-induced mental disorder). For example, if there is comorbid hallucinogen-induced psychotic disorder and hallucinogen use disorder, only the hallucinogen-induced psychotic disorder code is given, with the 4th character indicating whether the comorbid hallucinogen use disorder is mild, moderate, or severe: F16.159 for mild hallucinogen use disorder with hallucinogen-induced psychotic disorder or F16.259 for a moderate or severe hallucinogen use disorder with hallucinogen-induced psychotic disorder.

Specify current severity:
  305.30 (F16.10) Mild: Presence of 2–3 symptoms.
  304.50 (F16.20) Moderate: Presence of 4–5 symptoms.
  304.50 (F16.20) Severe: Presence of 6 or more symptoms.

Phencyclidine Intoxication and Other Hallucinogen Intoxication

Phencyclidine intoxication and other hallucinogen intoxication reflect the clinically significant behavioral or psychological changes that occur shortly after ingestion of a substance. Depending on the specific agent, intoxication lasts minutes to hours. Intoxication with phencyclidine differs from that with other hallucinogens. With phencyclidine intoxication, the individual may experience nystagmus, seizures, ataxia, dysarthria, hypertension, and hyperacusis. By contrast, individuals with other hallucinogen intoxication experience tachycardia, blurred vision, tremors, and sweating, among other symptoms. Behavioral changes such as belligerence, assaultiveness, unpredictability, and psychomotor agitation occur with phencyclidine intoxication, whereas other hallucinogen intoxication may present with marked anxiety or depression, ideas of reference, fear of "losing one's mind," and paranoid ideation. Additionally, other hallucinogen intoxication may result in perceptual changes such as depersonalization, derealization, hallucinations, and synesthesias that occur during, or shortly after, hallucinogen use.

Intoxication with either phencyclidine or other hallucinogens should be differentiated from intoxication with stimulants, anticholinergics, inhalants, or other drugs of abuse. Toxicological tests can be useful in making this distinction. Other conditions to consider include mood disorders, psychotic disorders, and withdrawal from other substances. The perceptual disturbances and impaired judgment associated with hallucinogen intoxication can result in injuries or fatalities from motor vehicle accidents, physical fights, or unintentional self-injury.

Diagnostic Criteria for Phencyclidine Intoxication

A. Recent use of phencyclidine (or a pharmacologically similar substance).

B. Clinically significant problematic behavioral changes (e.g., belligerence, assaultiveness, impulsiveness, unpredictability, psychomotor agitation, impaired judgment) that developed during, or shortly after, phencyclidine use.

C. Within 1 hour, two (or more) of the following signs or symptoms:

   Note: When the drug is smoked, "snorted," or used intravenously, the onset may be particularly rapid.

1. Vertical or horizontal nystagmus.
2. Hypertension or tachycardia.
3. Numbness or diminished responsiveness to pain.
4. Ataxia.
5. Dysarthria.
6. Muscle rigidity.
7. Seizures or coma.
8. Hyperacusis.

D. The signs or symptoms are not attributable to another medical condition and are not better explained by another mental disorder, including intoxication with another substance.

Coding note: The ICD-9-CM code is **292.89.** The ICD-10-CM code depends on whether there is a comorbid phencyclidine use disorder. If a mild phencyclidine use disorder is comorbid, the ICD-10-CM code is **F16.129,** and if a moderate or severe phencyclidine use disorder is comorbid, the ICD-10-CM code is **F16.229.** If there is no comorbid phencyclidine use disorder, then the ICD-10-CM code is **F16.929.**

Diagnostic Criteria for Other Hallucinogen Intoxication

A. Recent use of a hallucinogen (other than phencyclidine).
B. Clinically significant problematic behavioral or psychological changes (e.g., marked anxiety or depression, ideas of reference, fear of "losing one's mind," paranoid ideation, impaired judgment) that developed during, or shortly after, hallucinogen use.
C. Perceptual changes occurring in a state of full wakefulness and alertness (e.g., subjective intensification of perceptions, depersonalization, derealization, illusions, hallucinations, synesthesias) that developed during, or shortly after, hallucinogen use.
D. Two (or more) of the following signs developing during, or shortly after, hallucinogen use:

1. Pupillary dilation.
2. Tachycardia.
3. Sweating.
4. Palpitations.
5. Blurring of vision.
6. Tremors.
7. Incoordination.

E. The signs or symptoms are not attributable to another medical condition and are not better explained by another mental disorder, including intoxication with another substance.

Coding note: The ICD-9-CM code is **292.89.** The ICD-10-CM code depends on whether there is a comorbid hallucinogen use disorder. If a mild hallucinogen use disorder is comorbid, the ICD-10-CM code is **F16.129,** and if a moderate or severe hallucinogen use disorder is comorbid, the ICD-10-CM code is **F16.229**. If there is no comorbid hallucinogen use disorder, then the ICD-10-CM code is **F16.929**.

Hallucinogen Persisting Perception Disorder

Hallucinogen persisting perception disorder involves the reexperiencing of one or more of the perceptual symptoms that were experienced while intoxicated with the hallucinogen.

Diagnostic Criteria for Hallucinogen Persisting Perception Disorder 292.89 (F16.983)

A. Following cessation of use of a hallucinogen, the reexperiencing of one or more of the perceptual symptoms that were experienced while intoxicated with the hallucinogen (e.g., geometric hallucinations, false perceptions of movement in the peripheral visual fields, flashes of color, intensified colors, trails of images of moving objects, positive afterimages, halos around objects, macropsia and micropsia).
B. The symptoms in Criterion A cause clinically significant distress or impairment in social, occupational, or other important areas of functioning.
C. The symptoms are not attributable to another medical condition (e.g., anatomical lesions and infections of the brain, visual epilepsies) and are not better explained by another mental disorder (e.g., delirium, major neurocognitive disorder, schizophrenia) or hypnopompic hallucinations.

Other Phencyclidine- and Other Hallucinogen-Induced Disorders

Individuals are diagnosed with other phencyclidine- or other hallucinogen-induced disorder, such as phencyclidine-induced psychotic disorder, when the symptoms are sufficiently severe to warrant independent clinical attention.

Unspecified Phencyclidine- and Unspecified Hallucinogen-Related Disorders

Individuals are diagnosed with unspecified phencyclidine- or unspecified hallucinogen-related disorder if they have symptoms characteristic of a phencyclidine- or other hallucinogen-related disorder that are not classifiable as phencyclidine or other hallucinogen use disorder, intoxication, withdrawal, or induced disorder.

INHALANT-RELATED DISORDERS

Inhalant Use Disorder

Paint thinner, airplane glue, and gasoline are just a few of the inhalants that are commonplace. They enter the bloodstream quickly, have rapid onset of action, and can damage the central nervous system, kidneys, and liver.

People who regularly use hydrocarbon-based inhalants may develop most of the diagnostic features of a substance use disorder. One exception is withdrawal. Available scientific evidence does not support the diagnosis of inhalant withdrawal as a disorder.

Diagnostic Criteria for Inhalant Use Disorder

A. A problematic pattern of use of a hydrocarbon-based inhalant substance leading to clinically significant impairment or distress, as manifested by at least two of the following, occurring within a 12-month period:

1. The inhalant substance is often taken in larger amounts or over a longer period than was intended.
2. There is a persistent desire or unsuccessful efforts to cut down or control use of the inhalant substance.
3. A great deal of time is spent in activities necessary to obtain the inhalant substance, use it, or recover from its effects.
4. Craving, or a strong desire or urge to use the inhalant substance.
5. Recurrent use of the inhalant substance resulting in a failure to fulfill major role obligations at work, school, or home.
6. Continued use of the inhalant substance despite having persistent or recurrent social or interpersonal problems caused or exacerbated by the effects of its use.
7. Important social, occupational, or recreational activities are given up or reduced because of use of the inhalant substance.
8. Recurrent use of the inhalant substance in situations in which it is physically hazardous.
9. Use of the inhalant substance is continued despite knowledge of having a persistent or recurrent physical or psychological problem that is likely to have been caused or exacerbated by the substance.
10. Tolerance, as defined by either of the following:

    a. A need for markedly increased amounts of the inhalant substance to achieve intoxication or desired effect.
    b. A markedly diminished effect with continued use of the same amount of the inhalant substance.

Specify **the particular inhalant:** When possible, the particular substance involved should be named (e.g., "solvent use disorder").

Specify if:
> **In early remission:** After full criteria for inhalant use disorder were previously met, none of the criteria for inhalant use disorder have been met for at least 3 months but for less than 12 months (with the exception that Criterion A4, "Craving, or a strong desire or urge to use the inhalant substance," may be met).
>
> **In sustained remission:** After full criteria for inhalant use disorder were previously met, none of the criteria for inhalant use disorder have been met at any time during a period of 12 months or longer (with the exception that Criterion A4, "Craving, or a strong desire or urge to use the inhalant substance," may be met).

Specify if:
> **In a controlled environment:** This additional specifier is used if the individual is in an environment where access to inhalant substances is restricted.

Coding based on current severity: Note for ICD-10-CM codes: If an inhalant intoxication or another inhalant-induced mental disorder is also present, do not use the codes below for inhalant use disorder. Instead, the comorbid inhalant use disorder is indicated in the 4th character of the inhalant-induced disorder code (see the coding note for inhalant intoxication or a specific inhalant-induced mental disorder). For example, if there is comorbid inhalant-induced depressive disorder and inhalant use disorder, only the inhalant-induced depressive disorder code is given, with the 4th character indicating whether the comorbid inhalant use disorder is mild, moderate, or severe: F18.14 for mild inhalant use disorder with inhalant-induced depressive disorder or F18.24 for a moderate or severe inhalant use disorder with inhalant-induced depressive disorder.

Specify current severity:
> **305.90 (F18.10) Mild:** Presence of 2–3 symptoms.
> **304.60 (F18.20) Moderate:** Presence of 4–5 symptoms.
> **304.60 (F18.20) Severe:** Presence of 6 or more symptoms.

Inhalant Intoxication

Inhalant intoxication is a clinically significant disorder that develops during, or immediately after, intended or unintended inhalation of an inhalant substance. The intoxication clears within a few minutes to a few hours after exposure ends. Impairment from intoxication may have serious consequences with regard to job-related and social functioning. It may also lead to traffic accidents or unintentional self-injuries. Use of inhaled substances in a closed container, such as a plastic bag, may lead to unconsciousness, anoxia, and death.

Diagnostic Criteria for Inhalant Intoxication

A. Recent intended or unintended short-term, high-dose exposure to inhalant substances, including volatile hydrocarbons such as toluene or gasoline.
B. Clinically significant problematic behavioral or psychological changes (e.g., belligerence, assaultiveness, apathy, impaired judgment) that developed during, or shortly after, exposure to inhalants.

C. Two (or more) of the following signs or symptoms developing during, or shortly after, inhalant use or exposure:

1. Dizziness.
2. Nystagmus.
3. Incoordination.
4. Slurred speech.
5. Unsteady gait.
6. Lethargy.
7. Depressed reflexes.
8. Psychomotor retardation.
9. Tremor.
10. Generalized muscle weakness.
11. Blurred vision or diplopia.
12. Stupor or coma.
13. Euphoria.

D. The signs or symptoms are not attributable to another medical condition and are not better explained by another mental disorder, including intoxication with another substance.

Coding note: The ICD-9-CM code is **292.89.** The ICD-10-CM code depends on whether there is a comorbid inhalant use disorder. If a mild inhalant use disorder is comorbid, the ICD-10-CM code is **F18.129,** and if a moderate or severe inhalant use disorder is comorbid, the ICD-10-CM code is **F18.229.** If there is no comorbid inhalant use disorder, then the ICD-10-CM code is **F18.929.**

Other Inhalant-Induced Disorders and Unspecified Inhalant-Related Disorder

Individuals are diagnosed with other inhalant-induced disorders, such as inhalant-induced psychotic disorder, when the symptoms are sufficiently severe to warrant independent clinical attention.

Individuals are diagnosed with unspecified inhalant-related disorder if they have symptoms characteristic of an inhalant-related disorder that are not classifiable as inhalant use disorder, intoxication, or induced disorder.

OPIOID-RELATED DISORDERS

The opioids include natural and synthetic substances with morphine-like actions that are full agonists to the µ opioid receptor. Medications such as buprenorphine that have both opiate agonist and antagonist effects are also included in this class. Opioids are prescribed as analgesics, anesthetics, antidiarrheal agents, and cough suppressants. After heroin, opium is the most widely consumed illegal opiate in the world. In the United States, the nonmedical use of prescription opioids is a significant problem. Opioid users have a high likelihood of developing opioid use disorders and have an increased risk for HIV, as well as hepatitis B and C viruses; mortality rates are excessive.

Opioid Use Disorder

Opioid use disorder includes signs and symptoms that reflect compulsive, prolonged self-administration of opioid substances that are used for no legitimate medical purposes or that are used in doses that are greatly in excess of the amount needed to treat a medical condition requiring opioid treatment. Individuals with opioid use disorder tend to develop regular patterns of compulsive drug use, such that daily activities are planned around obtaining and administering the drugs. Opioids are usually purchased on the illegal market but may also be obtained from physicians by falsifying or exaggerating general medical problems or by receiving simultaneous prescriptions from several physicians ("doctor shopping"). Most individuals with this disorder have significant levels of tolerance and experience withdrawal on abrupt discontinuation of opioid substances.

Opioid use disorder can be associated with a history of drug-related crimes, usually related to attempts to obtain the drugs. Among health care professionals and individuals with ready access to controlled substances, there is often a different pattern of illegal activities, which might involve problems with state licensing boards. Marital difficulties and unemployment or other work-related problems are also associated with the disorder.

Many people with opioid use disorder are treated with agonist, partial agonist, or agonist/antagonist medication such as methadone, buprenorphine, or naltrexone. These individuals may have a presentation that meets none of the criteria for opioid use disorder (except perhaps tolerance or withdrawal). For these individuals, the additional specifier "on maintenance therapy" would be merited.

Diagnostic Criteria for Opioid Use Disorder

A. A problematic pattern of opioid use leading to clinically significant impairment or distress, as manifested by at least two of the following, occurring within a 12-month period:

1. Opioids are often taken in larger amounts or over a longer period than was intended.
2. There is a persistent desire or unsuccessful efforts to cut down or control opioid use.
3. A great deal of time is spent in activities necessary to obtain the opioid, use the opioid, or recover from its effects.
4. Craving, or a strong desire or urge to use opioids.
5. Recurrent opioid use resulting in a failure to fulfill major role obligations at work, school, or home.
6. Continued opioid use despite having persistent or recurrent social or interpersonal problems caused or exacerbated by the effects of opioids.
7. Important social, occupational, or recreational activities are given up or reduced because of opioid use.
8. Recurrent opioid use in situations in which it is physically hazardous.

9. Continued opioid use despite knowledge of having a persistent or recurrent physical or psychological problem that is likely to have been caused or exacerbated by the substance.
10. Tolerance, as defined by either of the following:
    a. A need for markedly increased amounts of opioids to achieve intoxication or desired effect.
    b. A markedly diminished effect with continued use of the same amount of an opioid.

    Note: This criterion is not considered to be met for those taking opioids solely under appropriate medical supervision.

11. Withdrawal, as manifested by either of the following:
    a. The characteristic opioid withdrawal syndrome (refer to Criteria A and B of the criteria set for opioid withdrawal).
    b. Opioids (or a closely related substance) are taken to relieve or avoid withdrawal symptoms.

    Note: This criterion is not considered to be met for those individuals taking opioids solely under appropriate medical supervision.

Specify if:

In early remission: After full criteria for opioid use disorder were previously met, none of the criteria for opioid use disorder have been met for at least 3 months but for less than 12 months (with the exception that Criterion A4, "Craving, or a strong desire or urge to use opioids," may be met).

In sustained remission: After full criteria for opioid use disorder were previously met, none of the criteria for opioid use disorder have been met at any time during a period of 12 months or longer (with the exception that Criterion A4, "Craving, or a strong desire or urge to use opioids," may be met).

Specify if:

On maintenance therapy: This additional specifier is used if the individual is taking a prescribed agonist medication such as methadone or buprenorphine and none of the criteria for opioid use disorder have been met for that class of medication (except tolerance to, or withdrawal from, the agonist). This category also applies to those individuals being maintained on a partial agonist, an agonist/antagonist, or a full antagonist such as oral naltrexone or depot naltrexone.

In a controlled environment: This additional specifier is used if the individual is in an environment where access to opioids is restricted.

Coding based on current severity: Note for ICD-10-CM codes: If an opioid intoxication, opioid withdrawal, or another opioid-induced mental disorder is also present, do not use the codes below for opioid use disorder. Instead, the comorbid opioid use disorder is indicated in the 4th character of the opioid-induced disorder code (see the coding note for opioid intoxication, opioid withdrawal, or a specific opioid-induced mental disorder). For example, if there is comorbid opioid-induced depressive disorder and opioid use disorder, only the opioid-induced depressive disorder code is given, with the 4th character indicating whether the comorbid opioid use disorder is mild, moderate, or severe: F11.14 for mild opioid use disorder with opioid-induced depressive disorder or F11.24 for a moderate or severe opioid use disorder with opioid-induced depressive disorder.

Specify current severity:
> **305.50 (F11.10) Mild:** Presence of 2–3 symptoms.
> **304.00 (F11.20) Moderate:** Presence of 4–5 symptoms.
> **304.00 (F11.20) Severe:** Presence of 6 or more symptoms.

Opioid Intoxication

The essential feature of opioid intoxication is the presence of abnormal behavioral or psychological changes that develop during or shortly after opioid use. Intoxication is accompanied by pupillary constriction and at least one of the following signs: drowsiness, slurred speech, or impairment in attention or memory. Drowsiness may progress to coma. People with opioid intoxication have demonstrated inattention to their environment, even to the point of ignoring potentially harmful events. The symptoms are not explained by another medical condition or another mental disorder.

Diagnostic Criteria for Opioid Intoxication

A. Recent use of an opioid.

B. Clinically significant problematic behavioral or psychological changes (e.g., initial euphoria followed by apathy, dysphoria, psychomotor agitation or retardation, impaired judgment) that developed during, or shortly after, opioid use.

C. Pupillary constriction (or pupillary dilation due to anoxia from severe overdose) and one (or more) of the following signs or symptoms developing during, or shortly after, opioid use:

1. Drowsiness or coma.
2. Slurred speech.
3. Impairment in attention or memory.

D. The signs or symptoms are not attributable to another medical condition and are not better explained by another mental disorder, including intoxication with another substance.

Specify if:
> **With perceptual disturbances:** This specifier may be noted in the rare instance in which hallucinations with intact reality testing or auditory, visual, or tactile illusions occur in the absence of a delirium.

Coding note: The ICD-9-CM code is **292.89.** The ICD-10-CM code depends on whether or not there is a comorbid opioid use disorder and whether or not there are perceptual disturbances.

> **For opioid intoxication without perceptual disturbances:** If a mild opioid use disorder is comorbid, the ICD-10-CM code is **F11.129,** and if a moderate or severe opioid use disorder is comorbid, the ICD-10-CM code is **F11.229.** If there is no comorbid opioid use disorder, then the ICD-10-CM code is **F11.929.**

> **For opioid intoxication with perceptual disturbances:** If a mild opioid use disorder is comorbid, the ICD-10-CM code is **F11.122,** and if a moderate or severe

opioid use disorder is comorbid, the ICD-10-CM code is **F11.222.** If there is no comorbid opioid use disorder, then the ICD-10-CM code is **F11.922.**

Opioid Withdrawal

The essential feature of opioid withdrawal is the presence of a characteristic withdrawal syndrome that develops after the cessation of or reduction in opioid use that has been heavy and prolonged. The syndrome can also be precipitated by administration of an opioid antagonist, such as naltrexone, after a period of opioid use. Symptoms include complaints of anxiety, restlessness, and muscle aches, along with irritability and increased sensitivity to pain. Other symptoms soon develop, ranging from cognitive (dysphoric mood) to physical (e.g., nausea and vomiting, lacrimation or rhinorrhea, piloerection, sweating) symptoms. Withdrawal may begin within 6–12 hours after the last dose of a short-acting drug such as heroin but within 2–4 days in the case of longer-acting drugs such as methadone.

Diagnostic Criteria for Opioid Withdrawal   292.0 (F11.23)

A. Presence of either of the following:
  1. Cessation of (or reduction in) opioid use that has been heavy and prolonged (i.e., several weeks or longer).
  2. Administration of an opioid antagonist after a period of opioid use.
B. Three (or more) of the following developing within minutes to several days after Criterion A:
  1. Dysphoric mood.
  2. Nausea or vomiting.
  3. Muscle aches.
  4. Lacrimation or rhinorrhea.
  5. Pupillary dilation, piloerection, or sweating.
  6. Diarrhea.
  7. Yawning.
  8. Fever.
  9. Insomnia.
C. The signs or symptoms in Criterion B cause clinically significant distress or impairment in social, occupational, or other important areas of functioning.
D. The signs or symptoms are not attributable to another medical condition and are not better explained by another mental disorder, including intoxication or withdrawal from another substance.

Coding note: The ICD-9-CM code is 292.0. The ICD-10-CM code for opioid withdrawal is F11.23. Note that the ICD-10-CM code indicates the comorbid presence of a moderate or severe opioid use disorder, reflecting the fact that opioid withdrawal can only occur in the presence of a moderate or severe opioid use disorder. It is not permissible to code a comorbid mild opioid use disorder with opioid withdrawal.

Other Opioid-Induced Disorders and Unspecified Opioid-Related Disorder

Individuals are diagnosed with other opioid-induced disorders, such as opioid-induced psychotic disorder, when the symptoms are sufficiently severe to warrant independent clinical attention.

Individuals are diagnosed with unspecified opioid-related disorder if they have symptoms characteristic of an opioid-related disorder that are not classifiable as opioid use disorder, intoxication, withdrawal, or induced disorder.

SEDATIVE-, HYPNOTIC-, OR ANXIOLYTIC-RELATED DISORDERS

Sedative, Hypnotic, or Anxiolytic Use Disorder

Sedative, hypnotic, or anxiolytic substances include benzodiazepines, benzodiazepine-like drugs, carbamates, barbiturates, and barbiturate-like hypnotics. This class includes all prescription sleeping medications and almost all prescription antianxiety medications. Nonbenzodiazepine antianxiety agents (e.g., buspirone) are not included in this class because they do not appear to be associated with significant misuse. At high doses, these drugs can be lethal, particularly when mixed with alcohol, although the lethal dose varies considerably among the specific drugs. Sedative, hypnotic, and anxiolytic substances are available both by prescription and on the black market. Very significant levels of tolerance to and withdrawal from these drugs can develop. The social and interpersonal consequences of sedative, hypnotic, or anxiolytic use disorder mimic those of alcohol in terms of the potential for disinhibited behavior. Accidents, interpersonal difficulties, and interference with work or school performance are all common.

Diagnostic Criteria for Sedative, Hypnotic, or Anxiolytic Use Disorder

A. A problematic pattern of sedative, hypnotic, or anxiolytic use leading to clinically significant impairment or distress, as manifested by at least two of the following, occurring within a 12-month period:

  1. Sedatives, hypnotics, or anxiolytics are often taken in larger amounts or over a longer period than was intended.
  2. There is a persistent desire or unsuccessful efforts to cut down or control sedative, hypnotic, or anxiolytic use.
  3. A great deal of time is spent in activities necessary to obtain the sedative, hypnotic, or anxiolytic; use the sedative, hypnotic, or anxiolytic; or recover from its effects.
  4. Craving, or a strong desire or urge to use the sedative, hypnotic, or anxiolytic.

5. Recurrent sedative, hypnotic, or anxiolytic use resulting in a failure to fulfill major role obligations at work, school, or home (e.g., repeated absences from work or poor work performance related to sedative, hypnotic, or anxiolytic use; sedative-, hypnotic-, or anxiolytic-related absences, suspensions, or expulsions from school; neglect of children or household).

6. Continued sedative, hypnotic, or anxiolytic use despite having persistent or recurrent social or interpersonal problems caused or exacerbated by the effects of sedatives, hypnotics, or anxiolytics (e.g., arguments with a spouse about consequences of intoxication; physical fights).

7. Important social, occupational, or recreational activities are given up or reduced because of sedative, hypnotic, or anxiolytic use.

8. Recurrent sedative, hypnotic, or anxiolytic use in situations in which it is physically hazardous (e.g., driving an automobile or operating a machine when impaired by sedative, hypnotic, or anxiolytic use).

9. Sedative, hypnotic, or anxiolytic use is continued despite knowledge of having a persistent or recurrent physical or psychological problem that is likely to have been caused or exacerbated by the sedative, hypnotic, or anxiolytic.

10. Tolerance, as defined by either of the following:

    a. A need for markedly increased amounts of the sedative, hypnotic, or anxiolytic to achieve intoxication or desired effect.

    b. A markedly diminished effect with continued use of the same amount of the sedative, hypnotic, or anxiolytic.

    Note: This criterion is not considered to be met for individuals taking sedatives, hypnotics, or anxiolytics under medical supervision.

11. Withdrawal, as manifested by either of the following:

    a. The characteristic withdrawal syndrome for sedatives, hypnotics, or anxiolytics (refer to Criteria A and B of the criteria set for sedative, hypnotic, or anxiolytic withdrawal).

    b. Sedatives, hypnotics, or anxiolytics (or a closely related substance, such as alcohol) are taken to relieve or avoid withdrawal symptoms.

    Note: This criterion is not considered to be met for individuals taking sedatives, hypnotics, or anxiolytics under medical supervision.

Specify if:

In early remission: After full criteria for sedative, hypnotic, or anxiolytic use disorder were previously met, none of the criteria for sedative, hypnotic, or anxiolytic use disorder have been met for at least 3 months but for less than 12 months (with the exception that Criterion A4, "Craving, or a strong desire or urge to use the sedative, hypnotic, or anxiolytic," may be met).

In sustained remission: After full criteria for sedative, hypnotic, or anxiolytic use disorder were previously met, none of the criteria for sedative, hypnotic, or anxiolytic use disorder have been met at any time during a period of 12 months or longer (with the exception that Criterion A4, "Craving, or a strong desire or urge to use the sedative, hypnotic, or anxiolytic," may be met).

Specify if:

In a controlled environment: This additional specifier is used if the individual is in an environment where access to sedatives, hypnotics, or anxiolytics is restricted.

Coding based on current severity: Note for ICD-10-CM codes: If a sedative, hypnotic, or anxiolytic intoxication; sedative, hypnotic, or anxiolytic withdrawal; or another sedative-, hypnotic-, or anxiolytic-induced mental disorder is also present, do not use the codes below for sedative, hypnotic, or anxiolytic use disorder. Instead the comorbid sedative, hypnotic, or anxiolytic use disorder is indicated in the 4th character of the sedative-, hypnotic-, or anxiolytic-induced disorder (see the coding note for sedative, hypnotic, or anxiolytic intoxication; sedative, hypnotic, or anxiolytic withdrawal; or specific sedative-, hypnotic-, or anxiolytic-induced mental disorder). For example, if there is comorbid sedative-, hypnotic-, or anxiolytic-induced depressive disorder and sedative, hypnotic, or anxiolytic use disorder, only the sedative-, hypnotic-, or anxiolytic-induced depressive disorder code is given with the 4th character indicating whether the comorbid sedative, hypnotic, or anxiolytic use disorder is mild, moderate, or severe: F13.14 for mild sedative, hypnotic, or anxiolytic use disorder with sedative-, hypnotic-, or anxiolytic-induced depressive disorder or F13.24 for a moderate or severe sedative, hypnotic, or anxiolytic use disorder with sedative-, hypnotic-, or anxiolytic-induced depressive disorder.

Specify current severity:

305.40 (F13.10) Mild: Presence of 2–3 symptoms.

304.10 (F13.20) Moderate: Presence of 4–5 symptoms.

304.10 (F13.20) Severe: Presence of 6 or more symptoms.

Sedative, Hypnotic, or Anxiolytic Intoxication

The essential feature of sedative, hypnotic, or anxiolytic intoxication is the presence of clinically significant maladaptive behavioral or psychological changes that develop during or shortly after use of a sedative, hypnotic, or anxiolytic drug. As occurs with other brain depressants, these behaviors may be accompanied by slurred speech, unsteady gait, nystagmus, memory or attentional problems, levels of incoordination that can interfere with driving, and stupor or coma. Memory impairment is a prominent feature and is most often characterized by an anterograde amnesia that resembles "alcoholic blackouts."

Diagnostic Criteria for Sedative, Hypnotic, or Anxiolytic Intoxication

A. Recent use of a sedative, hypnotic, or anxiolytic.

B. Clinically significant maladaptive behavioral or psychological changes (e.g., inappropriate sexual or aggressive behavior, mood lability, impaired judgment) that developed during, or shortly after, sedative, hypnotic, or anxiolytic use.

C. One (or more) of the following signs or symptoms developing during, or shortly after, sedative, hypnotic, or anxiolytic use:

1. Slurred speech.
2. Incoordination.

3. Unsteady gait.

4. Nystagmus.

5. Impairment in cognition (e.g., attention, memory).

6. Stupor or coma.

D. The signs or symptoms are not attributable to another medical condition and are not better explained by another mental disorder, including intoxication with another substance.

Coding note: The ICD-9-CM code is **292.89.** The ICD-10-CM code depends on whether there is a comorbid sedative, hypnotic, or anxiolytic use disorder. If a mild sedative, hypnotic, or anxiolytic use disorder is comorbid, the ICD-10-CM code is **F13.129,** and if a moderate or severe sedative, hypnotic, or anxiolytic use disorder is comorbid, the ICD-10-CM code is **F13.229.** If there is no comorbid sedative, hypnotic, or anxiolytic use disorder, then the ICD-10-CM code is **F13.929.**

Sedative, Hypnotic, or Anxiolytic Withdrawal

The essential feature of sedative, hypnotic, or anxiolytic withdrawal is the presence of a characteristic syndrome that develops after a marked cessation of (or decrease in) intake after several weeks or more of regular use. This syndrome is characterized by two or more symptoms that include, for example, autonomic hyperactivity, tremors, insomnia, anxiety, nausea sometimes accompanied by vomiting, and psychomotor agitation. Grand mal seizures occur in perhaps 20%–30% of people undergoing untreated withdrawal from these substances. In severe withdrawal, visual, tactile, or auditory hallucinations or illusions can occur, but are usually in the context of a delirium. The timing and severity of the syndrome will differ depending on specific substances and their pharmacokinetics and pharmacodynamics.

The time course of the syndrome is generally predicted by the half-life of the substance. Medications whose actions typically last about 10 hours or less produce withdrawal symptoms within 6–8 hours after levels in the blood begin decreasing. Intensity peaks on the second day, and symptoms improve markedly by day 4 or 5. For substances with longer half-lives, symptoms may not develop for more than 1 week, peak in intensity during the second week, and decrease in intensity during the third or fourth week. Additional long-term symptoms can persist at a much lower level of intensity for several months. Lingering withdrawal symptoms (e.g., anxiety, moodiness, trouble sleeping) can be mistaken for non-substance-induced anxiety or depressive disorders.

Diagnostic Criteria for Sedative, Hypnotic, or Anxiolytic Withdrawal

A. Cessation of (or reduction in) sedative, hypnotic, or anxiolytic use that has been prolonged.

B. Two (or more) of the following, developing within several hours to a few days after the cessation of (or reduction in) sedative, hypnotic, or anxiolytic use described in Criterion A:

1. Autonomic hyperactivity (e.g., sweating or pulse rate greater than 100 bpm).
2. Hand tremor.
3. Insomnia.
4. Nausea or vomiting.
5. Transient visual, tactile, or auditory hallucinations or illusions.
6. Psychomotor agitation.
7. Anxiety.
8. Grand mal seizures.

C. The signs or symptoms in Criterion B cause clinically significant distress or impairment in social, occupational, or other important areas of functioning.

D. The signs or symptoms are not attributable to another medical condition and are not better explained by another mental disorder, including intoxication or withdrawal from another substance.

Specify if:

With perceptual disturbances: This specifier may be noted when hallucinations with intact reality testing or auditory, visual, or tactile illusions occur in the absence of a delirium.

Coding note: The ICD-9-CM code is **292.0.** The ICD-10-CM code for sedative, hypnotic, or anxiolytic withdrawal depends on whether or not there is a comorbid moderate or severe sedative, hypnotic, or anxiolytic use disorder and whether or not there are perceptual disturbances. For sedative, hypnotic, or anxiolytic withdrawal without perceptual disturbances, the ICD-10-CM code is **F13.239.** For sedative, hypnotic, or anxiolytic withdrawal with perceptual disturbances, the ICD-10-CM code is **F13.232.** Note that the ICD-10-CM codes indicate the comorbid presence of a moderate or severe sedative, hypnotic, or anxiolytic use disorder, reflecting the fact that sedative, hypnotic, or anxiolytic withdrawal can only occur in the presence of a moderate or severe sedative, hypnotic, or anxiolytic use disorder. It is not permissible to code a comorbid mild sedative, hypnotic, or anxiolytic use disorder with sedative, hypnotic, or anxiolytic withdrawal.

Other Sedative-, Hypnotic-, or Anxiolytic-Induced Disorders and Unspecified Sedative-, Hypnotic-, or Anxiolytic-Related Disorder

Individuals are diagnosed with sedative-, hypnotic-, or anxiolytic-induced disorders, such as sedative-, hypnotic-, or anxiolytic-induced psychotic disorder, when the symptoms are sufficiently severe to warrant independent clinical attention.

Individuals are diagnosed with unspecified sedative-, hypnotic-, or anxiolytic-related disorder if they have symptoms characteristic of a sedative-, hypnotic-, or anxiolytic-related disorder that are not classifiable as sedative-, hypnotic-, or anxiolytic use disorder, intoxication, withdrawal, or induced disorder.

STIMULANT-RELATED DISORDERS

Stimulant-related disorders result from use of plant-derived stimulants such as cocaine; amphetamine and amphetamine-like drugs; and other stimulants, such as methylphenidate, that are structurally different from amphetamine but have action similar to amphetamine-type stimulants. Although cocaine and amphetamine-like stimulant drugs are different in some characteristics, such as their mechanisms of action, the clinical presentation related to these compounds is largely similar. Most of the effects of amphetamine-type stimulants are similar to those of cocaine, but there are some distinctions. For example, unlike cocaine, amphetamine-type stimulants do not have local anesthetic activity, and their risk for inducing certain medical conditions such as cardiac arrhythmias and seizures may be lower. The psychoactive effects of most amphetamine-like substances last longer than the effects of a dose of cocaine, and the peripheral sympathomimetic effects may be more potent. Cocaine and methamphetamine are almost always purchased illicitly, but amphetamine-type stimulants may also be obtained legally by prescription for the treatment of attention-deficit/hyperactivity disorder, narcolepsy, and other medical conditions.

Drugs in the amphetamine and cocaine categories have in common the production of intense stimulation in the user. This stimulation is the result of increases in biogenic amines in the central nervous system. The exact molecular mechanisms vary, but the results are similar, as is the clinical addiction syndrome for each. Thus, in DSM-5 all of the stimulant drugs are now described in one stimulant category rather than separately.

Stimulant Use Disorder

Stimulants have potent euphoric effects, and individuals exposed to cocaine or amphetamine-type stimulants can develop a use disorder after using the drug for short periods of time. Regardless of route of administration, tolerance occurs with repeated use. Withdrawal symptoms, particularly hypersomnia, increased appetite, and dysphoric mood, can be seen and are likely to enhance craving and the likelihood of relapse. People may spend large amounts of money for cocaine and amphetamine-type stimulants within a short period of time and may also engage in criminal activity to obtain money for stimulants.

Diagnostic Criteria for Stimulant Use Disorder

A. A pattern of amphetamine-type substance, cocaine, or other stimulant use leading to clinically significant impairment or distress, as manifested by at least two of the following, occurring within a 12-month period:

 1. The stimulant is often taken in larger amounts or over a longer period than was intended.

 2. There is a persistent desire or unsuccessful efforts to cut down or control stimulant use.

3. A great deal of time is spent in activities necessary to obtain the stimulant, use the stimulant, or recover from its effects.
4. Craving, or a strong desire or urge to use the stimulant.
5. Recurrent stimulant use resulting in a failure to fulfill major role obligations at work, school, or home.
6. Continued stimulant use despite having persistent or recurrent social or interpersonal problems caused or exacerbated by the effects of the stimulant.
7. Important social, occupational, or recreational activities are given up or reduced because of stimulant use.
8. Recurrent stimulant use in situations in which it is physically hazardous.
9. Stimulant use is continued despite knowledge of having a persistent or recurrent physical or psychological problem that is likely to have been caused or exacerbated by the stimulant.
10. Tolerance, as defined by either of the following:
    a. A need for markedly increased amounts of the stimulant to achieve intoxication or desired effect.
    b. A markedly diminished effect with continued use of the same amount of the stimulant.

    Note: This criterion is not considered to be met for those taking stimulant medications solely under appropriate medical supervision, such as medications for attention-deficit/hyperactivity disorder or narcolepsy.
11. Withdrawal, as manifested by either of the following:
    a. The characteristic withdrawal syndrome for the stimulant (refer to Criteria A and B of the criteria set for stimulant withdrawal).
    b. The stimulant (or a closely related substance) is taken to relieve or avoid withdrawal symptoms.

    Note: This criterion is not considered to be met for those taking stimulant medications solely under appropriate medical supervision, such as medications for attention-deficit/hyperactivity disorder or narcolepsy.

Specify if:

In early remission: After full criteria for stimulant use disorder were previously met, none of the criteria for stimulant use disorder have been met for at least 3 months but for less than 12 months (with the exception that Criterion A4, "Craving, or a strong desire or urge to use the stimulant," may be met).

In sustained remission: After full criteria for stimulant use disorder were previously met, none of the criteria for stimulant use disorder have been met at any time during a period of 12 months or longer (with the exception that Criterion A4, "Craving, or a strong desire or urge to use the stimulant," may be met).

Specify if:

In a controlled environment: This additional specifier is used if the individual is in an environment where access to stimulants is restricted.

Coding based on current severity: Note for ICD-10-CM codes: If an amphetamine intoxication, amphetamine withdrawal, or another amphetamine-induced mental disorder is also present, do not use the codes below for amphetamine use disorder. Instead, the comorbid amphetamine use disorder is indicated in the 4th character of the amphetamine-induced disorder code (see the coding note for amphetamine intoxication, amphetamine withdrawal, or a specific amphetamine-induced mental disorder). For example, if there is comorbid amphetamine-type or other stimulant-induced depressive disorder and amphetamine-type or other stimulant use disorder, only the amphetamine-type or other stimulant-induced depressive disorder code is given, with the 4th character indicating whether the comorbid amphetamine-type or other stimulant use disorder is mild, moderate, or severe: F15.14 for mild amphetamine-type or other stimulant use disorder with amphetamine-type or other stimulant-induced depressive disorder or F15.24 for a moderate or severe amphetamine-type or other stimulant use disorder with amphetamine-type or other stimulant-induced depressive disorder. Similarly, if there is comorbid cocaine-induced depressive disorder and cocaine use disorder, only the cocaine-induced depressive disorder code is given, with the 4th character indicating whether the comorbid cocaine use disorder is mild, moderate, or severe: F14.14 for mild cocaine use disorder with cocaine-induced depressive disorder or F14.24 for a moderate or severe cocaine use disorder with cocaine-induced depressive disorder.

Specify current severity:

Mild: Presence of 2–3 symptoms.

305.70 (F15.10) Amphetamine-type substance
305.60 (F14.10) Cocaine
305.70 (F15.10) Other or unspecified stimulant

Moderate: Presence of 4–5 symptoms.

304.40 (F15.20) Amphetamine-type substance
304.20 (F14.20) Cocaine
304.40 (F15.20) Other or unspecified stimulant

Severe: Presence of 6 or more symptoms.

304.40 (F15.20) Amphetamine-type substance
304.20 (F14.20) Cocaine
304.40 (F15.20) Other or unspecified stimulant

Stimulant Intoxication

Acute intoxication with high doses of stimulants is associated with increased autonomic activity, perceptual disturbances, behavioral changes (e.g., stereotyped behaviors such as picking at skin), and psychological changes (e.g., agitation, aggression).

Diagnostic Criteria for Stimulant Intoxication

A. Recent use of an amphetamine-type substance, cocaine, or other stimulant.
B. Clinically significant problematic behavioral or psychological changes (e.g., euphoria or affective blunting; changes in sociability; hypervigilance; interpersonal sensitivity; anxiety, tension, or anger; stereotyped behaviors; impaired judgment) that developed during, or shortly after, use of a stimulant.

C. Two (or more) of the following signs or symptoms, developing during, or shortly after, stimulant use:

1. Tachycardia or bradycardia.
2. Pupillary dilation.
3. Elevated or lowered blood pressure.
4. Perspiration or chills.
5. Nausea or vomiting.
6. Evidence of weight loss.
7. Psychomotor agitation or retardation.
8. Muscular weakness, respiratory depression, chest pain, or cardiac arrhythmias.
9. Confusion, seizures, dyskinesias, dystonias, or coma.

D. The signs or symptoms are not attributable to another medical condition and are not better explained by another mental disorder, including intoxication with another substance.

Specify **the specific intoxicant** (i.e., amphetamine-type substance, cocaine, or other stimulant).

Specify if:

With perceptual disturbances: This specifier may be noted when hallucinations with intact reality testing or auditory, visual, or tactile illusions occur in the absence of a delirium.

Coding note: The ICD-9-CM code is **292.89.** The ICD-10-CM code depends on whether the stimulant is an amphetamine, cocaine, or other stimulant; whether there is a comorbid amphetamine, cocaine, or other stimulant use disorder; and whether or not there are perceptual disturbances.

For amphetamine, cocaine, or other stimulant intoxication, without perceptual disturbances: If a mild amphetamine or other stimulant use disorder is comorbid, the ICD-10-CM code is **F15.129,** and if a moderate or severe amphetamine or other stimulant use disorder is comorbid, the ICD-10-CM code is **F15.229.** If there is no comorbid amphetamine or other stimulant use disorder, then the ICD-10-CM code is **F15.929.** Similarly, if a mild cocaine use disorder is comorbid, the ICD-10-CM code is **F14.129,** and if a moderate or severe cocaine use disorder is comorbid, the ICD-10-CM code is **F14.229.** If there is no comorbid cocaine use disorder, then the ICD-10-CM code is **F14.929.**

For amphetamine, cocaine, or other stimulant intoxication, with perceptual disturbances: If a mild amphetamine or other stimulant use disorder is comorbid, the ICD-10-CM code is **F15.122,** and if a moderate or severe amphetamine or other stimulant use disorder is comorbid, the ICD-10-CM code is **F15.222.** If there is no comorbid amphetamine or other stimulant use disorder, then the ICD-10-CM code is **F15.922.** Similarly, if a mild cocaine use disorder is comorbid, the ICD-10-CM code is **F14.122,** and if a moderate or severe cocaine use disorder is comorbid, the ICD-10-CM code is **F14.222.** If there is no comorbid cocaine use disorder, then the ICD-10-CM code is **F14.922.**

Stimulant Withdrawal

The essential feature of stimulant withdrawal is the presence of a characteristic withdrawal syndrome, which develops within a few hours after cessation of or reduction in use of a high-dose stimulant. Use has to have been prolonged. A withdrawal syndrome is characterized by the development of dysphoric mood accompanied by two or more of the following physiological changes: fatigue, vivid and unpleasant dreams, insomnia or hypersomnia, increased appetite, and psychomotor retardation or agitation. Acute withdrawal symptoms (a "crash") can be seen after periods of repetitive high-dose use. Depressive symptoms with suicidal ideation or behavior can occur.

Diagnostic Criteria for Stimulant Withdrawal

A. Cessation of (or reduction in) prolonged amphetamine-type substance, cocaine, or other stimulant use.

B. Dysphoric mood and two (or more) of the following physiological changes, developing within a few hours to several days after Criterion A:

1. Fatigue.
2. Vivid, unpleasant dreams.
3. Insomnia or hypersomnia.
4. Increased appetite.
5. Psychomotor retardation or agitation.

C. The signs or symptoms in Criterion B cause clinically significant distress or impairment in social, occupational, or other important areas of functioning.

D. The signs or symptoms are not attributable to another medical condition and are not better explained by another mental disorder, including intoxication or withdrawal from another substance.

Specify **the specific substance that causes the withdrawal syndrome** (i.e., amphetamine-type substance, cocaine, or other stimulant).

Coding note: The ICD-9-CM code is **292.0.** The ICD-10-CM code depends on whether the stimulant is an amphetamine, cocaine, or other stimulant. The ICD-10-CM code for amphetamine or an other stimulant withdrawal is **F15.23,** and the ICD-10-CM for cocaine withdrawal is **F14.23.** Note that the ICD-10-CM code indicates the comorbid presence of a moderate or severe amphetamine, cocaine, or other stimulant use disorder, reflecting the fact that amphetamine, cocaine, or other stimulant withdrawal can only occur in the presence of a moderate or severe amphetamine, cocaine, or other stimulant use disorder. It is not permissible to code a comorbid mild amphetamine, cocaine, or other stimulant use disorder with amphetamine, cocaine, or other stimulant withdrawal.

Other Stimulant-Induced Disorders and Unspecified Stimulant-Related Disorder

Individuals are diagnosed with other stimulant-induced disorders, such as stimulant-induced psychotic disorder, when the symptoms are sufficiently severe to warrant independent clinical attention.

Individuals are diagnosed with unspecified stimulant-related disorder if they have symptoms characteristic of a stimulant-related disorder that are not classifiable as stimulant use disorder, intoxication, withdrawal, or induced disorder.

TOBACCO-RELATED DISORDERS

Tobacco Use Disorder

The relative ability of tobacco products to produce a use disorder correlates with nicotine content, the rapidity of absorption, and associated conditioned features (e.g., oral gratification). Tobacco use disorder is common among daily cigarette and smokeless tobacco users but is uncommon among nondaily tobacco users or among users of nicotine medications. Tolerance to tobacco is exemplified by the disappearance of nausea and dizziness after its use is resumed. Cessation of tobacco use can produce a well-defined withdrawal syndrome. Many people with tobacco use disorder use tobacco to relieve or to avoid withdrawal symptoms. The large majority of tobacco users report craving when they do not smoke for several hours. Spending excessive time using tobacco can be exemplified by chain-smoking. Smoking within 30 minutes of waking, smoking daily, and awaking at night to smoke are associated with tobacco use disorder. Scientific evidence did not support the inclusion in DSM-5 of a tobacco intoxication disorder.

Diagnostic Criteria for Tobacco Use Disorder

A. A problematic pattern of tobacco use leading to clinically significant impairment or distress, as manifested by at least two of the following, occurring within a 12-month period:

1. Tobacco is often taken in larger amounts or over a longer period than was intended.
2. There is a persistent desire or unsuccessful efforts to cut down or control tobacco use.
3. A great deal of time is spent in activities necessary to obtain or use tobacco.
4. Craving, or a strong desire or urge to use tobacco.

5. Recurrent tobacco use resulting in a failure to fulfill major role obligations at work, school, or home (e.g., interference with work).

6. Continued tobacco use despite having persistent or recurrent social or interpersonal problems caused or exacerbated by the effects of tobacco (e.g., arguments with others about tobacco use).

7. Important social, occupational, or recreational activities are given up or reduced because of tobacco use.

8. Recurrent tobacco use in situations in which it is physically hazardous (e.g., smoking in bed).

9. Tobacco use is continued despite knowledge of having a persistent or recurrent physical or psychological problem that is likely to have been caused or exacerbated by tobacco.

10. Tolerance, as defined by either of the following:

    a. A need for markedly increased amounts of tobacco to achieve the desired effect.

    b. A markedly diminished effect with continued use of the same amount of tobacco.

11. Withdrawal, as manifested by either of the following:

    a. The characteristic withdrawal syndrome for tobacco (refer to Criteria A and B of the criteria set for tobacco withdrawal).

    b. Tobacco (or a closely related substance, such as nicotine) is taken to relieve or avoid withdrawal symptoms.

Specify if:

In early remission: After full criteria for tobacco use disorder were previously met, none of the criteria for tobacco use disorder have been met for at least 3 months but for less than 12 months (with the exception that Criterion A4, "Craving, or a strong desire or urge to use tobacco," may be met).

In sustained remission: After full criteria for tobacco use disorder were previously met, none of the criteria for tobacco use disorder have been met at any time during a period of 12 months or longer (with the exception that Criterion A4, "Craving, or a strong desire or urge to use tobacco," may be met).

Specify if:

On maintenance therapy: The individual is taking a long-term maintenance medication, such as nicotine replacement medication, and no criteria for tobacco use disorder have been met for that class of medication (except tolerance to, or withdrawal from, the nicotine replacement medication).

In a controlled environment: This additional specifier is used if the individual is in an environment where access to tobacco is restricted.

Coding based on current severity: Note for ICD-10-CM codes: If a tobacco withdrawal or tobacco-induced sleep disorder is also present, do not use the codes below for tobacco use disorder. Instead, the comorbid tobacco use disorder is indicated in the 4th character of the tobacco-induced disorder code (see the coding note for tobacco withdrawal or tobacco-induced sleep disorder). For example, if there is comorbid tobacco-induced sleep disorder and tobacco use disorder, only the tobacco-induced sleep disorder code is given, with the 4th character indicating whether the comorbid tobacco use disorder is moderate or severe: F17.208 for moderate or severe tobacco use disorder with tobacco-induced sleep disorder. It is not permissible to code a comorbid mild tobacco use disorder with a tobacco-induced sleep disorder.

Specify current severity:

305.1 (Z72.0) Mild: Presence of 2–3 symptoms.

305.1 (F17.200) Moderate: Presence of 4–5 symptoms.

305.1 (F17.200) Severe: Presence of 6 or more symptoms.

Tobacco Withdrawal

Tobacco withdrawal impairs the ability to stop tobacco use. The symptoms, which occur 24 hours after abstinence from tobacco, are much more intense among individuals who smoke cigarettes. This increased intensity is probably due to the more rapid onset of symptoms and higher levels of nicotine with cigarette smoking.

Diagnostic Criteria for Tobacco Withdrawal   **292.0 (F17.203)**

A. Daily use of tobacco for at least several weeks.

B. Abrupt cessation of tobacco use, or reduction in the amount of tobacco used, followed within 24 hours by four (or more) of the following signs or symptoms:

1. Irritability, frustration, or anger.
2. Anxiety.
3. Difficulty concentrating.
4. Increased appetite.
5. Restlessness.
6. Depressed mood.
7. Insomnia.

C. The signs or symptoms in Criterion B cause clinically significant distress or impairment in social, occupational, or other important areas of functioning.

D. The signs or symptoms are not attributed to another medical condition and are not better explained by another mental disorder, including intoxication or withdrawal from another substance.

Coding note: The ICD-9-CM code is 292.0. The ICD-10-CM code for tobacco withdrawal is F17.203. Note that the ICD-10-CM code indicates the comorbid presence of a moderate or severe tobacco use disorder, reflecting the fact that tobacco withdrawal can only occur in the presence of a moderate or severe tobacco use disorder. It is not permissible to code a comorbid mild tobacco use disorder with tobacco withdrawal.

Other Tobacco-Induced Disorders and Unspecified Tobacco-Related Disorder

Individuals are diagnosed with other tobacco-induced disorders, such as tobacco-induced sleep disorder, when the symptoms are sufficiently severe to warrant independent clinical attention.

Individuals are diagnosed with unspecified tobacco-related disorder if they have symptoms characteristic of a tobacco-related disorder that are not classifiable as tobacco use disorder, withdrawal, or induced disorder.

OTHER (OR UNKNOWN) SUBSTANCE–RELATED DISORDERS

When the substance or substances used are unknown, the individual is diagnosed with one of the other (or unknown) substance–related disorders. In addition to diagnoses for use disorder, intoxication, and withdrawal, two residual categories are available for other situations: other (or unknown) substance–induced disorders and unspecified other (or unknown) substance–related disorder.

NON-SUBSTANCE-RELATED DISORDERS

Gambling Disorder

Gambling is encountered in almost all cultures throughout recorded history. Although most individuals gamble responsibly, some become preoccupied with gambling and experience its multiple negative consequences. For these people, their gambling behavior has devastating consequences that impact the individual, his or her family, and society.

Disordered gambling behavior was first officially recognized in DSM-III, as *pathological gambling.* The disorder was categorized as one of the impulse-control disorders not elsewhere classified, along with disorders such as kleptomania, pyromania, and trichotillomania. In DSM-5, the disorder has been moved to the chapter on substance use disorders because of consistently high rates of comorbidity, similar presentations of some symptoms, and genetic and physiological overlap. Additionally, the placement of gambling disorder in the current chapter is likely to improve recognition of the disorder, especially among substance abusers, who are at high risk for gambling problems.

The criteria have had only minor changes from DSM-IV. Importantly, the name has changed from *pathological gambling* to *gambling disorder,* mainly to avoid the stigma attached to the word *pathological.* Also, the number of core symptoms required for the diagnosis has been reduced.

Diagnostic Criteria for Gambling Disorder 312.31 (F63.0)

A. Persistent and recurrent problematic gambling behavior leading to clinically significant impairment or distress, as indicated by the individual exhibiting four (or more) of the following in a 12-month period:

1. Needs to gamble with increasing amounts of money in order to achieve the desired excitement.

2. Is restless or irritable when attempting to cut down or stop gambling.
3. Has made repeated unsuccessful efforts to control, cut back, or stop gambling.
4. Is often preoccupied with gambling (e.g., having persistent thoughts of reliving past gambling experiences, handicapping or planning the next venture, thinking of ways to get money with which to gamble).
5. Often gambles when feeling distressed (e.g., helpless, guilty, anxious, depressed).
6. After losing money gambling, often returns another day to get even ("chasing" one's losses).
7. Lies to conceal the extent of involvement with gambling.
8. Has jeopardized or lost a significant relationship, job, or educational or career opportunity because of gambling.
9. Relies on others to provide money to relieve desperate financial situations caused by gambling.

B. The gambling behavior is not better explained by a manic episode.

Specify if:
Episodic: Meeting diagnostic criteria at more than one time point, with symptoms subsiding between periods of gambling disorder for at least several months.
Persistent: Experiencing continuous symptoms, to meet diagnostic criteria for multiple years.

Specify if:
In early remission: After full criteria for gambling disorder were previously met, none of the criteria for gambling disorder have been met for at least 3 months but for less than 12 months.
In sustained remission: After full criteria for gambling disorder were previously met, none of the criteria for gambling disorder have been met during a period of 12 months or longer.

Specify current severity:
Mild: 4–5 criteria met.
Moderate: 6–7 criteria met.
Severe: 8–9 criteria met.

Criterion A

The symptoms set forth mirror those of the substance addictions. Tolerance (needing to gamble with increasing amounts of money), withdrawal (restlessness or irritability when cutting back), and compulsive use (preoccupation with gambling, "chasing" of losses, repeated unsuccessful attempts to control gambling, and gambling as a way of escaping from problems) are the cardinal features of gambling disorder. The adverse consequences of addiction are also reflected in the remaining symptoms (lying to others, jeopardizing important relationships, and relying on others financially).

The DSM-5 diagnosis requires that four of nine symptoms be endorsed to qualify for the diagnosis of gambling disorder. This is a change from DSM-IV, in which five of 10 symptoms were required. DSM-IV Criterion A8 has been eliminated because the symptom "has committed illegal acts…to finance gambling" has been shown to have low prevalence; its elimination has little or no effect on prevalence. Also, the threshold of four symptoms was found to differentiate pathological from nonpathological forms of gambling.

Criterion B

Individuals with bipolar disorder may engage in multiple forms of impulsive behavior, including gambling, when hypomanic or manic. The diagnosis of gambling disorder requires that the gambling behavior not occur exclusively during a manic episode. It is possible, however, that someone may have both diagnoses, with the gambling worsening during mood instability, but this would require that the gambling behavior be also independent of manic episodes.

Specifiers

Gambling disorder can be episodic or persistent, and the course of the disorder can vary by type of gambling as well as life circumstances. For example, an individual who wagers problematically only on football games may have gambling disorder during football season and not wager at all, or not wager problematically, throughout the remainder of the year. Gambling disorder may also occur at one or more points in an individual's life but be absent during other periods. Alternatively, some individuals experience chronic gambling disorder throughout all or most of their lives.

Other specifiers, which are used for the other substance use disorders, include "in early remission" and "in sustained remission." Finally, a severity specifier has also been added to differentiate mild, moderate, and severe gambling disorder on the basis of the number of criteria the individual fulfills.

KEY POINTS

- The name of the diagnostic class has been changed from "substance-related disorders" to "substance-related and addictive disorders" to reflect emerging concepts regarding the addictions. Ten types of substance use disorders are listed, as well as gambling disorder, which is classified as a non-substance-related disorder.

- The major change is that the categories of abuse and dependence have been merged, creating a single category for a "use" disorder.

- DSM-IV's hallucinogen-related disorders and phencyclidine (or phencyclidine-like)–related disorders have been merged into a single category.

- The stimulant-related disorders category has replaced the categories for amphetamine and cocaine use disorders. Cannabis use disorder, cannabis withdrawal, and caffeine withdrawal are new. Nicotine-related disorders are now called *tobacco-related disorders*.

- Gambling disorder (formerly DSM-IV pathological gambling) has been moved to this chapter, reflecting emerging concepts regarding the addictions.

CHAPTER 17

Neurocognitive Disorders

Delirium
Delirium
Substance Intoxication Delirium
Substance Withdrawal Delirium
Medication-Induced Delirium
Delirium Due to Another Medical Condition
Delirium Due to Multiple Etiologies
Other Specified Delirium
Unspecified Delirium

Major and Mild Neurocognitive Disorders
Major Neurocognitive Disorder
Mild Neurocognitive Disorder

Major or Mild Neurocognitive Disorder Due to Alzheimer's Disease
Major or Mild Frontotemporal Neurocognitive Disorder
Major or Mild Neurocognitive Disorder With Lewy Bodies
Major or Mild Vascular Neurocognitive Disorder
Major or Mild Neurocognitive Disorder Due to Traumatic Brain Injury
Substance/Medication-Induced Major or Mild Neurocognitive Disorder
Major or Mild Neurocognitive Disorder Due to HIV Infection
Major or Mild Neurocognitive Disorder Due to Prion Disease
Major or Mild Neurocognitive Disorder Due to Parkinson's Disease
Major or Mild Neurocognitive Disorder Due to Huntington's Disease
Major or Mild Neurocognitive Disorder Due to Another Medical Condition
Major or Mild Neurocognitive Disorder Due to Multiple Etiologies
Unspecified Neurocognitive Disorder

The DSM-5 chapter on neurocognitive disorders encompasses disorders that have cognitive impairment as their presenting problem. In DSM-IV, the chapter was called "Delirium, Dementia, and Amnestic and Other Cognitive Disorders." The new title refers to disorders that are acquired (i.e., those attributed to medical conditions or the effects of drugs of abuse or medications) or are degenerative (i.e., those that reflect a decline from a previously attained level of cognitive functioning) rather than disorders that are congenital or apparent in childhood. The title was selected in part to avoid the stigma associated with the word *dementia* when categorizing deficits among younger people with progressive cognitive decline, such as that associated with HIV infection or traumatic brain injury. The neurocognitive disorders are divided into three broad syndromes: delirium, major neurocognitive disorders, and mild neurocognitive disorders. Disorders in this chapter are attributable to changes in brain structure, function, or chemistry.

Cognitive disorders have been recognized for centuries and have been an important category in DSM. In DSM-I, "acute" and "chronic" brain disorders constituted the two major divisions, each subcategorized by presumed cause (e.g., cerebral arteriosclerosis, convulsive disorder). In DSM-II, these disorders were listed as either "psychoses associated with organic brain syndromes" or "nonpsychotic organic brain syndromes." The term *psychosis* was used to denote severity (i.e., that the condition resulted in sufficiently impaired mental functioning to interfere grossly with the capacity to meet the ordinary demands of life) rather than the presence of hallucinations or delusions. What current practitioners might refer to as vascular dementia would have been classified in DSM-II as psychoses associated with organic brain syndromes with cerebral arteriosclerosis or other cerebrovascular disturbance. The term *organic mental disorders* continued to be used in DSM-III, although the term *psychosis* was no longer used to characterize severity. The word *organic* was finally omitted in DSM-IV; it was considered to be outdated because it implied that other disorders in the manual did not have an organic component.

The major change to this diagnostic class with DSM-5 is the introduction of the concept of "major" and "mild" neurocognitive disorders. The latter are less severe forms of cognitive impairment and can be a focus of care. The DSM-5 neurocognitive disorders are listed in Table 17–1.

DELIRIUM

Delirium

Delirium is a disturbance in level of awareness or attention, marked by the acute or subacute onset of cognitive changes attributable to a general medical condition; it tends to have an acute onset, relatively brief duration, and fluctuating course. Delirium is distinguished from major or mild neurocognitive disorders on the basis of its core characteristics: a disturbance in level of awareness and the reduced ability to direct, focus, sustain, and shift attention. Although some level of disturbance of awareness and attention can be observed in all neurocognitive disorders, these disturbances are not prominent in major or mild neurocognitive disorder (the relative absence of this disturbance was previously referred to as "clear consciousness"). Delirium can (and frequently does) coexist with major or mild neurocognitive disorder.

Diagnosing delirium is important because its underlying cause is often correctable, whereas untreated delirium is associated with a high mortality rate, serious medical complications, and irreversible cognitive impairments.

TABLE 17–1. Neurocognitive disorders

Delirium
  Delirium
    Substance intoxication delirium
    Substance withdrawal delirium
    Medication-induced delirium
    Delirium due to another medical condition
    Delirium due to multiple etiologies
  Other specified delirium
  Unspecified delirium
Major and mild neurocognitive disorders
  Major neurocognitive disorder
  Mild neurocognitive disorder

  Major or mild neurocognitive disorder due to Alzheimer's disease
  Major or mild frontotemporal neurocognitive disorder
  Major or mild neurocognitive disorder with Lewy bodies
  Major or mild vascular neurocognitive disorder
  Major or mild neurocognitive disorder due to traumatic brain injury
  Substance/medication-induced major or mild neurocognitive disorder
  Major or mild neurocognitive disorder due to HIV infection
  Major or mild neurocognitive disorder due to prion disease
  Major or mild neurocognitive disorder due to Parkinson's disease
  Major or mild neurocognitive disorder due to Huntington's disease
  Major or mild neurocognitive disorder due to another medical condition
  Major or mild neurocognitive disorder due to multiple etiologies
Unspecified neurocognitive disorder

Diagnostic Criteria for Delirium

A. A disturbance in attention (i.e., reduced ability to direct, focus, sustain, and shift attention) and awareness (reduced orientation to the environment).

B. The disturbance develops over a short period of time (usually hours to a few days), represents a change from baseline attention and awareness, and tends to fluctuate in severity during the course of a day.

C. An additional disturbance in cognition (e.g., memory deficit, disorientation, language, visuospatial ability, or perception).

D. The disturbances in Criteria A and C are not better explained by another preexisting, established, or evolving neurocognitive disorder and do not occur in the context of a severely reduced level of arousal, such as coma.

E. There is evidence from the history, physical examination, or laboratory findings that the disturbance is a direct physiological consequence of another medical condition, substance intoxication or withdrawal (i.e., due to a drug of abuse or to a medication), or exposure to a toxin, or is due to multiple etiologies.

Specify whether:

Substance intoxication delirium: This diagnosis should be made instead of substance intoxication when the symptoms in Criteria A and C predominate in the clinical picture and when they are sufficiently severe to warrant clinical attention.

Coding note: The ICD-9-CM and ICD-10-CM codes for the [specific substance] intoxication delirium are indicated in the table below. Note that the ICD-10-CM code depends on whether or not there is a comorbid substance use disorder present for the same class of substance. If a mild substance use disorder is comorbid with the substance intoxication delirium, the 4th position character is "1," and the clinician should record "mild [substance] use disorder" before the substance intoxication delirium (e.g., "mild cocaine use disorder with cocaine intoxication delirium"). If a moderate or severe substance use disorder is comorbid with the substance intoxication delirium, the 4th position character is "2," and the clinician should record "moderate [substance] use disorder" or "severe [substance] use disorder," depending on the severity of the comorbid substance use disorder. If there is no comorbid substance use disorder (e.g., after a one-time heavy use of the substance), then the 4th position character is "9," and the clinician should record only the substance intoxication delirium.

		ICD-10-CM		
	ICD-9-CM	With use disorder, mild	With use disorder, moderate or severe	Without use disorder
Alcohol	291.0	F10.121	F10.221	F10.921
Cannabis	292.81	F12.121	F12.221	F12.921
Phencyclidine	292.81	F16.121	F16.221	F16.921
Other hallucinogen	292.81	F16.121	F16.221	F16.921
Inhalant	292.81	F18.121	F18.221	F18.921
Opioid	292.81	F11.121	F11.221	F11.921
Sedative, hypnotic, or anxiolytic	292.81	F13.121	F13.221	F13.921
Amphetamine (or other stimulant)	292.81	F15.121	F15.221	F15.921
Cocaine	292.81	F14.121	F14.221	F14.921
Other (or unknown) substance	292.81	F19.121	F19.221	F19.921

Substance withdrawal delirium: This diagnosis should be made instead of substance withdrawal when the symptoms in Criteria A and C predominate in the clinical picture and when they are sufficiently severe to warrant clinical attention.

Code [specific substance] withdrawal delirium: **291.0 (F10.231)** alcohol; **292.0 (F11.23)** opioid; **292.0 (F13.231)** sedative, hypnotic, or anxiolytic; **292.0 (F19.231)** other (or unknown) substance/medication.

Medication-induced delirium: This diagnosis applies when the symptoms in Criteria A and C arise as a side effect of a medication taken as prescribed.

Coding note: The ICD-9-CM code for [specific medication]-induced delirium is **292.81.** The ICD-10-CM code depends on the type of medication. If the medication is an opioid taken as prescribed, the code is **F11.921.** If the medication is a sedative, hypnotic, or anxiolytic taken as prescribed, the code is **F13.921.** If the medication is an amphetamine-type or other stimulant taken as prescribed, the code is **F15.921.** For medications that do not fit into any of the classes (e.g., dexamethasone) and in cases in which a substance is judged to be an etiological factor but the specific class of substance is unknown, the code is **F19.921.**

293.0 (F05) Delirium due to another medical condition: There is evidence from the history, physical examination, or laboratory findings that the disturbance is attributable to the physiological consequences of another medical condition.

Coding note: Include the name of the other medical condition in the name of the delirium (e.g., 293.0 [F05] delirium due to hepatic encephalopathy). The other medical condition should also be coded and listed separately immediately before the delirium due to another medical condition (e.g., 572.2 [K72.90] hepatic encephalopathy; 293.0 [F05] delirium due to hepatic encephalopathy).

293.0 (F05) Delirium due to multiple etiologies: There is evidence from the history, physical examination, or laboratory findings that the delirium has more than one etiology (e.g., more than one etiological medical condition; another medical condition plus substance intoxication or medication side effect).

Coding note: Use multiple separate codes reflecting specific delirium etiologies (e.g., 572.2 [K72.90] hepatic encephalopathy, 293.0 [F05] delirium due to hepatic failure; 291.0 [F10.231] alcohol withdrawal delirium). Note that the etiological medical condition both appears as a separate code that precedes the delirium code and is substituted into the delirium due to another medical condition rubric.

Specify if:
Acute: Lasting a few hours or days.
Persistent: Lasting weeks or months.

Specify if:
Hyperactive: The individual has a hyperactive level of psychomotor activity that may be accompanied by mood lability, agitation, and/or refusal to cooperate with medical care.
Hypoactive: The individual has a hypoactive level of psychomotor activity that may be accompanied by sluggishness and lethargy that approaches stupor.
Mixed level of activity: The individual has a normal level of psychomotor activity even though attention and awareness are disturbed. Also includes individuals whose activity level rapidly fluctuates.

Criterion A

Delirium is a disturbance in level of awareness or attention, marked by the acute or subacute onset of cognitive changes. The individual's inability to appreciate or respond appropriately to the environment may be evidenced by problems with focus or sustained attention, apparent disorientation in familiar settings, and perseverating in responses. DSM-IV referred to these symptoms as a "disturbance of consciousness." *Consciousness,* however, was considered an imprecise term to describe the symptoms of delirium.

Criterion B

The course of delirium is usually short, developing over a few hours or a few days. The delirium usually remits when the underlying cause is identified and successfully treated.

Criterion C

Memory problems, disorientation, and language difficulties are usually present. Visuospatial impairment and impairment in executive function are also symptoms of delirium.

Criterion D

DSM-5 has also added a clarification that a preexisting neurocognitive disorder does not account for the cognitive changes. A severely reduced level of arousal, such as coma, would not provide a context adequate to assess orientation, attention, and cognitive functioning.

Criterion E

This criterion requires that the disturbance in attention and awareness be a direct physiological consequence of another medical condition, substance intoxication or withdrawal, or exposure to a toxin, or be due to multiple etiologies.

Subtypes and Specifiers

There are multiple subtypes for the diagnosis of delirium that address etiological issues. Two subtypes indicate whether the delirium is due to substance intoxication or substance withdrawal. These diagnoses should be made instead of substance intoxication or substance withdrawal when the symptoms in Criteria A and C predominate in the clinical picture and are sufficiently severe to warrant clinical attention. Substance intoxication or withdrawal delirium requires, in addition to the standard criteria for delirium, that the delirium have started during or after intoxication or withdrawal and that the substance be capable of producing delirium.

The following classes of substances can result in a substance intoxication delirium: cannabis; phencyclidine and other hallucinogens; stimulants; inhalants; opioids; and sedatives, hypnotics, and anxiolytics. During withdrawal, alcohol, opioids, and sedatives, hypnotics, and anxiolytics can be causes of delirium. Other (or unknown) substances can also be specified.

Another possible subtype is medication-induced delirium. Even in the absence of intoxication or withdrawal, a number of medications and toxins (e.g., benztropine, dexamethasone) can lead to delirium.

Other subtypes indicate whether the delirium is due to another medical condition (e.g., hepatic encephalopathy) or multiple etiologies (e.g., hepatic encephalopathy plus alcohol withdrawal).

Finally, there are specifiers to indicate whether the delirium is acute (lasting a few hours to a few days) or persistent (lasting weeks or months) and whether the delirium gives rise to hyperactive psychomotor activity (often accompanied by mood lability, agitation, and/or refusal to cooperate with medical care), hypoactive psychomotor activity (often accompanied by sluggishness and lethargy that approaches stupor), or a mixed level of activity (normal level of psychomotor activity even though attention and awareness are disturbed; includes individuals whose activity level rapidly fluctuates). Individuals with delirium may rapidly switch between hyperactive and hypoactive states. The hyperactive state may be more common or more frequently recognized and often is associated with medication side effects and drug withdrawal. The hypoactive state may be more frequent in older adults.

Other Specified Delirium and Unspecified Delirium

Other specified delirium or unspecified delirium is coded when it is not possible to establish an etiological subtype or when the disorder is subsyndromal (i.e., does not meet full criteria for delirium, such as in attenuated delirium syndrome). Examples include a clinical presentation of delirium that is suspected to be due to a general medical condition or substance use but for which there is insufficient evidence to establish a specific etiology. Such a diagnosis may also be appropriate when the delirium is due to causes not listed in this section (e.g., sensory deprivation).

Other Specified Delirium 780.09 (R41.0)

This category applies to presentations in which symptoms characteristic of delirium that cause clinically significant distress or impairment in social, occupational, or other important areas of functioning predominate but do not meet the full criteria for delirium or any of the disorders in the neurocognitive disorders diagnostic class. The other specified delirium category is used in situations in which the clinician chooses to communicate the specific reason that the presentation does not meet the criteria for delirium or any specific neurocognitive disorder. This is done by recording "other specified delirium" followed by the specific reason (e.g., "attenuated delirium syndrome").

An example of a presentation that can be specified using the "other specified" designation is the following:

Attenuated delirium syndrome: This syndrome applies in cases of delirium in which the severity of cognitive impairment falls short of that required for the diagnosis, or in which some, but not all, diagnostic criteria for delirium are met.

Unspecified Delirium   780.09 (R41.0)

This category applies to presentations in which symptoms characteristic of delirium that cause clinically significant distress or impairment in social, occupational, or other important areas of functioning predominate but do not meet the full criteria for delirium or any of the disorders in the neurocognitive disorders diagnostic class. The unspecified delirium category is used in situations in which the clinician chooses *not* to specify the reason that the criteria are not met for delirium, and includes presentations for which there is insufficient information to make a more specific diagnosis (e.g., in emergency room settings).

MAJOR AND MILD NEUROCOGNITIVE DISORDERS

Major Neurocognitive Disorder

Major neurocognitive disorder (including what was formerly known in DSM-IV as dementia) is an acquired disorder with significant cognitive decline in one or more (typically at least two) of the following domains:

- *Complex attention* (sustained attention, divided attention, selective attention, processing speed)
- *Executive function* (planning, decision making, working memory, responding to feedback/error correction, overriding habits, mental flexibility)
- *Learning and memory* (immediate memory, recent memory [including free recall, cued recall, and recognition memory])
- *Language* (expressive language [including naming, fluency, and grammar and syntax] and receptive language)
- *Perceptual-motor ability* (construction and visual perception)
- *Social cognition* (recognition of emotions, theory of mind, behavioral regulation)

The cognitive deficits must be sufficient to interfere with functional independence. Unlike the DSM-IV criteria for dementia, the DSM-5 major neurocognitive disorder criteria do not require memory to be one of the impaired domains and allow the cognitive deficit to be limited to one domain.

Although the word *dementia* is not precluded from use in the etiological subtypes, it is subsumed by the newly named entity *major neurocognitive disorder*. The term *dementia* was considered pejorative and stigmatizing by some, particularly among younger adults with cognitive deficits related to HIV infection, head injury, or other causes.

Diagnostic Criteria for Major Neurocognitive Disorder

A. Evidence of significant cognitive decline from a previous level of performance in one or more cognitive domains (complex attention, executive function, learning and memory, language, perceptual-motor, or social cognition) based on:

1. Concern of the individual, a knowledgeable informant, or the clinician that there has been a significant decline in cognitive function; and
2. A substantial impairment in cognitive performance, preferably documented by standardized neuropsychological testing or, in its absence, another quantified clinical assessment.

B. The cognitive deficits interfere with independence in everyday activities (i.e., at a minimum, requiring assistance with complex instrumental activities of daily living such as paying bills or managing medications).

C. The cognitive deficits do not occur exclusively in the context of a delirium.

D. The cognitive deficits are not better explained by another mental disorder (e.g., major depressive disorder, schizophrenia).

Specify whether due to:
 Alzheimer's disease (DSM-5, pp. 611–614)
 Frontotemporal lobar degeneration (DSM-5, pp. 614–618)
 Lewy body disease (DSM-5, pp. 618–621)
 Vascular disease (DSM-5, pp. 621–624)
 Traumatic brain injury (DSM-5, pp. 624–627)
 Substance/medication use (DSM-5, pp. 627–632)
 HIV infection (DSM-5, pp. 632–634)
 Prion disease (DSM-5, pp. 634–636)
 Parkinson's disease (DSM-5, pp. 636–638)
 Huntington's disease (DSM-5, pp. 638–641)
 Another medical condition (DSM-5, pp. 641–642)
 Multiple etiologies (DSM-5, pp. 642–643)
 Unspecified (DSM-5, p. 643)

Coding note: Code based on medical or substance etiology. In some cases, there is need for an additional code for the etiological medical condition, which must immediately precede the diagnostic code for major neurocognitive disorder, as follows:

Etiological subtype	Associated etiological medical code for major neurocognitive disorder[a]	Major neurocognitive disorder code[b]	Mild neurocognitive disorder code[c]
Alzheimer's disease	Probable: 331.0 (G30.9) Possible: no additional medical code	Probable: 294.1x (F02.8x) Possible: 331.9 (G31.9)[c]	331.83 (G31.84) (Do not use additional code for Alzheimer's disease.)

Etiological subtype	Associated etiological medical code for major neurocognitive disorder[a]	Major neurocognitive disorder code[b]	Mild neurocognitive disorder code[c]
Frontotemporal lobar degeneration	Probable: 331.19 (G31.09) Possible: no additional medical code	Probable: 294.1x (F02.8x) Possible: 331.9 (G31.9)[c]	331.83 (G31.84) (Do not use additional code for frontotemporal disease.)
Lewy body disease	Probable: 331.82 (G31.83) Possible: no additional medical code	Probable: 294.1x (F02.8x) Possible: 331.9 (G31.9)[c]	331.83 (G31.84) (Do not use additional code for Lewy body disease.)
Vascular disease	No additional medical code	Probable: 290.40 (F01.5x) Possible: 331.9 (G31.9)[c]	331.83 (G31.84) (Do not use additional code for the vascular disease.)
Traumatic brain injury	907.0 (S06.2X9S)	294.1x (F02.8x)	331.83 (G31.84) (Do not use additional code for the traumatic brain injury.)
Substance/ medication-induced	No additional medical code	Code based on the type of substance causing the major neurocognitive disorder[c,d]	Code based on the type of substance causing the mild neurocognitive disorder[d]
HIV infection	042 (B20)	294.1x (F02.8x)	331.83 (G31.84) (Do not use additional code for HIV infection.)
Prion disease	046.79 (A81.9)	294.1x (F02.8x)	331.83 (G31.84) (Do not use additional code for prion disease.)

Etiological subtype	Associated etiological medical code for major neurocognitive disorder[a]	Major neurocognitive disorder code[b]	Mild neurocognitive disorder code[c]
Parkinson's disease	Probable: 332.0 (G20) Possible: No additional medical code	Probable: 294.1x (F02.8x) Possible: 331.9 (G31.9)[c]	331.83 (G31.84) (Do not use additional code for Parkinson's disease.)
Huntington's disease	333.4 (G10)	294.1x (F02.8x)	331.83 (G31.84) (Do not use additional code for Huntington's disease.)
Due to another medical condition	Code the other medical condition first (e.g., 340 [G35] multiple sclerosis)	294.1x (F02.8x)	331.83 (G31.84) (Do not use additional codes for the presumed etiological medical conditions.)
Due to multiple etiologies	Code all of the etiological medical conditions first (with the exception of vascular disease)	294.1x (F02.8x) (Plus the code for the relevant substance/medication-induced major neurocognitive disorders if substances or medications play a role in the etiology.)	331.83 (G31.84) (Plus the code for the relevant substance/medication-induced mild neurocognitive disorders if substances or medications play a role in the etiology. Do not use additional codes for the presumed etiological medical conditions.)
Unspecified neurocognitive disorder	No additional medical code	799.59 (R41.9)	799.59 (R41.9)

[a]Code first, before code for major neurocognitive disorder.
[b]Code fifth character based on symptom specifier: .x0 without behavioral disturbance; .x1 with behavioral disturbance (e.g., psychotic symptoms, mood disturbance, agitation, apathy, or other behavioral symptoms).
[c]**Note:** Behavioral disturbance specifier cannot be coded but should still be indicated in writing.
[d]See "Substance/Medication-Induced Major or Mild Neurocognitive Disorder."

Specify:
> **Without behavioral disturbance:** If the cognitive disturbance is not accompanied by any clinically significant behavioral disturbance.
> **With behavioral disturbance** *(specify disturbance):* If the cognitive disturbance is accompanied by a clinically significant behavioral disturbance (e.g., psychotic symptoms, mood disturbance, agitation, apathy, or other behavioral symptoms).

Specify current severity:
> **Mild:** Difficulties with instrumental activities of daily living (e.g., housework, managing money).
> **Moderate:** Difficulties with basic activities of daily living (e.g., feeding, dressing).
> **Severe:** Fully dependent.

Criterion A

The DSM-5 wording focuses on "decline" from a previous level of performance, rather than "deficit" as in DSM-IV. The DSM-IV criteria for dementia used Alzheimer's disease as the prototype and thus required memory impairment for all dementias. There is growing recognition that in many of the neurocognitive disorders (e.g., those related to HIV infection, cerebrovascular disease, frontotemporal degeneration, traumatic brain injury), other domains such as language or executive functions may be impaired first, or exclusively, depending on the part of the brain affected and the natural history of the disease. The new definition also focuses first on performance rather than disability. The criterion encourages the use of objective measures, including formal neuropsychological testing where feasible, with less exclusive reliance on individual judgment. Observation of decline and objective assessment are both included to ensure specificity. Although this evidence is more critical for diagnosing mild neurocognitive disorder, similar statements are included for major neurocognitive disorder for parallel structure of Criterion A.

Criterion B

The DSM-5 language preserves the traditional function-based threshold for dementia but tries to operationalize it more clearly as a loss of independence.

Criteria C and D

The cognitive decline seen in major neurocognitive disorder affects some of the same cognitive domains as seen in delirium. Although it is clinically important to distinguish major neurocognitive disorder from delirium, the two may co-occur.

The cognitive deficits in major neurocognitive disorder are not better explained by another mental disorder (e.g., major depressive disorder, schizophrenia).

Subtypes and Specifiers

Subtypes and specifiers for major neurocognitive disorder are discussed under "Mild Neurocognitive Disorder" below.

Mild Neurocognitive Disorder

The mild neurocognitive disorder diagnosis is new and recognizes the substantial clinical needs of individuals who have mild cognitive deficits in one or more of the same domains as in major neurocognitive disorder but who can function independently (i.e., have intact instrumental activities of daily living) (Petersen and O'Brien 2006). Known in many settings as *mild cognitive impairment*, the disorder can be a focus of early intervention. This may enable the use of treatments that are ineffective at more severe levels of impairment and/or neuronal damage. In DSM-IV, mild cognitive disorder was subsumed under the category cognitive disorder not otherwise specified.

Examples of mild neurocognitive disorder are the prevalent neurocognitive disorders associated with such conditions as traumatic brain injury, HIV infection, substance use–related brain disorders, and early or mild stages of cerebrovascular disease or neurodegenerative disorders such as Alzheimer's disease. Because these conditions are increasingly being seen in clinical practice, clinicians have a need for reliable diagnostic criteria to assess their patients and provide services—tasks that include treatment of associated mood symptoms, further investigation of brain function, identification of treatable causes, and, for progressive disorders, selection of appropriate early interventions.

Diagnostic Criteria for Mild Neurocognitive Disorder

A. Evidence of modest cognitive decline from a previous level of performance in one or more cognitive domains (complex attention, executive function, learning and memory, language, perceptual-motor, or social cognition) based on:
  1. Concern of the individual, a knowledgeable informant, or the clinician that there has been a mild decline in cognitive function; and
  2. A modest impairment in cognitive performance, preferably documented by standardized neuropsychological testing or, in its absence, another quantified clinical assessment.
B. The cognitive deficits do not interfere with capacity for independence in everyday activities (i.e., complex instrumental activities of daily living such as paying bills or managing medications are preserved, but greater effort, compensatory strategies, or accommodation may be required).
C. The cognitive deficits do not occur exclusively in the context of a delirium.
D. The cognitive deficits are not better explained by another mental disorder (e.g., major depressive disorder, schizophrenia).

Specify whether due to:
  Alzheimer's disease (DSM-5, pp. 611–614)
  Frontotemporal lobar degeneration (DSM-5, pp. 614–618)
  Lewy body disease (DSM-5, pp. 618–621)
  Vascular disease (DSM-5, pp. 621–624)
  Traumatic brain injury (DSM-5, pp. 624–627)
  Substance/medication use (DSM-5, pp. 627–632)
  HIV infection (DSM-5, pp. 632–634)
  Prion disease (DSM-5, pp. 634–636)

Parkinson's disease (DSM-5, pp. 636–638)
Huntington's disease (DSM-5, pp. 638–641)
Another medical condition (DSM-5, pp. 641–642)
Multiple etiologies (DSM-5, pp. 642–643)
Unspecified (DSM-5, p. 643)

Coding note: For mild neurocognitive disorder due to any of the medical etiologies listed above, code **331.83 (G31.84).** Do *not* use additional codes for the presumed etiological medical conditions. For substance/medication-induced mild neurocognitive disorder, code based on type of substance; see "Substance/Medication-Induced Major or Mild Neurocognitive Disorder." For unspecified mild neurocognitive disorder, code **799.59 (R41.9).**

Specify:

Without behavioral disturbance: If the cognitive disturbance is not accompanied by any clinically significant behavioral disturbance.

With behavioral disturbance *(specify disturbance):* If the cognitive disturbance is accompanied by a clinically significant behavioral disturbance (e.g., psychotic symptoms, mood disturbance, agitation, apathy, or other behavioral symptoms).

Criterion A

The combination of symptoms and objective assessment is critical in mild neurocognitive disorder to maintain specificity. A report of a change in an individual's abilities protects against overdiagnosing the disorder in those with lifelong poor performance, whereas objective assessment protects against overdiagnosing the disorder among the "worried well."

Criterion B

Mild neurocognitive disorder is the diagnosis for people who are still independent but who must exert greater effort to carry out tasks or must use compensatory strategies.

Criteria C and D

The cognitive decline seen in mild neurocognitive disorder affects some of the same cognitive domains as seen in delirium. Although it is clinically important to distinguish mild neurocognitive disorder from delirium, the two may co-occur.

The cognitive deficits in mild neurocognitive disorder are not better explained by another mental disorder (e.g., major depressive disorder, schizophrenia).

Subtypes and Specifiers for Both Major and Mild Neurocognitive Disorders

Both major and mild neurocognitive disorders list subtypes by which the clinician can code the proposed etiology of the disorder. All of the following subtypes require that the diagnostic criteria for either mild or major neurocognitive disorder be met. The individual disorders are then differentiated on the basis of their etiology. In addition to the etiological subtypes (detailed below), major and mild neurocognitive disorders may be further delineated by the specifier "with behavioral disturbance" or "without behavioral disturbance" (e.g., psychotic symptoms, mood disturbance, agitation, apathy, or other behavioral symptoms). For major neurocognitive disorder, there are additional severity specifiers to document the functional effects of the neurocognitive disorder: "mild," reflecting difficulties with instrumental activities of daily living (e.g., housework, managing money); "moderate," reflecting difficulties with basic activities of daily living (e.g., feeding, dressing); and "severe," meaning the individual is fully dependent.

Major or Mild Neurocognitive Disorder Due to Alzheimer's Disease

Alzheimer's disease is a neurodegenerative disorder that typically occurs in late life but can occur earlier. It is marked by insidious onset, gradual decline, and typically an early prominent memory loss. Alzheimer's disease is also the most common cause of neurocognitive disorder. Because of the modest predictive value of the clinical picture alone and the significant social consequences of an Alzheimer's diagnosis, the mild variant of Alzheimer's disease subtype is not commonly diagnosed. Individuals seen in memory disorder clinics whose presentations meet criteria for mild neurocognitive disorder progress to dementia of the Alzheimer type at the rate of 12%–15% per year, while population-based studies show a much lower rate of progression. Research is ongoing into what specific features of mild neurocognitive disorder might reliably indicate the presence of prodromal Alzheimer's disease. The diagnosis of the Alzheimer's specifier must be made on clinical grounds in the absence of brain biopsy. Alzheimer's disease has a characteristic pattern of onset and progression of cognitive impairments.

Diagnostic Criteria for Major or Mild Neurocognitive Disorder Due to Alzheimer's Disease

---

A. The criteria are met for major or mild neurocognitive disorder.
B. There is insidious onset and gradual progression of impairment in one or more cognitive domains (for major neurocognitive disorder, at least two domains must be impaired).
C. Criteria are met for either probable or possible Alzheimer's disease as follows:

For major neurocognitive disorder:

Probable Alzheimer's disease is diagnosed if either of the following is present; otherwise, **possible Alzheimer's disease** should be diagnosed.

1. Evidence of a causative Alzheimer's disease genetic mutation from family history or genetic testing.
2. All three of the following are present:
   a. Clear evidence of decline in memory and learning and at least one other cognitive domain (based on detailed history or serial neuropsychological testing).

    b. Steadily progressive, gradual decline in cognition, without extended plateaus.

    c. No evidence of mixed etiology (i.e., absence of other neurodegenerative or cerebrovascular disease, or another neurological, mental, or systemic disease or condition likely contributing to cognitive decline).

For mild neurocognitive disorder:

Probable Alzheimer's disease is diagnosed if there is evidence of a causative Alzheimer's disease genetic mutation from either genetic testing or family history.

Possible Alzheimer's disease is diagnosed if there is no evidence of a causative Alzheimer's disease genetic mutation from either genetic testing or family history, and all three of the following are present:

1. Clear evidence of decline in memory and learning.
2. Steadily progressive, gradual decline in cognition, without extended plateaus.
3. No evidence of mixed etiology (i.e., absence of other neurodegenerative or cerebrovascular disease, or another neurological or systemic disease or condition likely contributing to cognitive decline).

D. The disturbance is not better explained by cerebrovascular disease, another neurodegenerative disease, the effects of a substance, or another mental, neurological, or systemic disorder.

Coding note: For probable major neurocognitive disorder due to Alzheimer's disease, with behavioral disturbance, code first **331.0 (G30.9)** Alzheimer's disease, followed by **294.11 (F02.81)** major neurocognitive disorder due to Alzheimer's disease. For probable neurocognitive disorder due to Alzheimer's disease, without behavioral disturbance, code first **331.0 (G30.9)** Alzheimer's disease, followed by **294.10 (F02.80)** major neurocognitive disorder due to Alzheimer's disease, without behavioral disturbance.

For possible major neurocognitive disorder due to Alzheimer's disease, code **331.9 (G31.9)** possible major neurocognitive disorder due to Alzheimer's disease. (**Note:** Do *not* use the additional code for Alzheimer's disease. Behavioral disturbance cannot be coded but should still be indicated in writing.)

For mild neurocognitive disorder due to Alzheimer's disease, code **331.83 (G31.84).** (**Note:** Do *not* use the additional code for Alzheimer's disease. Behavioral disturbance cannot be coded but should still be indicated in writing.)

Major or Mild Frontotemporal Neurocognitive Disorder

Frontotemporal lobar degeneration has been found to be an important cause of neurocognitive disorders. Frontotemporal neurocognitive disorder is characterized by behavioral and personality changes and language impairment. In fact, DSM-5 recognizes both a behavioral (e.g., apathy, stereotyped behaviors) and a language (e.g., word finding) variant. Frontotemporal neurocognitive disorder can be difficult to distinguish from primary psychiatric disorders (e.g., schizophrenia, bipolar disorder), and including them in the differential diagnosis will be helpful. Neuroimaging (e.g., atrophy in frontotemporal regions) and genetics (e.g., mutations in the gene coding for microtubule-associated protein tau) will be particularly useful in documenting anomalies in frontal and temporal regions.

Diagnostic Criteria for Major or Mild Frontotemporal Neurocognitive Disorder

A. The criteria are met for major or mild neurocognitive disorder.

B. The disturbance has insidious onset and gradual progression.

C. Either (1) or (2):

    1. Behavioral variant:

        a. Three or more of the following behavioral symptoms:

            i. Behavioral disinhibition.

            ii. Apathy or inertia.

            iii. Loss of sympathy or empathy.

            iv. Perseverative, stereotyped or compulsive/ritualistic behavior.

            v. Hyperorality and dietary changes.

        b. Prominent decline in social cognition and/or executive abilities.

    2. Language variant:

        a. Prominent decline in language ability, in the form of speech production, word finding, object naming, grammar, or word comprehension.

D. Relative sparing of learning and memory and perceptual-motor function.

E. The disturbance is not better explained by cerebrovascular disease, another neurodegenerative disease, the effects of a substance, or another mental, neurological, or systemic disorder.

Probable frontotemporal neurocognitive disorder is diagnosed if either of the following is present; otherwise, **possible frontotemporal neurocognitive disorder** should be diagnosed:

1. Evidence of a causative frontotemporal neurocognitive disorder genetic mutation, from either family history or genetic testing.
2. Evidence of disproportionate frontal and/or temporal lobe involvement from neuroimaging.

Possible frontotemporal neurocognitive disorder is diagnosed if there is no evidence of a genetic mutation, and neuroimaging has not been performed.

Coding note: For probable major neurocognitive disorder due to frontotemporal lobar degeneration, with behavioral disturbance, code first **331.19 (G31.09)** frontotemporal disease, followed by **294.11 (F02.81)** probable major neurocognitive disorder due to frontotemporal lobar degeneration, with behavioral disturbance. For probable major neurocognitive disorder due to frontotemporal lobar degeneration, without behavioral disturbance, code first **331.19 (G31.09)** frontotemporal disease, followed by **294.10 (F02.80)** probable major neurocognitive disorder due to frontotemporal lobar degeneration, without behavioral disturbance.

For possible major neurocognitive disorder due to frontotemporal lobar degeneration, code **331.9 (G31.9)** possible major neurocognitive disorder due to frontotemporal lobar degeneration. (**Note:** Do *not* use the additional code for frontotemporal disease. Behavioral disturbance cannot be coded but should still be indicated in writing.)

For mild neurocognitive disorder due to frontotemporal lobar degeneration, code **331.83 (G31.84).** (**Note:** Do *not* use the additional code for frontotemporal disease. Behavioral disturbance cannot be coded but should still be indicated in writing.)

Major or Mild Neurocognitive Disorder With Lewy Bodies

Lewy body disease is now recognized as the second most common degenerative dementia of older adults. The First International Consortium on Dementia With Lewy Bodies published consensus clinical and pathological criteria (McKeith et al. 1996). The DSM-5 diagnostic criteria are based on the third and most recent criteria (McKeith 2006). Prominent visual hallucinations and parkinsonian features tend to occur early in the illness. The course is often slightly more rapid than that in Alzheimer's disease. Individuals with this form of neurocognitive disorder are very sensitive to the extrapyramidal side effects of conventional antipsychotics.

Diagnostic Criteria for Major or Mild Neurocognitive Disorder With Lewy Bodies

A. The criteria are met for major or mild neurocognitive disorder.

B. The disorder has an insidious onset and gradual progression.

C. The disorder meets a combination of core diagnostic features and suggestive diagnostic features for either probable or possible neurocognitive disorder with Lewy bodies.

   For probable major or mild neurocognitive disorder with Lewy bodies, the individual has two core features, or one suggestive feature with one or more core features. For **possible major or mild neurocognitive disorder with Lewy bodies,** the individual has only one core feature, or one or more suggestive features.

   1. Core diagnostic features:

      a. Fluctuating cognition with pronounced variations in attention and alertness.
      b. Recurrent visual hallucinations that are well formed and detailed.
      c. Spontaneous features of parkinsonism, with onset subsequent to the development of cognitive decline.

   2. Suggestive diagnostic features:

      a. Meets criteria for rapid eye movement sleep behavior disorder.
      b. Severe neuroleptic sensitivity.

D. The disturbance is not better explained by cerebrovascular disease, another neurodegenerative disease, the effects of a substance, or another mental, neurological, or systemic disorder.

Coding note: For probable major neurocognitive disorder with Lewy bodies, with behavioral disturbance, code first **331.82 (G31.83)** Lewy body disease, followed by **294.11 (F02.81)** probable major neurocognitive disorder with Lewy bodies, with behavioral disturbance. For probable major neurocognitive disorder with Lewy bodies, without behavioral disturbance, code first **331.82 (G31.83)** Lewy body disease, followed by **294.10 (F02.80)** probable major neurocognitive disorder with Lewy bodies, without behavioral disturbance.

For possible major neurocognitive disorder with Lewy bodies, code **331.9 (G31.9)** possible major neurocognitive disorder with Lewy bodies. (**Note:** Do *not* use the additional code for Lewy body disease. Behavioral disturbance cannot be coded but should still be indicated in writing.)

For mild neurocognitive disorder with Lewy bodies, code **331.83 (G31.84)**. (**Note:** Do *not* use the additional code for Lewy body disease. Behavioral disturbance cannot be coded but should still be indicated in writing.)

Major or Mild Vascular Neurocognitive Disorder

The concept of vascular dementia has changed since the publication of DSM-IV. The former concept of multi-infarct dementia (i.e., DSM-IV vascular dementia) has been replaced by a much broader concept of dementia attributed to both small and large vessel disease. Assessment of cerebrovascular disease relies on history, physical examination, and neuroimaging. The new criteria are consistent with those of the other neurocognitive disorders as well as with the prevailing view among experts in this field that cognitive disorders caused by vascular disease lie on a continuum.

Diagnostic Criteria for Major or Mild Vascular Neurocognitive Disorder

A. The criteria are met for major or mild neurocognitive disorder.
B. The clinical features are consistent with a vascular etiology, as suggested by either of the following:
   1. Onset of the cognitive deficits is temporally related to one or more cerebrovascular events.
   2. Evidence for decline is prominent in complex attention (including processing speed) and frontal-executive function.
C. There is evidence of the presence of cerebrovascular disease from history, physical examination, and/or neuroimaging considered sufficient to account for the neurocognitive deficits.
D. The symptoms are not better explained by another brain disease or systemic disorder.

Probable vascular neurocognitive disorder is diagnosed if one of the following is present; otherwise **possible vascular neurocognitive disorder** should be diagnosed:

1. Clinical criteria are supported by neuroimaging evidence of significant parenchymal injury attributed to cerebrovascular disease (neuroimaging-supported).
2. The neurocognitive syndrome is temporally related to one or more documented cerebrovascular events.
3. Both clinical and genetic (e.g., cerebral autosomal dominant arteriopathy with subcortical infarcts and leukoencephalopathy) evidence of cerebrovascular disease is present.

Possible vascular neurocognitive disorder is diagnosed if the clinical criteria are met but neuroimaging is not available and the temporal relationship of the neurocognitive syndrome with one or more cerebrovascular events is not established.

Coding note: For probable major vascular neurocognitive disorder, with behavioral disturbance, code **290.40 (F01.51).** For probable major vascular neurocognitive disorder, without behavioral disturbance, code **290.40 (F01.50).** For possible major vascular neurocognitive disorder, with or without behavioral disturbance, code **331.9 (G31.9).** An additional medical code for the cerebrovascular disease is not needed.

For mild vascular neurocognitive disorder, code **331.83 (G31.84). (Note:** Do *not* use an additional code for the vascular disease. Behavioral disturbance cannot be coded but should still be indicated in writing.)

Major or Mild Neurocognitive Disorder Due to Traumatic Brain Injury

Neurocognitive disorder due to traumatic brain injury is caused by an impact to the head or with rapid movement or brain displacement within the skull. The clinical characteristics of the disorder depend on the location, severity, and duration of the trauma. This diagnosis may be difficult in individuals with alcohol use disorders because such individuals are at increased risk both for repeated head injuries and for substance-induced neurocognitive disorder. Posttraumatic stress may co-occur with the disorder.

Diagnostic Criteria for Major or Mild Neurocognitive Disorder Due to Traumatic Brain Injury

A. The criteria are met for major or mild neurocognitive disorder.
B. There is evidence of a traumatic brain injury—that is, an impact to the head or other mechanisms of rapid movement or displacement of the brain within the skull, with one or more of the following:
   1. Loss of consciousness.
   2. Posttraumatic amnesia.
   3. Disorientation and confusion.
   4. Neurological signs (e.g., neuroimaging demonstrating injury; a new onset of seizures; a marked worsening of a preexisting seizure disorder; visual field cuts; anosmia; hemiparesis).

C. The neurocognitive disorder presents immediately after the occurrence of the traumatic brain injury or immediately after recovery of consciousness and persists past the acute post-injury period.

Coding note: For major neurocognitive disorder due to traumatic brain injury, with behavioral disturbance: For ICD-9-CM, first code **907.0** late effect of intracranial injury without skull fracture, followed by **294.11** major neurocognitive disorder due to traumatic brain injury, with behavioral disturbance. For ICD-10-CM, first code **S06.2X9S** diffuse traumatic brain injury with loss of consciousness of unspecified duration, sequela; followed by **F02.81** major neurocognitive disorder due to traumatic brain injury, with behavioral disturbance.

For major neurocognitive disorder due to traumatic brain injury, without behavioral disturbance: For ICD-9-CM, first code **907.0** late effect of intracranial injury without skull fracture, followed by **294.10** major neurocognitive disorder due to traumatic brain injury, without behavioral disturbance. For ICD-10-CM, first code **S06.2X9S** diffuse traumatic brain injury with loss of consciousness of unspecified duration, sequela; followed by **F02.80** major neurocognitive disorder due to traumatic brain injury, without behavioral disturbance.

For mild neurocognitive disorder due to traumatic brain injury, code **331.83 (G31.84).** (**Note:** Do *not* use the additional code for traumatic brain injury. Behavioral disturbance cannot be coded but should still be indicated in writing.)

Substance/Medication-Induced Major or Mild Neurocognitive Disorder

Substance/medication-induced major or mild neurocognitive disorder needs to be distinguished from the cognitive impairments commonly seen with substance intoxication or withdrawal. The impairments seen in intoxication or withdrawal are usually reversible, whereas substance/medication-induced neurocognitive disorder is a persisting condition. This disorder results from the neurotoxic effects of a substance or medication, and the deficits are usually permanent. This disorder is more common in older individuals, with longer use of drugs or alcohol, and with other risk factors such as nutritional deficits.

Diagnostic Criteria for Substance/Medication-Induced Major or Mild Neurocognitive Disorder

A. The criteria are met for major or mild neurocognitive disorder.
B. The neurocognitive impairments do not occur exclusively during the course of a delirium and persist beyond the usual duration of intoxication and acute withdrawal.
C. The involved substance or medication and duration and extent of use are capable of producing the neurocognitive impairment.

D. The temporal course of the neurocognitive deficits is consistent with the timing of substance or medication use and abstinence (e.g., the deficits remain stable or improve after a period of abstinence).

E. The neurocognitive disorder is not attributable to another medical condition or is not better explained by another mental disorder.

Coding note: The ICD-9-CM and ICD-10-CM codes for the [specific substance/medication]-induced neurocognitive disorders are indicated in the table below. Note that the ICD-10-CM code depends on whether or not there is a comorbid substance use disorder present for the same class of substance. If a mild substance use disorder is comorbid with the substance-induced neurocognitive disorder, the 4th position character is "1," and the clinician should record "mild [substance] use disorder" before the substance-induced neurocognitive disorder (e.g., "mild inhalant use disorder with inhalant-induced major neurocognitive disorder"). If a moderate or severe substance use disorder is comorbid with the substance-induced neurocognitive disorder, the 4th position character is "2," and the clinician should record "moderate [substance] use disorder" or "severe [substance] use disorder," depending on the severity of the comorbid substance use disorder. If there is no comorbid substance use disorder, then the 4th position character is "9," and the clinician should record only the substance-induced neurocognitive disorder. For some classes of substances (i.e., alcohol; sedatives, hypnotics, anxiolytics), it is not permissible to code a comorbid mild substance use disorder with a substance-induced neurocognitive disorder; only a comorbid moderate or severe substance use disorder, or no substance use disorder, can be diagnosed. Behavioral disturbance cannot be coded but should still be indicated in writing.

		ICD-10-CM		
	ICD-9-CM	With use disorder, mild	With use disorder, moderate or severe	Without use disorder
Alcohol (major neurocognitive disorder), nonamnestic-confabulatory type	291.2	NA	F10.27	F10.97
Alcohol (major neurocognitive disorder), amnestic-confabulatory type	291.1	NA	F10.26	F10.96
Alcohol (mild neurocognitive disorder)	291.89	NA	F10.288	F10.988
Inhalant (major neurocognitive disorder)	292.82	F18.17	F18.27	F18.97
Inhalant (mild neurocognitive disorder)	292.89	F18.188	F18.288	F18.988

		ICD-10-CM		
	ICD-9-CM	With use disorder, mild	With use disorder, moderate or severe	Without use disorder
Sedative, hypnotic, or anxiolytic (major neurocognitive disorder)	292.82	NA	F13.27	F13.97
Sedative, hypnotic, or anxiolytic (mild neurocognitive disorder)	292.89	NA	F13.288	F13.988
Other (or unknown) substance (major neurocognitive disorder)	292.82	F19.17	F19.27	F19.97
Other (or unknown) substance (mild neurocognitive disorder)	292.89	F19.188	F19.288	F19.988

Specify if:
   Persistent: Neurocognitive impairment continues to be significant after an extended period of abstinence.

Major or Mild Neurocognitive Disorder Due to HIV Infection

Individuals with HIV infection are at increased risk of developing a neurocognitive disorder. The disorder could be due to any number of associated diseases, such as toxoplasmosis, cytomegalovirus, cryptococcosis, central nervous system lymphoma, or tuberculosis. This diagnosis should be given only when cognitive impairment is judged to be due to the direct central nervous system effects of HIV. This disorder is more common in individuals with prior episodes of severe immunosuppression, those with high viral loads in the cerebrospinal fluid, and those with HIV-related anemia or hypoalbuminemia.

Diagnostic Criteria for Major or Mild Neurocognitive Disorder Due to HIV Infection

A. The criteria are met for major or mild neurocognitive disorder.
B. There is documented infection with human immunodeficiency virus (HIV).

C. The neurocognitive disorder is not better explained by non-HIV conditions, including secondary brain diseases such as progressive multifocal leukoencephalopathy or cryptococcal meningitis.
D. The neurocognitive disorder is not attributable to another medical condition and is
   not better explained by a mental disorder.

Coding note: For major neurocognitive disorder due to HIV infection, with behavioral
disturbance, code first **042 (B20)** HIV infection, followed by **294.11 (F02.81)** major
neurocognitive disorder due to HIV infection, with behavioral disturbance. For major
neurocognitive disorder due to HIV infection, without behavioral disturbance, code first
042 (B20) HIV infection, followed by **294.10 (F02.80)** major neurocognitive disorder
due to HIV infection, without behavioral disturbance.

For mild neurocognitive disorder due to HIV infection, code **331.83 (G31.84)**. (**Note:**
Do *not* use the additional code for HIV infection. Behavioral disturbance cannot be
coded but should still be indicated in writing.)

Major or Mild Neurocognitive Disorder Due to Prion Disease

Neurocognitive disorder due to prion disease is rare, and the most common type is
Creutzfeldt-Jakob disease. The disease is accompanied by ataxia, myoclonus, chorea,
and dystonia. The course is typically rapidly progressive over as little as 6 months.
The diagnosis is confirmed with brain biopsy or autopsy.

Diagnostic Criteria for Major or Mild Neurocognitive Disorder Due to Prion Disease

A. The criteria are met for major or mild neurocognitive disorder.
B. There is insidious onset, and rapid progression of impairment is common.
C. There are motor features of prion disease, such as myoclonus or ataxia, or bio-
   marker evidence.
D. The neurocognitive disorder is not attributable to another medical condition and is
   not better explained by another mental disorder.

Coding note: For major neurocognitive disorder due to prion disease, with behavioral
disturbance, code first **046.79 (A81.9)** prion disease, followed by **294.11 (F02.81)** major neurocognitive disorder due to prion disease, with behavioral disturbance. For major neurocognitive disorder due to prion disease, without behavioral disturbance, code
first **046.79 (A81.9)** prion disease, followed by **294.10 (F02.80)** major neurocognitive
disorder due to prion disease, without behavioral disturbance.

For mild neurocognitive disorder due to prion disease, code **331.83 (G31.84)**. (**Note:** Do
not use the additional code for prion disease. Behavioral disturbance cannot be coded
but should still be indicated in writing.)

Major or Mild Neurocognitive Disorder Due to Parkinson's Disease

The essential feature of this disorder is cognitive decline after the onset of Parkinson's disease. As many as 75% of individuals with Parkinson's disease will develop a major neurocognitive disorder, and 27% will have a mild neurocognitive disorder. Individuals who are older at disease onset and those with increasing duration of disease appear more likely to develop a neurocognitive disorder.

Diagnostic Criteria for Major or Mild Neurocognitive Disorder Due to Parkinson's Disease

A. The criteria are met for major or mild neurocognitive disorder.
B. The disturbance occurs in the setting of established Parkinson's disease.
C. There is insidious onset and gradual progression of impairment.
D. The neurocognitive disorder is not attributable to another medical condition and is not better explained by another mental disorder.

Major or mild neurocognitive disorder probably due to Parkinson's disease should be diagnosed if 1 and 2 are both met. **Major or mild neurocognitive disorder possibly due to Parkinson's disease** should be diagnosed if 1 or 2 is met:

1. There is no evidence of mixed etiology (i.e., absence of other neurodegenerative or cerebrovascular disease or another neurological, mental, or systemic disease or condition likely contributing to cognitive decline).
2. The Parkinson's disease clearly precedes the onset of the neurocognitive disorder.

Coding note: For major neurocognitive disorder probably due to Parkinson's disease, with behavioral disturbance, code first **332.0 (G20)** Parkinson's disease, followed by **294.11 (F02.81)** major neurocognitive disorder probably due to Parkinson's disease, with behavioral disturbance. For major neurocognitive disorder probably due to Parkinson's disease, without behavioral disturbance, code first **332.0 (G20)** Parkinson's disease, followed by **294.10 (F02.80)** major neurocognitive disorder probably due to Parkinson's disease, without behavioral disturbance.

For major neurocognitive disorder possibly due to Parkinson's disease, code **331.9 (G31.9)** major neurocognitive disorder possibly due to Parkinson's disease. (**Note:** Do *not* use the additional code for Parkinson's disease. Behavioral disturbance cannot be coded but should still be indicated in writing.)

For mild neurocognitive disorder due to Parkinson's disease, code **331.83 (G31.84).** (**Note:** Do *not* use the additional code for Parkinson's disease. Behavioral disturbance cannot be coded but should still be indicated in writing.)

Major or Mild Neurocognitive Disorder Due to Huntington's Disease

Cognitive and behavioral changes often precede the motor abnormalities of bradykinesia and chorea. Diagnosis of Huntington's disease is based on the extrapyramidal motor abnormalities in a person with a family history of Huntington's, or genetic testing (CAG trinucleotide repeat expansion in the HTT gene on chromosome 4).

Diagnostic Criteria for Major or Mild Neurocognitive Disorder Due to Huntington's Disease

A. The criteria are met for major or mild neurocognitive disorder.
B. There is insidious onset and gradual progression.
C. There is clinically established Huntington's disease, or risk for Huntington's disease based on family history or genetic testing.
D. The neurocognitive disorder is not attributable to another medical condition and is not better explained by another mental disorder.

Coding note: For major neurocognitive disorder due to Huntington's disease, with behavioral disturbance, code first **333.4 (G10)** Huntington's disease, followed by **294.11 (F02.81)** major neurocognitive disorder due to Huntington's disease, with behavioral disturbance. For major neurocognitive disorder due to Huntington's disease, without behavioral disturbance, code first **333.4 (G10)** Huntington's disease, followed by **294.10 (F02.80)** major neurocognitive disorder due to Huntington's disease, without behavioral disturbance.

For mild neurocognitive disorder due to Huntington's disease, code **331.83 (G31.84)**. (**Note:** Do *not* use the additional code for Huntington's disease. Behavioral disturbance cannot be coded but should still be indicated in writing.)

Major or Mild Neurocognitive Disorder Due to Another Medical Condition

The diagnosis neurocognitive disorder due to another medical condition is used when an individual has a cause other than those listed specifically in DSM-5. Potential causes include brain tumors, subdural hematomas, multiple sclerosis, neurosyphilis, hypoglycemia, renal or hepatic failure, childhood and adult storage diseases, and vitamin deficiencies.

Diagnostic Criteria for Major or Mild Neurocognitive Disorder Due to Another Medical Condition

A. The criteria are met for major or mild neurocognitive disorder.
B. There is evidence from the history, physical examination, or laboratory findings

that the neurocognitive disorder is the pathophysiological consequence of another medical condition.

C. The cognitive deficits are not better explained by another mental disorder or another specific neurocognitive disorder (e.g., Alzheimer's disease, HIV infection).

Coding note: For major neurocognitive disorder due to another medical condition, with behavioral disturbance, code first the other medical condition, followed by the major neurocognitive disorder due to another medical condition, with behavioral disturbance (e.g., 340 [G35] multiple sclerosis, **294.11 [F02.81]** major neurocognitive disorder due to multiple sclerosis, with behavioral disturbance). For major neurocognitive disorder due to another medical condition, without behavioral disturbance, code first the other medical condition, followed by the major neurocognitive disorder due to another medical condition, without behavioral disturbance (e.g., 340 [G35] multiple sclerosis, **294.10 [F02.80]** major neurocognitive disorder due to multiple sclerosis, without behavioral disturbance).

For mild neurocognitive disorder due to another medical condition, code **331.83 (G31.84)**. (**Note:** Do *not* use the additional code for the other medical condition. Behavioral disturbance cannot be coded but should still be indicated in writing.)

Major or Mild Neurocognitive Disorder Due to Multiple Etiologies

If a major or mild neurocognitive disorder is of mixed etiology (e.g., Alzheimer's disease and cerebrovascular disease) and the multiple underlying diseases are known, the multiple etiological subtypes should all be diagnosed.

Diagnostic Criteria for Major or Mild Neurocognitive Disorder Due to Multiple Etiologies

A. The criteria are met for major or mild neurocognitive disorder.

B. There is evidence from the history, physical examination, or laboratory findings that the neurocognitive disorder is the pathophysiological consequence of more than one etiological process, excluding substances (e.g., neurocognitive disorder due to Alzheimer's disease with subsequent development of vascular neurocognitive disorder).

Note: Please refer to the diagnostic criteria for the various neurocognitive disorders due to specific medical conditions for guidance on establishing the particular etiologies.

C. The cognitive deficits are not better explained by another mental disorder and do not occur exclusively during the course of a delirium.

Coding note: For major neurocognitive disorder due to multiple etiologies, with behavioral disturbance, code **294.11 (F02.81)**; for major neurocognitive disorder due to multiple etiologies, without behavioral disturbance, code **294.10 (F02.80)**. All of the etiological medical conditions (with the exception of vascular disease) should be coded and listed separately immediately before major neurocognitive disorder due to multiple etiologies (e.g., **331.0 [G30.9]** Alzheimer's disease; **331.82 [G31.83]** Lewy body disease; **294.11 [F02.81]** major neurocognitive disorder due to multiple etiologies, with behavioral disturbance).

When a cerebrovascular etiology is contributing to the neurocognitive disorder, the diagnosis of vascular neurocognitive disorder should be listed in addition to major neurocognitive disorder due to multiple etiologies. For example, for a presentation of major neurocognitive disorder due to both Alzheimer's disease and vascular disease, with behavioral disturbance, code the following: **331.0 (G30.9)** Alzheimer's disease; **294.11 (F02.81)** major neurocognitive disorder due to multiple etiologies, with behavioral disturbance; **290.40 (F01.51)** major vascular neurocognitive disorder, with behavioral disturbance.

For mild neurocognitive disorder due to multiple etiologies, code **331.83 (G31.84).** (**Note:** Do *not* use the additional codes for the etiologies. Behavioral disturbance cannot be coded but should still be indicated in writing.)

Unspecified Neurocognitive Disorder

Neurocognitive disorders may be diagnosed as unspecified when there are symptoms of a neurocognitive disorder that cause distress or impairment but do not meet full criteria for any disorder in this diagnostic class. This diagnosis is used when the precise etiology cannot be determined.

Unspecified Neurocognitive Disorder	**799.59** (R41.9)

This category applies to presentations in which symptoms characteristic of a neurocognitive disorder that cause clinically significant distress or impairment in social, occupational, or other important areas of functioning predominate but do not meet the full criteria for any of the disorders in the neurocognitive disorders diagnostic class. The unspecified neurocognitive disorder category is used in situations in which the precise etiology cannot be determined with sufficient certainty to make an etiological attribution.

Coding note: For unspecified major or mild neurocognitive disorder, code 799.59 (R41.9). (**Note:** Do *not* use additional codes for any presumed etiological medical conditions. Behavioral disturbance cannot be coded but may be indicated in writing.)

KEY POINTS

- Called "delirium, dementia, and amnestic and other cognitive disorders" in DSM-IV, the diagnostic class has been renamed "neurocognitive disorders."

- DSM-5 recognizes both major neurocognitive disorders and a less severe level of cognitive impairment, referred to as *mild neurocognitive disorder.* The latter term is used for less disabling syndromes that may be a focus of concern.

- Examples of symptoms and assessments of the various neurocognitive domains (e.g., complex attention, executive function) are provided at both major and mild levels of impairment.

- Clinicians who diagnose either a major or mild neurocognitive disorder can specify an etiologic subtype (e.g., Alzheimer's disease).

CHAPTER 18

Personality Disorders

Cluster A Personality Disorders
301.0 (F60.0)   Paranoid Personality Disorder
301.20 (F60.1)   Schizoid Personality Disorder
301.22 (F21)   Schizotypal Personality Disorder

Cluster B Personality Disorders
301.7 (F60.2)   Antisocial Personality Disorder
301.83 (F60.3)   Borderline Personality Disorder
301.50 (F60.4)   Histrionic Personality Disorder
301.81 (F60.81) Narcissistic Personality Disorder

Cluster C Personality Disorders
301.82 (F60.6)   Avoidant Personality Disorder
301.6 (F60.7)   Dependent Personality Disorder
301.4 (F60.5)   Obsessive-Compulsive Personality Disorder

Other Personality Disorders
310.1 (F07.0)   Personality Change Due to Another Medical Condition
301.89 (F60.89) Other Specified Personality Disorder
301.9 (F60.9)   Unspecified Personality Disorder

Maladaptive character traits have been recognized for millennia. Formal attempts to list the variety of personality types took root with DSM-I, in which eight different types of personality disorders were enumerated. The list was expanded to 10 in DSM-II. In these early manuals, the disorders were briefly described but there were no criteria—for example, inadequate personality in DSM-II: "The behavior pattern is characterized by ineffectual responses to emotional, social, intellectual and physical demands. While the patient seems neither physically nor mentally deficient, he does manifest inadaptability, ineptness, poor judgment, social instability, and lack of physical and emotional stamina" (American Psychiatric Association 1968, p. 44).

In DSM-III, personality disorders were accorded new prominence by being coded on a separate axis (Axis II) in the new multiaxial system. Criteria for 11 different personality disorders were included, some retained from DSM-II and others newly created in response to clinical and research observations (e.g., schizotypal personality disorder, borderline personality disorder). DSM-III also introduced the concept of personality disorder "clusters," in which disorder types were grouped by their predominant symptom pattern: Cluster A for individuals considered odd or eccentric; Cluster B for individuals considered dramatic, emotional, or erratic; and Cluster C for individuals considered anxious or dependent.

In DSM-III-R and DSM-IV, the personality disorder diagnostic criteria were edited for clarity and in some cases simplified. The number of disorders was pared down to 10 in DSM-IV with the elimination of passive-aggressive personality disorder, which was thought to be insufficiently distinct.

During the development of DSM-5, the Personality and Personality Disorders Work Group developed a model that combined categorical diagnosis with optional dimensional ratings. Work group members had responded to the call by the DSM-5 Task Force to introduce dimensional measures that could be used to assess symptoms and syndromes and provide a more complete evaluation of an individual's disorder and level of functioning (Widiger et al. 2006) (See Chapter 1, "The March to DSM-5").

The work group recommended reducing the number of personality disorders to six by eliminating the dependent, histrionic, paranoid, and schizoid types; reformulating the diagnostic criteria for the remaining disorders to emphasize personality functioning and maladaptive personality traits; and describing five broad personality domains and 25 specific trait facets that could be dimensionally rated. The proposal received much criticism, in part because of its complexity and the perception that it would be overly time consuming for clinicians (Gunderson 2010). In December 2012, the American Psychiatric Association Board of Trustees voted to move the new scheme to Section III in DSM-5 and to include the 10 specific DSM-IV personality disorders in Section II. Thus, both versions are available to serve clinical practice and research initiatives (see Chapter 21, "Alternative DSM-5 Model for Personality Disorders").

There are several changes to highlight in the class. Perhaps the most important change is that the multiaxial evaluation system has been discontinued, and for that reason personality disorders are no longer coded on Axis II. The decision to discontinue the multiaxial system was largely due to its incompatibility with diagnostic systems in the rest of medicine, but there were other motivations as well. The scheme had been developed for DSM-III to help ensure that personality disorders and intellectual disability would receive greater recognition. An unintended consequence of placing personality disorders on an axis separate from the major disorders was to further marginalize them. Personality disorders are now coded at the same level as other mental disorders.

Next, the diagnosis personality disorder not otherwise specified has been replaced by other specified personality disorder and unspecified personality disorder. These two diagnostic categories are used in situations in which the individual's personality pattern meets general criteria for a personality disorder and traits of several different personality disorders are present but the criteria for any specific disorder are not met (e.g., the individual is considered to have a personality disorder that is not included in DSM-5, such as inadequate personality disorder). The unspecified personality disorder category is used in situations in which the clinician chooses not to specify the reason that the criteria are not met for a specific personality disorder and when there is insufficient information to make a more specific diagnosis.

Personality change due to another medical condition has been moved to this chapter from DSM-IV's "Mental Disorders Due to a General Medical Condition." The purpose of this change was to place the diagnosis within the class relevant to the predominant symptom pattern.

Additional changes to the class were prompted by discussions about the etiological relationship among disorders. Schizotypal personality disorder has been listed with the schizophrenia spectrum and other psychotic disorders, and antisocial personality disorder with the disruptive, impulse-control, and conduct disorders. The text and criteria for these two disorders remain in the personality disorders chapter.

GENERAL PERSONALITY DISORDER

DSM-IV introduced a general set of criteria for personality disorders that has not changed in DSM-5 except for minor edits. They address the question of whether or not an individual has a personality disorder. If present, the clinician should determine which of the ten specific disorders is present (the person's presentation may meet the criteria for more than one disorder). If the person's presentation meets the general diagnostic criteria but the criteria for any of the specific disorders are not met, then the diagnosis of either other specified personality disorder or unspecified personality disorder should be used.

The personality disorders continue to be grouped into three clusters on the basis of their descriptive similarity: Cluster A includes paranoid, schizoid, and schizotypal personality disorders. People with these disorders may appear odd or eccentric. Cluster B includes antisocial, borderline, histrionic, and narcissistic personality disorders. Individuals with these disorders may appear dramatic, emotional, or erratic. Cluster C includes avoidant, dependent, and obsessive-compulsive personality disorders. Individuals with these disorders may appear anxious or fearful. The ten personality disorders are described later in this chapter.

Diagnostic Criteria for General Personality Disorder

A. An enduring pattern of inner experience and behavior that deviates markedly from the expectations of the individual's culture. This pattern is manifested in two (or more) of the following areas:

1. Cognition (i.e., ways of perceiving and interpreting self, other people, and events).
2. Affectivity (i.e., the range, intensity, lability, and appropriateness of emotional response).

   3. Interpersonal functioning.
   4. Impulse control.

B. The enduring pattern is inflexible and pervasive across a broad range of personal and social situations.
C. The enduring pattern leads to clinically significant distress or impairment in social, occupational, or other important areas of functioning.
D. The pattern is stable and of long duration, and its onset can be traced back at least to adolescence or early adulthood.
E. The enduring pattern is not better explained as a manifestation or consequence of another mental disorder.
F. The enduring pattern is not attributable to the physiological effects of a substance (e.g., a drug of abuse, a medication) or another medical condition (e.g., head trauma).

Criterion A

This item ensures that the "pattern of inner experience" meets several conditions. First, the pattern is enduring and not transient. If it is of recent onset or is transient, it may well be attributable to another mental or medical disorder. Next, the pattern deviates "markedly" from the expectations of the individual's culture. This is a necessary and important distinction because some cultures encourage or tolerate individual expressions not tolerated in another culture. For example, in some non-Western societies the concepts of possession and magical experience are celebrated; in Western societies, these symptoms may be used to indicate a Cluster A personality disorder (e.g., schizotypal personality disorder).

The pattern must be manifested in two or more of four areas: cognition, affectivity, interpersonal functioning, and impulse control. This requirement means that the individual's symptoms or behaviors are not confined to a single domain. Typically, most individuals who meet criteria for a personality disorder have involvement in multiple symptom domains. For example, an individual with borderline personality disorder may have problems maintaining stable interpersonal relationships, have extreme difficulty regulating his or her emotions, have poor impulse control, and commit acts of self-harm.

Criteria B, C, and D

These criteria ensure that the pattern is "pervasive across a broad range of personal and social situations," is impairing, and is stable and enduring. In short, the personality difficulties are not confined to a single domain of functioning but affect most life domains (home, school, workplace). For example, the individual may have problems interacting not just with immediate family but with coworkers, friends and acquaintances, and even strangers. As might be expected, these problems are upsetting and distressing to individuals, even though they may be unaware of their own role in creating difficulties for themselves. Their personality disorder can prevent the formation or maintenance of stable interpersonal relationships, can contribute to job loss, and can contribute to overall unhappiness. Impairment occurs along a continuum as with most mental disorders. At the extreme end, the person may be unable to function without assistance because of near constant self-harm (borderline personality disorder) or because of uncontrolled criminal conduct that leads to incarceration (antisocial personality disorder). At the milder end, a person may function well in the workplace but be unable to maintain romantic attachments because of his or her rigidity and stubbornness (obsessive-compulsive personality disorder).

Criterion D requires that the pattern be stable and of long duration. A personality disorder is not considered time-limited or transitory. This requirement appears true for most individuals whose personality disorder is evident by late adolescence or early adulthood. Individuals with antisocial personality disorder have an even earlier onset, with behavioral problems having an onset prior to age 15 years (diagnosed in youth as conduct disorder). As a general rule, personality disorders tend to lessen in severity (or "burn out") with age. Longitudinal studies have shown, for instance, that persons with antisocial and borderline personality disorders have progressively fewer symptoms over time. At follow-up many will no longer meet full diagnostic criteria, yet symptoms remain that can nonetheless be impairing. This may be less true for other personality disorder types, such as obsessive-compulsive and schizotypal personality disorders. Further, because the problems associated with personality disorders tend to be at their most severe during formative periods in a person's life—when most people are completing their education, marrying and starting a family, and establishing a career—even when improved, many individuals with personality disorders never "catch up" educationally, socially, or economically with their peers who do not have personality disorders.

Criteria E and F

These are the "rule out" criteria meant to ensure that the clinician has ruled out other potential causes for the personality disturbance. Other mental disorders can induce personality changes. For instance, in the early phases of schizophrenia, individuals can develop symptoms that resemble those often attributed to a personality disorder, such as social withdrawal, magical thinking, impulsive acts, or mild suspiciousness, all occurring in the absence of frank hallucinations or delusions. The person with major depressive disorder can become socially withdrawn, develop low self-esteem, lack self-confidence, and become dependent on others even for simple decisions. These traits should be attributed to the major depression unless they clearly predate the onset of the depression and are part of an enduring pattern of experience and behavior.

In contrast, other medical disorders also must be ruled out as a cause of the personality pattern. Persons who use alcohol or other drugs excessively can develop symptoms suggesting a personality disorder—for example, drug-seeking behaviors that lead them to become irresponsible, to lie, or to commit crimes, or to become apathetic, erratic, or impulsive. Brain lesions, such as those caused by tumors or strokes, can contribute to the development of emotional lability, impulsive behavior, suspiciousness, or apathy.

Cluster A Personality Disorders

Paranoid Personality Disorder

Paranoid personality disorder describes individuals who are chronically suspicious and distrust others. In response to paranoid beliefs, they can be irritable, hostile, and avoidant. They can develop hypervigilance toward their environment, finding conspiracies against them wherever they look.

Paranoid personality disorder was introduced in DSM-I and has continued to be included in all subsequent DSM editions. Adolf Meyer is often credited with introducing the concept of paranoid personality, but other psychiatrists writing at the turn of the twentieth century, including Kraepelin, Bleuler, and Freud, provided early descriptions. Research suggests that paranoid personality disorder lies within the schizophrenia spectrum and results from a common genetic predisposition.

Diagnostic Criteria for Paranoid Personality Disorder   301.0 (F60.0)

A. A pervasive distrust and suspiciousness of others such that their motives are interpreted as malevolent, beginning by early adulthood and present in a variety of contexts, as indicated by four (or more) of the following:

1. Suspects, without sufficient basis, that others are exploiting, harming, or deceiving him or her.
2. Is preoccupied with unjustified doubts about the loyalty or trustworthiness of friends or associates.
3. Is reluctant to confide in others because of unwarranted fear that the information will be used maliciously against him or her.
4. Reads hidden demeaning or threatening meanings into benign remarks or events.
5. Persistently bears grudges (i.e., is unforgiving of insults, injuries, or slights).
6. Perceives attacks on his or her character or reputation that are not apparent to others and is quick to react angrily or to counterattack.
7. Has recurrent suspicions, without justification, regarding fidelity of spouse or sexual partner.

B. Does not occur exclusively during the course of schizophrenia, a bipolar disorder or depressive disorder with psychotic features, or another psychotic disorder and is not attributable to the physiological effects of another medical condition.

Note: If criteria are met prior to the onset of schizophrenia, add "premorbid," i.e., "paranoid personality disorder (premorbid)."

Schizoid Personality Disorder

Schizoid personality disorder describes people who have difficulty achieving intimacy or developing emotionally meaningful relationships. People with schizoid personality disorder choose solitary activities and tend to have no close relationships, including with family members. These individuals rarely experience strong emotions, express little desire for sexual intimacy with another person, tend to be indifferent to praise or criticism, and display a constricted affect. Individuals with schizoid personality disorder may come across to others as dull, emotionally constricted, and aloof.

Schizoid personality disorder was introduced in DSM-I and has continued to be included in all subsequent DSM editions. DSM-I and DSM-II emphasized the presence of autistic magical thinking, which is now considered a symptom of schizotypal personality disorder. The disorder is not diagnosed in persons with schizophrenia or other psychotic disorders because these conditions are typically accompanied by a seclusive lifestyle.

The disorder is uncommon in psychiatric settings because persons with this personality disorder rarely seek care. The distinction between schizoid and avoidant personality disorder can sometimes be difficult to make, but it rests on the motivation underlying the person's tendency to avoid interpersonal relationships.

Diagnostic Criteria for Schizoid Personality Disorder 301.20 (F60.1)

A. A pervasive pattern of detachment from social relationships and a restricted range of expression of emotions in interpersonal settings, beginning by early adulthood and present in a variety of contexts, as indicated by four (or more) of the following:

1. Neither desires nor enjoys close relationships, including being part of a family.
2. Almost always chooses solitary activities.
3. Has little, if any, interest in having sexual experiences with another person.
4. Takes pleasure in few, if any, activities.
5. Lacks close friends or confidants other than first-degree relatives.
6. Appears indifferent to the praise or criticism of others.
7. Shows emotional coldness, detachment, or flattened affectivity.

B. Does not occur exclusively during the course of schizophrenia, a bipolar disorder or depressive disorder with psychotic features, another psychotic disorder, or autism spectrum disorder and is not attributable to the physiological effects of another medical condition.

Note: If criteria are met prior to the onset of schizophrenia, add "premorbid," i.e., "schizoid personality disorder (premorbid)."

Schizotypal Personality Disorder

Schizotypal personality disorder is characterized by a pattern of peculiar behavior, odd speech and thinking, and unusual perceptual experiences. People with these symptoms may appear odd and unusual, but they are not psychotic. The disorder was new to DSM-III, its inclusion prompted by evidence that relatives of individuals with schizophrenia often displayed a cluster of schizophrenic-like traits, observations noted earlier by Kraepelin and Bleuler. Genetic and neurophysiological evidence later confirmed membership of this disorder within the schizophrenia spectrum.

Because a certain proportion of people diagnosed with schizotypal personality disorder develop schizophrenia, it may be more appropriate to understand their schizotypal traits as early (or prodromal) manifestations of schizophrenia. This can be coded by adding "(premorbid)" after the diagnosis in a person who has developed schizophrenia. Attenuated psychosis syndrome, described in Chapter 22, "Conditions for Further Study," and autism spectrum disorder, described in Chapter 3, "Neurodevelopmental Disorders," may be other diagnostic considerations.

The placement of schizotypal personality disorder alongside the psychotic disorders was debated during the development of DSM-IV. The decision at that time was to follow convention and keep schizotypal personality disorder in the personality disorders chapter, recognizing that other personality disorders also have spectrum relationships (e.g., avoidant personality disorder and anxiety disorders, borderline personality disorder and mood disorders). These arguments were revisited during DSM-5 deliberations, and the Psychotic Disorders Work Group recommended that the disorder be moved to the chapter "Schizophrenia Spectrum and Other Psychotic Disorders" as part of a general reorganization. As mentioned earlier, the text and criteria remain in this chapter and are unchanged from DSM-IV.

Schizotypal personality disorder is common and has a relatively stable course, with onset in childhood. It is often found in offspring of people with schizophrenia. Some individuals who meet this description in adolescence will go on to develop schizophrenia. After the age of risk for schizophrenia, typical individuals with schizotypal personality disorder rarely develop schizophrenia, and the symptoms may diminish with advancing age.

Diagnostic Criteria for Schizotypal Personality Disorder   301.22 (F21)

A. A pervasive pattern of social and interpersonal deficits marked by acute discomfort with, and reduced capacity for, close relationships as well as by cognitive or perceptual distortions and eccentricities of behavior, beginning by early adulthood and present in a variety of contexts, as indicated by five (or more) of the following:

1. Ideas of reference (excluding delusions of reference).
2. Odd beliefs or magical thinking that influences behavior and is inconsistent with subcultural norms (e.g., superstitiousness, belief in clairvoyance, telepathy, or "sixth sense"; in children and adolescents, bizarre fantasies or preoccupations).
3. Unusual perceptual experiences, including bodily illusions.
4. Odd thinking and speech (e.g., vague, circumstantial, metaphorical, overelaborate, or stereotyped).
5. Suspiciousness or paranoid ideation.
6. Inappropriate or constricted affect.

7. Behavior or appearance that is odd, eccentric, or peculiar.

8. Lack of close friends or confidants other than first-degree relatives.

9. Excessive social anxiety that does not diminish with familiarity and tends to be associated with paranoid fears rather than negative judgments about self.

B. Does not occur exclusively during the course of schizophrenia, a bipolar disorder or depressive disorder with psychotic features, another psychotic disorder, or autism spectrum disorder.

Note: If criteria are met prior to the onset of schizophrenia, add "premorbid," e.g., "schizotypal personality disorder (premorbid)."

CLUSTER B PERSONALITY DISORDERS

Antisocial Personality Disorder

Antisocial personality disorder is characterized by a pervasive pattern of poor social conformity, deceitfulness, impulsivity, criminality, and lack of remorse. The disorder is common, with a 12-month prevalence in the general population estimated at 3.3%. The disorder is more common in men than in women and is frequent in psychiatric and correctional settings.

Although descriptions of antisocial personality disorder date to the early nineteenth century, formal descriptions date to DSM-I, which included the category "sociopathic personality disturbance" to describe a variety of "reactions" (including antisocial reaction) that placed individuals in conflict with society. Antisocial personality disorder came into its own in DSM-II as a specific type of personality disorder, although it was only with DSM-III that diagnostic criteria were developed. The criteria were strongly influenced by the work of Lee Robins and her colleagues at Washington University (Black 2013). The disorder was described as consisting of an explicit set of irresponsible behaviors and antisocial acts, such as an inability to maintain consistent employment, illegal and aggressive behavior, and sexual promiscuity. The focus on behavioral traits has been a bone of contention ever since among clinicians and researchers who believe the criteria ignore the disorder's underlying psychological traits. Partly in response to these concerns, "lack of remorse" was added as a symptom in DSM-III-R. The criteria were simplified for DSM-IV, in part on the basis of results from data reanalyses and field trials, and are unchanged in DSM-5.

Individuals with this disorder may have little sense of responsibility, lack judgment, blame others, and rationalize their behaviors. Many people with antisocial personality disorder engage in criminal acts and are caught up in the criminal justice system. Domestic violence is common and divorce frequent. In the most severe cases, the individual may show a disturbing degree of callousness and amorality.

Diagnostic Criteria for Antisocial Personality Disorder 301.7 (F60.2)

A. A pervasive pattern of disregard for and violation of the rights of others, occurring since age 15 years, as indicated by three (or more) of the following:

1. Failure to conform to social norms with respect to lawful behaviors, as indicated by repeatedly performing acts that are grounds for arrest.
2. Deceitfulness, as indicated by repeated lying, use of aliases, or conning others for personal profit or pleasure.
3. Impulsivity or failure to plan ahead.
4. Irritability and aggressiveness, as indicated by repeated physical fights or assaults.
5. Reckless disregard for safety of self or others.
6. Consistent irresponsibility, as indicated by repeated failure to sustain consistent work behavior or honor financial obligations.
7. Lack of remorse, as indicated by being indifferent to or rationalizing having hurt, mistreated, or stolen from another.

B. The individual is at least age 18 years.
C. There is evidence of conduct disorder with onset before age 15 years.
D. The occurrence of antisocial behavior is not exclusively during the course of schizophrenia or bipolar disorder.

Borderline Personality Disorder

Although the term has a much longer history, borderline personality disorder was first included in DSM-III as a syndrome of profound identity disturbance, unstable moods, and difficult interpersonal relationships. Precursors were *emotionally unstable personality* in DSM-I and *explosive personality* in DSM-II. The criteria were slightly modified for DSM-III-R and DSM-IV and are unchanged in DSM-5. Core symptoms include a pervasive pattern of anger dyscontrol, affective instability, impulsive behavior, and unstable and overly intense interpersonal relationships.

Borderline personality disorder is one of the more common personality disorders, having a prevalence of 1.6%–5.9% in the general population; it is more frequent in women. Individuals with borderline personality disorder often hurt themselves—for example, by cutting or burning—and frequently attempt suicide. An estimated 8%–10% of persons with borderline personality disorder eventually commit suicide.

Diagnostic Criteria for Borderline Personality Disorder   301.83 (F60.3)

A pervasive pattern of instability of interpersonal relationships, self-image, and affects, and marked impulsivity, beginning by early adulthood and present in a variety of contexts, as indicated by five (or more) of the following:

1. Frantic efforts to avoid real or imagined abandonment. (**Note:** Do not include suicidal or self-mutilating behavior covered in Criterion 5.)
2. A pattern of unstable and intense interpersonal relationships characterized by alternating between extremes of idealization and devaluation.
3. Identity disturbance: markedly and persistently unstable self-image or sense of self.
4. Impulsivity in at least two areas that are potentially self-damaging (e.g., spending, sex, substance abuse, reckless driving, binge eating). (**Note:** Do not include suicidal or self-mutilating behavior covered in Criterion 5.)
5. Recurrent suicidal behavior, gestures, or threats, or self-mutilating behavior.
6. Affective instability due to a marked reactivity of mood (e.g., intense episodic dysphoria, irritability, or anxiety usually lasting a few hours and only rarely more than a few days).
7. Chronic feelings of emptiness.
8. Inappropriate, intense anger or difficulty controlling anger (e.g., frequent displays of temper, constant anger, recurrent physical fights).
9. Transient, stress-related paranoid ideation or severe dissociative symptoms.

Histrionic Personality Disorder

Histrionic personality disorder is characterized by a pattern of excessive emotionality and attention-seeking behavior and includes such symptoms as excessive concern with appearance and wanting to be the center of attention. Histrionic persons can be gregarious and charming but can also be manipulative, vain, and demanding.

The disorder takes its name from *hysteria*, a condition first described in the nineteenth century and associated with conversion, somatization, and dissociation symptoms. Self-dramatizing and attention-seeking behaviors were considered to be associated with hysteria. *Hysterical personality* was included in DSM-II and was renamed *histrionic personality disorder* in DSM-III so as not to be confused with hysteria (renamed *somatization disorder*). The disorder has a prevalence of nearly 2% in the general population and is more frequently diagnosed in women.

Diagnostic Criteria for Histrionic Personality Disorder   301.50 (F60.4)

A pervasive pattern of excessive emotionality and attention seeking, beginning by early adulthood and present in a variety of contexts, as indicated by five (or more) of the following:

1. Is uncomfortable in situations in which he or she is not the center of attention.
2. Interaction with others is often characterized by inappropriate sexually seductive or provocative behavior.
3. Displays rapidly shifting and shallow expression of emotions.
4. Consistently uses physical appearance to draw attention to self.
5. Has a style of speech that is excessively impressionistic and lacking in detail.

6. Shows self-dramatization, theatricality, and exaggerated expression of emotion.
7. Is suggestible (i.e., easily influenced by others or circumstances).
8. Considers relationships to be more intimate than they actually are.

Narcissistic Personality Disorder

Narcissistic personality disorder is named for Narcissus, from Greek mythology, who fell in love with his own reflection. Freud used the term to describe persons who were self-absorbed, and psychoanalysts have focused on the narcissist's need to bolster his or her self-esteem through grandiose fantasy, exaggerated ambition, exhibitionism, and feelings of entitlement. The disorder was first included in DSM-III, and the criteria were modified for DSM-III-R and DSM-IV. The criteria for narcissistic personality disorder are unchanged in DSM-5. The prevalence of this disorder may be as high as 6.2% in the general population, and most persons receiving the diagnosis are male.

Diagnostic Criteria for Narcissistic Personality Disorder   301.81 (F60.81)

A pervasive pattern of grandiosity (in fantasy or behavior), need for admiration, and lack of empathy, beginning by early adulthood and present in a variety of contexts, as indicated by five (or more) of the following:

1. Has a grandiose sense of self-importance (e.g., exaggerates achievements and talents, expects to be recognized as superior without commensurate achievements).
2. Is preoccupied with fantasies of unlimited success, power, brilliance, beauty, or ideal love.
3. Believes that he or she is "special" and unique and can only be understood by, or should associate with, other special or high-status people (or institutions).
4. Requires excessive admiration.
5. Has a sense of entitlement (i.e., unreasonable expectations of especially favorable treatment or automatic compliance with his or her expectations).
6. Is interpersonally exploitative (i.e., takes advantage of others to achieve his or her own ends).
7. Lacks empathy: is unwilling to recognize or identify with the feelings and needs of others.
8. Is often envious of others or believes that others are envious of him or her.
9. Shows arrogant, haughty behaviors or attitudes.

CLUSTER C PERSONALITY DISORDERS

Avoidant Personality Disorder

Avoidant personality disorder was introduced in DSM-III and was created to distinguish individuals who avoid social interaction because of fears of rejection, from individuals with either a schizoid or schizotypal personality disorder who have an impaired capacity for social relatedness. Predecessors include schizoid personality in DSM-I and DSM-II and inadequate personality in DSM-II. The latter term was used to describe individuals who had experienced failure in several important life domains, such as interpersonal relationships and occupations. The criteria for avoidant personality disorder are unchanged in DSM-5.

Avoidant personality disorder is characterized by low self-esteem, reluctance to engage in new activities, avoidance of social activities and interpersonal interactions, anxious preoccupation with social evaluation, and a general lack of positive engagement. Many of these traits are present from early childhood, and they typically persist into adulthood but become less evident with age. There is considerable overlap with several of the anxiety disorders, such as social anxiety disorder and agoraphobia. The disorder is equally prevalent in men and women, with an overall prevalence in the general population of 2.4%.

Diagnostic Criteria for Avoidant Personality Disorder 301.82 (F60.6)

A pervasive pattern of social inhibition, feelings of inadequacy, and hypersensitivity to negative evaluation, beginning by early adulthood and present in a variety of contexts, as indicated by four (or more) of the following:

1. Avoids occupational activities that involve significant interpersonal contact because of fears of criticism, disapproval, or rejection.
2. Is unwilling to get involved with people unless certain of being liked.
3. Shows restraint within intimate relationships because of the fear of being shamed or ridiculed.
4. Is preoccupied with being criticized or rejected in social situations.
5. Is inhibited in new interpersonal situations because of feelings of inadequacy.
6. Views self as socially inept, personally unappealing, or inferior to others.
7. Is unusually reluctant to take personal risks or to engage in any new activities because they may prove embarrassing.

Dependent Personality Disorder

Dependent personality disorder is characterized by a pattern of relying excessively on others for emotional support and making everyday decisions. The disorder was listed as a subtype of the DSM-I passive-aggressive personality, was omitted from DSM-II, and was subsequently reintroduced in DSM-III. Psychoanalytically oriented clinicians have linked dependency to fixation at the oral stage of development, which focuses on the biological gratification that arises from feeding. Other experts have tied dependent personality to the disruption of attachments early in life, or to overprotection and parental authoritarianism experienced in childhood. Dependent personality disorder has a prevalence of around 0.5% in the general population and is diagnosed more frequently in women.

There have been few empirical studies of dependent personality disorder. Some experts believe the disorder is not sufficiently distinctive to stand alone and point to the fact that dependency on others commonly occurs in people with other personality disorder types and in persons with chronic medical or mental disorders.

Diagnostic Criteria for Dependent Personality Disorder   301.6 (F60.7)

A pervasive and excessive need to be taken care of that leads to submissive and clinging behavior and fears of separation, beginning by early adulthood and present in a variety of contexts, as indicated by five (or more) of the following:

1. Has difficulty making everyday decisions without an excessive amount of advice and reassurance from others.
2. Needs others to assume responsibility for most major areas of his or her life.
3. Has difficulty expressing disagreement with others because of fear of loss of support or approval. (**Note:** Do not include realistic fears of retribution.)
4. Has difficulty initiating projects or doing things on his or her own (because of a lack of self-confidence in judgment or abilities rather than a lack of motivation or energy).
5. Goes to excessive lengths to obtain nurturance and support from others, to the point of volunteering to do things that are unpleasant.
6. Feels uncomfortable or helpless when alone because of exaggerated fears of being unable to care for himself or herself.
7. Urgently seeks another relationship as a source of care and support when a close relationship ends.
8. Is unrealistically preoccupied with fears of being left to take care of himself or herself.

Obsessive-Compulsive Personality Disorder

Obsessive-compulsive personality disorder is one of the older personality disorders, having originated with Freud's formulation of the anal character whose symptoms are orderliness, parsimony, and obstinacy. Compulsive personality was included in DSM-I, and the name was changed to obsessive compulsive personality in DSM-II. The description emphasized conformity and adherence to standards, rigidity, overconscientiousness, and inability to relax, which were thought to predispose to "obsessive compulsive neurosis" (i.e., obsessive-compulsive disorder). In DSM-II, the disorder was parenthetically called "anankastic personality." The criteria had minor modifications in DSM-III-R and DSM-IV; they are unchanged in DSM-5. Obsessive-compulsive personality disorder is conceptualized as a chronic maladaptive pattern of excessive perfectionism, preoccupation with orderliness and detail, and need for control of one's emotions and environment that contributes to significant distress or impairment, particularly in the areas of interpersonal functioning. The disorder is relatively common, having a prevalence in the general population that may be as high as 7.9%. It occurs more commonly in men than in women.

Diagnostic Criteria for Obsessive-Compulsive Personality Disorder
301.4 (F60.5)

A pervasive pattern of preoccupation with orderliness, perfectionism, and mental and interpersonal control, at the expense of flexibility, openness, and efficiency, beginning by early adulthood and present in a variety of contexts, as indicated by four (or more) of the following:

1. Is preoccupied with details, rules, lists, order, organization, or schedules to the extent that the major point of the activity is lost.
2. Shows perfectionism that interferes with task completion (e.g., is unable to complete a project because his or her own overly strict standards are not met).
3. Is excessively devoted to work and productivity to the exclusion of leisure activities and friendships (not accounted for by obvious economic necessity).
4. Is overconscientious, scrupulous, and inflexible about matters of morality, ethics, or values (not accounted for by cultural or religious identification).
5. Is unable to discard worn-out or worthless objects even when they have no sentimental value.
6. Is reluctant to delegate tasks or to work with others unless they submit to exactly his or her way of doing things.
7. Adopts a miserly spending style toward both self and others; money is viewed as something to be hoarded for future catastrophes.
8. Shows rigidity and stubbornness.

OTHER PERSONALITY DISORDERS

Personality Change Due to Another Medical Condition

This category was moved from DSM-IV's "Mental Disorders Due to a General Medical Condition." The predominant problem is a persistent personality disturbance, or change, that is attributed to another medical condition such as a frontal lobe lesion. With this condition, the disturbance represents a change from the individual's usual personality pattern. (In children, the period of change lasts at least 1 year.) Medical evaluation has established that the personality change has been brought about by a medical condition, and the change does not occur exclusively during the course of a delirium. Finally, the change causes distress or impairment in social, occupational, or other important areas of functioning.

Commonly observed manifestations consistent with the personality change include mood instability, poor impulse control, aggressive outbursts, apathy, suspiciousness, and paranoid ideations. Others may see the person as being not himself or herself. The nature of the symptoms may differ markedly from person to person depending on the location of the brain lesion or the pathophysiological process underlying the disturbance. Clinicians may specify the predominant pattern or symptoms (e.g., labile type).

Diagnostic Criteria for Personality Change Due to Another Medical Condition   310.1 (F07.0)

A. A persistent personality disturbance that represents a change from the individual's previous characteristic personality pattern.

   Note: In children, the disturbance involves a marked deviation from normal development or a significant change in the child's usual behavior patterns, lasting at least 1 year.

B. There is evidence from the history, physical examination, or laboratory findings that the disturbance is the direct pathophysiological consequence of another medical condition.

C. The disturbance is not better explained by another mental disorder (including another mental disorder due to another medical condition).

D. The disturbance does not occur exclusively during the course of a delirium.

E. The disturbance causes clinically significant distress or impairment in social, occupational, or other important areas of functioning.

Specify whether:

   Labile type: If the predominant feature is affective lability.
   Disinhibited type: If the predominant feature is poor impulse control as evidenced by sexual indiscretions, etc.
   Aggressive type: If the predominant feature is aggressive behavior.
   Apathetic type: If the predominant feature is marked apathy and indifference.
   Paranoid type: If the predominant feature is suspiciousness or paranoid ideation.
   Other type: If the presentation is not characterized by any of the above subtypes.
   Combined type: If more than one feature predominates in the clinical picture.
   Unspecified type

Coding note: Include the name of the other medical condition (e.g., 310.1 [F07.0] personality change due to temporal lobe epilepsy). The other medical condition should be coded and listed separately immediately before the personality disorder due to another medical condition (e.g., 345.40 [G40.209] temporal lobe epilepsy; 310.1 [F07.0] personality change due to temporal lobe epilepsy).

Other Specified Personality Disorder and Unspecified Personality Disorder

These categories are used when an individual has symptoms of a personality disorder that cause distress and impairment but do not meet the full criteria for any of the more specific disorders in the class. In these situations, the clinician has judged that the general personality disorder criteria have been met.

The category other specified personality disorder is used when the clinician chooses to communicate the specific reason that the presentation does not meet the criteria. Clinicians are encouraged to record the specific reason (e.g., mixed personality features).

Other Specified Personality Disorder   301.89 (F60.89)

This category applies to presentations in which symptoms characteristic of a personality disorder that cause clinically significant distress or impairment in social, occupational, or other important areas of functioning predominate but do not meet the full criteria for any of the disorders in the personality disorders diagnostic class. The other specified personality disorder category is used in situations in which the clinician chooses to communicate the specific reason that the presentation does not meet the criteria for any specific personality disorder. This is done by recording "other specified personality disorder" followed by the specific reason (e.g., "mixed personality features").

The category unspecified personality disorder is used when the clinician chooses not to specify the reason why the criteria are not met for a specific personality disorder and when there is insufficient information to make a more specific diagnosis.

Unspecified Personality Disorder   301.9 (F60.9)

This category applies to presentations in which symptoms characteristic of a personality disorder that cause clinically significant distress or impairment in social, occupational, or other important areas of functioning predominate but do not meet the full criteria for any of the disorders in the personality disorders diagnostic class. The unspecified personality disorder category is used in situations in which the clinician chooses *not* to specify the reason that the criteria are not met for a specific personality disorder, and includes presentations in which there is insufficient information to make a more specific diagnosis.

KEY POINTS

- The DSM-IV criteria for a general personality disorder and the ten specific disorder types are unchanged in DSM-5. An alternative diagnostic scheme developed by the DSM-5 Personality and Personality Disorders Work Group that combines categorical diagnosis with dimensional ratings of personality domains and traits is included in Section III ("Alternative DSM-5 Model for Personality Disorders").

- The multiaxial diagnostic system introduced in DSM-III has been discontinued. Personality disorders are now coded at the same level as other mental disorders. The three personality disorder clusters (i.e., Clusters A, B, C) are unchanged.

- Personality change due to another medical condition has been moved to this class from DSM-IV's "Mental Disorders Due to a General Medical Condition." In DSM-5, disorders judged due to another medical disorder are placed in the class with which they share the predominant symptom pattern.

- The diagnosis personality disorder not otherwise specified has been replaced by other specified personality disorder and unspecified personality disorder. These residual diagnoses can be used when an individual who otherwise meets the general personality disorder criteria does not meet criteria for one of the 10 specific disorders and, in the case of unspecified personality disorder, when there is insufficient information to make a more specific diagnosis.

CHAPTER 19

Medication-Induced Movement Disorders and Other Conditions That May Be a Focus of Clinical Attention

Medication-Induced Movement Disorders and Other Adverse Effects of Medications

332.1 (G21.11)	Neuroleptic-Induced Parkinsonism
332.1 (G21.19)	Other Medication-Induced Parkinsonism
333.92 (G21.0)	Neuroleptic Malignant Syndrome
333.72 (G24.02)	Medication-Induced Acute Dystonia
333.99 (G25.71)	Medication-Induced Acute Akathisia
333.85 (G24.01)	Tardive Dyskinesia
333.72 (G24.09)	Tardive Dystonia
333.99 (G25.71)	Tardive Akathisia
333.1 (G25.1)	Medication-Induced Postural Tremor
333.99 (G25.79)	Other Medication-Induced Movement Disorder
995.29 (T43.205_)	Antidepressant Discontinuation Syndrome
995.20 (T50.905_)	Other Adverse Effect of Medication

Other Conditions That May Be a Focus of Clinical Attention
Relational Problems
Abuse and Neglect
Educational and Occupational Problems
Housing and Economic Problems
Other Problems Related to the Social Environment
Problems Related to Crime or Interaction With the Legal System
Other Health Service Encounters for Counseling and Medical Advice
Problems Related to Other Psychosocial, Personal, and Environmental Circumstances
Other Circumstances of Personal History

This chapter includes conditions of clinical importance that may be a focus of diagnosis and treatment but are not considered mental disorders. These include 1) medication-induced movement disorders and other adverse effects of medication, and 2) other conditions that may be a focus of clinical attention (V/Z codes). All of these conditions have the potential to cause great distress to patients or their family members. While these conditions are common, their codes are underutilized by clinicians.

The use of these codes is important because they represent conditions that either are important in their own right or can adversely affect the course of a mental disorder. For example, when a patient with schizophrenia refuses medication or takes it sporadically because of lack of insight or denial, that condition (V15.81/Z91.19 nonadherence to medical treatment) complicates the individual's treatment and should be coded in addition to the diagnosis of schizophrenia. Recording the codes for conditions not thought to be mental disorders may also be useful simply to enable clinicians to note the individual's reason for contact with the mental health care system.

MEDICATION-INDUCED MOVEMENT DISORDERS AND OTHER ADVERSE EFFECTS OF MEDICATION

DSM-IV introduced the subcategory medication-induced movement disorders because of the importance of such disorders to treatment and differential diagnosis. DSM-5 has given them their own chapter and expanded the title. These diagnoses can be used to describe problems that patients sometimes develop with medications. Antipsychotic medications are the most common offenders, and they are widely known to induce movement disorders in some patients. Movement disorders range from troublesome but reversible (akathisia), to disabling and irreversible (tardive dyskinesia), to even fatal in some cases (neuroleptic malignant syndrome [NMS]). Their inclusion in DSM-5 may help boost their recognition and treatment, and help with differential diagnosis. For example, medication-induced acute akathisia needs to be distinguished from anxiety disorders, whereas NMS needs to be distinguished from catatonia. Many of the symptoms reported in patients with an akathisia (e.g., anxiety, jitteriness) are indistinguishable from symptoms of an anxiety disorder. Therefore, the clinician must take a thorough history to determine the temporal relationship between medication and symptom onset and consider other possible causes.

The term *neuroleptic* was introduced in the 1950s to highlight the antipsychotic and extrapyramidal side effects of chlorpromazine, and was soon used to describe any antipsychotic medication. With the introduction of the "atypical," or second-generation, antipsychotics (e.g., clozapine, risperidone, quetiapine), which have a lower propensity to cause extrapyramidal side effects, the term has become outdated, although it remains appropriate when describing medication-induced abnormal movements. Neuroleptic medications include both conventional (e.g., chlorpromazine, haloperidol, fluphenazine) and atypical antipsychotics; certain dopamine receptor–blocking drugs used to treat nausea and gastroparesis (e.g., prochlorperazine, promethazine, trimethobenzamide, thiethylperazine, metoclopramide); and amoxapine, which is marketed as an antidepressant.

A listing of DSM-5 medication-induced movement disorders and other adverse effects of medication, along with ICD-9-CM/ICD-10-CM codes, is given in Table 19–1.

TABLE 19–1. Medication-induced movement disorders and other adverse effects of medication

ICD-9-CM code	ICD-10-CM code	Description
332.1	G21.11	Neuroleptic-induced parkinsonism
332.1	G21.19	Other medication-induced parkinsonism
333.92	G21.0	Neuroleptic malignant syndrome
333.72	G24.02	Medication-induced acute dystonia
333.99	G25.71	Medication-induced acute akathisia
333.85	G24.01	Tardive dyskinesia
333.72	G24.09	Tardive dystonia
333.99	G25.71	Tardive akathisia
333.1	G25.1	Medication-induced postural tremor
333.99	G25.79	Other medication-induced movement disorder
		Antidepressant discontinuation syndrome
995.29	T43.205A	Initial encounter
995.29	T43.205D	Subsequent encounter
995.29	T43.205S	Sequelae
		Other adverse effect of medication
995.20	T50.905A	Initial encounter
995.20	T50.905D	Subsequent encounter
995.20	T50.905S	Sequelae

Source. Reprinted from Nussbaum AM: *The Pocket Guide to the DSM-5^TM Diagnostic Exam.* Washington, DC, American Psychiatric Publishing, 2013. Copyright 2013, American Psychiatric Association. Used with permission.

Neuroleptic-Induced Parkinsonism and Other Medication-Induced Parkinsonism

Parkinsonian tremor, muscular rigidity, akinesia (i.e., loss of movement or difficulty initiating movement), or bradykinesia (i.e., slowing movement) developing within a few weeks of starting or raising the dosage of a medication (e.g., a neuroleptic) or after reducing the dosage of a medication used to treat extrapyramidal symptoms.

Neuroleptic Malignant Syndrome

Although neuroleptic malignant syndrome is easily recognized in its classic full-blown form, it is often heterogeneous in onset, presentation, progression, and outcome. The clinical features described below are those considered most important in making the diagnosis of neuroleptic malignant syndrome based on consensus recommendations.

Patients have generally been exposed to a dopamine antagonist within 72 hours prior to symptom development. Hyperthermia (>100.4°F or >38.0°C on at least two occasions, measured orally), associated with profuse diaphoresis, is a distinguishing feature of neuroleptic malignant syndrome, setting it apart from other neurological side effects of antipsychotic medications. Extreme elevations in temperature, reflecting a breakdown in central thermoregulation, are more likely to support the diagnosis of neuroleptic malignant syndrome. Generalized rigidity, described as "lead pipe" in its most severe form and usually unresponsive to antiparkinsonian agents, is a cardinal feature of the disorder and may be associated with other neurological symptoms (e.g., tremor, sialorrhea, akinesia, dystonia, trismus, myoclonus, dysarthria, dysphagia, rhabdomyolysis). Creatine kinase elevation of at least four times the upper limit of normal is commonly seen. Changes in mental status, characterized by delirium or altered consciousness ranging from stupor to coma, are often an early sign. Affected individuals may appear alert but dazed and unresponsive, consistent with catatonic stupor. Autonomic activation and instability—manifested by tachycardia (rate>25% above baseline), diaphoresis, blood pressure elevation (systolic or diastolic ≥25% above baseline) or fluctuation (≥20 mmHg diastolic change or ≥25 mmHg systolic change within 24 hours), urinary incontinence, and pallor—may be seen at any time but provide an early clue to the diagnosis. Tachypnea (rate >50% above baseline) is common, and respiratory distress—resulting from metabolic acidosis, hypermetabolism, chest wall restriction, aspiration pneumonia, or pulmonary emboli—can occur and lead to sudden respiratory arrest.

A workup, including laboratory investigation, to exclude other infectious, toxic, metabolic, and neuropsychiatric etiologies or complications is essential. Although several laboratory abnormalities are associated with neuroleptic malignant syndrome, no single abnormality is specific to the diagnosis. Individuals with neuroleptic malignant syndrome may have leukocytosis, metabolic acidosis, hypoxia, decreased serum iron concentrations, and elevations in serum muscle enzymes and catecholamines. Findings from cerebrospinal fluid analysis and neuroimaging studies are generally normal, whereas electroencephalography shows generalized slowing. Autopsy findings in fatal cases have been nonspecific and variable, depending on complications.

Medication-Induced Acute Dystonia

Abnormal and prolonged contraction of the muscles of the eyes (oculogyric crisis), head, neck (torticollis or retrocollis), limbs, or trunk developing within a few days of starting or raising the dosage of a medication (such as a neuroleptic) or after reducing the dosage of a medication used to treat extrapyramidal symptoms.

Medication-Induced Acute Akathisia

Subjective complaints of restlessness, often accompanied by observed excessive movements (e.g., fidgety movements of the legs, rocking from foot to foot, pacing, inability to sit or stand still), developing within a few weeks of starting or raising the dosage of a medication (such as a neuroleptic) or after reducing the dosage of a medication used to treat extrapyramidal symptoms.

Tardive Dyskinesia

Involuntary athetoid or choreiform movements (lasting at least a few weeks) generally of the tongue, lower face and jaw, and extremities (but sometimes involving the pharyngeal, diaphragmatic, or trunk muscles) developing in association with the use of a neuroleptic medication for at least a few months.

Symptoms may develop after a shorter period of medication use in older persons. In some patients, movements of this type may appear after discontinuation, or after change or reduction in dosage, of neuroleptic medications, in which case the condition is called *neuroleptic withdrawal-emergent dyskinesia*. Because withdrawal-emergent dyskinesia is usually time-limited, lasting less than 4–8 weeks, dyskinesia that persists beyond this window is considered to be tardive dyskinesia.

Tardive Dystonia and Tardive Akathisia

Tardive syndrome involving other types of movement problems, such as dystonia or akathisia, which are distinguished by their late emergence in the course of treatment and their potential persistence for months to years, even in the face of neuroleptic discontinuation or dosage reduction.

Medication-Induced Postural Tremor

Fine tremor (usually in the range of 8–12 Hz) occurring during attempts to maintain a posture and developing in association with the use of medication (e.g., lithium, antidepressants, valproate). This tremor is very similar to the tremor seen with anxiety, caffeine, and other stimulants.

Other Medication-Induced Movement Disorder

This category is for medication-induced movement disorders not captured by any of the specific disorders listed above. Examples include 1) presentations resembling neuroleptic malignant syndrome that are associated with medications other than neuroleptics and 2) other medication-induced tardive conditions.

Antidepressant Discontinuation Syndrome

Initial Encounter
Subsequent Encounter
Sequelae

Antidepressant discontinuation syndrome is a set of symptoms that can occur after an abrupt cessation (or marked reduction in dose) of an antidepressant medication that was taken continuously for at least 1 month. Symptoms generally begin within 2–4 days and typically include specific sensory, somatic, and cognitive-emotional manifestations. Frequently reported sensory and somatic symptoms include flashes of light, "electric shock" sensations, nausea, and hyperresponsivity to noises or lights. Nonspecific anxiety and feelings of dread may also be reported. Symptoms are alleviated by restarting the same medication or starting a different medication that has a similar mechanism of action—for example, discontinuation symptoms after withdrawal from a serotonin-norepinephrine reuptake inhibitor may be alleviated by starting a tricyclic antidepressant. To qualify as antidepressant discontinuation syndrome, the symptoms should not have been present before the antidepressant dosage was reduced and are not better explained by another mental disorder (e.g., manic or hypomanic episode, substance intoxication, substance withdrawal, somatic symptom disorder).

Discontinuation symptoms may occur following treatment with tricyclic antidepressants (e.g., imipramine, amitriptyline, desipramine), serotonin reuptake inhibitors (e.g., fluoxetine, paroxetine, sertraline), and monoamine oxidase inhibitors (e.g., phenelzine, selegiline, pargyline). The incidence of this syndrome depends on the dosage and half-life of the medication being taken, as well as the rate at which the medication is tapered. Short-acting medications that are stopped abruptly rather than tapered gradually may pose the greatest risk. The short-acting selective serotonin reuptake inhibitor (SSRI) paroxetine is the agent most commonly associated with discontinuation symptoms, but such symptoms occur for all types of antidepressants.

Unlike withdrawal syndromes associated with opioids, alcohol, and other substances of abuse, antidepressant discontinuation syndrome has no pathognomonic symptoms. Instead, the symptoms tend to be vague and variable and typically begin 2–4 days after the last dose of the antidepressant. For SSRIs (e.g., paroxetine), symptoms such as dizziness, ringing in the ears, "electric shocks in the head," an inability to sleep, and acute anxiety are described. The antidepressant use prior to discontinuation must not have incurred hypomania or euphoria (i.e., there should be confidence that the discontinuation syndrome is not the result of fluctuations in mood stability associated with the previous treatment). The antidepressant discontinuation syndrome is based solely on pharmacological factors and is not related to the reinforcing effects of an antidepressant. Also, in the case of stimulant augmentation of an antidepressant, abrupt cessation may result in stimulant withdrawal symptoms (see "Stimulant Withdrawal" in Chapter 16, "Substance-Related and Addictive Disorders") rather than the antidepressant discontinuation syndrome described here.

Other Adverse Effect of Medication

Initial Encounter
Subsequent Encounter
Sequelae

This category is available for optional use by clinicians to code side effects of medication (other than movement symptoms) when these adverse effects become a main focus of clinical attention. Examples include severe hypotension, cardiac arrhythmias, and priapism.

OTHER CONDITIONS THAT MAY BE
A FOCUS OF CLINICAL ATTENTION

DSM authors have long recognized that certain problems may motivate people to seek psychiatric care but that these conditions are not mental illnesses. In DSM-II, problems experienced by people who were considered psychiatrically healthy that were sufficiently severe to warrant a visit to a psychiatrist were assigned to the category "conditions without manifest psychiatric disorder and non-specific conditions." This category included, for instance, marital maladjustment, occupational maladjustment, and dyssocial behavior (e.g., for professional criminals who did not have antisocial personality disorder). In DSM-III, the authors expanded the list and provided greater specificity for the various problems not considered attributable to a mental disorder. These were "V code" diagnoses, using wording taken from ICD-9-CM, which includes the codes listed in a section called "Supplementary Classification of Factors Influencing Health Status and Contact With Health Services." (The letter *V* has no special significance when used in this context.)

In DSM-IV, V code diagnoses were grouped as 1) relational problems; 2) problems related to abuse or neglect (including the physical and sexual abuse of children and adults and neglect of a child); and 3) additional conditions, including noncompliance with treatment, malingering, adult antisocial behavior, child or adolescent antisocial behavior, borderline intellectual functioning, age-related cognitive decline, bereavement, academic problem, occupational problem, identity problem, religious or spiritual problem, acculturation problem, and phase of life problem. Boundaries were created to distinguish bereavement from major depressive disorder.

In addition to the subcategories relational problems and abuse and neglect, new subcategories in DSM-5 are educational and occupational problems; housing and economic problems; other problems related to the social environment; problems related to crime or interaction with the legal system; other health service encounters for counseling or medical advice; problems related to other psychosocial, personal, and environmental circumstances; and other circumstances of personal history. In DSM-5, the term *uncomplicated bereavement* has been restored (V62.82/Z63.4), but those who develop a major depressive episode in response to the death of a loved one should receive the diagnosis of major depressive disorder (see Chapter 5, "Mood Disorders," for further discussion).

With DSM-5, several additional changes have been made. First, each disorder has also been provided with a dual "Z code" diagnosis, the letter used in the coding for these conditions in ICD-10-CM, expected to become operational in October 2014. As with the letter *V*, the letter *Z* has no special significance in this context. Hence, in this chapter, and throughout the book, we refer to these conditions as "V/Z code" diagnoses. In confirmed or suspected cases of child, spouse/partner, or adult neglect, or psychological, physical, or sexual violence, a 995 code is used (a T code in the ICD-10-CM system).

With the discontinuation of the multiaxial diagnostic scheme, stressors that formerly would have been recorded on Axis IV may now be recognized by using the V/Z codes. The expanded list in DSM-5 allows for a more complete description of situations that are relevant to seeking care but are not attributable to a mental illness, such as homelessness, extreme poverty, or being the victim of a crime.

A listing of other conditions that may be a focus of clinical attention, along with ICD-9-CM/ICD-10-CM codes, is given in Table 19–2.

Relational Problems

To encourage the use of these diagnoses by clinicians, the section was reorganized and expanded for DSM-5. Relational problems are accorded much greater specificity, and instead of five diagnoses as in DSM-IV, there are now eight. This category concerns patterns of interaction between members of a relational unit. The patterns are associated with symptoms or significant impairment in functioning in one or more individual members or with significant impairment of the relational unit itself. The category should be of special interest to clinicians engaged in family and couples therapy.

Key relationships, especially intimate adult partner relationships and parent/caregiver–child relationships have a significant impact on the health of the individuals in these relationships. These relationships can be health promoting and protective, neutral, or detrimental to health outcomes. In the extreme, these close relationships can be associated with maltreatment or neglect, which has significant medical and psychological consequences for the affected individual. A relational problem may come to clinical attention either as the reason that the individual seeks health care or as a problem that affects the course, prognosis, or treatment of the individual's mental or other medical disorder.

Problems Related to Family Upbringing

V61.20 (Z62.820) Parent-Child Relational Problem
V61.8 (Z62.891)   Sibling Relational Problem
V61.8 (Z62.29)   Upbringing Away From Parents
V61.29 (Z62.898)   Child Affected by Parental Relationship Distress

Other Problems Related to Primary Support Group

V61.10 (Z63.0)   Relationship Distress With Spouse or Intimate Partner
V61.03 (Z63.5)   Disruption of Family by Separation or Divorce

TABLE 19–2. Other conditions that may be a focus of clinical attention

ICD-9-CM code	ICD-10-CM code	Description
V61.20	Z62.820	Parent-child relational problem
V61.8	Z62.891	Sibling relational problem
V61.8	Z62.29	Upbringing away from parents
V61.29	Z62.898	Child affected by parental relationship distress
V61.10	Z63.0	Relationship distress with spouse or intimate partner
V61.03	Z63.5	Disruption of family by separation or divorce
V61.8	Z63.8	High expressed emotion level within family
V62.82	Z63.4	Uncomplicated bereavement
		Child physical abuse, confirmed
995.54	T74.12XA	Initial encounter
995.54	T74.12XD	Subsequent encounter
		Child physical abuse, suspected
995.54	T76.12XA	Initial encounter
995.54	T76.12XD	Subsequent encounter
		Other circumstances related to child physical abuse
V61.21	Z69.010	Encounter for mental health services for victim of child abuse by parent
V61.21	Z69.020	Encounter for mental health services for victim of nonparental child abuse
V15.41	Z62.810	Personal history (past history) of physical abuse in childhood
V61.22	Z69.011	Encounter for mental health services for perpetrator of parental child abuse
V62.83	Z69.021	Encounter for mental health services for perpetrator of nonparental child abuse
		Child sexual abuse, confirmed
995.53	T74.22XA	Initial encounter
995.53	T74.22XD	Subsequent encounter
		Child sexual abuse, suspected
995.53	T76.22XA	Initial encounter
995.53	T76.22XD	Subsequent encounter

TABLE 19–2.　**Other conditions that may be a focus of clinical attention** *(continued)*

ICD-9-CM code	ICD-10-CM code	Description
		Other circumstances related to child sexual abuse
V61.21	Z69.010	Encounter for mental health services for victim of child sexual abuse by parent
V61.21	Z69.020	Encounter for mental health services for victim of nonparental child sexual abuse
V15.41	Z62.810	Personal history (past history) of sexual abuse in childhood
V61.22	Z69.011	Encounter for mental health services for perpetrator of parental child sexual abuse
V62.83	Z69.021	Encounter for mental health services for perpetrator of nonparental child sexual abuse
		Child neglect, confirmed
995.52	T74.02XA	Initial encounter
995.52	T74.02XD	Subsequent encounter
		Child neglect, suspected
995.52	T76.02XA	Initial encounter
995.52	T76.02XD	Subsequent encounter
		Other circumstances related to child neglect
V61.21	Z69.010	Encounter for mental health services for victim of child neglect by parent
V61.21	Z69.020	Encounter for mental health services for victim of nonparental child neglect
V15.42	Z62.812	Personal history (past history) of neglect in childhood
V61.22	Z69.011	Encounter for mental health services for perpetrator of parental child neglect
V62.83	Z69.021	Encounter for mental health services for perpetrator of nonparental child neglect
		Child psychological abuse, confirmed
995.51	T74.32XA	Initial encounter
995.51	T74.32XD	Subsequent encounter
		Child psychological abuse, suspected
995.51	T76.32XA	Initial encounter
995.51	T76.32XD	Subsequent encounter

TABLE 19–2. **Other conditions that may be a focus of clinical attention** *(continued)*

ICD-9-CM code	ICD-10-CM code	Description
		Other circumstances related to child psychological abuse
V61.21	Z69.010	Encounter for mental health services for victim of child psychological abuse by parent
V61.21	Z69.020	Encounter for mental health services for victim of nonparental child psychological abuse
V15.42	Z62.811	Personal history (past history) of psychological abuse in childhood
V61.22	Z69.011	Encounter for mental health services for perpetrator of parental child psychological abuse
V62.83	Z69.021	Encounter for mental health services for perpetrator of nonparental child psychological abuse
		Spouse or partner violence, physical, confirmed
995.81	T74.11XA	Initial encounter
995.81	T74.11XD	Subsequent encounter
		Spouse or partner violence, physical, suspected
995.81	T76.11XA	Initial encounter
995.81	T76.11XD	Subsequent encounter
		Other circumstances related to spouse or partner violence, physical
V61.11	Z69.11	Encounter for mental health services for victim of spouse or partner violence, physical
V15.41	Z91.410	Personal history (past history) of spouse or partner violence, physical
V61.12	Z69.12	Encounter for mental health services for perpetrator of spouse or partner violence, physical
		Spouse or partner violence, sexual, confirmed
995.83	T74.21XA	Initial encounter
995.83	T74.21XD	Subsequent encounter
		Spouse or partner violence, sexual, suspected
995.83	T76.21XA	Initial encounter
995.83	T76.21XD	Subsequent encounter

TABLE 19–2. Other conditions that may be a focus of clinical attention (*continued*)

ICD-9-CM code	ICD-10-CM code	Description
		Other circumstances related to spouse or partner violence, sexual
V61.11	Z69.81	Encounter for mental health services for victim of spouse or partner violence, sexual
V15.41	Z91.410	Personal history (past history) of spouse or partner violence, sexual
V61.12	Z69.12	Encounter for mental health services for perpetrator of spouse or partner violence, sexual
		Spouse or partner neglect, confirmed
995.85	T74.01XA	Initial encounter
995.85	T74.01XD	Subsequent encounter
		Spouse or partner neglect, suspected
995.85	T76.01XA	Initial encounter
995.85	T76.01XD	Subsequent encounter
		Other circumstances related to spouse or partner neglect
V61.11	Z69.11	Encounter for mental health services for victim of spouse or partner neglect
V15.42	Z91.412	Personal history (past history) of spouse or partner neglect
V61.12	Z69.12	Encounter for mental health services for perpetrator of spouse or partner neglect
		Spouse or partner abuse, psychological, confirmed
995.82	T74.31XA	Initial encounter
995.82	T74.31XD	Subsequent encounter
		Spouse or partner abuse, psychological, suspected
995.82	T76.31XA	Initial encounter
995.82	T76.31XD	Subsequent encounter
		Other circumstances related to spouse or partner abuse, psychological
V61.11	Z69.11	Encounter for mental health services for victim of spouse or partner psychological abuse
V15.42	Z91.411	Personal history (past history) of spouse or partner psychological abuse
V61.12	Z69.12	Encounter for mental health services for perpetrator of spouse or partner psychological abuse

TABLE 19–2. Other conditions that may be a focus of clinical attention *(continued)*

ICD-9-CM code	ICD-10-CM code	Description
		Adult physical abuse by nonspouse or nonpartner, confirmed
995.81	T74.11XA	Initial encounter
995.81	T74.11XD	Subsequent encounter
		Adult physical abuse by nonspouse or nonpartner, suspected
995.81	T76.11XA	Initial encounter
995.81	T76.11XD	Subsequent encounter
		Adult sexual abuse by nonspouse or nonpartner, confirmed
995.83	T74.21XA	Initial encounter
995.83	T74.21XD	Subsequent encounter
		Adult sexual abuse by nonspouse or nonpartner, suspected
995.83	T76.21XA	Initial encounter
995.83	T76.21XD	Subsequent encounter
		Adult psychological abuse by nonspouse or nonpartner, confirmed
995.82	T74.31XA	Initial encounter
995.82	T74.31XD	Subsequent encounter
		Adult psychological abuse by nonspouse or nonpartner, suspected
995.82	T76.31XA	Initial encounter
995.82	T76.31XD	Subsequent encounter
		Other circumstances related to adult abuse by nonspouse or nonpartner
V65.49	Z69.81	Encounter for mental health services for victim of nonspousal or nonpartner adult abuse
V62.83	Z69.82	Encounter for mental health services for perpetrator of nonspousal or nonpartner adult abuse
V62.3	Z55.9	Academic or educational problem
V62.21	Z56.82	Problem related to current military deployment status
V62.29	Z56.9	Other problem related to employment
V60.0	Z59.0	Homelessness

TABLE 19–2. **Other conditions that may be a focus of clinical attention** *(continued)*

ICD-9-CM code	ICD-10-CM code	Description
V60.1	Z59.1	Inadequate housing
V60.89	Z59.2	Discord with neighbor, lodger, or landlord
V60.6	Z59.3	Problem related to living in a residential institution
V60.2	Z59.4	Lack of adequate food or safe drinking water
V60.2	Z59.5	Extreme poverty
V60.2	Z59.6	Low income
V60.2	Z59.7	Insufficient social insurance or welfare support
V60.9	Z59.9	Unspecified housing or economic problem
V62.89	Z60.0	Phase of life problem
V60.3	Z60.2	Problem related to living alone
V62.4	Z60.3	Acculturation difficulty
V62.4	Z60.4	Social exclusion or rejection
V62.4	Z60.5	Target of (perceived) adverse discrimination or persecution
V62.9	Z60.9	Unspecified problem related to social environment
V62.89	Z65.4	Victim of crime
V62.5	Z65.0	Conviction in civil or criminal proceedings without imprisonment
V62.5	Z65.1	Imprisonment or other incarceration
V62.5	Z65.2	Problems related to release from prison
V62.5	Z65.3	Problems related to other legal circumstances
V65.49	Z70.9	Sex counseling
V65.40	Z71.9	Other counseling or consultation
V62.89	Z65.8	Religious or spiritual problem
V61.7	Z64.0	Problems related to unwanted pregnancy
V61.5	Z64.1	Problems related to multiparity
V62.89	Z64.4	Discord with social service provider, including probation officer, case manager, or social services worker
V62.89	Z65.4	Victim of terrorism or torture
V62.22	Z65.5	Exposure to disaster, war, or other hostilities
V62.89	Z65.8	Other problem related to psychosocial circumstances

TABLE 19–2. Other conditions that may be a focus of clinical attention *(continued)*

ICD-9-CM code	ICD-10-CM code	Description
V62.9	Z65.9	Unspecified problem related to unspecified psychosocial circumstances
V15.49	Z91.49	Other personal history of psychological trauma
V15.59	Z91.5	Personal history of self-harm
V62.22	Z91.82	Personal history of military deployment
V15.89	Z91.89	Other personal risk factors
V69.9	Z72.9	Problem related to lifestyle
V71.01	Z72.811	Adult antisocial behavior
V71.02	Z72.810	Child or adolescent antisocial behavior
V63.9	Z75.3	Unavailability or inaccessibility of health care facilities
V63.8	Z75.4	Unavailability or inaccessibility of other helping agencies
V15.81	Z91.19	Nonadherence to medical treatment
278.00	E66.9	Overweight or obesity
V65.2	Z76.5	Malingering
V40.31	Z91.83	Wandering associated with a mental disorder
V62.89	R41.83	Borderline intellectual functioning

Source. Reprinted from Nussbaum AM: *The Pocket Guide to the DSM-5™ Diagnostic Exam.* Washington, DC, American Psychiatric Publishing, 2013. Copyright 2013, American Psychiatric Association. Used with permission.

V61.8 (Z63.8)   High Expressed Emotion Level Within Family
V62.82 (Z63.4)   Uncomplicated Bereavement

Abuse and Neglect

The section on problems related to abuse or neglect was added in DSM-IV in part due to the clinical and public health significance of the conditions. This section has been further expanded in DSM-5. Readers should note that different diagnostic codes are given on the basis of the focus of clinical attention. If the problem is addressed in the context of the family or relational unit, the V/Z code is used. If the focus is on the victim, the 995 code (or a T code in ICD-10-CM) is used.

Maltreatment by a family member (e.g., caregiver, intimate adult partner) or by a nonrelative can be the area of current clinical focus, or such maltreatment can be an important factor in the assessment and treatment of patients with mental or other medical disorders. Because of the legal implications of abuse and neglect, care should be used in assessing these conditions and assigning these codes. Having a past history of abuse or neglect can influence diagnosis and treatment response in a number of mental disorders, and may also be noted along with the diagnosis.

Child Maltreatment and Neglect Problems

Child Physical Abuse

Child physical abuse is nonaccidental physical injury to a child—ranging from minor bruises to severe fractures or death—occurring as a result of punching, beating, kicking, biting, shaking, throwing, stabbing, choking, hitting (with a hand, stick, strap, or other object), burning, or any other method that is inflicted by a parent, caregiver, or other individual who has responsibility for the child. Such injury is considered abuse regardless of whether the caregiver intended to hurt the child. Physical discipline, such as spanking or paddling, is not considered abuse as long as it is reasonable and causes no bodily injury to the child.

Child Physical Abuse, Confirmed
995.54 (T74.12XA) Initial encounter
995.54 (T74.12XD) Subsequent encounter

Child Physical Abuse, Suspected
995.54 (T76.12XA) Initial encounter
995.54 (T76.12XD) Subsequent encounter

Other Circumstances Related to Child Physical Abuse
V61.21 (Z69.010)   Encounter for mental health services for victim of child abuse by parent
V61.21 (Z69.020)   Encounter for mental health services for victim of nonparental child abuse
V15.41 (Z62.810)   Personal history (past history) of physical abuse in childhood
V61.22 (Z69.011)   Encounter for mental health services for perpetrator of parental child abuse
V62.83 (Z69.021)   Encounter for mental health services for perpetrator of nonparental child abuse

Child Sexual Abuse

Child sexual abuse encompasses any sexual act involving a child that is intended to provide sexual gratification to a parent, caregiver, or other individual who has responsibility for the child. Sexual abuse includes activities such as fondling a child's genitals, penetration, incest, rape, sodomy, and indecent exposure. Sexual abuse also includes noncontact exploitation of a child by a parent or caregiver—for example, forcing, tricking, enticing, threatening, or pressuring a child to participate in acts for the sexual gratification of others, without direct physical contact between child and abuser.

Child Sexual Abuse, Confirmed
995.53 (T74.22XA) Initial encounter
995.53 (T74.22XD) Subsequent encounter

Child Sexual Abuse, Suspected
995.53 (T76.22XA) Initial encounter
995.53 (T76.22XD) Subsequent encounter

Other Circumstances Related to Child Sexual Abuse
V61.21 (Z69.010) Encounter for mental health services for victim of child sexual abuse by parent
V61.21 (Z69.020) Encounter for mental health services for victim of nonparental child sexual abuse
V15.41 (Z62.810) Personal history (past history) of sexual abuse in childhood
V61.22 (Z69.011) Encounter for mental health services for perpetrator of parental child sexual abuse
V62.83 (Z69.021) Encounter for mental health services for perpetrator of nonparental child sexual abuse

Child Neglect

Child neglect is defined as any confirmed or suspected egregious act or omission by a child's parent or other caregiver that deprives the child of basic age-appropriate needs and thereby results, or has reasonable potential to result, in physical or psychological harm to the child. Child neglect encompasses abandonment; lack of appropriate supervision; failure to attend to necessary emotional or psychological needs; and failure to provide necessary education, medical care, nourishment, shelter, and/or clothing.

Child Neglect, Confirmed
995.52 (T74.02XA) Initial encounter
995.52 (T74.02XD) Subsequent encounter

Child Neglect, Suspected
995.52 (T76.02XA) Initial encounter
995.52 (T76.02XD) Subsequent encounter

Other Circumstances Related to Child Neglect
V61.21 (Z69.010) Encounter for mental health services for victim of child neglect by parent
V61.21 (Z69.020) Encounter for mental health services for victim of nonparental child neglect
V15.42 (Z62.812) Personal history (past history) of neglect in childhood
V61.22 (Z69.011) Encounter for mental health services for perpetrator of parental child neglect
V62.83 (Z69.021) Encounter for mental health services for perpetrator of nonparental child neglect

Child Psychological Abuse

Child psychological abuse is nonaccidental verbal or symbolic acts by a child's parent or caregiver that result, or have reasonable potential to result, in significant psychological harm to the child. (Physical and sexual abusive acts are not included in this category.) Examples of psychological abuse of a child include berating, disparaging, or humiliating the child; threatening the child; harming/abandoning—or indicating that the alleged offender will harm/abandon—people or things that the child cares about; confining the child (as by tying a child's arms or legs together or binding a child to furniture or another object, or confining a child to a small enclosed area [e.g., a closet]); egregious scapegoating of the child; coercing the child to inflict pain on himself or herself; and disciplining the child excessively (i.e., at an extremely high frequency or duration, even if not at a level of physical abuse) through physical or nonphysical means.

Child Psychological Abuse, Confirmed
995.51 (T74.32XA) Initial encounter
995.51 (T74.32XD) Subsequent encounter

Child Psychological Abuse, Suspected
995.51 (T76.32XA) Initial encounter
995.51 (T76.32XD) Subsequent encounter

Other Circumstances Related to Child Psychological Abuse
V61.21 (Z69.010)   Encounter for mental health services for victim of child psychological abuse by parent
V61.21 (Z69.020)   Encounter for mental health services for victim of nonparental child psychological abuse
V15.42 (Z62.811)   Personal history (past history) of psychological abuse in childhood
V61.22 (Z69.011)   Encounter for mental health services for perpetrator of parental child psychological abuse
V62.83 (Z69.021)   Encounter for mental health services for perpetrator of nonparental child psychological abuse

Adult Maltreatment and Neglect Problems

Spouse or Partner Violence, Physical

This category should be used when nonaccidental acts of physical force that result, or have reasonable potential to result, in physical harm to an intimate partner or that evoke significant fear in the partner have occurred during the past year. Nonaccidental acts of physical force include shoving, slapping, hair pulling, pinching, restraining, shaking, throwing, biting, kicking, hitting with the fist or an object, burning, poisoning, applying force to the throat, cutting off the air supply, holding the head under water, and using a weapon. Acts for the purpose of physically protecting oneself or one's partner are excluded.

Spouse or Partner Violence, Physical, Confirmed
995.81 (T74.11XA) Initial encounter
995.81 (T74.11XD) Subsequent encounter

Spouse or Partner Violence, Physical, Suspected
995.81 (T76.11XA) Initial encounter
995.81 (T76.11XD) Subsequent encounter

Other Circumstances Related to Spouse or Partner Violence, Physical

V61.11 (Z69.11)	Encounter for mental health services for victim of spouse or partner violence, physical
V15.41 (Z91.410)	Personal history (past history) of spouse or partner violence, physical
V61.12 (Z69.12)	Encounter for mental health services for perpetrator of spouse or partner violence, physical

Spouse or Partner Violence, Sexual

This category should be used when forced or coerced sexual acts with an intimate partner have occurred during the past year. Sexual violence may involve the use of physical force or psychological coercion to compel the partner to engage in a sexual act against his or her will, whether or not the act is completed. Also included in this category are sexual acts with an intimate partner who is unable to consent.

Spouse or Partner Violence, Sexual, Confirmed

995.83 (T74.21XA) Initial encounter
995.83 (T74.21XD) Subsequent encounter

Spouse or Partner Violence, Sexual, Suspected

995.83 (T76.21XA) Initial encounter
995.83 (T76.21XD) Subsequent encounter

Other Circumstances Related to Spouse or Partner Violence, Sexual

V61.11 (Z69.81)	Encounter for mental health services for victim of spouse or partner violence, sexual
V15.41 (Z91.410)	Personal history (past history) of spouse or partner violence, sexual
V61.12 (Z69.12)	Encounter for mental health services for perpetrator of spouse or partner violence, sexual

Spouse or Partner Neglect

Partner neglect is any egregious act or omission in the past year by one partner that deprives a dependent partner of basic needs and thereby results, or has reasonable potential to result, in physical or psychological harm to the dependent partner. This category is used in the context of relationships in which one partner is extremely dependent on the other partner for care or for assistance in navigating ordinary daily activities—for example, a partner who is incapable of self-care owing to substantial physical, psychological/intellectual, or cultural limitations (e.g., inability to communicate with others and manage everyday activities due to living in a foreign culture).

Spouse or Partner Neglect, Confirmed

995.85 (T74.01XA) Initial encounter
995.85 (T74.01XD) Subsequent encounter

Spouse or Partner Neglect, Suspected

995.85 (T76.01XA) Initial encounter
995.85 (T76.01XD) Subsequent encounter

Other Circumstances Related to Spouse or Partner Neglect

V61.11 (Z69.11)   Encounter for mental health services for victim of spouse or part-
                    ner neglect
V15.42 (Z91.412)   Personal history (past history) of spouse or partner neglect
V61.12 (Z69.12)   Encounter for mental health services for perpetrator of spouse or
                    partner neglect

Spouse or Partner Abuse, Psychological

Partner psychological abuse encompasses nonaccidental verbal or symbolic acts by
one partner that result, or have reasonable potential to result, in significant harm to
the other partner. This category should be used when such psychological abuse has
occurred during the past year. Acts of psychological abuse include berating or humiliating the victim; interrogating the victim; restricting the victim's ability to come and
go freely; obstructing the victim's access to assistance (e.g., law enforcement; legal,
protective, or medical resources); threatening the victim with physical harm or sexual
assault; harming, or threatening to harm, people or things that the victim cares about;
unwarranted restriction of the victim's access to or use of economic resources; isolating the victim from family, friends, or social support resources; stalking the victim; and
trying to make the victim think that he or she is crazy.

Spouse or Partner Abuse, Psychological, Confirmed

995.82 (T74.31XA) Initial encounter
995.82 (T74.31XD) Subsequent encounter

Spouse or Partner Abuse, Psychological, Suspected

995.82 (T76.31XA) Initial encounter
995.82 (T76.31XD) Subsequent encounter

Other Circumstances Related to Spouse or Partner Abuse, Psychological

V61.11 (Z69.11)   Encounter for mental health services for victim of spouse or part-
                    ner psychological abuse
V15.42 (Z91.411)   Personal history (past history) of spouse or partner psychological
                    abuse
V61.12 (Z69.12)   Encounter for mental health services for perpetrator of spouse or
                    partner psychological abuse

Adult Abuse by Nonspouse or Nonpartner

This category should be used when an adult has been abused by another adult who
is not an intimate partner. Such maltreatment may involve acts of physical, sexual, or
emotional abuse. Examples of adult abuse include nonaccidental acts of physical
force (e.g., pushing/shoving, scratching, slapping, throwing something that could
hurt, punching, biting) that have resulted—or have reasonable potential to result—in
physical harm or have caused significant fear; forced or coerced sexual acts; and verbal or symbolic acts with the potential to cause psychological harm (e.g., berating or
humiliating the person; interrogating the person; restricting the person's ability to come
and go freely; obstructing the person's access to assistance; threatening the person;
harming or threatening to harm people or things that the person cares about; restrict-

ing the person's access to or use of economic resources; isolating the person from family, friends, or social support resources; stalking the person; trying to make the person think that he or she is crazy). Acts for the purpose of physically protecting oneself or the other person are excluded.

Adult Physical Abuse by Nonspouse or Nonpartner, Confirmed
995.81 (T74.11XA) Initial encounter
995.81 (T74.11XD) Subsequent encounter

Adult Physical Abuse by Nonspouse or Nonpartner, Suspected
995.81 (T76.11XA) Initial encounter
995.81 (T76.11XD) Subsequent encounter

Adult Sexual Abuse by Nonspouse or Nonpartner, Confirmed
995.83 (T74.21XA) Initial encounter
995.83 (T74.21XD) Subsequent encounter

Adult Sexual Abuse by Nonspouse or Nonpartner, Suspected
995.83 (T76.21XA) Initial encounter
995.83 (T76.21XD) Subsequent encounter

Adult Psychological Abuse by Nonspouse or Nonpartner, Confirmed
995.82 (T74.31XA) Initial encounter
995.82 (T74.31XD) Subsequent encounter

Adult Psychological Abuse by Nonspouse or Nonpartner, Suspected
995.82 (T76.31XA) Initial encounter
995.82 (T76.31XD) Subsequent encounter

Other Circumstances Related to Adult Abuse by Nonspouse or Nonpartner
V65.49 (Z69.81) Encounter for mental health services for victim of nonspousal or nonpartner adult abuse
V62.83 (Z69.82) Encounter for mental health services for perpetrator of nonspousal or nonpartner adult abuse

Educational and Occupational Problems

This is a new category that allows the clinician to record whether the individual has an academic or educational problem, a problem related to current military deployment status, or a problem related to employment.

Educational Problems

V62.3 (Z55.9) Academic or Educational Problem

Occupational Problems

V62.21 (Z56.82) Problem Related to Current Military Deployment Status
V62.29 (Z56.9) Other Problem Related to Employment

Housing and Economic Problems

This is a new category created to acknowledge housing and economic problems that many individuals experience. There are nine codes available to help describe the individual's problem(s): homelessness; inadequate housing; discord with neighbor, lodger, or landlord; problem related to living in a residential institution; lack of adequate food or safe drinking water; extreme poverty; low income; insufficient social insurance or welfare support; and unspecified housing or economic problem.

Housing Problems

V60.0 (Z59.0)   Homelessness
V60.1 (Z59.1)   Inadequate Housing
V60.89 (Z59.2) Discord With Neighbor, Lodger, or Landlord
V60.6 (Z59.3)   Problem Related to Living in a Residential Institution

Economic Problems

V60.2 (Z59.4)   Lack of Adequate Food or Safe Drinking Water
V60.2 (Z59.5)   Extreme Poverty
V60.2 (Z59.6)   Low Income
V60.2 (Z59.7)   Insufficient Social Insurance or Welfare Support
V60.9 (Z59.9)   Unspecified Housing or Economic Problem

Other Problems Related to the Social Environment

There are six codes available in this category to better describe the individual's life transition, social, and living problems: phase of life problem; problem related to living alone; acculturation difficulty; social exclusion or rejection; target of (perceived) adverse discrimination or persecution; and unspecified problem related to social environment.

V62.89 (Z60.0) Phase of Life Problem
V60.3 (Z60.2)   Problem Related to Living Alone
V62.4 (Z60.3)   Acculturation Difficulty
V62.4 (Z60.4)   Social Exclusion or Rejection
V62.4 (Z60.5)   Target of (Perceived) Adverse Discrimination or Persecution
V62.9 (Z60.9)   Unspecified Problem Related to Social Environment

Problems Related to Crime or Interaction With the Legal System

This category is new and can be used to describe the individual's problem(s) with the legal system: victim of crime; conviction in civil or criminal proceedings without imprisonment; imprisonment or other incarceration; problems related to release from prison; and problems related to other legal circumstances.

V62.89 (Z65.4) Victim of Crime
V62.5 (Z65.0)   Conviction in Civil or Criminal Proceedings Without Imprisonment
V62.5 (Z65.1)   Imprisonment or Other Incarceration
V62.5 (Z65.2)   Problems Related to Release From Prison
V62.5 (Z65.3)   Problems Related to Other Legal Circumstances

Other Health Service Encounters for Counseling and Medical Advice

There are two codes available for use in individuals who seek sex counseling or other counseling or consultation. While they may not have a mental illness, some persons will seek counseling to receive sex education, to discuss problems related to their sexual orientation (or their partners'), and other issues. Many people will also seek counseling for various reasons unrelated to mental health, such as spiritual counseling or dietary counseling.

V65.49 (Z70.9) Sex Counseling
V65.40 (Z71.9) Other Counseling or Consultation

Problems Related to Other Psychosocial, Personal, and Environmental Circumstances

Eight codes are available in this category that includes problems related to psychosocial, personal, and environmental concerns: religious or spiritual problem; problems related to unwanted pregnancy; problems related to multiparity; discord with social service provider, including probation officer, case manager, or social services worker; victim of terrorism or torture; exposure to disaster, war, or other hostilities; other problem related to psychosocial circumstances; and unspecified problem related to unspecified psychosocial circumstances.

V62.89 (Z65.8) Religious or Spiritual Problem
V61.7 (Z64.0)   Problems Related to Unwanted Pregnancy
V61.5 (Z64.1)   Problems Related to Multiparity
V62.89 (Z64.4) Discord With Social Service Provider, Including Probation Officer, Case Manager, or Social Services Worker
V62.89 (Z65.4) Victim of Terrorism or Torture
V62.22 (Z65.5) Exposure to Disaster, War, or Other Hostilities
V62.89 (Z65.8) Other Problem Related to Psychosocial Circumstances
V62.9 (Z65.9)   Unspecified Problem Related to Unspecified Psychosocial Circumstances

Other Circumstances of Personal History

This category includes 14 codes to further describe problems related to personal history: other personal history of psychological trauma; personal history of self-harm; personal history of military deployment; other personal risk factors; problem related to lifestyle; adult antisocial behavior; child or adolescent antisocial behavior; unavailability or inaccessibility of health care facilities; unavailability or inaccessibility of other helping agencies; nonadherence to medical treatment; overweight or obesity; malingering; wandering associated with a mental disorder; and borderline intellectual functioning.

Of the seven conditions listed below, adult antisocial behavior has the longest history. Although such behavior is troublesome to the individual and the community, it is not considered a mental disorder. Some individuals engage in antisocial acts, but their behavior does not meet the criteria for antisocial personality disorder or conduct disorder. Examples include people who pursue criminal careers, prostitutes, and professional thieves. In the process of differential diagnosis, the clinician will need to distinguish adult antisocial behavior from antisocial personality disorder. The person with antisocial personality disorder will have a history of conduct disorder.

V15.49 (Z91.49)   Other Personal History of Psychological Trauma
V15.59 (Z91.5)   Personal History of Self-Harm
V62.22 (Z91.82)   Personal History of Military Deployment
V15.89 (Z91.89)   Other Personal Risk Factors
V69.9 (Z72.9)   Problem Related to Lifestyle
V71.01 (Z72.811) Adult Antisocial Behavior
V71.02 (Z72.810) Child or Adolescent Antisocial Behavior

Problems Related to Access to Medical and Other Health Care

Two codes are used to describe the unavailability or inaccessibility of health care facilities, or the unavailability or inaccessibility of other helping agencies. These problems may be particularly problematic in rural areas or remote regions where health care facilities are inadequate or lacking altogether.

V63.9 (Z75.3) Unavailability or Inaccessibility of Health Care Facilities
V63.8 (Z75.4) Unavailability or Inaccessibility of Other Helping Agencies

Nonadherence to Medical Treatment

Nonadherence to medical treatment is common and interferes with the clinician's ability to help a patient. Although nonadherence per se is not considered a mental disorder, clinicians need to have an understanding of treatment adherence in general, and more specifically in individual patients, whose motivations, concerns, and other issues affect adherence, such as an individual's denial of illness or lack of insight or possibly patient concerns about treatment side effects.

Overweight or obesity is new to DSM-5 and is a significant problem for many individuals who seek mental health care. Research has long shown a relationship between overweight/obesity and mental disorders, and the problem is gaining in importance as this condition becomes more frequent in the general population. Many psychotropic medications are known to contribute to obesity and its associated metabolic problems such as diabetes and hyperlipidemia. Including this category may lead to better recognition and reporting of overweight and obesity. This problem is coded as 278.00 (E66.9) rather than with a V/Z code.

Malingering is another problem clinicians encounter, and it involves the intentional production of false or grossly exaggerated physical or psychological symptoms motivated by external incentives (e.g., avoiding military conscription or duty, avoiding work, evading criminal prosecution). Malingering is important to consider in the process of differential diagnosis and should be suspected when any of the following clues are present: medicolegal context of presentation (e.g., the person is referred by an attorney); marked discrepancy between the person's claimed disability and objective findings; lack of cooperation during the diagnostic evaluation and noncompliance with the treatment regimen; and the presence of an antisocial personality disorder.

Wandering associated with a mental disorder is new to DSM-5, and is a category used to describe people whose tendency to walk about leads to significant clinical management or safety concerns. For example, individuals with major neurocognitive or neurodevelopmental disorders may experience a restless urge to wander that places them at risk for falls and causes them to leave supervised settings without needed accompaniment. This category is not meant to be used in those individuals whose intent is to escape an unwanted housing situation (e.g., children who are running away from home, patients who no longer wish to remain in the hospital) or those who walk or pace as a result of medication-induced akathisia. Nor should this category used to describe the individual with antisocial personality disorder whose *wanderlust* leads him to move from place to place without any particular goal or destination other than to perhaps dodge past crimes and identities.

The category *borderline intellectual functioning* can be used when the individual's subnormal cognitive performance is the focus of clinical attention or has an impact on the individual's treatment or prognosis. Differentiating between borderline intellectual functioning and an intellectual disability requires careful assessment that must take into account both intellectual and adaptive functioning. Unlike DSM-IV, there is no longer an IQ range specified to help identify borderline intellectual functioning. This condition is important to acknowledge because an individual may benefit from efforts to optimize academic achievement; to address difficulties with school, as well as social and work relationships; and to develop functional skills and guidance in vocational training.

V15.81 (Z91.19)   Nonadherence to Medical Treatment
278.00 (E66.9)   Overweight or Obesity
V65.2 (Z76.5)   Malingering
V40.31 (Z91.83)   Wandering Associated With a Mental Disorder
V62.89 (R41.83)   Borderline Intellectual Functioning

KEY POINTS

- The DSM-IV chapter "Other Conditions That May Be a Focus of Clinical Attention," which included the V/Z/T code diagnoses, has been expanded for DSM-5, and the medication-induced movement disorders and other adverse effects of medication have been moved to their own chapter.

- The codes included in this chapter are available to describe or denote conditions that are of clinical interest or concern but that are not considered mental disorders.

- Many of these conditions would have been listed on Axis IV of the multiaxial system in DSM-IV as "stressors" relevant to the care of the individual.

- Uncomplicated bereavement is available for use in bereaved individuals whose symptoms do not meet criteria for major depressive disorder.

- Overweight or obesity is a new category that may help lead to better recognition and reporting of this condition.

CHAPTER 20

Assessment Measures

Level 1 and Level 2 Cross-Cutting Symptom Measures
Clinician-Rated Dimensions of Psychosis Symptom Severity
World Health Organization Disability Assessment Schedule 2.0
Cultural Formulation Interview

Section III of DSM-5, "Emerging Measures and Models," includes new assessments and models that can be used by clinicians and researchers to provide a more thorough evaluation of the patient. The measures and models, all of which are optional, include the Level 1 Cross-Cutting Symptom Measure, a list of Level 2 Cross-Cutting Symptom Measures, the Clinician-Rated Dimensions of Psychosis Symptom Severity scale, and the World Health Organization Disability Assessment Schedule 2.0 (WHODAS 2.0). Level 2 severity measures are available online and may be used to explore significant responses to the Level 1 screen. The Cultural Formulation Interview, a comprehensive review of the cultural context of mental disorders, is also provided.

The authors of DSM-5 aimed to integrate dimensional measures into the manual. The goal was to enhance the assessment of symptom variation and severity, enabling the clinician to provide a more complete evaluation of the patient to assist with treatment decisions and in monitoring outcome. The goal was largely achieved with regard to several major categories. For example, intellectual disability (intellectual developmental disorder) no longer is linked to specific IQ ranges; rather, the diagnosis depends on a dimensional assessment of adaptive functioning, which is anchored to conceptual, social, and practical domains (see Chapter 3, "Neurodevelopmental Disorders," of this guidebook). Another example is the decision to merge substance abuse and dependence into a single "use" disorder rated according to severity, which ranges from mild (two to three symptoms) to severe (six or more symptoms). The most ambitious plan to incorporate dimensions was developed by the Personality and Personality Disorders Work Group. Although their hybrid categorical-dimensional diagnostic system was not accepted for inclusion in Section II, the scheme is included in Section III (and described in Chapter 21, "Alternative DSM-5 Model for Personality Disorders," of this guidebook). Thus, DSM-5 places greater emphasis on dimensional measures compared with its predecessors, yet categorical diagnosis remains its fundamental goal.

Level 1 and Level 2 Cross-Cutting Symptom Measures

Cross-cutting symptom measures can serve as an approach for reviewing important psychopathological domains, and they function as the equivalent of general medicine's review of systems. (*Cross-cutting* refers to the measure "cutting across" various psychopathological domains.) A similar review of various mental functions can provide a more complete mental status evaluation by drawing attention to symptoms that may not be suggested by the individual's presenting symptoms but are important to the individual's care. In DSM-5, cross-cutting measures have two levels: Level 1 questions are a brief survey of 13 symptom domains for adult patients and 12 domains for child and adolescent patients. Level 2 questions provide a more in-depth assessment of certain domains. The measures were developed to be administered initially and over time to track the patient's symptoms and treatment response.

New to DSM-5 is the Level 1 Cross-Cutting Symptom Measure. This patient- or informant-rated measure can be used to assess mental health domains that are important across psychiatric diagnoses. The adult version has 23 questions that assess 13 domains: depression, anger, mania, anxiety, somatic symptoms, suicidal ideation, psychosis, sleep problems, memory, repetitive thoughts and behaviors, dissociation, personality functioning, and substance use. Each domain consists of one to three questions. Each item inquires about how much (or how often) the individual has been bothered by the specific symptoms during the past 2 weeks. The measure was found to be clinically useful and to have good reliability in the DSM-5 field trials. A similar instrument for children ages 6–17 years consisting of 25 questions assessing 12 psychiatric domains was tested and found to have good reliability. The adult version of the measure is included on the following pages and, along with the analogous child measure, is available at www.psychiatry.org/dsm5.

Achieving threshold scores on the Level 1 Cross-Cutting Symptom Measure can indicate a need for a more detailed inquiry. Level 2 Cross-Cutting Symptom Measures can provide one way of obtaining more in-depth information on potentially significant symptoms to inform diagnosis and treatment planning. These measures are available online at www.psychiatry.org/dsm5. They include well-validated measures such as the Patient Health Questionnaire 15-Item Somatic Symptom Severity Scale and the Florida Obsessive-Compulsive Inventory Severity Scale.

DSM-5 Self-Rated Level 1 Cross-Cutting Symptom Measure—Adult

Name: _____   Age: _____   Sex: [ ] Male [ ] Female   Date: _____

If the measure is being completed by an informant, what is your relationship with the individual?: _____

In a typical week, approximately how much time do you spend with the individual? _____ **hours/week**

Instructions: The questions below ask about things that might have bothered you. For each question, circle the number that best describes how much (or how often) you have been bothered by each problem during the **past TWO (2) WEEKS.**

		During the past **TWO (2) WEEKS,** how much (or how often) have you been bothered by the following problems?	**None** Not at all	**Slight** Rare, less than a day or two	**Mild** Several days	**Moderate** More than half the days	**Severe** Nearly every day	**Highest Domain Score** (clinician)
I.	1.	Little interest or pleasure in doing things?	0	1	2	3	4	
	2.	Feeling down, depressed, or hopeless?	0	1	2	3	4	
II.	3.	Feeling more irritated, grouchy, angry than usual?	0	1	2	3	4	
III.	4.	Sleeping less than usual, but still have a lot of energy?	0	1	2	3	4	
	5.	Starting lots more projects than usual or doing more risky things than usual?	0	1	2	3	4	
IV.	6.	Feeling nervous, anxious, frightened, worried, or on edge?	0	1	2	3	4	
	7.	Feeling panic or being frightened?	0	1	2	3	4	
	8.	Avoiding situations that make you anxious?	0	1	2	3	4	
V.	9.	Unexplained aches and pains (e.g., head, back, joints, abdomen, legs)?	0	1	2	3	4	
	10.	Feeling that your illnesses are not being taken seriously enough?	0	1	2	3	4	
VI.	11.	Thoughts of actually hurting yourself?	0	1	2	3	4	

			0	1	2	3	4
VII.	12.	Hearing things other people couldn't hear, such as voices even when no one was around?	0	1	2	3	4
	13.	Feeling that someone could hear your thoughts, or that you could hear what another person was thinking?	0	1	2	3	4
VIII.	14.	Problems with sleep that affected your sleep quality over all?	0	1	2	3	4
IX.	15.	Problems with memory (e.g., learning new information) or with location (e.g., finding your way home)?	0	1	2	3	4
X.	16.	Unpleasant thoughts, urges, or images that repeatedly enter your mind?	0	1	2	3	4
	17.	Feeling driven to perform certain behaviors or mental acts over and over again?	0	1	2	3	4
XI.	18.	Feeling detached or distant from yourself, your body, your physical surroundings, or your memories?	0	1	2	3	4
XII.	19.	Not knowing who you really are or what you want out of life?	0	1	2	3	4
	20.	Not feeling close to other people or enjoying your relationships with them?	0	1	2	3	4
XIII.	21.	Drink at least 4 drinks of any kind of alcohol in a single day?	0	1	2	3	4
	22.	Smoke any cigarettes, a cigar, or pipe, or use snuff or chewing tobacco?	0	1	2	3	4
	23.	Use any of the following medicines ON YOUR OWN, that is, without a doctor's prescription, in greater amounts or longer than prescribed [e.g., painkillers (like Vicodin), stimulants (like Ritalin or Adderall), sedatives or tranquilizers (like sleeping pills or Valium), or drugs like marijuana, cocaine or crack, club drugs (like ecstasy), hallucinogens (like LSD), heroin, inhalants or solvents (like glue), or methamphetamine (like speed)]?	0	1	2	3	4

Clinician-Rated Dimensions of Psychosis Symptom Severity

Because psychotic disorders are heterogeneous and symptom severity can predict important aspects of the illness, dimensional assessments can help capture meaningful variation in symptom presentations. This can help with treatment planning, prognostic decision-making, and research on pathophysiological mechanisms. The Clinician-Rated Dimensions of Psychosis Symptom Severity can be used in the dimensional assessment of the primary symptoms of psychosis, such as hallucinations, delusions, and disorganized speech. The scale also assesses depression and mania. This eight-item measure can be completed by the clinician or researcher at the time of assessment. Each symptom is rated for current severity (past 7 days) on a 5-point scale (0: "Not present" to 4: "Present and severe"). The scale can be used to rate any of the psychotic disorders. The time frame is the past 7 days. The scale is shown below.

Clinician-Rated Dimensions of Psychosis Symptom Severity

Name: _____ **Age:** _____ **Sex:** [ ] Male [ ] Female **Date:** _____

Instructions: Based on all the information you have on the individual and using your clinical judgment, please rate (with checkmark) the presence and severity of the following symptoms as experienced by the individual in the past seven (7) days.

Domain	0	1	2	3	4	Score
I. Hallucinations	☐ Not present	☐ Equivocal (severity or duration not sufficient to be considered psychosis)	☐ Present, but mild (little pressure to act upon voices, not very bothered by voices)	☐ Present and moderate (some pressure to respond to voices, or is somewhat bothered by voices)	☐ Present and severe (severe pressure to respond to voices, or is very bothered by voices)	
II. Delusions	☐ Not present	☐ Equivocal (severity or duration not sufficient to be considered psychosis)	☐ Present, but mild (little pressure to act upon delusional beliefs, not very bothered by beliefs)	☐ Present and moderate (some pressure to act upon beliefs, or is somewhat bothered by beliefs)	☐ Present and severe (severe pressure to act upon beliefs, or is very bothered by beliefs)	
III. Disorganized speech	☐ Not present	☐ Equivocal (severity or duration not sufficient to be considered disorganization)	☐ Present, but mild (some difficulty following speech)	☐ Present and moderate (speech often difficult to follow)	☐ Present and severe (speech almost impossible to follow)	
IV. Abnormal psychomotor behavior	☐ Not present	☐ Equivocal (severity or duration not sufficient to be considered abnormal psychomotor behavior)	☐ Present, but mild (occasional abnormal or bizarre motor behavior or catatonia)	☐ Present and moderate (frequent abnormal or bizarre motor behavior or catatonia)	☐ Present and severe (abnormal or bizarre motor behavior or catatonia almost constant)	
V. Negative symptoms (restricted emotional expression or avolition)	☐ Not present	☐ Equivocal decrease in facial expressivity, prosody, gestures, or self-initiated behavior	☐ Present, but mild decrease in facial expressivity, prosody, gestures, or self-initiated behavior	☐ Present and moderate decrease in facial expressivity, prosody, gestures, or self-initiated behavior	☐ Present and severe decrease in facial expressivity, prosody, gestures, or self-initiated behavior	

Domain	0	1	2	3	4	Score
VI. Impaired cognition	☐ Not present	☐ Equivocal (cognitive function not clearly outside the range expected for age or SES; i.e., within 0.5 SD of mean)	☐ Present, but mild (some reduction in cognitive function; below expected for age and SES, 0.5–1 SD from mean)	☐ Present and moderate (clear reduction in cognitive function; below expected for age and SES, 1–2 SD from mean)	☐ Present and severe (severe reduction in cognitive function; below expected for age and SES, >2 SD from mean)	
VII. Depression	☐ Not present	☐ Equivocal (occasionally feels sad, down, depressed, or hopeless; concerned about having failed someone or at something but not preoccupied)	☐ Present, but mild (frequent periods of feeling very sad, down, moderately depressed, or hopeless; concerned about having failed someone or at something, with some preoccupation)	☐ Present and moderate (frequent periods of deep depression or hopelessness; preoccupation with guilt, having done wrong)	☐ Present and severe (deeply depressed or hopeless daily; delusional guilt or unreasonable self-reproach grossly out of proportion to circumstances)	
VIII. Mania	☐ Not present	☐ Equivocal (occasional elevated, expansive, or irritable mood or some restlessness)	☐ Present, but mild (frequent periods of somewhat elevated, expansive, or irritable mood or restlessness)	☐ Present and moderate (frequent periods of extensively elevated, expansive, or irritable mood or restlessness)	☐ Present and severe (daily and extensively elevated, expansive, or irritable mood or restlessness)	

Note. SD=standard deviation; SES=socioeconomic status.

World Health Organization Disability Assessment Schedule 2.0

The adult self-administered version of the World Health Organization Disability Assessment Schedule 2.0 (WHODAS 2.0) is a 36-item measure that assesses disability in adults age 18 years and older. Six domains are assessed: understanding and communication; getting around; self-care; getting along with people; life activities (e.g., household activities); and participation in society. If the person is unable to complete the form, a knowledgeable informant may complete the proxy-administered version. Both are available at www.psychiatry.org/dsm5. Each version asks the individual to rate how much difficulty he or she has had in the specific areas in the past 30 days.

There are two options for scoring. In a simple version of scoring, the scores assigned to each item (none = 1, mild = 2, moderate = 3, severe = 4, and extreme = 5) are summed. There is no weighting of individual items. A more complex scoring method, called "item-response-theory"–based scoring, takes into account multiple levels of difficulty for each item. A computer program is available from the World Health Organization Web site. The authors of DSM-5, in part on the basis of the findings from field trials in adult samples, recommend the calculation and use of average scores for each domain (e.g., understanding and communication) and for general disability. These scores were found to be reliable and clinically useful to the clinicians participating in the field trials. The average domain score is calculated by dividing the raw domain score by the number of items in the domain. The average general disability score is calculated by dividing the raw overall score by the number of items in the measure (i.e., 36). The measure may be repeated at regular intervals to track change in the individual's level of disability over time. Consistently high scores on a particular domain may indicate significant and problematic areas for the individual that might warrant further assessment and intervention.

WHODAS 2.0
World Health Organization Disability Assessment Schedule 2.0
36-item version, self-administered

Patient Name: _____ **Age:** _____   **Sex:** ❑ Male ❑ Female   **Date:** _____

This questionnaire asks about <u>difficulties due to health/mental health conditions</u>. Health conditions include **diseases or illnesses, other health problems that may be short or long lasting, injuries, mental or emotional problems, and problems with alcohol or drugs.** Think back over the **<u>past 30 days</u>** and answer these questions thinking about how much difficulty you had doing the following activities. For each question, please circle only **<u>one</u>** response.

		1	2	3	4	5	Raw Item Score	Raw Domain Score	Average Domain Score
Numeric scores assigned to each of the items:								*Clinician Use Only*	
In the <u>last 30 days</u>, how much difficulty did you have in:									
Understanding and communicating									
D1.1	<u>Concentrating</u> on doing something for <u>ten minutes?</u>	None	Mild	Moderate	Severe	Extreme or cannot do			
D1.2	<u>Remembering</u> to do <u>important things?</u>	None	Mild	Moderate	Severe	Extreme or cannot do			
D1.3	<u>Analyzing and finding solutions to problems</u> in day-to-day life?	None	Mild	Moderate	Severe	Extreme or cannot do			
D1.4	<u>Learning</u> a <u>new task</u>, for example, learning how to get to a new place?	None	Mild	Moderate	Severe	Extreme or cannot do		30	5
D1.5	<u>Generally understanding</u> what people say?	None	Mild	Moderate	Severe	Extreme or cannot do			
D1.6	<u>Starting and maintaining</u> a <u>conversation?</u>	None	Mild	Moderate	Severe	Extreme or cannot do			
Getting around									
D2.1	<u>Standing</u> for <u>long periods</u>, such as <u>30 minutes?</u>	None	Mild	Moderate	Severe	Extreme or cannot do			
D2.2	<u>Standing up</u> from sitting down?	None	Mild	Moderate	Severe	Extreme or cannot do			
D2.3	<u>Moving</u> around <u>inside your home?</u>	None	Mild	Moderate	Severe	Extreme or cannot do		25	5
D2.4	<u>Getting out</u> of your <u>home?</u>	None	Mild	Moderate	Severe	Extreme or cannot do			
D2.5	<u>Walking a long distance</u>, such as a kilometer (or equivalent)?	None	Mild	Moderate	Severe	Extreme or cannot do			
Self-care									
D3.1	<u>Washing</u> your <u>whole body?</u>	None	Mild	Moderate	Severe	Extreme or cannot do			
D3.2	Getting <u>dressed?</u>	None	Mild	Moderate	Severe	Extreme or cannot do			
D3.3	<u>Eating?</u>	None	Mild	Moderate	Severe	Extreme or cannot do		20	5
D3.4	Staying <u>by yourself</u> for a <u>few days?</u>	None	Mild	Moderate	Severe	Extreme or cannot do			
Getting along with people									
D4.1	<u>Dealing</u> with people <u>you do not know?</u>	None	Mild	Moderate	Severe	Extreme or cannot do			
D4.2	<u>Maintaining a friendship?</u>	None	Mild	Moderate	Severe	Extreme or cannot do			
D4.3	<u>Getting along</u> with people who are <u>close</u> to you?	None	Mild	Moderate	Severe	Extreme or cannot do		25	5
D4.4	<u>Making new friends?</u>	None	Mild	Moderate	Severe	Extreme or cannot do			
D4.5	<u>Sexual</u> activities?	None	Mild	Moderate	Severe	Extreme or cannot do			

	Numeric scores assigned to each of the items:	1	2	3	4	5	Raw Item Score	Raw Domain Score	Average Domain Score
	In the last 30 days, how much difficulty did you have in:								
	Life activities—Household								
D5.1	Taking care of your household responsibilities?	None	Mild	Moderate	Severe	Extreme or cannot do			
D5.2	Doing most important household tasks well?	None	Mild	Moderate	Severe	Extreme or cannot do			
D5.3	Getting all of the household work done that you needed to do?	None	Mild	Moderate	Severe	Extreme or cannot do		20	5
D5.4	Getting your household work done as quickly as needed?	None	Mild	Moderate	Severe	Extreme or cannot do			
	Life activities—School/Work								
	If you work (paid, non-paid, self-employed) or go to school, complete questions D5.5–D5.8, below. Otherwise, skip to D6.1.								
	Because of your health condition, in the past 30 days, how much difficulty did you have in:								
D5.5	Your day-to-day work/school?	None	Mild	Moderate	Severe	Extreme or cannot do			
D5.6	Doing your most important work/school tasks well?	None	Mild	Moderate	Severe	Extreme or cannot do			
D5.7	Getting all of the work done that you need to do?	None	Mild	Moderate	Severe	Extreme or cannot do		20	5
D5.8	Getting your work done as quickly as needed?	None	Mild	Moderate	Severe	Extreme or cannot do			
	Participation in society								
	In the past 30 days:								
D6.1	How much of a problem did you have in joining in community activities (for example, festivities, religious, or other activities) in the same way as anyone else can?	None	Mild	Moderate	Severe	Extreme or cannot do			
D6.2	How much of a problem did you have because of barriers or hindrances around you?	None	Mild	Moderate	Severe	Extreme or cannot do			
D6.3	How much of a problem did you have living with dignity because of the attitudes and actions of others?	None	Mild	Moderate	Severe	Extreme or cannot do			
D6.4	How much time did you spend on your health condition or its consequences?	None	Some	Moderate	A Lot	Extreme or cannot do		40	5
D6.5	How much have you been emotionally affected by your health condition?	None	Mild	Moderate	Severe	Extreme or cannot do			
D6.6	How much has your health been a drain on the financial resources of you or your family?	None	Mild	Moderate	Severe	Extreme or cannot do			
D6.7	How much of a problem did your family have because of your health problems?	None	Mild	Moderate	Severe	Extreme or cannot do			
D6.8	How much of a problem did you have in doing things by yourself for relaxation or pleasure?	None	Mild	Moderate	Severe	Extreme or cannot do			
	General Disability Score (Total):							180	5

Clinician Use Only

Cultural Formulation Interview

The Cultural Formulation Interview (CFI) consists of 16 questions clinicians can use to obtain information about the impact of a patient's culture on key aspects of care. In the CFI, *culture* refers primarily to the values, orientations, and assumptions that individuals derive from membership in diverse social groups (e.g., ethnic groups, the military, faith communities), which may conform or differ from medical explanations. The term *culture* also refers to aspects of a person's background that may affect his or her perspective, such as ethnicity, race, language, or religion.

The CFI focuses on the patient's perspectives on the problem, the role of others in influencing the course of the problem, the impact of the patient's cultural background, the patient's help-seeking experiences, and current expectations about treatment and other forms of care. The CFI follows a person-centered approach to cultural assessment by asking the patient to address these topics on the basis of his or her own views rather than inquiring about the views of the person's cultural group(s) of origin. This is intended to avoid stereotyping, as individuals vary substantially in how they combine and interpret cultural information and perspectives. Because the CFI concerns the patient's views, there are no right or wrong answers. The interview is available online at www.psychiatry.org/dsm5.

The CFI can be used at the beginning of an initial assessment interview with all adult patients in all clinical settings, regardless of the patient's background or that of the clinician. Patients and clinicians who appear to share the same cultural background may in fact differ on a number of perspectives relevant to care. Alternatively, individual questions may be used at any point in the interview, as necessary. During later stages in care, the CFI may be particularly helpful when there is difficulty in making a diagnostic judgment, owing to a significant difference in cultural, religious, or socioeconomic background of clinician and patient; when there is uncertainty about the match between culturally expressed symptoms and diagnostic criteria; when it is difficult to make a dimensional judgment of severity; when patients and clinicians disagree on the course of treatment; or in cases of limited engagement and adherence. This interview process and the information it elicits are expected to enhance the cultural validity of the diagnostic assessment, facilitate treatment planning, and promote patient engagement and satisfaction.

The CFI emphasizes four main domains:

1. **Cultural Definition of the Problem:** The presenting issues that led to the current illness episode, cast within the patient's worldview. In this section, the patient describes the problem and focuses on its most troubling aspects. This information starts to address what is most at stake for the patient with respect to the current presentation, including nonmedical aspects.
2. **Cultural Perceptions of Cause, Context, and Support:** The patient's explanations for the circumstances of illness, including the cause of the problem. The patient also clarifies factors that improve or worsen the problem, with particular attention to the role of family, friends, and cultural background. The clinician seeks to obtain a holistic picture of the patient in his or her social environment with emphasis on how cultural elements affect the presentation.

3. **Cultural Factors Affecting Self-Coping and Past Help Seeking:** The strategies employed by the patient to improve the situation, including those that have been most and least helpful. The patient also identifies past barriers to care. This information helps clarify the patient's perspective on the nature of the problem, his or her mental health treatment expectations as opposed to expectations regarding other forms of help, and current resources to address the situation.

4. **Cultural Factors Affecting Current Help Seeking:** The patient's perception of the relationship with the clinician, current potential treatment barriers, and preferences for care. In this section, the patient specifies how the clinician may facilitate current treatment and what may interfere with the clinical relationship. Treatment preferences are elicited that may be incorporated into the treatment plan.

Supplementary modules have been developed that expand each domain of the CFI and may help guide clinicians who wish to probe these domains in greater depth. Supplementary modules have also been developed for populations with unique needs, such as children and adolescents, elderly patients, and immigrants and refugees.

Cultural Formulation Interview (CFI)

Supplementary modules used to expand each CFI subtopic are noted in parentheses.

| *GUIDE TO INTERVIEWER* | INSTRUCTIONS TO THE INTERVIEWER ARE *ITALICIZED.* |

The following questions aim to clarify key aspects of the presenting clinical problem from the point of view of the individual and other members of the individual's social network (i.e., family, friends, or others involved in current problem). This includes the problem's meaning, potential sources of help, and expectations for services.

INTRODUCTION FOR THE INDIVIDUAL:
I would like to understand the problems that bring you here so that I can help you more effectively. I want to know about *your* experience and ideas. I will ask some questions about what is going on and how you are dealing with it. Please remember there are no right or wrong answers.

CULTURAL DEFINITION OF THE PROBLEM

CULTURAL DEFINITION OF THE PROBLEM

(Explanatory Model, Level of Functioning)

Elicit the individual's view of core problems and key concerns.

Focus on the individual's own way of understanding the problem.

Use the term, expression, or brief description elicited in question 1 to identify the problem in subsequent questions (e.g., "your conflict with your son").

1. What brings you here today?
   IF INDIVIDUAL GIVES FEW DETAILS OR ONLY MENTIONS SYMPTOMS OR A MEDICAL DIAGNOSIS, PROBE:
   People often understand their problems in their own way, which may be similar to or different from how doctors describe the problem. How would *you* describe your problem?

Ask how individual frames the problem for members of the social network.

2. Sometimes people have different ways of describing their problem to their family, friends, or others in their community. How would you describe your problem to them?

Focus on the aspects of the problem that matter most to the individual.

3. What troubles you most about your problem?

CULTURAL PERCEPTIONS OF CAUSE, CONTEXT, AND SUPPORT

CAUSES

(Explanatory Model, Social Network, Older Adults)

This question indicates the meaning of the condition for the individual, which may be relevant for clinical care.

Note that individuals may identify multiple causes, depending on the facet of the problem they are considering.

4. Why do you think this is happening to you? What do you think are the causes of your [PROBLEM]?

   PROMPT FURTHER IF REQUIRED:
   Some people may explain their problem as the result of bad things that happen in their life, problems with others, a physical illness, a spiritual reason, or many other causes.

Focus on the views of members of the individual's social network. These may be diverse and vary from the individual's.

5. What do others in your family, your friends, or others in your community think is causing your [PROBLEM]?

Cultural Formulation Interview (CFI) *(continued)*

Supplementary modules used to expand each CFI subtopic are noted in parentheses.

GUIDE TO INTERVIEWER	INSTRUCTIONS TO THE INTERVIEWER ARE *ITALICIZED.*

Stressors and Supports

(Social Network, Caregivers, Psychosocial Stressors, Religion and Spirituality, Immigrants and Refugees, Cultural Identity, Older Adults, Coping and Help Seeking)

Elicit information on the individual's life context, focusing on resources, social supports, and resilience. May also probe other supports (e.g., from coworkers, from participation in religion or spirituality).	6. Are there any kinds of support that make your [PROBLEM] better, such as support from family, friends, or others?
Focus on stressful aspects of the individual's environment. Can also probe, e.g., relationship problems, difficulties at work or school, or discrimination.	7. Are there any kinds of stresses that make your [PROBLEM] worse, such as difficulties with money, or family problems?

Role of Cultural Identity

(Cultural Identity, Psychosocial Stressors, Religion and Spirituality, Immigrants and Refugees, Older Adults, Children and Adolescents)

	Sometimes, aspects of people's background or identity can make their [PROBLEM] better or worse. By **background** or **identity**, I mean, for example, the communities you belong to, the languages you speak, where you or your family are from, your race or ethnic background, your gender or sexual orientation, or your faith or religion.
Ask the individual to reflect on the most salient elements of his or her cultural identity. Use this information to tailor questions 9–10 as needed.	8. For you, what are the most important aspects of your background or identity?
Elicit aspects of identity that make the problem better or worse. *Probe as needed (e.g., clinical worsening as a result of discrimination due to migration status, race/ ethnicity, or sexual orientation).*	9. Are there any aspects of your background or identity that make a difference to your [PROBLEM]?
Probe as needed (e.g., migration-related problems; conflict across generations or due to gender roles).	10. Are there any aspects of your background or identity that are causing other concerns or difficulties for you?

CULTURAL FACTORS AFFECTING SELF-COPING AND PAST HELP SEEKING

Self-Coping

(Coping and Help Seeking, Religion and Spirituality, Older Adults, Caregivers, Psychosocial Stressors)

Clarify self-coping for the problem.	11. Sometimes people have various ways of dealing with problems like [PROBLEM]. What have you done on your own to cope with your [PROBLEM]?

Cultural Formulation Interview (CFI) *(continued)*

Supplementary modules used to expand each CFI subtopic are noted in parentheses.

GUIDE TO INTERVIEWER

INSTRUCTIONS TO THE INTERVIEWER ARE ITALICIZED.

PAST HELP SEEKING

(Coping and Help Seeking, Religion and Spirituality, Older Adults, Caregivers, Psychosocial Stressors, Immigrants and Refugees, Social Network, Clinician-Patient Relationship)

Elicit various sources of help (e.g., medical care, mental health treatment, support groups, work-based counseling, folk healing, religious or spiritual counseling, other forms of traditional or alternative healing).

Probe as needed (e.g., "What other sources of help have you used?").

Clarify the individual's experience and regard for previous help.

12. Often, people look for help from many different sources, including different kinds of doctors, helpers, or healers. In the past, what kinds of treatment, help, advice, or healing have you sought for your [PROBLEM]? *PROBE IF DOES NOT DESCRIBE USEFULNESS OF HELP RECEIVED:* What types of help or treatment were most useful? Not useful?

BARRIERS

(Coping and Help Seeking, Religion and Spirituality, Older Adults, Psychosocial Stressors, Immigrants and Refugees, Social Network, Clinician-Patient Relationship)

Clarify the role of social barriers to help seeking, access to care, and problems engaging in previous treatment.

Probe details as needed (e.g., "What got in the way?").

13. Has anything prevented you from getting the help you need? *PROBE AS NEEDED:* For example, money, work or family commitments, stigma or discrimination, or lack of services that understand your language or background?

CULTURAL FACTORS AFFECTING CURRENT HELP SEEKING

PREFERENCES

(Social Network, Caregivers, Religion and Spirituality, Older Adults, Coping and Help Seeking)

Clarify individual's current perceived needs and expectations of help, broadly defined.

Probe if individual lists only one source of help (e.g., "What other kinds of help would be useful to you at this time?").

Focus on the views of the social network regarding help seeking.

Now let's talk some more about the help you need.

14. What kinds of help do you think would be most useful to you at this time for your [PROBLEM]?

15. Are there other kinds of help that your family, friends, or other people have suggested would be helpful for you now?

CLINICIAN-PATIENT RELATIONSHIP

(Clinician-Patient Relationship, Older Adults)

Elicit possible concerns about the clinic or the clinician-patient relationship, including perceived racism, language barriers, or cultural differences that may undermine goodwill, communication, or care delivery.

Probe details as needed (e.g., "In what way?").

Address possible barriers to care or concerns about the clinic and the clinician-patient relationship raised previously.

Sometimes doctors and patients misunderstand each other because they come from different backgrounds or have different expectations.

16. Have you been concerned about this and is there anything that we can do to provide you with the care you need?

Alternative DSM-5 Model for Personality Disorders

General Criteria for Personality Disorder

Specific Personality Disorders
Antisocial Personality Disorder
Avoidant Personality Disorder
Borderline Personality Disorder
Narcissistic Personality Disorder
Obsessive-Compulsive Personality Disorder
Schizotypal Personality Disorder
Personality Disorder—Trait Specified

The Personality and Personality Disorders Work Group developed a new model for the assessment of personality disorders and traits that included both categorical diagnoses and dimensional approaches. Although the proposal was not accepted by the American Psychiatric Association Board of Trustees for inclusion in Section II, the board chose to include it in Section III (as the chapter "Alternative DSM-5 Model for Personality Disorders"). According to DSM-5, this approach "preserve[s] continuity with current clinical practice, while also introducing a new approach that aims to address numerous shortcomings of the current approach to personality disorders" (American Psychiatric Association 2013, p. 761).

The work group proposed a wholesale reformulation of the personality disorder class. This involved the elimination of 4 of 10 personality disorders and the introduction of a hybrid assessment scheme combining categorical diagnosis with the optional dimensional assessment of personality impairment and pathological traits. Work group members were influenced by many factors and considered the time ripe for a new approach to personality assessment. Among their many concerns: 1) the number (10) of personality disorders, some of which were rarely used and poorly supported by the literature; 2) diagnostic criteria that failed to tap important psychological dimensions in favor of behavioral traits; 3) frequent comorbidity that made it uncommon for a person to be diagnosed with a single personality disorder type; 4) polythetic criteria (i.e., the "Chinese menu" approach) that contributed to the heterogeneity seen with some disorders, such as borderline personality disorder, which requires at least five of nine symptoms, leading to 151 ways to satisfy the criteria, with none required (Sanislow et al. 2002); and, finally, 5) the fact that clinicians had little opportunity to fully describe the extent of a person's personality pathology because of the lack of dimensional approaches. The work group concluded that the two approaches were complementary and offered advantages over the DSM-IV approach, and they developed a new model to address these concerns.

Their model came under critical fire from both clinicians and researchers almost from the outset. Although critics generally acknowledged the value of dimensional assessments, the proposed model was considered too complicated for busy clinicians, many of whom—it was thought—would never have time to use it. Further, many psychiatrists are unfamiliar with the personality domains and traits assessed (which came largely from the field of academic psychology) and expressed discomfort with the model. Many were concerned that use of the model for dimensionally rating personality domains and traits would be mandatory and not optional. Interestingly, the use of dimensional ratings was considered during the development of DSM-III but was rejected mainly because of the relative lack of familiarity that psychiatrists have with such systems and the concern that the systems provide more information than clinicians would use (Spitzer et al. 1980). The use of any new system involves a learning curve, and this was especially true when DSM-III was rolled out and required that clinicians rethink their approach to assessment and diagnosis.

In the alternative model, categorical diagnosis has been preserved. The number of personality disorders has been reduced from 10 to 6. It was thought that reducing the number of diagnoses would help minimize the problem of frequent comorbidity. Because there have been very few empirical studies of the paranoid, schizoid, histrionic, and dependent types, these disorders were thought appropriate for exclusion. Although there had been some initial discussion about deleting narcissistic personality disorder as well, the work group decided to retain it in their model (Ronningstam 2011).

The rationale for retaining the six disorders was based on evidence of disorder prevalence, degree of psychosocial impairment, and other research supporting the validity of the diagnoses. For example, the antisocial, borderline, and schizotypal types have extensive evidence regarding validity and clinical usefulness. The narcissistic type was retained largely on the basis of the substantial clinician interest in the disorder despite its infrequent use.

The criteria for the six personality disorders were revised to make them uniform and to ensure that they were based on a standard set of empirically tested personality domains and traits. The criteria are not polythetic, in order to address concerns about heterogeneity. Diagnosis of any of the six personality disorders requires that the individual have impairments in personality functioning (Criterion A) and pathological personality traits specific to the disorder (Criterion B). Although not part of the disorder-specific criteria (but part of the general personality disorder criteria), the individual also must have impairment of functioning that is stable across time (Criterion D) and consistent across situations (Criterion C), and the impairments must not be normative for the person's developmental stage or sociocultural environment (Criterion G) and must not be due to a substance or another medical condition (Criterion F). For individuals who do not fit within these diagnoses, the new category personality disorder—trait specified is used (replacing the DSM-IV category personality disorder not otherwise specified).

Categorical diagnosis is combined with an optional dimensional assessment of the individual's level of personality impairment and pathological personality traits (Krueger and Eaton 2010; Krueger et al. 2011). When impairments are present, the Level of Personality Functioning Scale can be used to assess degree of disturbance in self- and interpersonal functioning. Components of self-functioning involve identity and self-direction, whereas components of interpersonal functioning involve empathy and intimacy. Impairment is rated on a 5-point scale, ranging from 0 (healthy functioning) to 4 (poor functioning). Ratings can also be made for a broad range of adaptive and maladaptive personality trait domains and facets, to identify the nature and extent of personality pathology, information that may be helpful for treatment planning. The personality domains and trait facets can be used to describe the personality characteristics of any individual, even those without a personality disorder.

The work group drew on existing models of maladaptive personality traits and reached consensus on the broad domains of personality that the new system should encompass, influenced by McCrae and Costa's (1987) five-factor model. The five domains are negative affectivity, detachment, antagonism, disinhibition, and psychoticism. Each comprises a lower order of specific traits called *facets*. Trait facets are useful for representing personality variation *within* domains. For this reason, there are many more facets (25) than domains (which compares to the 79 personality disorder criteria in DSM-IV). One aim of the work group had been to condense this somewhat unwieldy number into a more manageable and reliable set of traits. Trait domains and facets are rated on a 4-point dimensional scale, ranging from 0 (very little or not descriptive at all) to 3 (extremely descriptive). Trait domains and their relevant trait facets are as follows:

- **Negative affectivity** (experiences negative emotions frequently and intensely): emotional lability, anxiousness, separation insecurity, perseveration, submissiveness, hostility, depressivity, suspiciousness, (lack of) restricted affectivity
- **Detachment** (withdrawal from other people and from social interactions): restricted affectivity, depressivity, suspiciousness, withdrawal, anhedonia, intimacy avoidance
- **Antagonism** (engaging in behaviors that put the person at odds with other people): manipulativeness, deceitfulness, grandiosity, attention seeking, callousness, hostility
- **Disinhibition** (engaging in behaviors on impulse, without reflecting on potential future consequences): irresponsibility, impulsivity, distractibility, risk taking, (lack of) rigid perfectionism
- **Psychoticism** (unusual and bizarre experiences): unusual beliefs and experiences, eccentricity, cognitive and perceptual dysregulation

The alternative model is designed to be flexible to suit the clinician's needs and interests. Clinicians can diagnose categorical personality disorders, diagnose personality disorder—trait specified for individuals who do not meet one of the six specified types, describe the heterogeneity at both the level of personality functioning and the level of pathological traits within personality disorder types, or describe personality trait profiles for all patients.

GENERAL CRITERIA FOR PERSONALITY DISORDER

A personality disorder diagnosis requires an assessment of level of personality impairment in two or more of four areas: identity, self-direction, empathy, and intimacy (Criterion A). The impairments must be "moderate or greater" as assessed with the Level of Personality Functioning Scale (Table 21–1). Pathological personality traits must be present that are disorder specific (Criterion B). The impairments in personality functioning and personality traits are relatively inflexible and pervasive across a broad range of personal and social situations (Criterion C); relatively stable across time, with onsets that can be traced back to at least adolescence or early adulthood (Criterion D); not better accounted for by another mental disorder (Criterion E); not attributable to the effects of a substance or of another medical condition (Criterion F); and not better understood as normal for an individual's developmental stage or sociocultural environment (Criterion G).

General Criteria for Personality Disorder

The essential features of a personality disorder are

A. Moderate or greater impairment in personality (self/interpersonal) functioning.
B. One or more pathological personality traits.
C. The impairments in personality functioning and the individual's personality trait expression are relatively inflexible and pervasive across a broad range of personal and social situations.
D. The impairments in personality functioning and the individual's personality trait expression are relatively stable across time, with onsets that can be traced back to at least adolescence or early adulthood.
E. The impairments in personality functioning and the individual's personality trait expression are not better explained by another mental disorder.
F. The impairments in personality functioning and the individual's personality trait expression are not solely attributable to the physiological effects of a substance or another medical condition (e.g., severe head trauma).
G. The impairments in personality functioning and the individual's personality trait expression are not better understood as normal for an individual's developmental stage or sociocultural environment.

All Section III personality disorders described by the criteria sets below also meet the general definition.

TABLE 21–1. **Level of Personality Functioning Scale**

Level of impairment	SELF		INTERPERSONAL	
	Identity	Self-direction	Empathy	Intimacy
0—Little or no impairment	Has ongoing awareness of a unique self; maintains role-appropriate boundaries. Has consistent and self-regulated positive self-esteem, with accurate self-appraisal. Is capable of experiencing, tolerating, and regulating a full range of emotions.	Sets and aspires to reasonable goals based on a realistic assessment of personal capacities. Utilizes appropriate standards of behavior, attaining fulfillment in multiple realms. Can reflect on, and make constructive meaning of, internal experience.	Is capable of accurately understanding others' experiences and motivations in most situations. Comprehends and appreciates others' perspectives, even if disagreeing. Is aware of the effect of own actions on others.	Maintains multiple satisfying and enduring relationships in personal and community life. Desires and engages in a number of caring, close, and reciprocal relationships. Strives for cooperation and mutual benefit and flexibly responds to a range of others' ideas, emotions, and behaviors.
1—Some impairment	Has relatively intact sense of self, with some decrease in clarity of boundaries when strong emotions and mental distress are experienced. Self-esteem diminished at times, with overly critical or somewhat distorted self-appraisal. Strong emotions may be distressing, associated with a restriction in range of emotional experience.	Is excessively goal-directed, somewhat goal-inhibited, or conflicted about goals. May have an unrealistic or socially inappropriate set of personal standards, limiting some aspects of fulfillment. Is able to reflect on internal experiences, but may overemphasize a single (e.g., intellectual, emotional) type of self-knowledge.	Is somewhat compromised in ability to appreciate and understand others' experiences; may tend to see others as having unreasonable expectations or a wish for control. Although capable of considering and understanding different perspectives, resists doing so. Has inconsistent awareness of effect of own behavior on others.	Is able to establish enduring relationships in personal and community life, with some limitations on degree of depth and satisfaction. Is capable of forming and desires to form intimate and reciprocal relationships, but may be inhibited in meaningful expression and sometimes constrained if intense emotions or conflicts arise. Cooperation may be inhibited by unrealistic standards; somewhat limited in ability to respect or respond to others' ideas, emotions, and behaviors.

TABLE 21–1. Level of Personality Functioning Scale (*continued*)

Level of impairment	SELF		INTERPERSONAL	
	Identity	Self-direction	Empathy	Intimacy
2—Moderate impairment	Depends excessively on others for identity definition, with compromised boundary delineation. Has vulnerable self-esteem controlled by exaggerated concern about external evaluation, with a wish for approval. Has sense of incompleteness or inferiority, with compensatory inflated, or deflated, self-appraisal. Emotional regulation depends on positive external appraisal. Threats to self-esteem may engender strong emotions such as rage or shame.	Goals are more often a means of gaining external approval than self-generated, and thus may lack coherence and/or stability. Personal standards may be unreasonably high (e.g., a need to be special or please others) or low (e.g., not consonant with prevailing social values). Fulfillment is compromised by a sense of lack of authenticity. Has impaired capacity to reflect on internal experience.	Is hyperattuned to the experience of others, but only with respect to perceived relevance to self. Is excessively self-referential; significantly compromised ability to appreciate and understand others' experiences and to consider alternative perspectives. Is generally unaware of or unconcerned about effect of own behavior on others, or unrealistic appraisal of own effect.	Is capable of forming and desires to form relationships in personal and community life, but connections may be largely superficial. Intimate relationships are predominantly based on meeting self-regulatory and self-esteem needs, with an unrealistic expectation of being perfectly understood by others. Tends not to view relationships in reciprocal terms, and cooperates predominantly for personal gain.

TABLE 21–1. Level of Personality Functioning Scale (*continued*)

Level of impairment	SELF		INTERPERSONAL	
	Identity	Self-direction	Empathy	Intimacy
3—Severe impairment	Has a weak sense of autonomy/agency; experience of a lack of identity, or emptiness. Boundary definition is poor or rigid: may show overidentification with others, overemphasis on independence from others, or vacillation between these. Fragile self-esteem is easily influenced by events, and self-image lacks coherence. Self-appraisal is un-nuanced: self-loathing, self-aggrandizing, or an illogical, unrealistic combination. Emotions may be rapidly shifting or a chronic, unwavering feeling of despair.	Has difficulty establishing and/or achieving personal goals. Internal standards for behavior are unclear or contradictory. Life is experienced as meaningless or dangerous. Has significantly compromised ability to reflect on and understand own mental processes.	Ability to consider and understand the thoughts, feelings, and behavior of other people is significantly limited; may discern very specific aspects of others' experience, particularly vulnerabilities and suffering. Is generally unable to consider alternative perspectives; highly threatened by differences of opinion or alternative viewpoints. Is confused about or unaware of impact of own actions on others; often bewildered about people's thoughts and actions, with destructive motivations frequently misattributed to others.	Has some desire to form relationships in community and personal life is present, but capacity for positive and enduring connections is significantly impaired. Relationships are based on a strong belief in the absolute need for the intimate other(s), and/or expectations of abandonment or abuse. Feelings about intimate involvement with others alternate between fear/rejection and desperate desire for connection. Little mutuality: others are conceptualized primarily in terms of how they affect the self (negatively or positively); cooperative efforts are often disrupted due to the perception of slights from others.

TABLE 21–1. Level of Personality Functioning Scale (continued)

Level of impairment	SELF		INTERPERSONAL	
	Identity	Self-direction	Empathy	Intimacy
4—Extreme impairment	Experience of a unique self and sense of agency/autonomy are virtually absent, or are organized around perceived external persecution. Boundaries with others are confused or lacking. Has weak or distorted self-image easily threatened by interactions with others; significant distortions and confusion around self-appraisal. Emotions not congruent with context or internal experience. Hatred and aggression may be dominant affects, although they may be disavowed and attributed to others.	Has poor differentiation of thoughts from actions, so goal-setting ability is severely compromised, with unrealistic or incoherent goals. Internal standards for behavior are virtually lacking. Genuine fulfillment is virtually inconceivable. Is profoundly unable to constructively reflect on own experience. Personal motivations may be unrecognized and/or experienced as external to self.	Has pronounced inability to consider and understand others' experience and motivation. Attention to others' perspectives is virtually absent (attention is hypervigilant, focused on need fulfillment and harm avoidance). Social interactions can be confusing and disorienting.	Desire for affiliation is limited because of profound disinterest or expectation of harm. Engagement with others is detached, disorganized, or consistently negative. Relationships are conceptualized almost exclusively in terms of their ability to provide comfort or inflict pain and suffering. Social/interpersonal behavior is not reciprocal; rather, it seeks fulfillment of basic needs or escape from pain.

SPECIFIC PERSONALITY DISORDERS

Section III includes diagnostic criteria for antisocial, avoidant, borderline, narcissistic, obsessive-compulsive, and schizotypal personality disorders. Each is defined by specific impairments in personality functioning (Criterion A) and characteristic pathological personality traits (Criterion B).

Antisocial Personality Disorder

Antisocial personality disorder is characterized by a failure to conform to lawful and ethical behavior and/or an egocentric, callous lack of concern for others, accompanied by deceitfulness, irresponsibility, manipulativeness, and/or risk taking.

Proposed Diagnostic Criteria for Antisocial Personality Disorder

---

A. Moderate or greater impairment in personality functioning, manifested by characteristic difficulties in two or more of the following four areas:

1. **Identity:** Egocentrism; self-esteem derived from personal gain, power, or pleasure.
2. **Self-direction:** Goal setting based on personal gratification; absence of prosocial internal standards, associated with failure to conform to lawful or culturally normative ethical behavior.
3. **Empathy:** Lack of concern for feelings, needs, or suffering of others; lack of remorse after hurting or mistreating another.
4. **Intimacy:** Incapacity for mutually intimate relationships, as exploitation is a primary means of relating to others, including by deceit and coercion; use of dominance or intimidation to control others.

B. Six or more of the following seven pathological personality traits:

1. **Manipulativeness** (an aspect of **Antagonism**): Frequent use of subterfuge to influence or control others; use of seduction, charm, glibness, or ingratiation to achieve one's ends.
2. **Callousness** (an aspect of **Antagonism**): Lack of concern for feelings or problems of others; lack of guilt or remorse about the negative or harmful effects of one's actions on others; aggression; sadism.
3. **Deceitfulness** (an aspect of **Antagonism**): Dishonesty and fraudulence; misrepresentation of self; embellishment or fabrication when relating events.
4. **Hostility** (an aspect of **Antagonism**): Persistent or frequent angry feelings; anger or irritability in response to minor slights and insults; mean, nasty, or vengeful behavior.
5. **Risk taking** (an aspect of **Disinhibition**): Engagement in dangerous, risky, and potentially self-damaging activities, unnecessarily and without regard for consequences; boredom proneness and thoughtless initiation of activities to counter

boredom; lack of concern for one's limitations and denial of the reality of personal danger.

6. ***Impulsivity*** (an aspect of **Disinhibition**): Acting on the spur of the moment in response to immediate stimuli; acting on a momentary basis without a plan or consideration of outcomes; difficulty establishing and following plans.

7. ***Irresponsibility*** (an aspect of **Disinhibition**): Disregard for—and failure to honor—financial and other obligations or commitments; lack of respect for—and lack of follow-through on—agreements and promises.

Note: The individual is at least 18 years of age.

Specify if:
   With psychopathic features.

Criterion A

The individual must have moderate or greater impairment in personality functioning in two or more of four areas: identity, self-direction, empathy, and intimacy. Individuals with antisocial personality disorder may exhibit a notable egocentrism bordering on grandiosity that may not be evident initially, and a concomitant sense of entitlement and invulnerability (A1). Self-esteem may be disproportionately high, leading to selfishness and overt or covert disregard for legal, moral, or cultural restrictions (A2). These individuals may show a lack of concern for others' feelings or needs or a frank lack of remorse (A3). Sometimes a form of indifference or emotional detachment emerges that is accompanied by the absence of empathy and inability to establish genuine intimacy (A4), although these characteristics may not be immediately noticeable in everyday social transactions or during an initial assessment.

Criterion B

This item requires endorsement of six or more of seven pathological personality traits. These include manipulativeness (B1), which can manifest as the deliberate use of subterfuge to control or influence others; callousness (B2), which can include lack of remorse or guilt and/or a lack of concern for the feelings of others; deceitfulness (B3), manifested as dishonesty and fraudulence, as well as misrepresentation of self and also embellishment and fabrication; hostility (B4), which includes persistent or frequent angry feelings or vengeful behavior; risk taking (B5), which includes participating in risky or dangerous behaviors; impulsivity (B6), which involves acting on the spur of the moment without regard for consequences; and irresponsibility (B7), which entails a disregard for financial and other commitments.

The individual must be at least 18 years old. The specifier "with psychopathic features" can be used to denote the presence of psychopathy, which describes a subset of persons with antisocial personality disorder characterized by "a lack of anxiety or fear and by a bold interpersonal style that may mask maladaptive behaviors" (American Psychiatric Association 2013, p. 765).

Avoidant Personality Disorder

Typical features of avoidant personality disorder are the avoidance of social situations and inhibition in interpersonal relationships related to feelings of ineptitude and inadequacy, anxious preoccupation with negative evaluation and rejection, and fears of ridicule or embarrassment.

Proposed Diagnostic Criteria for Avoidant Personality Disorder

A. Moderate or greater impairment in personality functioning, manifested by characteristic difficulties in two or more of the following four areas:

1. **Identity:** Low self-esteem associated with self-appraisal as socially inept, personally unappealing, or inferior; excessive feelings of shame.
2. **Self-direction:** Unrealistic standards for behavior associated with reluctance to pursue goals, take personal risks, or engage in new activities involving interpersonal contact.
3. **Empathy:** Preoccupation with, and sensitivity to, criticism or rejection, associated with distorted inference of others' perspectives as negative.
4. **Intimacy:** Reluctance to get involved with people unless being certain of being liked; diminished mutuality within intimate relationships because of fear of being shamed or ridiculed.

B. Three or more of the following four pathological personality traits, one of which must be (1) Anxiousness:

1. **Anxiousness** (an aspect of **Negative Affectivity**): Intense feelings of nervousness, tenseness, or panic, often in reaction to social situations; worry about the negative effects of past unpleasant experiences and future negative possibilities; feeling fearful, apprehensive, or threatened by uncertainty; fears of embarrassment.
2. **Withdrawal** (an aspect of **Detachment**): Reticence in social situations; avoidance of social contacts and activity; lack of initiation of social contact.
3. **Anhedonia** (an aspect of **Detachment**): Lack of enjoyment from, engagement in, or energy for life's experiences; deficits in the capacity to feel pleasure or take interest in things.
4. **Intimacy avoidance** (an aspect of **Detachment**): Avoidance of close or romantic relationships, interpersonal attachments, and intimate sexual relationships.

Criterion A

The individual must have moderate or greater impairment in personality functioning in two or more of four areas: identity, self-direction, empathy, and intimacy. Individuals with avoidant personality disorder may have low self-esteem and see themselves as socially inept, personally unappealing, or inferior and sometimes have excessive feelings of shame or inadequacy (A1). These individuals may be averse to taking personal risk or engaging in new activities that involve interpersonal contact. This can lead them to avoid engaging in anything new or challenging that is outside their comfort zone (A2). They may be so preoccupied with the potential for negative social evaluation that they find it difficult to empathize with the actual feelings or perspectives of others (A3). These individuals may avoid even casual involvement with others and rarely develop close personal relationships because of their conviction that anyone who came to know them well would recognize their inadequacy and reject them (A4).

Criterion B

This item requires endorsement of three or more of four items. Individuals with avoidant personality disorder are often very anxious in social situations and worry about the negative effects of past unpleasant experiences (B1). This may lead them to avoid social situations or other activities that involve dealing with others. They may prefer to spend time alone rather than with others, and may prefer to maintain emotional distance from others and have minimal engagement with others when social contact is necessary (B2). Avoidance extends to positive emotions as well. Individuals with avoidant personality disorder may lack interest in and claim not to derive pleasure from activities that most people do. They may see themselves as unenergetic and unenthusiastic, and they may acknowledge that they do not try to live full lives and do not enjoy their day-to-day activities or even life itself (B3). Intimate relationships in particular are avoided. Such people may disavow interest in romantic attachments and sexual relationships and often distance themselves from any relationship that begins to get close (B4).

Borderline Personality Disorder

Borderline personality disorder is characterized by instability of self-image, personal goals, interpersonal relationships, and affects, accompanied by impulsivity, risk-taking, and/or hostility.

Proposed Diagnostic Criteria for Borderline Personality Disorder

---

A. Moderate or greater impairment in personality functioning, manifested by characteristic difficulties in two or more of the following four areas:

1. **Identity:** Markedly impoverished, poorly developed, or unstable self-image, often associated with excessive self-criticism; chronic feelings of emptiness; dissociative states under stress.
2. **Self-direction:** Instability in goals, aspirations, values, or career plans.
3. **Empathy:** Compromised ability to recognize the feelings and needs of others associated with interpersonal hypersensitivity (i.e., prone to feel slighted or insulted); perceptions of others selectively biased toward negative attributes or vulnerabilities.

4. ***Intimacy:*** Intense, unstable, and conflicted close relationships, marked by mistrust, neediness, and anxious preoccupation with real or imagined abandonment; close relationships often viewed in extremes of idealization and devaluation and alternating between overinvolvement and withdrawal.

B. Four or more of the following seven pathological personality traits, at least one of which must be (5) Impulsivity, (6) Risk taking, or (7) Hostility:

1. ***Emotional lability*** (an aspect of **Negative Affectivity**): Unstable emotional experiences and frequent mood changes; emotions that are easily aroused, intense, and/or out of proportion to events and circumstances.

2. ***Anxiousness*** (an aspect of **Negative Affectivity**): Intense feelings of nervousness, tenseness, or panic, often in reaction to interpersonal stresses; worry about the negative effects of past unpleasant experiences and future negative possibilities; feeling fearful, apprehensive, or threatened by uncertainty; fears of falling apart or losing control.

3. ***Separation insecurity*** (an aspect of **Negative Affectivity**): Fears of rejection by—and/or separation from—significant others, associated with fears of excessive dependency and complete loss of autonomy.

4. ***Depressivity*** (an aspect of **Negative Affectivity**): Frequent feelings of being down, miserable, and/or hopeless; difficulty recovering from such moods; pessimism about the future; pervasive shame; feelings of inferior self-worth; thoughts of suicide and suicidal behavior.

5. ***Impulsivity*** (an aspect of **Disinhibition**): Acting on the spur of the moment in response to immediate stimuli; acting on a momentary basis without a plan or consideration of outcomes; difficulty establishing or following plans; a sense of urgency and self-harming behavior under emotional distress.

6. ***Risk taking*** (an aspect of **Disinhibition**): Engagement in dangerous, risky, and potentially self-damaging activities, unnecessarily and without regard to consequences; lack of concern for one's limitations and denial of the reality of personal danger.

7. ***Hostility*** (an aspect of **Antagonism**): Persistent or frequent angry feelings; anger or irritability in response to minor slights and insults.

Criterion A

The individual must have moderate or greater impairment in personality functioning in two or more of four areas: identity, self-direction, empathy, and intimacy. Individuals with borderline personality disorder may have a markedly unstable and often negative self-image (Criterion A1), with dramatic shifts in self-direction, including goals, values, and aspirations (A2). These individuals are often interpersonally hypersensitive and have difficulty trusting others, yet they have an intolerance of being alone. They may appear to have empathy for others, but the apparent empathy may quickly evaporate if they feel their own needs are not being met (A3). Interpersonal relationships are often unstable and intense. This may lead these individuals to overidealize romantic partners on the first or second meeting, leading to demands to spend a lot of time together and to share the most intimate details of their own lives very early in a relationship (A4).

Criterion B

This item requires endorsement of four or more of seven items, at least one of which must be impulsivity, risk taking, or hostility. Individuals with borderline personality disorder may experience a marked affective instability due to marked reactivity of mood that is out of proportion to actual events or circumstances (B1). These individuals may experience intense feelings of anxiety, often in response to personal stresses (B2). They often experience intense fears of rejection by or separation from significant others that may be associated with significant despondency (B3). Dysphoric mood is common, with frequent feelings of despair and hopelessness that may lead to suicidal thoughts or behaviors (B4). Recurrent suicidality may be the reason these individuals seek help. Individuals with this disorder are often impulsive, acting on the spur of the moment, often in response to immediate stimuli (B5). This can lead them to abuse substances, engage in unsafe sex, drive dangerously, or engage in other risky behaviors (B6). They have difficulty controlling their anger and may display extreme sarcasm, bitterness, or verbal outbursts, even in response to minor slights or insults (B7).

Narcissistic Personality Disorder

Narcissistic personality disorder is typically characterized by variable and vulnerable self-esteem, with attempts at regulation through attention seeking and approval seeking and either overt or covert grandiosity.

Proposed Diagnostic Criteria for Narcissistic Personality Disorder

A. Moderate or greater impairment in personality functioning, manifested by characteristic difficulties in two or more of the following four areas:
1. **Identity:** Excessive reference to others for self-definition and self-esteem regulation; exaggerated self-appraisal inflated or deflated, or vacillating between extremes; emotional regulation mirrors fluctuations in self-esteem.
2. **Self-direction:** Goal setting based on gaining approval from others; personal standards unreasonably high in order to see oneself as exceptional, or too low based on a sense of entitlement; often unaware of own motivations.
3. **Empathy:** Impaired ability to recognize or identify with the feelings and needs of others; excessively attuned to reactions of others, but only if perceived as relevant to self; over- or underestimation of own effect on others.
4. **Intimacy:** Relationships largely superficial and exist to serve self-esteem regulation; mutuality constrained by little genuine interest in others' experiences and predominance of a need for personal gain.
B. Both of the following pathological personality traits:
1. **Grandiosity** (an aspect of **Antagonism**): Feelings of entitlement, either overt or covert; self-centeredness; firmly holding to the belief that one is better than others; condescension toward others.

2. ***Attention seeking*** (an aspect of **Antagonism**): Excessive attempts to attract and be the focus of the attention of others; admiration seeking.

Criterion A

The individual must have moderate or greater impairment in personality functioning in two or more of four areas: identity, self-direction, empathy, and intimacy. There may be a pervasive sense of exaggerated self-importance and appraisal (A1). Individuals with this disorder may exhibit a sense of entitlement (A2) and have little ability to recognize the feelings of others (A3). Relationships may seem very superficial and self-serving (A4).

Criterion B

This item requires endorsement of two pathological personality traits: grandiosity and attention seeking. A core characteristic of individuals with narcissistic personality disorder is the regulation of self-esteem by resorting to grandiose strategies of overcompensation, which may include feelings of entitlement, self-centeredness, and the belief that one is better than others (B1). These individuals display an overreliance on seeking attention and admiration from others or seeking to be the focus of attention by others (B2).

Obsessive-Compulsive Personality Disorder

Obsessive-compulsive personality disorder is typically characterized by difficulties in establishing and sustaining close relationships, associated with a rigid perfectionism, inflexibility, and restricted emotional expression.

Proposed Diagnostic Criteria for Obsessive-Compulsive Personality Disorder

A. Moderate or greater impairment in personality functioning, manifested by characteristic difficulties in two or more of the following four areas:

1. ***Identity:*** Sense of self derived predominantly from work or productivity; constricted experience and expression of strong emotions.
2. ***Self-direction:*** Difficulty completing tasks and realizing goals, associated with rigid and unreasonably high and inflexible internal standards of behavior; overly conscientious and moralistic attitudes.
3. ***Empathy:*** Difficulty understanding and appreciating the ideas, feelings, or behaviors of others.
4. ***Intimacy:*** Relationships seen as secondary to work and productivity; rigidity and stubbornness negatively affect relationships with others.

B. Three or more of the following four pathological personality traits, one of which must be (1) Rigid perfectionism:

1. ***Rigid perfectionism*** (an aspect of extreme Conscientiousness [the opposite pole of Detachment]): Rigid insistence on everything being flawless, perfect,

and without errors or faults, including one's own and others' performance; sacrificing of timeliness to ensure correctness in every detail; believing that there is only one right way to do things; difficulty changing ideas and/or viewpoint; preoccupation with details, organization, and order.

2. *Perseveration* (an aspect of **Negative Affectivity**): Persistence at tasks long after the behavior has ceased to be functional or effective; continuance of the same behavior despite repeated failures.

3. *Intimacy avoidance* (an aspect of **Detachment**): Avoidance of close or romantic relationships, interpersonal attachments, and intimate sexual relationships.

4. *Restricted affectivity* (an aspect of **Detachment**): Little reaction to emotionally arousing situations; constricted emotional experience and expression; indifference or coldness.

Criterion A

The individual must have moderate or greater impairment in personality functioning in two or more of four areas: identity, self-direction, empathy, and intimacy. Individuals with this disorder may have an excessive devotion to work or productivity, with constricted expression of emotions (A1). These individuals may attempt to maintain a sense of control through a rigid preoccupation with order and detail, to the extent that the major goal of attempted activities is often not achieved (A2). They may have difficulty understanding and appreciating the feelings of others (A3). These traits may lead these individuals to value work and productivity over personal relationships, which are viewed as of secondary importance (A4).

Criterion B

This item requires endorsement of three or more of four items, one of which must be rigid perfectionism. The individual may be overly focused on achieving perfection, often believing that there is only one right way to do things (B1). Activities are often overly methodical because the individual is overly concerned with time, punctuality, schedules, and rules. The individual may persist at tasks despite repeated failures, even when a behavior has ceased to be functional or effective (B2). The rigid approach to tasks, problems, and people results in limited capacity to adapt to changing demands or circumstances. The need to complete tasks perfectly may result in a paralysis of indecision, such that important tasks may never be completed. These individuals lack appreciation of the impact of their own behaviors on the thoughts and emotions of other people, which may contribute to their avoidance or lack of romantic relationships, friendships, or even sexual intimacy (B3, B4).

Schizotypal Personality Disorder

Schizotypal personality disorder is typically characterized by impairments in the capacity for social and close relationships and eccentricities in cognition, perception, and behavior that are associated with distorted self-image and incoherent personal goals and accompanied by suspiciousness and restricted emotional expression.

Proposed Diagnostic Criteria for Schizotypal Personality Disorder

A. Moderate or greater impairment in personality functioning, manifested by characteristic difficulties in two or more of the following four areas:

1. ***Identity:*** Confused boundaries between self and others; distorted self-concept; emotional expression often not congruent with context or internal experience.
2. ***Self-direction:*** Unrealistic or incoherent goals; no clear set of internal standards.
3. ***Empathy:*** Pronounced difficulty understanding impact of own behaviors on others; frequent misinterpretations of others' motivations and behaviors.
4. ***Intimacy:*** Marked impairments in developing close relationships, associated with mistrust and anxiety.

B. Four or more of the following six pathological personality traits:

1. ***Cognitive and perceptual dysregulation*** (an aspect of **Psychoticism**): Odd or unusual thought processes; vague, circumstantial, metaphorical, over-elaborate, or stereotyped thought or speech; odd sensations in various sensory modalities.
2. ***Unusual beliefs and experiences*** (an aspect of **Psychoticism**): Thought content and views of reality that are viewed by others as bizarre or idiosyncratic; unusual experiences of reality.
3. ***Eccentricity*** (an aspect of **Psychoticism**): Odd, unusual, or bizarre behavior or appearance; saying unusual or inappropriate things.
4. ***Restricted affectivity*** (an aspect of **Detachment**): Little reaction to emotionally arousing situations; constricted emotional experience and expression; indifference or coldness.
5. ***Withdrawal*** (an aspect of **Detachment**): Preference for being alone to being with others; reticence in social situations; avoidance of social contacts and activity; lack of initiation of social contact.
6. ***Suspiciousness*** (an aspect of **Detachment**): Expectations of—and heightened sensitivity to—signs of interpersonal ill-intent or harm; doubts about loyalty and fidelity of others; feelings of persecution.

Criterion A

The individual must have moderate or greater impairment in personality functioning in two or more of four areas: identity, self-direction, empathy, and intimacy. Individuals with schizotypal personality disorder may have confused boundaries between self and others, distorted self-concept, and emotional expression that is not congruent with context or internal experience (A1). Impairments in self-direction include unrealistic or incoherent goals and having no clear set of internal standards (A2). Problems with empathy may include pronounced difficulty understanding the impact of their own behaviors on others and misinterpretations of others' motivations and behaviors (A3). Problems with intimacy may include marked impairments in developing close relationships, associated with mistrust and anxiety (A4).

Criterion B

This item requires endorsement of four or more of six items. Individuals with schizotypal personality disorder often have pronounced pathological personality traits in the area of psychoticism because they are prone to psychotic-like experiences such as having unusual thought processes or magical beliefs or they may display vague or digressive speech (B1, B2). These individuals are considered by others to be odd or eccentric, and they may display bizarre behaviors or make odd statements (B3). Restricted affectivity can be of concern, and the individual may have little reaction to emotionally stimulating events (B4). Social withdrawal is common; the individual displays reticence in social situations or simply prefers to be alone (B5). Suspiciousness is commonly experienced. The individual may be hypervigilant and suspect others as having negative or harmful intentions toward him or her (B6).

Personality Disorder—Trait Specified

Personality disorder—trait specified replaces the DSM-IV diagnosis personality disorder not otherwise specified. This is a residual category for persons with personality disorders that do not meet criteria for one of the specific disorders. Rather than leaving the nature of the personality disorder unspecified, the clinician can specify the individual's personality disorder. Both the personality domain and trait facet levels allow a detailed assessment of the individual's personality features. For example, two people may be similar because they both have extreme disinhibition, but they may differ in that only one of them also manifests psychoticism with unusual beliefs and experiences.

Proposed Diagnostic Criteria for Personality Disorder—Trait Specified

---

A. Moderate or greater impairment in personality functioning, manifested by difficulties in two or more of the following four areas:
   1. *Identity*
   2. *Self-direction*
   3. *Empathy*
   4. *Intimacy*

B. One or more pathological personality trait domains OR specific trait facets within domains, considering ALL of the following domains:
   1. **Negative Affectivity** (vs. Emotional Stability): Frequent and intense experiences of high levels of a wide range of negative emotions (e.g., anxiety, de-

pression, guilt/shame, worry, anger), and their behavioral (e.g., self-harm) and interpersonal (e.g., dependency) manifestations.

2. **Detachment** (vs. Extraversion): Avoidance of socioemotional experience, including both withdrawal from interpersonal interactions, ranging from casual, daily interactions to friendships to intimate relationships, as well as restricted affective experience and expression, particularly limited hedonic capacity.

3. **Antagonism** (vs. Agreeableness): Behaviors that put the individual at odds with other people, including an exaggerated sense of self-importance and a concomitant expectation of special treatment, as well as a callous antipathy toward others, encompassing both unawareness of others' needs and feelings, and a readiness to use others in the service of self-enhancement.

4. **Disinhibition** (vs. Conscientiousness): Orientation toward immediate gratification, leading to impulsive behavior driven by current thoughts, feelings, and external stimuli, without regard for past learning or consideration of future consequences.

5. **Psychoticism** (vs. Lucidity): Exhibiting a wide range of culturally incongruent odd, eccentric, or unusual behaviors and cognitions, including both process (e.g., perception, dissociation) and content (e.g., beliefs).

Criteria A and B

The individual must have moderate or greater impairment in two or more of four areas: identity, self-direction, empathy, and intimacy (Criterion A). The clinician should endorse one or more of five pathological trait domains or specific trait facets within domains (Criterion B). This approach allows the clinician to take a broad perspective and record the person's prominent maladaptive personality features. He or she can simply record which of the five personality trait domains characterize an individual, or choose to specify more detailed features and record which of the trait facets (within the domains) are most characteristic. The decision to use this category depends on the needs of the clinical situation.

CHAPTER 22

Conditions for Further Study

Attenuated Psychosis Syndrome
Depressive Episodes With Short-Duration Hypomania
Persistent Complex Bereavement Disorder
Caffeine Use Disorder
Internet Gaming Disorder
Neurobehavioral Disorder Associated With Prenatal Alcohol Exposure
Suicidal Behavior Disorder
Nonsuicidal Self-Injury

Section III of DSM-5 includes eight proposed disorders that may be included in future DSM editions (Table 22–1). In this section, the DSM-5 authors provide an opportunity for establishing standardized criteria to facilitate research that might indicate whether a disorder should eventually be included as an official diagnosis. Inclusion of these criteria sets is "intended to provide a common language for researchers and clinicians who are interested in studying these disorders" (American Psychiatric Association 2013, p. 783). It is hoped that this will stimulate research that may allow the field to better understand these conditions and inform decisions about their placement in future DSM editions.

Placing provisional disorders in the manual began with DSM-III-R, which included Appendix A, "Proposed Diagnostic Categories Needing Further Study." Three criteria sets were included: late luteal phase dysphoric disorder, sadistic personality disorder, and self-defeating personality disorder. Of these three, only late luteal phase dysphoric disorder has gained the requisite recognition and research support. It is included (with modification) in DSM-5 as premenstrual dysphoric disorder.

DSM-IV included 26 criteria sets, revised criteria, and axes in a much expanded Appendix B ("Criteria Sets and Axes Provided for Further Study"). Each had been recommended for inclusion in DSM-IV, but the task force concluded that insufficient

---

TABLE 22–1. DSM-5 criteria sets for conditions for further study

---

Attenuated psychosis syndrome

Depressive episodes with short-duration hypomania

Persistent complex bereavement disorder

Caffeine use disorder

Internet gaming disorder

Neurobehavioral disorder associated with prenatal alcohol exposure

Suicidal behavior disorder

Nonsuicidal self-injury

---

data existed to warrant their inclusion as official categories or axes. These included proposed diagnoses (e.g., postconcussional disorder, dissociative trance disorder), criteria (e.g., alternative Criterion B for dysthymic disorder), and axes (Defensive Functioning Scale).

Of the conditions included in DSM-IV Appendix B, several have become standalone diagnoses in DSM-5, a fact that demonstrates the utility of providing criteria to stimulate research. Postconcussional disorder and mild neurocognitive disorder are included in DSM-5, although the former has been reformulated as neurocognitive disorder due to traumatic brain injury. Caffeine withdrawal, premenstrual dysphoric disorder, factitious disorder by proxy (now factitious disorder imposed on another), and binge-eating disorder are also included, in each instance with edits to their respective criteria. On the other hand, several proposed disorders did not make the cut: postpsychotic depressive disorder of schizophrenia, simple deteriorative disorder (simple schizophrenia), minor depressive disorder, recurrent brief depressive disorder, mixed anxiety-depressive disorder, dissociative trance disorder, depressive personality disorder, and passive-aggressive personality disorder (negativistic personality disorder).

Attenuated Psychosis Syndrome

The Psychotic Disorders Work Group proposed the new diagnosis attenuated psychosis syndrome. The rationale is to identify persons at risk for schizophrenia in order to facilitate early identification and treatment to improve outcomes. The syndrome consists of mild psychotic-like symptoms and clinically relevant distress and impairment. Conversion to schizophrenia or some other full-blown psychosis is a possible outcome and occurs in a significant minority of individuals. Because the syndrome is most often seen as a comorbid disorder, it is not clear whether it represents a distinct disorder or rather a trait or state vulnerability for increased risk of development of a psychotic disorder. Another concern is that it appears to overlap with schizotypal personality disorder, and it is not clear how the conditions relate.

The proposed diagnosis became a focus of controversy during the development of DSM-5. Critics within and outside the field expressed concern that the diagnosis would result in psychiatric labeling of persons who are not ill and who in most cases would never develop a psychotic disorder, and would lead to unnecessary and costly interventions. This could include the increased use of off-label antipsychotics, putting patients at risk for iatrogenic complications (e.g., weight gain, metabolic disorders, movement disorders).

Proposed Criteria for Attenuated Psychosis Syndrome

A. At least one of the following symptoms is present in attenuated form, with relatively intact reality testing, and is of sufficient severity or frequency to warrant clinical attention:
   1. Delusions.
   2. Hallucinations.
   3. Disorganized speech.
B. Symptom(s) must have been present at least once per week for the past month.
C. Symptom(s) must have begun or worsened in the past year.
D. Symptom(s) is sufficiently distressing and disabling to the individual to warrant clinical attention.
E. Symptom(s) is not better explained by another mental disorder, including a depressive or bipolar disorder with psychotic features, and is not attributable to the physiological effects of a substance or another medical condition.
F. Criteria for any psychotic disorder have never been met.

Depressive Episodes With Short-Duration Hypomania

Individuals with short-duration hypomania have experienced at least one major depressive episode as well as at least two episodes of 2–3 days' duration in which criteria for a hypomanic episode were met except for symptom duration. The symptoms represent a noticeable change in the individual's normal behavior.

The Mood Disorders Work Group proposed the diagnosis to recognize that people who have experienced short-duration hypomania and a major depressive episode, with their increased comorbidity with substance use disorders and greater history of bipolar disorder, more closely resembles individuals with bipolar disorder that those with major depressive disorder. It is estimated that 2.8% of the general population experience short-duration hypomania, and the prevalence seems greater in women.

While the proposed criteria would fill a diagnostic gap for those with short-duration hypomania, the diagnosis could lead to confusion with bipolar II disorder, major depressive disorder with mixed features, or cyclothymic disorder. The condition could also be confused with borderline personality disorder, in which affective instability is a common symptom.

Proposed Criteria for Depressive Episodes With Short-Duration Hypomania

Lifetime experience of at least one major depressive episode meeting the following criteria:

A. Five (or more) of the following criteria have been present during the same 2-week period and represent a change from previous functioning; at least one of the symptoms is either (1) depressed mood or (2) loss of interest or pleasure. (**Note:** Do not include symptoms that are clearly attributable to a medical condition.)

   1. Depressed mood most of the day, nearly every day, as indicated by either subjective report (e.g., feels sad, empty, or hopeless) or observation made by others (e.g., appears tearful). (**Note:** In children and adolescents, can be irritable mood.)
   2. Markedly diminished interest or pleasure in all, or almost all, activities most of the day, nearly every day (as indicated by either subjective account or observation).
   3. Significant weight loss when not dieting or weight gain (e.g., a change of more than 5% of body weight in a month), or decrease or increase in appetite nearly every day. (**Note:** In children, consider failure to make expected weight gain.)
   4. Insomnia or hypersomnia nearly every day.
   5. Psychomotor agitation or retardation nearly every day (observable by others, not merely subjective feelings of restlessness or being slowed down).
   6. Fatigue or loss of energy nearly every day.
   7. Feelings of worthlessness or excessive or inappropriate guilt (which may be delusional) nearly every day (not merely self-reproach or guilt about being sick).
   8. Diminished ability to think or concentrate, or indecisiveness, nearly every day (either by subjective account or as observed by others).
   9. Recurrent thoughts of death (not just fear of dying), recurrent suicidal ideation without a specific plan, or a suicide attempt or a specific plan for committing suicide.

B. The symptoms cause clinically significant distress or impairment in social, occupational, or other important areas of functioning.

C. The disturbance is not attributable to the physiological effects of a substance or another medical condition.

D. The disturbance is not better explained by schizoaffective disorder and is not superimposed on schizophrenia, schizophreniform disorder, delusional disorder, or other specified or unspecified schizophrenia spectrum and other psychotic disorder.

At least two lifetime episodes of hypomanic periods that involve the required criterion symptoms below but are of insufficient duration (at least 2 days but less than 4 consecutive days) to meet criteria for a hypomanic episode. The criterion symptoms are as follows:

A. A distinct period of abnormally and persistently elevated, expansive, or irritable mood and abnormally and persistently increased activity or energy.

B. During the period of mood disturbance and increased energy and activity, three (or more) of the following symptoms have persisted (four if the mood is only irritable), represent a noticeable change from usual behavior, and have been present to a significant degree:

1. Inflated self-esteem or grandiosity.
2. Decreased need for sleep (e.g., feels rested after only 3 hours of sleep).
3. More talkative than usual or pressured to keep talking.
4. Flight of ideas or subjective experience that thoughts are racing.
5. Distractibility (i.e., attention too easily drawn to unimportant or irrelevant external stimuli), as reported or observed.
6. Increase in goal-directed activity (either socially, at work or school, or sexually) or psychomotor agitation.
7. Excessive involvement in activities that have a high potential for painful consequences (e.g., the individual engages in unrestrained buying sprees, sexual indiscretions, or foolish business investments).

C. The episode is associated with an unequivocal change in functioning that is uncharacteristic of the individual when not symptomatic.
D. The disturbance in mood and the change in functioning are observable by others.
E. The episode is not severe enough to cause marked impairment in social or occupational functioning or to necessitate hospitalization. If there are psychotic features, the episode is, by definition, manic.
F. The episode is not attributable to the physiological effects of a substance (e.g., a drug of abuse, a medication or other treatment).

Persistent Complex Bereavement Disorder

The Anxiety, Obsessive-Compulsive Spectrum, Posttraumatic, and Dissociative Disorders Work Group proposed persistent complex bereavement disorder as a new diagnosis on the basis of research showing that people who experience "prolonged" or "complicated" grief after loss of a close family member or friend have significant distress or functional impairment compared with persons who experience normal grief reactions. The work group believes that such conditions are not adequately covered in DSM.

Proposed Criteria for Persistent Complex Bereavement Disorder

A. The individual experienced the death of someone with whom he or she had a close relationship.
B. Since the death, at least one of the following symptoms is experienced on more days than not and to a clinically significant degree and has persisted for at least 12 months after the death in the case of bereaved adults and 6 months for bereaved children:

1. Persistent yearning/longing for the deceased. In young children, yearning may be expressed in play and behavior, including behaviors that reflect being separated from, and also reuniting with, a caregiver or other attachment figure.
2. Intense sorrow and emotional pain in response to the death.
3. Preoccupation with the deceased.
4. Preoccupation with the circumstances of the death. In children, this preoccupation with the deceased may be expressed through the themes of play and behavior and may extend to preoccupation with possible death of others close to them.

C. Since the death, at least six of the following symptoms are experienced on more days than not and to a clinically significant degree, and have persisted for at least 12 months after the death in the case of bereaved adults and 6 months for bereaved children:

Reactive distress to the death

1. Marked difficulty accepting the death. In children, this is dependent on the child's capacity to comprehend the meaning and permanence of death.
2. Experiencing disbelief or emotional numbness over the loss.
3. Difficulty with positive reminiscing about the deceased.
4. Bitterness or anger related to the loss.
5. Maladaptive appraisals about oneself in relation to the deceased or the death (e.g., self-blame).
6. Excessive avoidance of reminders of the loss (e.g., avoidance of individuals, places, or situations associated with the deceased; in children, this may include avoidance of thoughts and feelings regarding the deceased).

Social/identity disruption

7. A desire to die in order to be with the deceased.
8. Difficulty trusting other individuals since the death.
9. Feeling alone or detached from other individuals since the death.
10. Feeling that life is meaningless or empty without the deceased, or the belief that one cannot function without the deceased.
11. Confusion about one's role in life, or a diminished sense of one's identity (e.g., feeling that a part of oneself died with the deceased).
12. Difficulty or reluctance to pursue interests since the loss or to plan for the future (e.g., friendships, activities).

D. The disturbance causes clinically significant distress or impairment in social, occupational, or other important areas of functioning.
E. The bereavement reaction is out of proportion to or inconsistent with cultural, religious, or age-appropriate norms.

Specify if:

With traumatic bereavement: Bereavement due to homicide or suicide with persistent distressing preoccupations regarding the traumatic nature of the death (often in response to loss reminders), including the deceased's last moments, degree of suffering and mutilating injury, or the malicious or intentional nature of the death.

Caffeine Use Disorder

The Substance-Related Disorders Work Group proposed inclusion of caffeine use disorder. Data show that a substantial proportion of chronic caffeine users develop features of substance dependence: continued use despite physical or psychological harm, unsuccessful efforts to cut down or quit, and continued use to avoid withdrawal symptoms. Establishing a caffeine use disorder diagnosis would increase recognition of the syndrome among health care providers and the general population. Recognition could lead to the development of specific cessation strategies and interventions that could benefit a large number of individuals. On the other hand, critics suggest that recognizing this disorder might trivialize substance use disorders in general because its prevalence would potentially include a large proportion of the adult general population.

Proposed Criteria for Caffeine Use Disorder

A problematic pattern of caffeine use leading to clinically significant impairment or distress, as manifested by at least the first three of the following criteria occurring within a 12-month period:

1. A persistent desire or unsuccessful efforts to cut down or control caffeine use.
2. Continued caffeine use despite knowledge of having a persistent or recurrent physical or psychological problem that is likely to have been caused or exacerbated by caffeine.
3. Withdrawal, as manifested by either of the following:
    a. The characteristic withdrawal syndrome for caffeine.
    b. Caffeine (or a closely related) substance is taken to relieve or avoid withdrawal symptoms.
4. Caffeine is often taken in larger amounts or over a longer period than was intended.
5. Recurrent caffeine use resulting in a failure to fulfill major role obligations at work, school, or home (e.g., repeated tardiness or absences from work or school related to caffeine use or withdrawal).
6. Continued caffeine use despite having persistent or recurrent social or interpersonal problems caused or exacerbated by the effects of caffeine (e.g., arguments with spouse about consequences of use, medical problems, cost).
7. Tolerance, as defined by either of the following:
    a. A need for markedly increased amounts of caffeine to achieve desired effect.
    b. Markedly diminished effect with continued use of the same amount of caffeine.
8. A great deal of time is spent in activities necessary to obtain caffeine, use caffeine, or recover from its effects.
9. Craving or a strong desire or urge to use caffeine.

Internet Gaming Disorder

Criteria were proposed by the Substance-Related Disorders Work Group to recognize a new and rapidly expanding condition made possible by modern technology. Internet gaming disorder consists of excessive and/or inappropriate use of the Internet to engage in games, often with other players. Although this condition is relatively common, with many reports from Asian countries, work group members argued that it is not adequately represented DSM. Internet gaming disorder is possible only in societies where computers are available and the Internet is accessible. For this reason, it shows the clear influence of cultural and technological change on socially sanctioned behavior taken to its extreme. Despite its newness, the disorder captures the same common clinical features that link it to the substance addictions: repetitive and driven behaviors despite negative consequences, diminished control over the behaviors, cravings for the behavior, and experiencing a pleasurable response while engaged in the behavior. Symptoms of tolerance and withdrawal, similar to those seen with substance use disorders, have also been reported.

Discussion regarding including this syndrome during the development of DSM-5 sparked debate among professionals and the lay public. Some believe that its inclusion would medicalize bad behavior and potentially lead to including other so-called behavioral addictions in future editions of DSM (e.g., compulsive shopping, overeating, hypersexual behavior). Others suggest that the concept is overly narrow, and a broader category of "Internet addiction" or "compulsive computer use" should have been proposed.

Proposed Criteria for Internet Gaming Disorder

Persistent and recurrent use of the Internet to engage in games, often with other players, leading to clinically significant impairment or distress as indicated by five (or more) of the following in a 12-month period:

1. Preoccupation with Internet games. (The individual thinks about previous gaming activity or anticipates playing the next game; Internet gaming becomes the dominant activity in daily life).
   Note: This disorder is distinct from Internet gambling, which is included under gambling disorder.
2. Withdrawal symptoms when Internet gaming is taken away. (These symptoms are typically described as irritability, anxiety, or sadness, but there are no physical signs of pharmacological withdrawal.)
3. Tolerance—the need to spend increasing amounts of time engaged in Internet games.
4. Unsuccessful attempts to control the participation in Internet games.
5. Loss of interests in previous hobbies and entertainment as a result of, and with the exception of, Internet games.
6. Continued excessive use of Internet games despite knowledge of psychosocial problems.
7. Has deceived family members, therapists, or others regarding the amount of Internet gaming.

8. Use of Internet games to escape or relieve a negative mood (e.g., feelings of help-lessness, guilt, anxiety).
9. Has jeopardized or lost a significant relationship, job, or educational or career op-portunity because of participation in Internet games.

Note: Only nongambling Internet games are included in this disorder. Use of the In-ternet for required activities in a business or profession is not included; nor is the dis-order intended to include other recreational or social Internet use. Similarly, sexual Internet sites are excluded.

Specify current severity:

Internet gaming disorder can be mild, moderate, or severe depending on the degree of disruption of normal activities. Individuals with less severe Internet gaming disorder may exhibit fewer symptoms and less disruption of their lives. Those with severe Inter-net gaming disorder will have more hours spent on the computer and more severe loss of relationships or career or school opportunities.

Neurobehavioral Disorder Associated With Prenatal Alcohol Exposure

The Substance-Related Disorders Work Group proposed criteria for neurobehavioral disorder associated with prenatal alcohol exposure to encompass a full range of de-velopmental disabilities associated with in utero exposure to alcohol. The proposed condition is a behavioral and psychological syndrome that creates clinically signifi-cant distress and impairment.

The rationale for including this condition is to boost the recognition of persons nega-tively impacted by prenatal alcohol exposure and to facilitate treatment referral. These in-dividuals are overrepresented, although generally unrecognized, in the child welfare system, juvenile detention and correctional facilities, and both outpatient and inpatient psychiatric settings. Including this condition in DSM could boost recognition and referral for appropriate care by mental health, educational, and criminal justice systems. On the downside, some would argue that its symptoms are adequately captured in DSM and that clinicians simply need to be alert to the symptoms. Another concern is that the diag-nosis presumes a causal association with alcohol, which is difficult to prove. The symp-toms are wide ranging and overlap with those of many disorders—including conduct disorder and antisocial personality disorder—that are not specifically excluded.

Proposed Criteria for Neurobehavioral Disorder Associated With Prenatal Alcohol Exposure

A. More than minimal exposure to alcohol during gestation, including prior to preg-nancy recognition. Confirmation of gestational exposure to alcohol may be ob-tained from maternal self-report of alcohol use in pregnancy, medical or other records, or clinical observation.
B. Impaired neurocognitive functioning as manifested by one or more of the following:

1. Impairment in global intellectual performance (i.e., IQ of 70 or below, or a standard score of 70 or below on a comprehensive developmental assessment).
2. Impairment in executive functioning (e.g., poor planning and organization; inflexibility; difficulty with behavioral inhibition).
3. Impairment in learning (e.g., lower academic achievement than expected for intellectual level; specific learning disability).
4. Memory impairment (e.g., problems remembering information learned recently; repeatedly making the same mistakes; difficulty remembering lengthy verbal instructions).
5. Impairment in visual-spatial reasoning (e.g., disorganized or poorly planned drawings or constructions; problems differentiating left from right).

C. Impaired self-regulation as manifested by one or more of the following:

1. Impairment in mood or behavioral regulation (e.g., mood lability; negative affect or irritability; frequent behavioral outbursts).
2. Attention deficit (e.g., difficulty shifting attention; difficulty sustaining mental effort).
3. Impairment in impulse control (e.g., difficulty waiting turn; difficulty complying with rules).

D. Impairment in adaptive functioning as manifested by two or more of the following, one of which must be (1) or (2):

1. Communication deficit (e.g., delayed acquisition of language; difficulty understanding spoken language).
2. Impairment in social communication and interaction (e.g., overly friendly with strangers; difficulty reading social cues; difficulty understanding social consequences).
3. Impairment in daily living skills (e.g., delayed toileting, feeding, or bathing; difficulty managing daily schedule).
4. Impairment in motor skills (e.g., poor fine motor development; delayed attainment of gross motor milestones or ongoing deficits in gross motor function; deficits in coordination and balance).

E. Onset of the disorder (symptoms in Criteria B, C, and D) occurs in childhood.
F. The disturbance causes clinically significant distress or impairment in social, academic, occupational, or other important areas of functioning.
G. The disorder is not better explained by the direct physiological effects associated with postnatal use of a substance (e.g., a medication, alcohol or other drugs), a general medical condition (e.g., traumatic brain injury, delirium, dementia), another known teratogen (e.g., fetal hydantoin syndrome), a genetic condition (e.g., Williams syndrome, Down syndrome, Cornelia de Lange syndrome), or environmental neglect.

Suicidal Behavior Disorder

The rationale supporting the inclusion of suicidal behavior disorder, offered by the Mood Disorders Work Group, has mainly to do with coding. Although suicidal behavior causes significant morbidity and leads to high utilization of mental health resources, DSM codes reflecting suicidal behavior are limited to E (external cause of

injury) codes drawn from ICD-9-CM (E950–E959) that differentiate between accidental and self-inflicted injury. The codes are often assigned by administrative personnel
and are frequently ignored. Although suicidal behavior and ideation are listed as
symptoms of major depressive disorder and borderline personality disorder, these
symptoms are not codable and misrepresent the independent associations that these
behaviors have with many other psychiatric disorders. Furthermore, research suggests that suicidal behaviors share similar pathological features, regardless of comorbidity. Thus, the absence of an approved code leads to incomplete and misleading
information in clinical records, and the availability of a codable condition might help
with prevention and safety monitoring efforts.

Proposed Criteria for Suicidal Behavior Disorder

A. Within the last 24 months, the individual has made a suicide attempt.
   Note: A suicide attempt is a self-initiated sequence of behaviors by an individual
   who, at the time of initiation, expected that the set of actions would lead to his or
   her own death. (The "time of initiation" is the time when a behavior took place that
   involved applying the method.)
B. The act does not meet criteria for nonsuicidal self-injury—that is, it does not involve self-injury directed to the surface of the body undertaken to induce relief from
   a negative feeling/cognitive state or to achieve a positive mood state.
C. The diagnosis is not applied to suicidal ideation or to preparatory acts.
D. The act was not initiated during a state of delirium or confusion.
E. The act was not undertaken solely for a political or religious objective.

Specify if:
   Current: Not more than 12 months since the last attempt.
   In early remission: 12–24 months since the last attempt.

Nonsuicidal Self-Injury

The Childhood and Adolescent Disorders Work Group proposed nonsuicidal self-injury with the rationale that these symptoms are poorly represented in DSM. The closest approximation is Item 5 in the criteria set for DSM-IV borderline personality
disorder: "recurrent suicidal behavior, gestures, or threats, or self-mutilating behavior." Research shows that repeated self-injury co-occurs in both adolescents and
adults with a variety of diagnoses, and many of these individuals do not meet criteria
for borderline personality disorder. The criteria correct the following misinformation
regarding self-injury: 1) that it is pathognomonic of borderline personality disorder,
and 2) that it is a form of attempted suicide. Neither statement is true, yet both have
the potential to lead to overly restrictive or inappropriate clinical management (e.g.,
inpatient hospitalization, lengthy and complex psychotherapies). These criteria help
distinguish nonsuicidal self-injury and attempted suicide. For most individuals, the
former is not designed to result in death but rather to bring relief from tension and

other negative affects. These behaviors (e.g., cutting, burning) tend to have low lethality. The proposed definition requires that injuries be superficial and frequently repeated. Most individuals who engage in these behaviors are aware of their non-life-threatening nature. Nevertheless, recurrent self-injurious behaviors are associated with an elevated risk for attempted and completed suicide.

One concern about the criteria for nonsuicidal self-injury is that borderline personality disorder is not specifically excluded. Although self-harm is not specific for the diagnosis of borderline personality disorder, the two are tightly linked, so the exclusion should be clear.

Proposed Criteria for Nonsuicidal Self-Injury

A. In the last year, the individual has, on 5 or more days, engaged in intentional self-inflicted damage to the surface of his or her body of a sort likely to induce bleeding, bruising, or pain (e.g., cutting, burning, stabbing, hitting, excessive rubbing), with the expectation that the injury will lead to only minor or moderate physical harm (i.e., there is no suicidal intent).

Note: The absence of suicidal intent has either been stated by the individual or can be inferred by the individual's repeated engagement in a behavior that the individual knows, or has learned, is not likely to result in death.

B. The individual engages in the self-injurious behavior with one or more of the following expectations:

  1. To obtain relief from a negative feeling or cognitive state.
  2. To resolve an interpersonal difficulty.
  3. To induce a positive feeling state.

Note: The desired relief or response is experienced during or shortly after the self-injury, and the individual may display patterns of behavior suggesting a dependence on repeatedly engaging in it.

C. The intentional self-injury is associated with at least one of the following:

  1. Interpersonal difficulties or negative feelings or thoughts, such as depression, anxiety, tension, anger, generalized distress, or self-criticism, occurring in the period immediately prior to the self-injurious act.
  2. Prior to engaging in the act, a period of preoccupation with the intended behavior that is difficult to control.
  3. Thinking about self-injury that occurs frequently, even when it is not acted upon.

D. The behavior is not socially sanctioned (e.g., body piercing, tattooing, part of a religious or cultural ritual) and is not restricted to picking a scab or nail biting.

E. The behavior or its consequences cause clinically significant distress or interference in interpersonal, academic, or other important areas of functioning.

F. The behavior does not occur exclusively during psychotic episodes, delirium, substance intoxication, or substance withdrawal. In individuals with a neurodevelopmental disorder, the behavior is not part of a pattern of repetitive stereotypies. The behavior is not better explained by another mental disorder or medical condition (e.g., psychotic disorder, autism spectrum disorder, intellectual disability, Lesch-Nyhan syndrome, stereotypic movement disorder with self-injury, trichotillomania [hair-pulling disorder], excoriation [skin-picking] disorder).

KEY POINTS

- This chapter includes proposed disorders that may be included in future editions of DSM. Their inclusion in DSM-5 provides an opportunity for establishing standardized criteria to facilitate research.

- To achieve full disorder status, the condition should be "unrepresented" (or not well represented in DSM); have clinical value; have the potential to improve accurate identification and/or treatment; and be prevalent, impairing, and distinctive.

- DSM-5 includes eight criteria sets in Section III in the chapter "Conditions for Further Study." For each condition, it was concluded that insufficient data are currently available to warrant inclusion as an official DSM diagnosis. The conditions include attenuated psychosis syndrome, which became a lightning rod in the DSM-5 deliberations; depressive episodes with short-duration hypomania; persistent complex bereavement disorder; caffeine use disorder; Internet gaming disorder; neurobehavioral disorder associated with prenatal alcohol exposure; suicidal behavior disorder; and nonsuicidal self-injury.

References

Alexander FG, Selesnick ST: The History of Psychiatry: An Evaluation of Psychiatric Thought and Practice From Prehistoric Times. New York, Harper & Row, 1966

Allen RP, Walters AS, Montplaisir J, et al: Restless legs syndrome prevalence and impact: REST general population study. Arch Intern Med 165:1286–1292, 2005

American Academy of Sleep Medicine: International Classification of Sleep Disorders. Chicago, IL, American Academy of Sleep Medicine, 2005

American Medical Association: A Standard Classified Nomenclature of Disease. Chicago, IL, American Medical Association, 1933

American Medico-Psychological Association: Statistical Manual for the Use of Institutions for the Insane. New York, National Committee for Mental Hygiene, 1918

American Psychiatric Association: Diagnostic and Statistical Manual: Mental Disorders. Washington, DC, American Psychiatric Association, 1952

American Psychiatric Association: Diagnostic and Statistical Manual of Mental Disorders, 2nd Edition. Washington, DC, American Psychiatric Association, 1968

American Psychiatric Association: Diagnostic and Statistical Manual of Mental Disorders, 3rd Edition. Washington, DC, American Psychiatric Association, 1980

American Psychiatric Association: Diagnostic and Statistical Manual of Mental Disorders, 3rd Edition, Revised. Washington, DC, American Psychiatric Association, 1987

American Psychiatric Association: Diagnostic and Statistical Manual of Mental Disorders, 4th Edition. Washington, DC, American Psychiatric Association, 1994

American Psychiatric Association: Diagnostic and Statistical Manual of Mental Disorders, 4th Edition, Text Revision. Washington, DC, American Psychiatric Association, 2000

American Psychiatric Association: Diagnostic and Statistical Manual of Mental Disorders, 5th Edition. Arlington, VA, American Psychiatric Association, 2013

Andlauer O, Moore H, Jouhier L, et al: Nocturnal rapid eye movement sleep latency for identifying patients with narcolepsy/hypocretin deficiency. JAMA Neurol 6:1–12, 2013

Andrews G, Charney DS, Sirovatka PJ, et al: Stress-Induced and Fear Circuitry Disorders: Refining the Research Agenda for DSM-V. Arlington, VA, American Psychiatric Association, 2009

Andrews G, Goldberg DP, Krueger RF, et al: Exploring the feasibility of a meta-structure for DSM-V and ICD-11: could it improve utility and validity? Psychol Med 39:1993–2000, 2009

Angst J, Azorin JM, Bowden CL, et al: Prevalence and characteristics of undiagnosed bipolar disorders in patients with a major depressive episode: the BRIDGE study. Arch Gen Psychiatry 68:791–798, 2011

Angst J, Gamma A, Bowden CL, et al: Diagnostic criteria for bipolarity based on an international sample of 5,635 patients with DSM-IV major depressive episodes. Eur Arch Psychiatry Clin Neurosci 262:3–11, 2012

Applegate B, Lahey BB, Hart EL, et al: Validity of the age-of-onset criterion for ADHD: a report from the DSM-IV field trials. J Am Acad Child Adolesc Psychiatry 36:1211–1221, 1997

Axelson D, Birmaher B, Strober M, et al: Phenomenology of children and adolescents with bipolar spectrum disorders. Arch Gen Psychiatry 63:1139–1148, 2006

Bell V, Halligan PW, Ellis HD: Diagnosing delusions: a review of inter-rater reliability. Schizophr Res 86:76–79, 2006

Bishop DVM: Pragmatic language impairment: a correlate of SLI, a distinct subgroup, or part of the autistic continuum? in Speech and Language Impairments in Children: Causes, Characteristics, Intervention, and Outcome. Edited by Bishop DVM, Leonard LB. East Sussex, UK, Psychology Press, 2000, pp 99–113

Bishop DV, Norbury CF: Exploring the borderlands of autistic disorder and specific language impairment: a study using standardised diagnostic instruments. J Child Psychol Psychiatry 43:917–929, 2002

Black DW: Bad Boys, Bad Men: Confronting Antisocial Personality Disorder (Sociopathy), Revised and Updated. New York, Oxford University Press, 2013

Bleuler E: Dementia Praecox or the Group of Schizophrenias. Translated by Zinken J. New York, International Universities Press, 1950

Brotto LA: The DSM diagnostic criteria for hypoactive sexual desire disorder. Arch Sex Behav 39:221–239, 2010

Bryant RA, Friedman MJ, Spiegel D, et al: A review of acute stress disorder in DSM-5. Depress Anxiety 28:802–817, 2011

Burgess CR, Scammell TE: Narcolepsy: neural mechanisms of sleepiness and cataplexy. J Neurosci 32:12305–12311, 2012

Burke JD, Loeber R, Birmaher B: Oppositional defiant disorder and conduct disorder: a review of the past 10 years, part II. J Am Acad Child Adolesc Psychiatry 41:1275–1293, 2002

Cassano GB, Rucci P, Frank E, et al: The mood spectrum in unipolar and bipolar disorder: arguments for a unitary approach. Am J Psychiatry 161:1264–1269, 2004

Cermolacce M, Sass L, Parnas J: What is bizarre in bizarre delusions? A critical review. Schizophr Bull 36:667–679, 2010

Coccaro EF: Intermittent explosive disorder as a disorder of impulsive aggression for DSM-5. Am J Psychiatry 169:577–588, 2012

Cosgrove L, Krimsky S: A comparison of DSM-IV and DSM-5 panel members' financial associations with industry: a pernicious problem persists. PLoS Med 9(3):e1001190, 2012 (doi:10.1371/journal.pmed.1001190)

Dauvilliers Y, Arnulf I, Mignot E: Narcolepsy with cataplexy. Lancet 369:499–511, 2007

Dement WC: A history of narcolepsy and other sleep disorders. J Hist Neurosci 2:121–134, 1993

Dement W, Rechtschaffen A, Gulevich G: The nature of the narcoleptic sleep attack. Neurology 16:18–33, 1966

Dimsdale JE, Creed F: The proposed diagnosis of somatic symptom disorders in DSM-V to replace somatoform disorders in DSM-IV—a preliminary report. J Psychosom Res 76:473–476, 2009

Dimsdale JE, Xin Y, Kleinman A, et al (eds): Somatic Presentations of Mental Disorders: Refining the Research Agenda for DSM-5. Arlington, VA, American Psychiatric Association, 2009

Drossman DA, Dumitrascu DL: Rome III: new standard for functional gastrointestinal disorders. J Gastrointestin Liver Dis 15:237–241, 2006

Endicott J, Spitzer RL, Fleiss JL, et al: The Global Assessment Scale: a procedure for measuring overall severity of psychiatric disturbance. Arch Gen Psychiatry 33:766–771, 1976

Esquirol JE: Des maladies mentales. Paris, Baillière, 1838

Feighner JP, Robins E, Guze SB, et al: Diagnostic criteria for use in psychiatric research. Arch Gen Psychiatry 26:57–63, 1972

Foote B, Smolin Y, Kaplan M, et al: Prevalence of dissociative disorders in psychiatric outpatients. Am J Psychiatry 163:623–629, 2006

Ford DE, Kamerow DB: Epidemiologic study of sleep disturbances and psychiatric disorders: an opportunity for prevention? JAMA 262:1479–1484, 1989

Frances A, Pincus HA, Widiger TA, et al: DSM-IV: work in progress. Am J Psychiatry 147:1439–1448, 1990

Freud S: Obsessions and phobias: their psychical mechanism and their aetiology (1895), in The Standard Edition of the Complete Psychological Works of Sigmund Freud, Vol 3. Translated and edited by Strachey J. London, Hogarth Press, 1962, pp 74–82

Friedman MJ, Resick PA, Bryant RA, et al: Considering PTSD for DSM-5. Depress Anxiety 28:750–769, 2011

Frost RO, Steketee G, Tolin DF: Diagnosis and assessment of hoarding disorder. Annu Rev Clin Psychol 8:219–242, 2012

Goldberg JF, Perlis RH, Bowden CL, et al: Manic symptoms during depressive episodes in 1,380 patients with bipolar disorder: findings from the STEP-BD. Am J Psychiatry 166:173–181, 2009

Goodwin D, Guze S: Psychiatric Diagnosis, 4th Edition. New York, Oxford University Press, 1989

Grant JE, Levine L, Kim D, et al: Impulse control disorders in adult psychiatric inpatients. Am J Psychiatry. 162:2184–2188, 2005

Gunderson JG: Commentary on "Personality traits and the classification of mental disorders: toward a more complete integration in DSM-5 and an empirical model of psychopathology." Personal Disord 1:119–122, 2010

Hasler B, Germain A: Correlates and treatments of nightmares in adults. Sleep Med Clin 4:507–517, 2009

Helmes E, Landmark J: Subtypes of schizophrenia: a cluster analytic approach. Can J Psychiatry 48:702–708, 2003

Helzer JE, van den Brink W, Guth SE: Should there be both categorical and dimensional criteria for the substance use disorders in DSM-V? Addiction 101:17–22, 2006

Helzer R, Kraemer H, Krueger R, et al: Dimensional Approaches in Diagnostic Classification: Refining the Research Agenda for DSM-V. Arlington, VA, American Psychiatric Association, 2008

Hollander E, Zohar J, Sirovatka PJ, et al: Obsessive-Compulsive Spectrum Disorders: Refining the Research Agenda for DSM-V. Arlington, VA, American Psychiatric Association, 2011

Joinson C, Heron J, Butler U, et al: Psychological differences between children with and without soiling problems. Pediatrics 117:1575–1584, 2006

Kanner L: Child Psychiatry, 2nd Edition. Springfield, IL, Charles C Thomas, 1948

Kasanin J: The acute schizoaffective psychoses. Am J Psychiatry 90:97–126, 1933

Kendler KS, Muñoz RA, Murphy G: The development of the Feighner criteria: a historical perspective. Am J Psychiatry 167:134–142, 2010

Kieling C, Kieling RR, Rohde LA, et al: The age at onset of attention deficit hyperactivity disorder. Am J Psychiatry 167:14–16, 2010

Klein DN, Shankman SA, Lewinsohn PM, et al: Family study of chronic depression in a community sample of young adults. Am J Psychiatry 161:646–653, 2004

Kraemer HC, Kupfer DJ, Narrow WE, et al: Moving toward DSM-5: the field trials. Am J Psychiatry 167:1158–1159, 2010

Kraemer HC, Kupfer DJ, Clarke DE, et al: DSM-5: how reliable is reliable enough? Am J Psychiatry 169:13–15, 2012

Kraepelin E: Dementia Praecox and Paraphrenia. Translated by Barclay RM, Robertson GM. Edinburgh, E & S Livingstone, 1919

Krueger RF, Eaton NR: Personality traits and the classification of mental disorders: toward a more complete integration in DSM-5 and an empirical model of psychopathology. Personal Disord 1:97–118, 2010

Krueger RF, Eaton NR, Clark LA, et al: Deriving an empirical structure of personality pathology for DSM-5. J Pers Disord 25:170–191, 2011

Kupfer DJ, Regier DA: Neuroscience, clinical evidence, and the future of psychiatric classification. Am J Psychiatry 168:1–3, 2011

Kupfer DJ, First MB, Regier DA (eds): A Research Agenda for DSM-V. Washington, DC, American Psychiatric Publishing, 2002

Kupfer DJ, Kuhl EA, Regier DA: DSM-5—the future arrived. JAMA 309(16):1691–1692, 2013

Langfeldt G: The Schizophreniform States: A Katamnestic Study Based on Individual Reexaminations. Copenhagen, Denmark, Munksgaard, 1939

Lanius R, Brand B, Vermetten E, et al: The dissociative subtype of posttraumatic stress disorder: rationale, clinical and neurobiological evidence, and implications. Depress Anxiety 29:701–708, 2012

Leckman JF, Denys D, Simpson HB, et al: Obsessive-compulsive disorder: a review of the diagnostic criteria and possible subtypes and dimensional specifiers for DSM-V. Depress Anxiety 27:507–527, 2010

Mataix-Cols D, Frost RO, Pertusa A, et al: Hoarding disorder: a new diagnosis for DSM-V? Depress Anxiety 27:556–572, 2010

Matte B, Rohde LA, Grevet EH: ADHD in adults: a concept in evolution. Atten Defic Hyperact Disord 4:53–62, 2012

McCrae RR, Costa PT Jr: Validation of the five-factor model of personality across instruments and observers. J Person Soc Psychol 52:81–90, 1987

McCullough JP Jr, Klein DN, Keller MB, et al: Comparison of DSM-III-R chronic major depression and major depression superimposed on dysthymia (double depression): validity of the distinction. J Abnorm Psychol 109:419–427, 2000

McGlashan T, Fenton W: Classical Subtypes of Schizophrenia. Washington, DC, American Psychiatric Association, 1994

McKeith IG: Consensus guidelines for the clinical and pathologic diagnosis of dementia with Lewy bodies (DLB): report of the Consortium on DLB International Workshop. J Alzheimers Dis 9:417–423, 2006

McKeith IG, Galasko D, Kosaka K, et al: Consensus guidelines for the clinical and pathologic diagnosis of dementia with Lewy bodies (DLB): report of the Consortium on DLB International Workshop. Neurology 47:1113–1124, 1996

Morin CM, Edinger JD: Sleep/wake disorders, in Oxford Textbook of Psychopathology, 2nd Edition. Edited by Blaney PH, Millon T. New York, Oxford University Press, 2009, pp 506–526

Murray CJL, Lopez AD: The Global Burden of Disease. Boston, MA, Harvard University Press, 1996

Narrow W, First MB, Sirovatka PJ, et al: Age and General Considerations in Psychiatric Diagnosis: A Research Agenda for DSM-V. Arlington, VA, American Psychiatric Association, 2007

National Institutes of Health: National Institutes of Health State of the Science Conference statement on Manifestations and Management of Chronic Insomnia in Adults, June 13–15, 2005. Sleep 28:1049–1057, 2005

National Sleep Foundation: 2005 adult sleep habits and styles (Sleep in America polls). Available at: http://www.sleepfoundation.org/article/sleep-america-polls/2005-adult-sleep-habits-and-styles. Accessed July 12, 2013.

Nielsen T, Zadra A: Idiopathic nightmares and dream disturbances associated with sleep-wake transitions, in Principles and Practice of Sleep Medicine, 5th Edition. Edited by Kryger MH, Roth T, Dement WC. New York, Elsevier, 2010, pp 1106–1115

Nordgaard J, Arnfred SM, Handest P, et al: The diagnostic status of first-rank symptoms. Schizophr Bull 34:137–154, 2008

Ohayon MM, Dauvilliers Y, Reynolds CF: Operational definitions and algorithms for excessive sleepiness in the general population: implications for DSM-5 nosology. Arch Gen Psychiatry 69:71–79, 2012

Petersen RC, O'Brien J: Mild cognitive impairment should be considered for DSM-V. J Geriatr Psychiatry Neurol 19:147–154, 2006

Phillips KA, Wilhelm S, Koran LM, et al: Body dysmorphic disorder: some key issues for DSM-V. Depress Anxiety 27:573–591, 2010

Potenza MN: Should addictive disorders include non-substance-related conditions? Addiction 101:142–151, 2006

Regier DA: Dimensional approaches to psychiatric classification: refining the research agenda for DSM-V: an introduction. Int J Methods Psychiatr Res 16(suppl):S1–S5, 2007

Regier DA, Narrow WE, Kuhl EA, et al (eds): The Conceptual Evolution of DSM-5. Arlington, VA, American Psychiatric Association, 2011

Robins E, Guze SB: Establishment of diagnostic validity in psychiatric illness: its application to schizophrenia. Am J Psychiatry 126:983–987, 1970

Ronningstam E: Narcissistic personality disorder in DSM-V—in support of retaining a significant diagnosis. J Pers Disord 25:248–259, 2011

Roth B, Nevsimalova S, Rechtschaffen A: Hypersomnia with "sleep drunkenness." Arch Gen Psychiatry 26:456–462, 1972

Russell G: Bulimia nervosa: an ominous variant of anorexia nervosa. Psychol Med 9:429–448, 1979

Sanislow CA , Gillo CM, Morey LC, et al: Confirmatory factor analysis of the DSM-IV criteria for borderline personality disorder: findings from the Collaborative Longitudinal Personality Disorders Study. Am J Psychiatry 159:284–290, 2002

Sar V, Akyuz G, Dogan O: Prevalence of dissociative disorders among women in the general population. Psychiatry Res 149:169–176, 2007

Scheeringa MS, Zeanah CH, Cohen JA: PTSD in children and adolescents: toward an empirically based algorithm. Depress Anxiety 28:770–782, 2011

Schneider K: Clinical Psychopathology. New York, Grune & Stratton, 1959

Segraves RT: Considerations for diagnostic criteria for erectile dysfunction in DSM V. J Sex Med 7:654–660, 2010

Shorter E: A History of Psychiatry: From the Era of the Asylum to the Age of Prozac. New York, Wiley, 1997

Spiegel D, Loewenstein RJ, Lewis-Fernandez R, et al: Dissociative disorders in DSM-5. Depress Anxiety 28:824–852, 2011

Spitzer RL, Endicott J, Robins E: Research diagnostic criteria (RDC). New York, Biometrics Research, New York State Psychiatric Institute, 1975

Spitzer RL, Williams JB, Skodol AE: DSM-III: the major achievements and an overview. Am J Psychiatry 137:151–164, 1980

Stein DJ, Grant JE, Franklin ME, et al: Trichotillomania (hair pulling disorder), skin picking disorder, and stereotypic movement disorder: toward DSM-V. Depress Anxiety 27:611–626, 2010

Strain JJ, Friedman MJ: Considering adjustment disorders as stress response syndromes for DSM-5. Depress Anxiety 28:818–823, 2011

Walkup JT, Ferrao Y, Leckman JF, et al: Tic disorders: some key issues for DSM-V. Depress Anxiety 27:600–610, 2010

Widiger T, Simonsen E, Sirovatka P, et al (eds): Dimensional Models of Personality Disorders: Refining the Research Agenda for DSM-V. Arlington, VA, American Psychiatric Association, 2006

Wittchen HU, Gloster AT, Beesdo-Baum K, et al: Agoraphobia: a review of the diagnostic classificatory position and criteria. Depress Anxiety 27:113–133, 2010

World Health Organization: Manual of International Statistical Classification of Diseases, Injuries, and Causes of Death, 6th Revision. Geneva, World Health Organization, 1948

World Health Organization: International Classification of Diseases, 8th Revision. Geneva, World Health Organization, 1967

World Health Organization: International Classification of Diseases, 9th Revision. Geneva, World Health Organization, 1977

World Health Organization: International Classification of Diseases, 9th Revision, Clinical Modification. Ann Arbor, MI, Commission on Professional and Hospital Activities, 1978

World Health Organization: International Statistical Classification of Diseases and Related Health Problems, 10th Revision. Geneva, World Health Organization, 1992

World Health Organization: The World Health Report 2001—Mental Health: New Understanding, New Hope. Geneva, World Health Organization, 2001. Available at: http://www.who.int/whr/2001/en/index.html. Accessed July 12, 2013.

Appendix

DSM-5 Classification

Before each disorder name, ICD-9-CM codes are provided, followed by ICD-10-CM codes in parentheses. Blank lines indicate that either the ICD-9-CM or the ICD-10-CM code is not applicable. For some disorders, the code can be indicated only according to the subtype or specifier.

ICD-9-CM codes are to be used for coding purposes in the United States through September 30, 2014. ICD-10-CM codes are to be used starting October 1, 2014.

Note for all mental disorders due to another medical condition: Indicate the name of the other medical condition in the name of the mental disorder due to [the medical condition]. The code and name for the other medical condition should be listed first immediately before the mental disorder due to the medical condition.

Neurodevelopmental Disorders

Intellectual Disabilities

___.__ (__.__)		Intellectual Disability (Intellectual Developmental Disorder)
		Specify current severity:
317	(F70)	Mild
318.0	(F71)	Moderate
318.1	(F72)	Severe
318.2	(F73)	Profound

315.8 **(F88)**   Global Developmental Delay

319   **(F79)**   Unspecified Intellectual Disability (Intellectual Developmental
                              Disorder)

Communication Disorders

315.32 **(F80.2)**   Language Disorder

315.39 **(F80.0)**   Speech Sound Disorder

315.35 **(F80.81)**   Childhood-Onset Fluency Disorder (Stuttering)
                              Note: Later-onset cases are diagnosed as 307.0 (F98.5) adult-onset fluency
                              disorder.

315.39 **(F80.89)**   Social (Pragmatic) Communication Disorder

307.9 **(F80.9)**   Unspecified Communication Disorder

Autism Spectrum Disorder

299.00 **(F84.0)**   Autism Spectrum Disorder
                              Specify if: Associated with a known medical or genetic condition or environ-
                              mental factor; Associated with another neurodevelopmental, mental, or
                              behavioral disorder
                              Specify current severity for Criterion A and Criterion B: Requiring very sub-
                              stantial support, Requiring substantial support, Requiring support
                              Specify if: With or without accompanying intellectual impairment, With or
                              without accompanying language impairment, With catatonia (use addi-
                              tional code 293.89 [F06.1])

Attention-Deficit/Hyperactivity Disorder

___.__ (___.__)   Attention-Deficit/Hyperactivity Disorder
                              Specify whether:

314.01 **(F90.2)**   Combined presentation

314.00 **(F90.0)**   Predominantly inattentive presentation

314.01 **(F90.1)**   Predominantly hyperactive/impulsive presentation
                              Specify if: In partial remission
                              Specify current severity: Mild, Moderate, Severe

314.01 **(F90.8)**   Other Specified Attention-Deficit/Hyperactivity Disorder

314.01 **(F90.9)**   Unspecified Attention-Deficit/Hyperactivity Disorder

Specific Learning Disorder

___.__ (___.__)   Specific Learning Disorder
                              Specify if:

315.00 **(F81.0)**   With impairment in reading (*specify* if with word reading
                                  accuracy, reading rate or fluency, reading comprehension)

315.2 **(F81.81)**   With impairment in written expression (*specify* if with spelling
                                  accuracy, grammar and punctuation accuracy, clarity or
                                  organization of written expression)

315.1 (F81.2)   With impairment in mathematics (*specify* if with number sense, memorization of arithmetic facts, accurate or fluent calculation, accurate math reasoning)
Specify current severity: Mild, Moderate, Severe

Motor Disorders

315.4 (F82)   Developmental Coordination Disorder

307.3 (F98.4)   Stereotypic Movement Disorder
Specify if: With self-injurious behavior, Without self-injurious behavior
Specify if: Associated with a known medical or genetic condition, neurodevelopmental disorder, or environmental factor
Specify current severity: Mild, Moderate, Severe

Tic Disorders

307.23 (F95.2)   Tourette's Disorder

307.22 (F95.1)   Persistent (Chronic) Motor or Vocal Tic Disorder
Specify if: With motor tics only, With vocal tics only

307.21 (F95.0)   Provisional Tic Disorder

307.20 (F95.8)   Other Specified Tic Disorder

307.20 (F95.9)   Unspecified Tic Disorder

Other Neurodevelopmental Disorders

315.8 (F88)   Other Specified Neurodevelopmental Disorder

315.9 (F89)   Unspecified Neurodevelopmental Disorder

Schizophrenia Spectrum and Other Psychotic Disorders

The following specifiers apply to Schizophrenia Spectrum and Other Psychotic Disorders where indicated:
[a]*Specify* if: The following course specifiers are only to be used after a 1-year duration of the disorder: First episode, currently in acute episode; First episode, currently in partial remission; First episode, currently in full remission; Multiple episodes, currently in acute episode; Multiple episodes, currently in partial remission; Multiple episodes, currently in full remission; Continuous; Unspecified
[b]*Specify* if: With catatonia (use additional code 293.89 [F06.1])
[c]*Specify* current severity of delusions, hallucinations, disorganized speech, abnormal psychomotor behavior, negative symptoms, impaired cognition, depression, and mania symptoms

301.22 (F21)   Schizotypal (Personality) Disorder

297.1 (F22)   Delusional Disorder[a, c]
Specify whether: Erotomanic type, Grandiose type, Jealous type, Persecutory type, Somatic type, Mixed type, Unspecified type
Specify if: With bizarre content

298.8 (F23)   Brief Psychotic Disorder[b, c]
Specify if: With marked stressor(s), Without marked stressor(s), With postpartum onset

295.40 (F20.81)	Schizophreniform Disorder[b, c]
	Specify if: With good prognostic features, Without good prognostic features
295.90 (F20.9)	Schizophrenia[a, b, c]
___.__ (___.__)	Schizoaffective Disorder[a, b, c]
	Specify whether:
295.70 (F25.0)	Bipolar type
295.70 (F25.1)	Depressive type
___.__ (___.__)	Substance/Medication-Induced Psychotic Disorder[c]
	Note: See the criteria set and corresponding recording procedures for substance-specific codes and ICD-9-CM and ICD-10-CM coding.
	Specify if: With onset during intoxication, With onset during withdrawal
___.__ (___.__)	Psychotic Disorder Due to Another Medical Condition[c]
	Specify whether:
293.81 (F06.2)	With delusions
293.82 (F06.0)	With hallucinations
293.89 (F06.1)	Catatonia Associated With Another Mental Disorder (Catatonia Specifier)
293.89 (F06.1)	Catatonic Disorder Due to Another Medical Condition
293.89 (F06.1)	Unspecified Catatonia
	Note: Code first **781.99 (R29.818)** other symptoms involving nervous and musculoskeletal systems.
298.8 (F28)	Other Specified Schizophrenia Spectrum and Other Psychotic Disorder
298.9 (F29)	Unspecified Schizophrenia Spectrum and Other Psychotic Disorder

Bipolar and Related Disorders

The following specifiers apply to Bipolar and Related Disorders where indicated:

[a]*Specify:* With anxious distress (*specify* current severity: mild, moderate, moderate-severe, severe); With mixed features; With rapid cycling; With melancholic features; With atypical features; With mood-congruent psychotic features; With mood-incongruent psychotic features; With catatonia (use additional code 293.89 [F06.1]); With peripartum onset; With seasonal pattern

___.__ (___.__)	Bipolar I Disorder[a]
___.__ (___.__)	Current or most recent episode manic
296.41 (F31.11)	Mild
296.42 (F31.12)	Moderate
296.43 (F31.13)	Severe
296.44 (F31.2)	With psychotic features
296.45 (F31.73)	In partial remission
296.46 (F31.74)	In full remission
296.40 (F31.9)	Unspecified
296.40 (F31.0)	Current or most recent episode hypomanic
296.45 (F31.71)	In partial remission

296.46 (F31.72)		In full remission
296.40 (F31.9)		Unspecified
___.__ (__.__)		Current or most recent episode depressed
296.51 (F31.31)		Mild
296.52 (F31.32)		Moderate
296.53 (F31.4)		Severe
296.54 (F31.5)		With psychotic features
296.55 (F31.75)		In partial remission
296.56 (F31.76)		In full remission
296.50 (F31.9)		Unspecified
296.7 (F31.9)		Current or most recent episode unspecified

296.89 (F31.81) Bipolar II Disorder[a]
Specify current or most recent episode: Hypomanic, Depressed
Specify course if full criteria for a mood episode are not currently met: In partial remission, In full remission
Specify severity if full criteria for a mood episode are currently met: Mild, Moderate, Severe

301.13 (F34.0) Cyclothymic Disorder
Specify if: With anxious distress

___.__ (__.__) Substance/Medication-Induced Bipolar and Related Disorder
Note: See the criteria set and corresponding recording procedures for substance-specific codes and ICD-9-CM and ICD-10-CM coding.
Specify if: With onset during intoxication, With onset during withdrawal

293.83 (__.__) Bipolar and Related Disorder Due to Another Medical Condition
Specify if:

(F06.33)	With manic features
(F06.33)	With manic- or hypomanic-like episode
(F06.34)	With mixed features

296.89 (F31.89) Other Specified Bipolar and Related Disorder

296.80 (F31.9) Unspecified Bipolar and Related Disorder

Depressive Disorders

The following specifiers apply to Depressive Disorders where indicated:
[a]*Specify:* With anxious distress (*specify* current severity: mild, moderate, moderate-severe, severe); With mixed features; With melancholic features; With atypical features; With mood-congruent psychotic features; With mood-incongruent psychotic features; With catatonia (use additional code 293.89 [F06.1]); With peripartum onset; With seasonal pattern

296.99 (F34.8)	Disruptive Mood Dysregulation Disorder
___.__ (__.__)	Major Depressive Disorder[a]
___.__ (__.__)	Single episode
296.21 (F32.0)	Mild
296.22 (F32.1)	Moderate
296.23 (F32.2)	Severe
296.24 (F32.3)	With psychotic features

296.25	(F32.4)	In partial remission
296.26	(F32.5)	In full remission
296.20	(F32.9)	Unspecified
__._	(__._)	Recurrent episode
296.31	(F33.0)	Mild
296.32	(F33.1)	Moderate
296.33	(F33.2)	Severe
296.34	(F33.3)	With psychotic features
296.35	(F33.41)	In partial remission
296.36	(F33.42)	In full remission
296.30	(F33.9)	Unspecified

300.4 (F34.1) Persistent Depressive Disorder (Dysthymia)[a]
Specify if: In partial remission, In full remission
Specify if: Early onset, Late onset
Specify if: With pure dysthymic syndrome; With persistent major depressive episode; With intermittent major depressive episodes, with current episode; With intermittent major depressive episodes, without current episode
Specify current severity: Mild, Moderate, Severe

625.4 (N94.3) Premenstrual Dysphoric Disorder

__._ (__._) Substance/Medication-Induced Depressive Disorder
Note: See the criteria set and corresponding recording procedures for substance-specific codes and ICD-9-CM and ICD-10-CM coding.
Specify if: With onset during intoxication, With onset during withdrawal

293.83 (__._) Depressive Disorder Due to Another Medical Condition
Specify if:
(F06.31)   With depressive features
(F06.32)   With major depressive-like episode
(F06.34)   With mixed features

311 (F32.8) Other Specified Depressive Disorder

311 (F32.9) Unspecified Depressive Disorder

Anxiety Disorders

309.21 (F93.0) Separation Anxiety Disorder

313.23 (F94.0) Selective Mutism

300.29 (__._) Specific Phobia
Specify if:
(F40.218)   Animal
(F40.228)   Natural environment
(__._)   Blood-injection-injury
(F40.230)   Fear of blood
(F40.231)   Fear of injections and transfusions
(F40.232)   Fear of other medical care
(F40.233)   Fear of injury

(F40.248)   Situational

(F40.298)   Other

300.23 (F40.10)   Social Anxiety Disorder (Social Phobia)
Specify if: Performance only

300.01 (F41.0)   Panic Disorder

___.__ (___.__)   Panic Attack Specifier

300.22 (F40.00)   Agoraphobia

300.02 (F41.1)   Generalized Anxiety Disorder

___.__ (___.__)   Substance/Medication-Induced Anxiety Disorder
Note: See the criteria set and corresponding recording procedures for sub-
stance-specific codes and ICD-9-CM and ICD-10-CM coding.
Specify if: With onset during intoxication, With onset during withdrawal,
With onset after medication use

293.84 (F06.4)   Anxiety Disorder Due to Another Medical Condition

300.09 (F41.8)   Other Specified Anxiety Disorder

300.00 (F41.9)   Unspecified Anxiety Disorder

Obsessive-Compulsive and Related Disorders

The following specifier applies to Obsessive-Compulsive and Related Disorders where indicated:
[a]*Specify* if: With good or fair insight, With poor insight, With absent insight/delusional beliefs

300.3 (F42)   Obsessive-Compulsive Disorder[a]
Specify if: Tic-related

300.7 (F45.22)   Body Dysmorphic Disorder[a]
Specify if: With muscle dysmorphia

300.3 (F42)   Hoarding Disorder[a]
Specify if: With excessive acquisition

312.39 (F63.3)   Trichotillomania (Hair-Pulling Disorder)

698.4 (L98.1)   Excoriation (Skin-Picking) Disorder

___.__ (___.__)   Substance/Medication-Induced Obsessive-Compulsive and Related
Disorder
Note: See the criteria set and corresponding recording procedures for sub-
stance-specific codes and ICD-9-CM and ICD-10-CM coding.
Specify if: With onset during intoxication, With onset during withdrawal,
With onset after medication use

294.8 (F06.8)   Obsessive-Compulsive and Related Disorder Due to Another
Medical Condition
Specify if: With obsessive-compulsive disorder–like symptoms, With
appearance preoccupations, With hoarding symptoms, With hair-pulling
symptoms, With skin-picking symptoms

300.3 (F42)   Other Specified Obsessive-Compulsive and Related Disorder

300.3 (F42)   Unspecified Obsessive-Compulsive and Related Disorder

Trauma- and Stressor-Related Disorders

313.89 (F94.1)   Reactive Attachment Disorder
Specify if: Persistent
Specify current severity: Severe

313.89 (F94.2)   Disinhibited Social Engagement Disorder
Specify if: Persistent
Specify current severity: Severe

309.81 (F43.10)   Posttraumatic Stress Disorder (includes Posttraumatic Stress
Disorder for Children 6 Years and Younger)
Specify whether: With dissociative symptoms
Specify if: With delayed expression

308.3   (F43.0)   Acute Stress Disorder

___.__   (___.__)   Adjustment Disorders
Specify whether:
309.0   (F43.21)   With depressed mood
309.24 (F43.22)   With anxiety
309.28 (F43.23)   With mixed anxiety and depressed mood
309.3   (F43.24)   With disturbance of conduct
309.4   (F43.25)   With mixed disturbance of emotions and conduct
309.9   (F43.20)   Unspecified

309.89 (F43.8)   Other Specified Trauma- and Stressor-Related Disorder

309.9   (F43.9)   Unspecified Trauma- and Stressor-Related Disorder

Dissociative Disorders

300.14 (F44.81)   Dissociative Identity Disorder

300.12 (F44.0)   Dissociative Amnesia
Specify if:
300.13 (F44.1)   With dissociative fugue

300.6   (F48.1)   Depersonalization/Derealization Disorder

300.15 (F44.89)   Other Specified Dissociative Disorder

300.15 (F44.9)   Unspecified Dissociative Disorder

Somatic Symptom and Related Disorders

300.82 (F45.1)   Somatic Symptom Disorder
Specify if: With predominant pain
Specify if: Persistent
Specify current severity: Mild, Moderate, Severe

300.7	(F45.21)	Illness Anxiety Disorder

Specify whether: Care seeking type, Care avoidant type

300.11	(___.__)	Conversion Disorder (Functional Neurological Symptom Disorder)

Specify symptom type:

(F44.4)	With weakness or paralysis
(F44.4)	With abnormal movement
(F44.4)	With swallowing symptoms
(F44.4)	With speech symptom
(F44.5)	With attacks or seizures
(F44.6)	With anesthesia or sensory loss
(F44.6)	With special sensory symptom
(F44.7)	With mixed symptoms

Specify if: Acute episode, Persistent
Specify if: With psychological stressor (specify stressor), Without psychological stressor

316	(F54)	Psychological Factors Affecting Other Medical Conditions

Specify current severity: Mild, Moderate, Severe, Extreme

300.19	(F68.10)	Factitious Disorder (includes Factitious Disorder Imposed on Self, Factitious Disorder Imposed on Another)

Specify Single episode, Recurrent episodes

300.89	(F45.8)	Other Specified Somatic Symptom and Related Disorder
300.82	(F45.9)	Unspecified Somatic Symptom and Related Disorder

Feeding and Eating Disorders

The following specifiers apply to Feeding and Eating Disorders where indicated:
[a]*Specify* if: In remission
[b]*Specify* if: In partial remission, In full remission
[c]*Specify* current severity: Mild, Moderate, Severe, Extreme

307.52	(___.__)	Pica[a]
	(F98.3)	In children
	(F50.8)	In adults
307.53	(F98.21)	Rumination Disorder[a]
307.59	(F50.8)	Avoidant/Restrictive Food Intake Disorder[a]
307.1	(___.__)	Anorexia Nervosa[b, c]

Specify whether:

	(F50.01)	Restricting type
	(F50.02)	Binge-eating/purging type
307.51	(F50.2)	Bulimia Nervosa[b, c]
307.51	(F50.8)	Binge-Eating Disorder[b, c]
307.59	(F50.8)	Other Specified Feeding or Eating Disorder
307.50	(F50.9)	Unspecified Feeding or Eating Disorder

Elimination Disorders

307.6 (F98.0)   Enuresis
Specify whether: Nocturnal only, Diurnal only, Nocturnal and diurnal

307.7 (F98.1)   Encopresis
Specify whether: With constipation and overflow incontinence, Without constipation and overflow incontinence

___.__ (___.__)   Other Specified Elimination Disorder
788.39 (N39.498)   With urinary symptoms
787.60 (R15.9)   With fecal symptoms

___.__ (___.__)   Unspecified Elimination Disorder
788.30 (R32)   With urinary symptoms
787.60 (R15.9)   With fecal symptoms

Sleep-Wake Disorders

The following specifiers apply to Sleep-Wake Disorders where indicated:
[a]_Specify_ if: Episodic, Persistent, Recurrent
[b]_Specify_ if: Acute, Subacute, Persistent
[c]_Specify_ current severity: Mild, Moderate, Severe

307.42 (F51.01)   Insomnia Disorder[a]
Specify if: With non–sleep disorder mental comorbidity, With other medical comorbidity, With other sleep disorder

307.44 (F51.11)   Hypersomnolence Disorder[b, c]
Specify if: With mental disorder, With medical condition, With another sleep disorder

___.__ (___.__)   Narcolepsy[c]
Specify whether:
347.00 (G47.419)   Narcolepsy without cataplexy but with hypocretin deficiency
347.01 (G47.411)   Narcolepsy with cataplexy but without hypocretin deficiency
347.00 (G47.419)   Autosomal dominant cerebellar ataxia, deafness, and narcolepsy
347.00 (G47.419)   Autosomal dominant narcolepsy, obesity, and type 2 diabetes
347.10 (G47.429)   Narcolepsy secondary to another medical condition

Breathing-Related Sleep Disorders

327.23 (G47.33)   Obstructive Sleep Apnea Hypopnea[c]

___.__ (___.__)   Central Sleep Apnea
Specify whether:
327.21 (G47.31)   Idiopathic central sleep apnea
786.04 (R06.3)   Cheyne-Stokes breathing
780.57 (G47.37)   Central sleep apnea comorbid with opioid use
Note: First code opioid use disorder, if present.
Specify current severity

___.___ (___.___)	Sleep-Related Hypoventilation	
	Specify whether:	
327.24 (G47.34)	Idiopathic hypoventilation	
327.25 (G47.35)	Congenital central alveolar hypoventilation	
327.26 (G47.36)	Comorbid sleep-related hypoventilation	
	Specify current severity	

Circadian Rhythm Sleep-Wake Disorders

___.___ (___.___)	Circadian Rhythm Sleep-Wake Disorders[a]	
	Specify whether:	
307.45 (G47.21)	Delayed sleep phase type	
	Specify if: Familial, Overlapping with non-24-hour sleep-wake type	
307.45 (G47.22)	Advanced sleep phase type	
	Specify if: Familial	
307.45 (G47.23)	Irregular sleep-wake type	
307.45 (G47.24)	Non-24-hour sleep-wake type	
307.45 (G47.26)	Shift work type	
307.45 (G47.20)	Unspecified type	

Parasomnias

___.___ (___.___)	Non–Rapid Eye Movement Sleep Arousal Disorders	
	Specify whether:	
307.46 (F51.3)	Sleepwalking type	
	Specify if: With sleep-related eating, With sleep-related sexual behavior (sexsomnia)	
307.46 (F51.4)	Sleep terror type	
307.47 (F51.5)	Nightmare Disorder[b, c]	
	Specify if: During sleep onset	
	Specify if: With associated non–sleep disorder, With associated other medical condition, With associated other sleep disorder	
327.42 (G47.52)	Rapid Eye Movement Sleep Behavior Disorder	
333.94 (G25.81)	Restless Legs Syndrome	
___.___ (___.___)	Substance/Medication-Induced Sleep Disorder	
	Note: See the criteria set and corresponding recording procedures for substance-specific codes and ICD-9-CM and ICD-10-CM coding.	
	Specify whether: Insomnia type, Daytime sleepiness type, Parasomnia type, Mixed type	
	Specify if: With onset during intoxication, With onset during discontinuation/withdrawal	
780.52 (G47.09)	Other Specified Insomnia Disorder	
780.52 (G47.00)	Unspecified Insomnia Disorder	
780.54 (G47.19)	Other Specified Hypersomnolence Disorder	
780.54 (G47.10)	Unspecified Hypersomnolence Disorder	
780.59 (G47.8)	Other Specified Sleep-Wake Disorder	
780.59 (G47.9)	Unspecified Sleep-Wake Disorder	

Sexual Dysfunctions

The following specifiers apply to Sexual Dysfunctions where indicated:
[a]*Specify* whether: Lifelong, Acquired
[b]*Specify* whether: Generalized, Situational
[c]*Specify* current severity: Mild, Moderate, Severe

302.74 (F52.32)	Delayed Ejaculation[a, b, c]	
302.72 (F52.21)	Erectile Disorder[a, b, c]	
302.73 (F52.31)	Female Orgasmic Disorder[a, b, c]	
	Specify if: Never experienced an orgasm under any situation	
302.72 (F52.22)	Female Sexual Interest/Arousal Disorder[a, b, c]	
302.76 (F52.6)	Genito-Pelvic Pain/Penetration Disorder[a, c]	
302.71 (F52.0)	Male Hypoactive Sexual Desire Disorder[a, b, c]	
302.75 (F52.4)	Premature (Early) Ejaculation[a, b, c]	
___.__ (___.__)	Substance/Medication-Induced Sexual Dysfunction[c]	

Note: See the criteria set and corresponding recording procedures for substance-specific codes and ICD-9-CM and ICD-10-CM coding.
Specify if: With onset during intoxication, With onset during withdrawal, With onset after medication use

302.79 (F52.8)	Other Specified Sexual Dysfunction
302.70 (F52.9)	Unspecified Sexual Dysfunction

Gender Dysphoria

___.__ (___.__)	Gender Dysphoria
302.6 (F64.2)	Gender Dysphoria in Children

Specify if: With a disorder of sex development

302.85 (F64.1)	Gender Dysphoria in Adolescents and Adults

Specify if: With a disorder of sex development
Specify if: Posttransition
Note: Code the disorder of sex development if present, in addition to gender dysphoria.

302.6 (F64.8)	Other Specified Gender Dysphoria
302.6 (F64.9)	Unspecified Gender Dysphoria

Disruptive, Impulse-Control, and Conduct Disorders

313.81 (F91.3)	Oppositional Defiant Disorder

Specify current severity: Mild, Moderate, Severe

312.34 (F63.81)	Intermittent Explosive Disorder

___.__	(___.__)	Conduct Disorder
		Specify whether:
312.81	(F91.1)	Childhood-onset type
312.82	(F91.2)	Adolescent-onset type
312.89	(F91.9)	Unspecified onset

Specify if: With limited prosocial emotions
Specify current severity: Mild, Moderate, Severe

301.7	(F60.2)	Antisocial Personality Disorder
312.33	(F63.1)	Pyromania
312.32	(F63.2)	Kleptomania
312.89	(F91.8)	Other Specified Disruptive, Impulse-Control, and Conduct Disorder
312.9	(F91.9)	Unspecified Disruptive, Impulse-Control, and Conduct Disorder

Substance-Related and Addictive Disorders

The following specifiers and note apply to Substance-Related and Addictive Disorders where indicated:
[a]*Specify* if: In early remission, In sustained remission
[b]*Specify* if: In a controlled environment
[c]*Specify* if: With perceptual disturbances
[d]The ICD-10-CM code indicates the comorbid presence of a moderate or severe substance use disorder, which must be present in order to apply the code for substance withdrawal.

Substance-Related Disorders

Alcohol-Related Disorders

___.__	(___.__)	Alcohol Use Disorder[a, b]
		Specify current severity:
305.00	(F10.10)	Mild
303.90	(F10.20)	Moderate
303.90	(F10.20)	Severe
303.00	(___.__)	Alcohol Intoxication
	(F10.129)	With use disorder, mild
	(F10.229)	With use disorder, moderate or severe
	(F10.929)	Without use disorder
291.81	(___.__)	Alcohol Withdrawal[c, d]
	(F10.239)	Without perceptual disturbances
	(F10.232)	With perceptual disturbances
___.__	(___.__)	Other Alcohol-Induced Disorders
291.9	(F10.99)	Unspecified Alcohol-Related Disorder

Caffeine-Related Disorders

305.90	(F15.929)	Caffeine Intoxication

292.0	(F15.93)	Caffeine Withdrawal
___.__	(___.__)	Other Caffeine-Induced Disorders
292.9	(F15.99)	Unspecified Caffeine-Related Disorder

Cannabis-Related Disorders

___.__	(___.__)	Cannabis Use Disorder[a, b]
		Specify current severity:
305.20	(F12.10)	Mild
304.30	(F12.20)	Moderate
304.30	(F12.20)	Severe
292.89	(___.__)	Cannabis Intoxication[c]
		Without perceptual disturbances
	(F12.129)	With use disorder, mild
	(F12.229)	With use disorder, moderate or severe
	(F12.929)	Without use disorder
		With perceptual disturbances
	(F12.122)	With use disorder, mild
	(F12.222)	With use disorder, moderate or severe
	(F12.922)	Without use disorder
292.0	(F12.288)	Cannabis Withdrawal[d]
___.__	(___.__)	Other Cannabis-Induced Disorders
292.9	(F12.99)	Unspecified Cannabis-Related Disorder

Hallucinogen-Related Disorders

___.__	(___.__)	Phencyclidine Use Disorder[a, b]
		Specify current severity:
305.90	(F16.10)	Mild
304.60	(F16.20)	Moderate
304.60	(F16.20)	Severe
___.__	(___.__)	Other Hallucinogen Use Disorder[a, b]
		Specify the particular hallucinogen
		Specify current severity:
305.30	(F16.10)	Mild
304.50	(F16.20)	Moderate
304.50	(F16.20)	Severe
292.89	(___.__)	Phencyclidine Intoxication
	(F16.129)	With use disorder, mild
	(F16.229)	With use disorder, moderate or severe
	(F16.929)	Without use disorder
292.89	(___.__)	Other Hallucinogen Intoxication
	(F16.129)	With use disorder, mild

	(F16.229)	With use disorder, moderate or severe
	(F16.929)	Without use disorder
292.89	(F16.983)	Hallucinogen Persisting Perception Disorder
___.__	(___.__)	Other Phencyclidine-Induced Disorders
___.__	(___.__)	Other Hallucinogen-Induced Disorders
292.9	(F16.99)	Unspecified Phencyclidine-Related Disorder
292.9	(F16.99)	Unspecified Hallucinogen-Related Disorder

Inhalant-Related Disorders

___.__	(___.__)	Inhalant Use Disorder[a, b]
		Specify the particular inhalant
		Specify current severity:
305.90	(F18.10)	Mild
304.60	(F18.20)	Moderate
304.60	(F18.20)	Severe
292.89	(___.__)	Inhalant Intoxication
	(F18.129)	With use disorder, mild
	(F18.229)	With use disorder, moderate or severe
	(F18.929)	Without use disorder
___.__	(___.__)	Other Inhalant-Induced Disorders
292.9	(F18.99)	Unspecified Inhalant-Related Disorder

Opioid-Related Disorders

___.__	(___.__)	Opioid Use Disorder[a]
		Specify if: On maintenance therapy, In a controlled environment
		Specify current severity:
305.50	(F11.10)	Mild
304.00	(F11.20)	Moderate
304.00	(F11.20)	Severe
292.89	(___.__)	Opioid Intoxication[c]
		Without perceptual disturbances
	(F11.129)	With use disorder, mild
	(F11.229)	With use disorder, moderate or severe
	(F11.929)	Without use disorder
		With perceptual disturbances
	(F11.122)	With use disorder, mild
	(F11.222)	With use disorder, moderate or severe
	(F11.922)	Without use disorder
292.0	(F11.23)	Opioid Withdrawal[d]
___.__	(___.__)	Other Opioid-Induced Disorders
292.9	(F11.99)	Unspecified Opioid-Related Disorder

Sedative-, Hypnotic-, or Anxiolytic-Related Disorders

___._ (__._)		Sedative, Hypnotic, or Anxiolytic Use Disorder[a, b]
		Specify current severity:
305.40 (F13.10)		Mild
304.10 (F13.20)		Moderate
304.10 (F13.20)		Severe
292.89 (__._)		Sedative, Hypnotic, or Anxiolytic Intoxication
	(F13.129)	With use disorder, mild
	(F13.229)	With use disorder, moderate or severe
	(F13.929)	Without use disorder
292.0 (__._)		Sedative, Hypnotic, or Anxiolytic Withdrawal[c, d]
	(F13.239)	Without perceptual disturbances
	(F13.232)	With perceptual disturbances
___._ (__._)		Other Sedative-, Hypnotic-, or Anxiolytic-Induced Disorders
292.9 (F13.99)		Unspecified Sedative-, Hypnotic-, or Anxiolytic-Related Disorder

Stimulant-Related Disorders

___._ (__._)		Stimulant Use Disorder[a, b]
		Specify current severity:
___._ (__._)		Mild
305.70 (F15.10)		Amphetamine-type substance
305.60 (F14.10)		Cocaine
305.70 (F15.10)		Other or unspecified stimulant
___._ (__._)		Moderate
304.40 (F15.20)		Amphetamine-type substance
304.20 (F14.20)		Cocaine
304.40 (F15.20)		Other or unspecified stimulant
___._ (__._)		Severe
304.40 (F15.20)		Amphetamine-type substance
304.20 (F14.20)		Cocaine
304.40 (F15.20)		Other or unspecified stimulant
292.89 (__._)		Stimulant Intoxication[c]
		Specify the specific intoxicant
292.89 (__._)		Amphetamine or other stimulant, Without perceptual disturbances
	(F15.129)	With use disorder, mild
	(F15.229)	With use disorder, moderate or severe
	(F15.929)	Without use disorder
292.89 (__._)		Cocaine, Without perceptual disturbances
	(F14.129)	With use disorder, mild

(F14.229)	With use disorder, moderate or severe
(F14.929)	Without use disorder
292.89 (__._)	Amphetamine or other stimulant, With perceptual disturbances
(F15.122)	With use disorder, mild
(F15.222)	With use disorder, moderate or severe
(F15.922)	Without use disorder
292.89 (__._)	Cocaine, With perceptual disturbances
(F14.122)	With use disorder, mild
(F14.222)	With use disorder, moderate or severe
(F14.922)	Without use disorder
292.0 (__._)	Stimulant Withdrawal[d]
	Specify the specific substance causing the withdrawal syndrome
(F15.23)	Amphetamine or other stimulant
(F14.23)	Cocaine
__.__ (__._)	Other Stimulant-Induced Disorders
292.9 (__._)	Unspecified Stimulant-Related Disorder
(F15.99)	Amphetamine or other stimulant
(F14.99)	Cocaine

Tobacco-Related Disorders

__.__ (__._)	Tobacco Use Disorder[a]
	Specify if: On maintenance therapy, In a controlled environment
	Specify current severity:
305.1 (Z72.0)	Mild
305.1 (F17.200)	Moderate
305.1 (F17.200)	Severe
292.0 (F17.203)	Tobacco Withdrawal[d]
__.__ (__._)	Other Tobacco-Induced Disorders
292.9 (F17.209)	Unspecified Tobacco-Related Disorder

Other (or Unknown) Substance–Related Disorders

__.__ (__._)	Other (or Unknown) Substance Use Disorder[a, b]
	Specify current severity:
305.90 (F19.10)	Mild
304.90 (F19.20)	Moderate
304.90 (F19.20)	Severe
292.89 (__._)	Other (or Unknown) Substance Intoxication
(F19.129)	With use disorder, mild
(F19.229)	With use disorder, moderate or severe
(F19.929)	Without use disorder
292.0 (F19.239)	Other (or Unknown) Substance Withdrawal[d]

___.__ (___.__)   Other (or Unknown) Substance–Induced Disorders

292.9 (F19.99)   Unspecified Other (or Unknown) Substance–Related Disorder

Non-Substance-Related Disorders

312.31 (F63.0)   Gambling Disorder[a]
                      Specify if: Episodic, Persistent
                      Specify current severity: Mild, Moderate, Severe

Neurocognitive Disorders

___.__ (___.__)   Delirium
                      [a]**Note:** See the criteria set and corresponding recording procedures for sub-
                         stance-specific codes and ICD-9-CM and ICD-10-CM coding.
                      Specify whether:

___.__ (___.__)   Substance intoxication delirium[a]

___.__ (___.__)   Substance withdrawal delirium[a]

292.81 (___.__)   Medication-induced delirium[a]

293.0 (F05)   Delirium due to another medical condition

293.0 (F05)   Delirium due to multiple etiologies
                      Specify if: Acute, Persistent
                      Specify if: Hyperactive, Hypoactive, Mixed level of activity

780.09 (R41.0)   Other Specified Delirium

780.09 (R41.0)   Unspecified Delirium

Major and Mild Neurocognitive Disorders

Specify whether due to: Alzheimer's disease, Frontotemporal lobar degeneration, Lewy body disease, Vascular disease, Traumatic brain injury, Substance/medication use, HIV infection, Prion
disease, Parkinson's disease, Huntington's disease, Another medical condition, Multiple etiologies, Unspecified

[a]*Specify* Without behavioral disturbance, With behavioral disturbance. *For possible major neurocognitive disorder and for mild neurocognitive disorder, behavioral disturbance cannot be coded but should
still be indicated in writing.*

[b]*Specify* current severity: Mild, Moderate, Severe. *This specifier applies only to major neurocognitive
disorders (including probable and possible).*

Note: As indicated for each subtype, an additional medical code is needed for probable major neurocognitive disorder or major neurocognitive disorder. An additional medical code should *not* be
used for possible major neurocognitive disorder or mild neurocognitive disorder.

Major or Mild Neurocognitive Disorder Due to Alzheimer's Disease

___.__ (___.__)   Probable Major Neurocognitive Disorder Due to Alzheimer's
                         Disease[b]
                      Note: Code first **331.0 (G30.9)** Alzheimer's disease.

294.11 (F02.81)   With behavioral disturbance

294.10 (F02.80)   Without behavioral disturbance

331.9   (G31.9)   Possible Major Neurocognitive Disorder Due to Alzheimer's
                         Disease[a, b]

331.83 (G31.84)   Mild Neurocognitive Disorder Due to Alzheimer's Disease[a]

Major or Mild Frontotemporal Neurocognitive Disorder

___.__   (___.__)   Probable Major Neurocognitive Disorder Due to Frontotemporal
                         Lobar Degeneration[b]
                         Note: Code first **331.19 (G31.09)** frontotemporal disease.
294.11 (F02.81)   With behavioral disturbance
294.10 (F02.80)   Without behavioral disturbance
331.9   (G31.9)   Possible Major Neurocognitive Disorder Due to Frontotemporal
                         Lobar Degeneration[a, b]

331.83 (G31.84)   Mild Neurocognitive Disorder Due to Frontotemporal Lobar
                         Degeneration[a]

Major or Mild Neurocognitive Disorder With Lewy Bodies

___.__   (___.__)   Probable Major Neurocognitive Disorder With Lewy Bodies[b]
                         Note: Code first **331.82 (G31.83)** Lewy body disease.
294.11 (F02.81)   With behavioral disturbance
294.10 (F02.80)   Without behavioral disturbance
331.9   (G31.9)   Possible Major Neurocognitive Disorder With Lewy Bodies[a, b]

331.83 (G31.84)   Mild Neurocognitive Disorder With Lewy Bodies[a]

Major or Mild Vascular Neurocognitive Disorder

___.__   (___.__)   Probable Major Vascular Neurocognitive Disorder[b]
                         Note: No additional medical code for vascular disease.
290.40 (F01.51)   With behavioral disturbance
290.40 (F01.50)   Without behavioral disturbance
331.9   (G31.9)   Possible Major Vascular Neurocognitive Disorder[a, b]

331.83 (G31.84)   Mild Vascular Neurocognitive Disorder[a]

Major or Mild Neurocognitive Disorder Due to Traumatic Brain Injury

___.__   (___.__)   Major Neurocognitive Disorder Due to Traumatic Brain Injury[b]
                         Note: For ICD-9-CM, code first **907.0** late effect of intracranial injury without
                         skull fracture. For ICD-10-CM, code first **S06.2X9S** diffuse traumatic brain
                         injury with loss of consciousness of unspecified duration, sequela.
294.11 (F02.81)   With behavioral disturbance
294.10 (F02.80)   Without behavioral disturbance
331.83 (G31.84)   Mild Neurocognitive Disorder Due to Traumatic Brain Injury[a]

Substance/Medication-Induced Major or Mild Neurocognitive Disorder[a]

Note: No additional medical code. See the criteria set and corresponding recording procedures for
substance-specific codes and ICD-9-CM and ICD-10-CM coding.
Specify if: Persistent

Major or Mild Neurocognitive Disorder Due to HIV Infection

___.__ (___.__)   Major Neurocognitive Disorder Due to HIV Infection[b]
                  Note: Code first **042 (B20)** HIV infection.
294.11 (F02.81)   With behavioral disturbance
294.10 (F02.80)   Without behavioral disturbance
331.83 (G31.84)   Mild Neurocognitive Disorder Due to HIV Infection[a]

Major or Mild Neurocognitive Disorder Due to Prion Disease

___.__ (___.__)   Major Neurocognitive Disorder Due to Prion Disease[b]
                  Note: Code first **046.79 (A81.9)** prion disease.
294.11 (F02.81)   With behavioral disturbance
294.10 (F02.80)   Without behavioral disturbance
331.83 (G31.84)   Mild Neurocognitive Disorder Due to Prion Disease[a]

Major or Mild Neurocognitive Disorder Due to Parkinson's Disease

___.__ (___.__)   Major Neurocognitive Disorder Probably Due to Parkinson's Disease[b]
                  Note: Code first **332.0 (G20)** Parkinson's disease.
294.11 (F02.81)   With behavioral disturbance
294.10 (F02.80)   Without behavioral disturbance
331.9 (G31.9)   Major Neurocognitive Disorder Possibly Due to Parkinson's
                  Disease[a, b]

331.83 (G31.84)   Mild Neurocognitive Disorder Due to Parkinson's Disease[a]

Major or Mild Neurocognitive Disorder Due to Huntington's Disease

___.__ (___.__)   Major Neurocognitive Disorder Due to Huntington's Disease[b]
                  Note: Code first **333.4 (G10)** Huntington's disease.
294.11 (F02.81)   With behavioral disturbance
294.10 (F02.80)   Without behavioral disturbance
331.83 (G31.84)   Mild Neurocognitive Disorder Due to Huntington's Disease[a]

Major or Mild Neurocognitive Disorder Due to Another Medical Condition

___.__ (___.__)   Major Neurocognitive Disorder Due to Another Medical Condition[b]
                  Note: Code first the other medical condition.
294.11 (F02.81)   With behavioral disturbance
294.10 (F02.80)   Without behavioral disturbance
331.83 (G31.84)   Mild Neurocognitive Disorder Due to Another Medical Condition[a]

Major or Mild Neurocognitive Disorder Due to Multiple Etiologies

___.__ (___.__)   Major Neurocognitive Disorder Due to Multiple Etiologies[b]
                  Note: Code first all the etiological medical conditions (with the exception of
                  vascular disease).
294.11 (F02.81)   With behavioral disturbance
294.10 (F02.80)   Without behavioral disturbance

331.83 (G31.84)   Mild Neurocognitive Disorder Due to Multiple Etiologies[a]

Unspecified Neurocognitive Disorder

799.59 (R41.9)   Unspecified Neurocognitive Disorder[a]

Personality Disorders

Cluster A Personality Disorders

301.0   (F60.0)   Paranoid Personality Disorder

301.20 (F60.1)   Schizoid Personality Disorder

301.22 (F21)   Schizotypal Personality Disorder

Cluster B Personality Disorders

301.7   (F60.2)   Antisocial Personality Disorder

301.83 (F60.3)   Borderline Personality Disorder

301.50 (F60.4)   Histrionic Personality Disorder

301.81 (F60.81)   Narcissistic Personality Disorder

Cluster C Personality Disorders

301.82 (F60.6)   Avoidant Personality Disorder

301.6   (F60.7)   Dependent Personality Disorder

301.4   (F60.5)   Obsessive-Compulsive Personality Disorder

Other Personality Disorders

310.1   (F07.0)   Personality Change Due to Another Medical Condition
Specify whether: Labile type, Disinhibited type, Aggressive type, Apathetic type, Paranoid type, Other type, Combined type, Unspecified type

301.89 (F60.89)   Other Specified Personality Disorder

301.9   (F60.9)   Unspecified Personality Disorder

Paraphilic Disorders

The following specifier applies to Paraphilic Disorders where indicated:
[a]*Specify* if: In a controlled environment, In full remission

302.82 (F65.3)   Voyeuristic Disorder[a]

302.4   (F65.2)   Exhibitionistic Disorder[a]
Specify whether: Sexually aroused by exposing genitals to prepubertal children, Sexually aroused by exposing genitals to physically mature individuals, Sexually aroused by exposing genitals to prepubertal children and to physically mature individuals

302.89 (F65.81)   Frotteuristic Disorder[a]

302.83	(F65.51)	Sexual Masochism Disorder[a]

Specify if: With asphyxiophilia

302.84	(F65.52)	Sexual Sadism Disorder[a]

302.2	(F65.4)	Pedophilic Disorder

Specify whether: Exclusive type, Nonexclusive type
Specify if: Sexually attracted to males, Sexually attracted to females, Sexually attracted to both
Specify if: Limited to incest

302.81	(F65.0)	Fetishistic Disorder[a]

Specify: Body part(s), Nonliving object(s), Other

302.3	(F65.1)	Transvestic Disorder[a]

Specify if: With fetishism, With autogynephilia

302.89	(F65.89)	Other Specified Paraphilic Disorder
302.9	(F65.9)	Unspecified Paraphilic Disorder

Other Mental Disorders

294.8	(F06.8)	Other Specified Mental Disorder Due to Another Medical Condition
294.9	(F09)	Unspecified Mental Disorder Due to Another Medical Condition
300.9	(F99)	Other Specified Mental Disorder
300.9	(F99)	Unspecified Mental Disorder

Medication-Induced Movement Disorders and Other Adverse Effects of Medication

332.1	(G21.11)	Neuroleptic-Induced Parkinsonism
332.1	(G21.19)	Other Medication-Induced Parkinsonism
333.92	(G21.0)	Neuroleptic Malignant Syndrome
333.72	(G24.02)	Medication-Induced Acute Dystonia
333.99	(G25.71)	Medication-Induced Acute Akathisia
333.85	(G24.01)	Tardive Dyskinesia
333.72	(G24.09)	Tardive Dystonia
333.99	(G25.71)	Tardive Akathisia
333.1	(G25.1)	Medication-Induced Postural Tremor
333.99	(G25.79)	Other Medication-Induced Movement Disorder
__.__	(__.__)	Antidepressant Discontinuation Syndrome
995.29	(T43.205A)	Initial encounter
995.29	(T43.205D)	Subsequent encounter
995.29	(T43.205S)	Sequelae

___.__ (___.__)   Other Adverse Effect of Medication
995.20 (T50.905A)   Initial encounter
995.20 (T50.905D)   Subsequent encounter
995.20 (T50.905S)   Sequelae

Other Conditions That May Be a Focus of Clinical Attention

Relational Problems

Problems Related to Family Upbringing

V61.20 (Z62.820)   Parent-Child Relational Problem

V61.8 (Z62.891)   Sibling Relational Problem

V61.8 (Z62.29)   Upbringing Away From Parents

V61.29 (Z62.898)   Child Affected by Parental Relationship Distress

Other Problems Related to Primary Support Group

V61.10 (Z63.0)   Relationship Distress With Spouse or Intimate Partner

V61.03 (Z63.5)   Disruption of Family by Separation or Divorce

V61.8 (Z63.8)   High Expressed Emotion Level Within Family

V62.82 (Z63.4)   Uncomplicated Bereavement

Abuse and Neglect

Child Maltreatment and Neglect Problems

Child Physical Abuse

Child Physical Abuse, Confirmed
995.54 (T74.12XA)   Initial encounter
995.54 (T74.12XD)   Subsequent encounter

Child Physical Abuse, Suspected
995.54 (T76.12XA)   Initial encounter
995.54 (T76.12XD)   Subsequent encounter

Other Circumstances Related to Child Physical Abuse
V61.21 (Z69.010)   Encounter for mental health services for victim of child abuse by parent

V61.21 (Z69.020)   Encounter for mental health services for victim of nonparental child abuse

V15.41 (Z62.810)   Personal history (past history) of physical abuse in childhood

V61.22 (Z69.011)   Encounter for mental health services for perpetrator of parental child abuse

V62.83 (Z69.021)   Encounter for mental health services for perpetrator of nonparental child abuse

Child Sexual Abuse

Child Sexual Abuse, Confirmed
995.53 (T74.22XA)   Initial encounter
995.53 (T74.22XD)   Subsequent encounter

Child Sexual Abuse, Suspected
995.53 (T76.22XA)   Initial encounter
995.53 (T76.22XD)   Subsequent encounter

Other Circumstances Related to Child Sexual Abuse
V61.21 (Z69.010)   Encounter for mental health services for victim of child sexual
                                        abuse by parent
V61.21 (Z69.020)   Encounter for mental health services for victim of nonparental
                                        child sexual abuse
V15.41 (Z62.810)   Personal history (past history) of sexual abuse in childhood
V61.22 (Z69.011)   Encounter for mental health services for perpetrator of parental
                                        child sexual abuse
V62.83 (Z69.021)   Encounter for mental health services for perpetrator of
                                        nonparental child sexual abuse

Child Neglect

Child Neglect, Confirmed
995.52 (T74.02XA)   Initial encounter
995.52 (T74.02XD)   Subsequent encounter

Child Neglect, Suspected
995.52 (T76.02XA)   Initial encounter
995.52 (T76.02XD)   Subsequent encounter

Other Circumstances Related to Child Neglect
V61.21 (Z69.010)   Encounter for mental health services for victim of child neglect by
                                        parent
V61.21 (Z69.020)   Encounter for mental health services for victim of nonparental
                                        child neglect
V15.42 (Z62.812)   Personal history (past history) of neglect in childhood
V61.22 (Z69.011)   Encounter for mental health services for perpetrator of parental
                                        child neglect
V62.83 (Z69.021)   Encounter for mental health services for perpetrator of
                                        nonparental child neglect

Child Psychological Abuse

Child Psychological Abuse, Confirmed
995.51 (T74.32XA)   Initial encounter
995.51 (T74.32XD)   Subsequent encounter

Child Psychological Abuse, Suspected
995.51 (T76.32XA)   Initial encounter
995.51 (T76.32XD)   Subsequent encounter

Other Circumstances Related to Child Psychological Abuse

V61.21 (Z69.010)   Encounter for mental health services for victim of child psychological abuse by parent

V61.21 (Z69.020)   Encounter for mental health services for victim of nonparental child psychological abuse

V15.42 (Z62.811)   Personal history (past history) of psychological abuse in childhood

V61.22 (Z69.011)   Encounter for mental health services for perpetrator of parental child psychological abuse

V62.83 (Z69.021)   Encounter for mental health services for perpetrator of nonparental child psychological abuse

Adult Maltreatment and Neglect Problems

Spouse or Partner Violence, Physical

Spouse or Partner Violence, Physical, Confirmed

995.81 (T74.11XA)   Initial encounter

995.81 (T74.11XD)   Subsequent encounter

Spouse or Partner Violence, Physical, Suspected

995.81 (T76.11XA)   Initial encounter

995.81 (T76.11XD)   Subsequent encounter

Other Circumstances Related to Spouse or Partner Violence, Physical

V61.11 (Z69.11)   Encounter for mental health services for victim of spouse or partner violence, physical

V15.41 (Z91.410)   Personal history (past history) of spouse or partner violence, physical

V61.12 (Z69.12)   Encounter for mental health services for perpetrator of spouse or partner violence, physical

Spouse or Partner Violence, Sexual

Spouse or Partner Violence, Sexual, Confirmed

995.83 (T74.21XA)   Initial encounter

995.83 (T74.21XD)   Subsequent encounter

Spouse or Partner Violence, Sexual, Suspected

995.83 (T76.21XA)   Initial encounter

995.83 (T76.21XD)   Subsequent encounter

Other Circumstances Related to Spouse or Partner Violence, Sexual

V61.11 (Z69.81)   Encounter for mental health services for victim of spouse or partner violence, sexual

V15.41 (Z91.410)   Personal history (past history) of spouse or partner violence, sexual

V61.12 (Z69.12)   Encounter for mental health services for perpetrator of spouse or partner violence, sexual

Spouse or Partner, Neglect

Spouse or Partner Neglect, Confirmed
995.85 (T74.01XA)   Initial encounter
995.85 (T74.01XD)   Subsequent encounter

Spouse or Partner Neglect, Suspected
995.85 (T76.01XA)   Initial encounter
995.85 (T76.01XD)   Subsequent encounter

Other Circumstances Related to Spouse or Partner Neglect
V61.11 (Z69.11)   Encounter for mental health services for victim of spouse or
                        partner neglect
V15.42 (Z91.412)   Personal history (past history) of spouse or partner neglect
V61.12 (Z69.12)   Encounter for mental health services for perpetrator of spouse or
                        partner neglect

Spouse or Partner Abuse, Psychological

Spouse or Partner Abuse, Psychological, Confirmed
995.82 (T74.31XA)   Initial encounter
995.82 (T74.31XD)   Subsequent encounter

Spouse or Partner Abuse, Psychological, Suspected
995.82 (T76.31XA)   Initial encounter
995.82 (T76.31XD)   Subsequent encounter

Other Circumstances Related to Spouse or Partner Abuse, Psychological
V61.11 (Z69.11)   Encounter for mental health services for victim of spouse or
                        partner psychological abuse
V15.42 (Z91.411)   Personal history (past history) of spouse or partner psychological
                        abuse
V61.12 (Z69.12)   Encounter for mental health services for perpetrator of spouse or
                        partner psychological abuse

Adult Abuse by Nonspouse or Nonpartner

Adult Physical Abuse by Nonspouse or Nonpartner, Confirmed
995.81 (T74.11XA)   Initial encounter
995.81 (T74.11XD)   Subsequent encounter

Adult Physical Abuse by Nonspouse or Nonpartner, Suspected
995.81 (T76.11XA)   Initial encounter
995.81 (T76.11XD)   Subsequent encounter

Adult Sexual Abuse by Nonspouse or Nonpartner, Confirmed
995.83 (T74.21XA)   Initial encounter
995.83 (T74.21XD)   Subsequent encounter

Adult Sexual Abuse by Nonspouse or Nonpartner, Suspected
995.83 (T76.21XA)   Initial encounter
995.83 (T76.21XD)   Subsequent encounter

Adult Psychological Abuse by Nonspouse or Nonpartner, Confirmed
995.82 (T74.31XA)   Initial encounter
995.82 (T74.31XD)   Subsequent encounter

Adult Psychological Abuse by Nonspouse or Nonpartner, Suspected
99 5.82 (T76.31XA)   Initial encounter
995.82 (T76.31XD)   Subsequent encounter

Other Circumstances Related to Adult Abuse by Nonspouse or Nonpartner
V65.49 (Z69.81)   Encounter for mental health services for victim of nonspousal adult abuse
V62.83 (Z69.82)   Encounter for mental health services for perpetrator of nonspousal adult abuse

Educational and Occupational Problems

Educational Problems
V62.3 (Z55.9)   Academic or Educational Problem

Occupational Problems
V62.21 (Z56.82)   Problem Related to Current Military Deployment Status
V62.29 (Z56.9)   Other Problem Related to Employment

Housing and Economic Problems

Housing Problems
V60.0 (Z59.0)   Homelessness
V60.1 (Z59.1)   Inadequate Housing
V60.89 (Z59.2)   Discord With Neighbor, Lodger, or Landlord
V60.6 (Z59.3)   Problem Related to Living in a Residential Institution

Economic Problems
V60.2 (Z59.4)   Lack of Adequate Food or Safe Drinking Water
V60.2 (Z59.5)   Extreme Poverty
V60.2 (Z59.6)   Low Income
V60.2 (Z59.7)   Insufficient Social Insurance or Welfare Support
V60.9 (Z59.9)   Unspecified Housing or Economic Problem

Other Problems Related to the Social Environment

V62.89 (Z60.0)   Phase of Life Problem
V60.3 (Z60.2)   Problem Related to Living Alone
V62.4 (Z60.3)   Acculturation Difficulty
V62.4 (Z60.4)   Social Exclusion or Rejection
V62.4 (Z60.5)   Target of (Perceived) Adverse Discrimination or Persecution
V62.9 (Z60.9)   Unspecified Problem Related to Social Environment

Problems Related to Crime or Interaction With the Legal System

V62.89 (Z65.4)	Victim of Crime
V62.5 (Z65.0)	Conviction in Civil or Criminal Proceedings Without Imprisonment
V62.5 (Z65.1)	Imprisonment or Other Incarceration
V62.5 (Z65.2)	Problems Related to Release From Prison
V62.5 (Z65.3)	Problems Related to Other Legal Circumstances

Other Health Service Encounters for Counseling and Medical Advice

V65.49 (Z70.9)	Sex Counseling
V65.40 (Z71.9)	Other Counseling or Consultation

Problems Related to Other Psychosocial, Personal, and Environmental Circumstances

V62.89 (Z65.8)	Religious or Spiritual Problem
V61.7 (Z64.0)	Problems Related to Unwanted Pregnancy
V61.5 (Z64.1)	Problems Related to Multiparity
V62.89 (Z64.4)	Discord With Social Service Provider, Including Probation Officer, Case Manager, or Social Services Worker
V62.89 (Z65.4)	Victim of Terrorism or Torture
V62.22 (Z65.5)	Exposure to Disaster, War, or Other Hostilities
V62.89 (Z65.8)	Other Problem Related to Psychosocial Circumstances
V62.9 (Z65.9)	Unspecified Problem Related to Unspecified Psychosocial Circumstances

Other Circumstances of Personal History

V15.49 (Z91.49)	Other Personal History of Psychological Trauma
V15.59 (Z91.5)	Personal History of Self-Harm
V62.22 (Z91.82)	Personal History of Military Deployment
V15.89 (Z91.89)	Other Personal Risk Factors
V69.9 (Z72.9)	Problem Related to Lifestyle
V71.01 (Z72.811)	Adult Antisocial Behavior
V71.02 (Z72.810)	Child or Adolescent Antisocial Behavior

Problems Related to Access to Medical and Other Health Care

V63.9 (Z75.3)	Unavailability or Inaccessibility of Health Care Facilities
V63.8 (Z75.4)	Unavailability or Inaccessibility of Other Helping Agencies

Nonadherence to Medical Treatment

V15.81 (Z91.19)	Nonadherence to Medical Treatment
278.00 (E66.9)	Overweight or Obesity
V65.2 (Z76.5)	Malingering

V40.31 (Z91.83)   Wandering Associated With a Mental Disorder

V62.89 (R41.83)   Borderline Intellectual Functioning

Index

Page numbers printed in **boldface** type refer to tables.
Page numbers followed by *n* indicate note numbers.

Abuse and neglect, 421–427, 511–515
  adult maltreatment and neglect
    problems, 424–427
  child maltreatment and neglect
    problems, 422–424
  description of, 421–422
Acute akathisia, medication induced, 411
Acute dystonia, medication-induced, 410
Acute stress disorder, 20, 21, 124, 183–186
  description of, 183–184
  diagnostic criteria for, 184–186
  DSM-5 classification, 496
Adaptive functioning, definition of, 34
Addictive disorders. *See also* Substance-
  related and addictive disorders
  changes to diagnostic category, 24
ADHD. See Attention-deficit/hyperactivity
  disorder
Adjustment disorders, 21, 186–188
  description of, 186
  diagnostic criteria for, 186–188
  DSM-5 classification, 496
  specifiers, 188
Adult abuse by nonspouse or nonpartner,
  426–427
  coding, 427
  description of, 426–427
  DSM-5 classification, 514–515
Adult maltreatment and neglect problems,
  424–427
  adult abuse by nonspouse or nonpartner,
    426–427
  DSM-5 classification, 513
  spouse or partner abuse, psychological,
    426
  spouse or partner neglect, 425–426

spouse or partner violence, physical,
  424–425
spouse or partner violence, sexual, 425
Advanced sleep phase type, 23
Affect
  description of, 90
  negative affectivity, 451
Affective disorders, 90. *See also* Mood
  disorders
*Age and Gender Considerations in Psychiatric
  Diagnosis,* 2
Agoraphobia, 20, 137–139
  description of, 137
  diagnostic criteria for, 137–139
  DSM-5 classification, 495
Alcohol, **81, 100, 117,** 141, **143, 268, 282, 362,
  380**
  diagnoses associated with substance
    class, **314**
Alcohol intoxication, 320–321
  description of, 320–321
  diagnostic criteria for, 321
  DSM-5 classification, 501
Alcohol-related disorders, 316–323
  alcohol intoxication, 320–321
  alcohol use disorder, 318–320
  alcohol withdrawal, 321–322
  description of, 322–323
  DSM-5 classification, 501
  other alcohol-induced disorders, 322–323
  unspecified alcohol-related disorder,
    322–323
Alcohol use disorder, 318–320
  description of, 318–319
  diagnostic criteria for, 319–320
  DSM-5 classification, 501

Alcohol withdrawal, 321–322
  description of, 321–322
  diagnostic criteria for, 322
  DSM-5 classification, 501
Alzheimer's disease
  coding with etiological medical
      condition, **367**
  major or mild neurocognitive disorder
      due to, 373–374
Amenorrhea, 224
American Psychiatric Institute for Research
    and Education (APIRE), 1–2
Amnestic disorder, 24
Amphetamines, **81, 100, 117,** 141, **143,** 152,
    164, 268, 282, 362
Anhedonia, description of, 459
Anorexia nervosa, 22, 223–226
  atypical, 231
  description of, 223–224
  diagnostic criteria for, 224–225
  DSM-5 classification, 497
  specifiers, 225–226
"Another medical condition," 25–26
Antagonism, description of, 451, 467
Antidepressant discontinuation syndrome,
    25, 412
  description of, 412
  DSM-5 classification, 510
Antisocial personality disorder, 24, 397–398,
    457–458
  description of, 306, 397
  diagnostic criteria for, 398
  DSM-5 classification, 501
  proposed description of, 457
  proposed diagnostic criteria for, 457–458
Anxiety, description of, 123–124
Anxiety disorder due to another medical
      condition, 142–144
  coding, **143**
  description of, 142–143
  diagnostic criteria for, 143–144
  DSM-5 classification, 495
Anxiety disorders, 123–145
  agoraphobia, 137–139
  anxiety disorder due to another medical
      condition, 142–144, **143**
  changes to diagnostic category, 20,
      123–125, **124**
  DSM-5 classification, 494–495

generalized anxiety disorder, 139–141
  other specified anxiety disorder, 144
  panic attack specifier, 135–137
  panic disorder, 133–135
  selective mutism, 127–128
  separation anxiety disorder, 125–126
  social anxiety disorder (social phobia),
      131–133
  specific phobia, 128–131
  substance/medication-induced anxiety
      disorder, 141–142
  unspecified anxiety disorder, 144, 145
Anxiety neurosis, 123–124
Anxiousness, description of, 459, 461
APIRE. *See* American Psychiatric Institute
    for Research and Education
Apnea episode, 252. *See also* Obstructive
    sleep apnea hypopnea
Asperger's disorder, 18, 40
Asphyxiophilia, 290
Assessment measures, 433–447
  clinician-rated dimensions of psychosis
      symptom severity, 437, **438–439**
  cultural formulation interview, 443–444,
      445–447
  description of, 433
  Level 1 Cross-Cutting Symptom
      Measures, 434, **435–436**
  Level 2 Cross-Cutting Symptom
      Measures, 434,
  World Health Organization disability
      assessment schedule 2.0, 440,
      441–442
Ataque de nervios, 188, 189
Attention-deficit/hyperactivity disorder
    (ADHD), 18, 44–49, 302
  description of, 44
  diagnostic criteria for, 45–48
  DSM-5 classification, 490
  essential features of, 47
  other specified attention-deficit/
      hyperactivity disorder, 48
  unspecified attention-deficit/
      hyperactivity disorder, 48–49
Attention seeking, description of, 463
Attenuated delirium syndrome, 366
Attenuated psychosis syndrome, 25, 87
  proposed disorder for further study,
      470–471

proposed criteria for, 471
proposed description of, 470–471
Autism spectrum disorder, 18, 40–44
    changes to diagnostic category, 31
    description of, 40–41
    diagnostic criteria for, 41–44
    differentiated from intellectual disability
        disorder, 43
    DSM-5 classification, 490
    essential features of, 43
Autistic disorder, 18
Autogynephilia, 293
Avoidant personality disorder, 400–401,
    459–460
    description of, 400–401
    diagnostic criteria for, 401
    proposed description of, 459
    proposed diagnostic criteria for, 459–460
Avoidant/restrictive food intake disorder,
    18, 22, 221–223
    description of, 221–222
    diagnostic criteria for, 222–223
    DSM-5 classification, 497

"Baby blues," 70
Behavioral addictions, 313. *See also*
    Substance-related and addictive
    disorders
Bereavement, 103–104. *See also* Persistent
    complex bereavement disorder
Binge-eating disorder, 22, 228–230
    versus bulimia nervosa, 228
    description of, 228
    diagnostic criteria for, 228–230
    DSM-5 classification, 497
    of low frequency and/or limited
        duration, 231
Bipolar and related disorder due to another
    medical condition, 100–101
    changes to diagnostic category, 19
    coding, 101
    diagnostic criteria, 101
    DSM-5 classification, 493
Bipolar and related disorders, 90–103
    bipolar and related disorder due to
        another medical condition, 100–101
    bipolar I disorder, 95–96, **96**
    bipolar II disorder, 97–98
    changes to diagnostic category, 90–91

cyclothymic disorder, 98–99
DSM-5 classification, **91,** 492–493
hypomanic episode, 94–95
major depressive episode, 95
manic episode, 92–94
other specified bipolar and related
    disorder, 101–103
substance/medication-induced bipolar
    and related disorder, 99–100, **100**
unspecified bipolar and related disorder,
    101–102, 103
Bipolar I disorder, 95–96
    coding and recording procedures, 95–96
        96
    diagnostic criteria for, 95–96
    DSM-5 classification, 492–493
    most recent episode mixed, 19
Bipolar II disorder, 97–98
    coding and recording procedures, 97–98
    diagnostic criteria for, 97–98
    DSM-5 classification, 493
Bleuler, Eugen, xix, 72
Body dysmorphic disorder, 19, 20, 21, 22,
    153–156
    description of, 153–154
    diagnostic criteria for, 154–155
    DSM-5 classification, 495
    specifiers, 155–156
Body dysmorphic–like disorder with actual
    flaws, 166
Body dysmorphic–like disorder without
    repetitive behaviors, 166
Body-focused repetitive behavior disorder,
    166
Boissier de Sauvages, François, xviii
Borderline personality disorder, 398–399,
    460–462
    description of, 398
    diagnostic criteria for, 398–399
    proposed description of, 460
    proposed diagnostic criteria for, 460–462
Breathing-related sleep disorders, 23,
    252–257
    central sleep apnea, 254–255
    changes to diagnostic category, 252
    DSM-5 classification, 498–499
    obstructive sleep apnea hypopnea, 252–
        254
    sleep-related hypoventilation, 256–257

Brief psychotic disorder, 68–70. *See also*
   Stressor-related disorders
   description of, 68
   diagnostic criteria for, 68–69
   DSM-5 classification, 491
   specifiers, 69–70
Briquet's syndrome, 201
Bulimia nervosa, 22, 226–228
   versus binge-eating disorder, 228
   description of, 226
   diagnostic criteria for, 226–228
   DSM-5 classification, 497
   of low frequency and/or limited
      duration, 231

Caffeine, 141, **143**
Caffeine intoxication, 323–324
   description of, 323
   diagnostic criteria for, 323–324
   DSM-5 classification, 501
Caffeine-related disorders, **268,** 323–325
   caffeine intoxication, 323–324
   caffeine withdrawal, 24, 324–325
   description of, 323
   diagnoses associated with substance
      class, **314**
   DSM-5 classification, 501–502
   other caffeine-induced disorders, 325
   unspecified caffeine-related disorder,
      325
Caffeine use disorder, 475
   proposed disorder for further study,
      475
         proposed description of, 475
         proposed diagnostic criteria for, 475
Caffeine withdrawal, 24, 324–325
   description of, 324
   diagnostic criteria for, 324–325
   DSM-5 classification, 502
Callousness, description of, 457
Cannabis, **143, 268, 362**
   coding, **81**
   diagnoses associated with substance
      class, **314**
   withdrawal, 24
Cannabis intoxication, 327–328
   description of, 327
   diagnostic criteria for, 328
   DSM-5 classification, 502

Cannabis-related disorders, 325–329
   cannabis intoxication, 327–328
   cannabis use disorder, 325–327
   cannabis withdrawal, 328–329
   description of, 325
   DSM-5 classification, 502
   other cannabis-induced disorders,
      329
   unspecified cannabis-related disorder,
      329
Cannabis use disorder, 325–327
   description of, 325–326
   diagnostic criteria for, 326–327
   DSM-5 classification, 502
Cannabis withdrawal, 328–329
   description of, 328–329
   diagnostic criteria for, 329
   DSM-5 classification, 502
Cataplexy, 250
Catatonia associated with another mental
      disorder (catatonia specifier), 83
   description of, 83
   diagnostic criteria for, 83
   DSM-5 classification, 492
Catatonia specifier, 19. *See also* Catatonia
      associated with another mental
      disorder
Catatonic disorder due to another medical
      condition, 84–85
   description of, 84
   diagnostic criteria for, 84–85
   DSM-5 classification, 492
Central sleep apnea, 23, 254–255
   comorbid with opioid use, 255
   description of, 254
   diagnostic criteria for, 255
   DSM-5 classification, 498
   specifiers, 255
   subtypes, 255
Cerebrospinal fluid (CSF), 251–252
CFI. *See* Cultural formulation interview
Charcot, Jean-Martin, 208
Cheyne-Stokes breathing, 255
Childhood disintegrative disorder, 18, 40
   diagnostic criteria for, 38
Childhood-onset fluency disorder
      (stuttering), 38
   description of, 38
   DSM-5 classification, 490

Child maltreatment and neglect problems, 422–424
   child physical abuse, 422
   child sexual abuse, 422–423
   DSM-5 classification, 511
Child physical abuse, 422
   coding, 422
   description of, 422
   DSM-5 classification, 511
Child sexual abuse, 422–423
   coding, 424
   description of, 423–424
   DSM-5 classification, 512
Circadian rhythm, description of, 257
Circadian rhythm sleep-wake disorders, 23, 257–260
   description of, 257
   diagnostic criteria for, 258–259
   DSM-5 classification, 499
   specifiers, 259–260
   subtypes, 259–260
Clinician-rated dimensions of psychosis symptom severity, 87, 437, **438–439**
Cluster A personality disorders, 394–397
   DSM-5 classification, 509
   paranoid personality disorder, 394
   schizoid personality disorder, 394–395
   schizotypal personality disorder, 395–397
Cluster B personality disorders, 397–400
   antisocial personality disorder, 397–398
   borderline personality disorder, 398–399
   DSM-5 classification, 509
   histrionic personality disorder, 399–400
   narcissistic personality disorder, 400
Cluster C personality disorders, 400–403
   avoidant personality disorder, 400–401
   dependent personality disorder, 401–402
   DSM-5 classification, 509
   obsessive-compulsive personality disorder, 402–403
Cocaine, **81,100**, **117**, 141, **143**, **164**, **268**, **282**, **362**
Coding. *See also under diagnostic criteria for each disorder*
   DSM-5, 15–16
   ICD-9-CM, 15–16
   specifiers, 16
   V/Z codes, 16

Communication disorders, 18, 36–40
   changes to diagnostic category, 31
   childhood-onset fluency disorder (stuttering), 38
   description of, 36
   DSM-5 classification, 490
   language disorder, 36–37
   social (pragmatic) communication disorder, 39
   speech sound disorder, 37–38
   unspecified communication disorder, 40
Comorbid sleep-related hypoventilation, 256
Conduct disorders, 18, 302–306. *See also* Disruptive, impulse-control, and conduct disorders
   changes to diagnostic category, 24
   description of, 302–303
   diagnostic criteria for, 303–305
   DSM-5 classification, 501
   specifiers, 305–306
   subtypes, 305–306
Congenital central alveolar hypoventilation, 256
Constipation. *See* Encopresis
Conversion disorder (functional neurological symptom disorder), 22, 207–210
   description of, 207–208
   diagnostic criteria for, 208–210
   DSM-5 classification, 497
   specifiers, 210
Coprophilia, 293
Craving, description of, 316
Creutzfeldt-Jakob disease, 382
Cross-cutting, description of, 434
CSF. *See* Cerebrospinal fluid
Cultural formulation interview (CFI), 443–444, **445–447**
   cultural definition of the problem, 443
   cultural factors affecting current help seeking, 444
   cultural factors affecting self-coping and past help seeking, 444
   cultural perceptions of cause, context, and support, 443–444
Cyclothymic disorder, 98–99
   description of, 98
   diagnostic criteria for, 98–99
   DSM-5 classification, 493

Deceitfulness, description of, 457
Delayed ejaculation, 276–277
    description of, 278
    diagnostic criteria for, 276–277
    DSM-5 classification, 500
Delirium, 360–366
    coding, **362**
    description of, 360
    diagnostic criteria for, 361–364
    DSM-5 classification, 506
    due to another medical condition, 363
    due to multiple etiologies, 363
    medication-induced, 363
    other specified delirium, 365–366
    specifiers, 364–365
    substance withdrawal, 363
    unspecified delirium, 365, 366
Delusional disorder, 19, 64–67
    description of, 64
    diagnostic criteria for, 65–67
    DSM-5 classification, 491
    subtypes and specifiers, 67
Delusional parasitosis, 66
Delusions, 86–87
Dementia, 24, 360. *See also* Neurocognitive
    disorders
Dementia praecox, xviii–xix, 64, 71–72
Dependent personality disorder, 401–402
    description of, 401–402
    diagnostic criteria for, 402
Depersonalization, description of, 196
Depersonalization/derealization disorder,
    21, 196–198
    description of, 196
    diagnostic criteria for, 196–198
    DSM-5 classification, 496
Depressive disorder due to another medical
    condition, 118–119
    coding, 119
    description of, 118
    diagnostic criteria for, 118–119
    DSM-5 classification, 494
Depressive disorders, 103–120
    changes to diagnostic category, 19–20,
        103–105
    depressive disorder due to another
        medical condition, 118–119
    disruptive mood dysregulation disorder,
        105–108

DSM-5 classification, **104,** 493–494
    major depressive disorder, recurrent
        episode, 112
    major depressive disorder, single
        episode, 112
    major depressive episode, 108–112
    other specified depressive disorder,
        119–120
    persistent depressive disorder
        (dysthymia), 112–115
    premenstrual dysphoric disorder, 115–116
    substance/medication-induced
        depressive disorder, 116–118, **117**
    unspecified depressive disorder, 119–120
Depressive episodes with short-duration
    hypomania, 471–473
    proposed disorder for further study,
        471–473
        proposed description of, 471
        proposed diagnostic criteria for,
            472–473
Depressivity, description of, 461
Derealization, description of, 192, 197
Detachment, description of, 451, 467
Developmental coordination disorder, 51–52
    description of, 51–52
    diagnostic criteria for, 52
    DSM-5 classification, 491
Dhat syndrome, 166
Diagnostic Spectra and DSM/ICD
    Harmonization Study Group, 9
*Diagnostic and Statistical Manual of Mental
    Disorders* (DSM)
    conditions for further study, 25
    development of, xix–xxii
    DSM-I, xvii
    DSM-II, xx
    DSM-III, xiii, xx–xxii
    DSM-III-R, xxii
    DSM-IV, xii, xiii, xxii
        Task Force, 2
    DSM-IV-R, xxii
    DSM-5, 1–8
        alternative model for personality
            disorders, 449–467
        "another medical condition" category,
            25–26
        arrangement of disorders, 9–10
        bipolar and related disorders, **91**

changes to each diagnostic category, 18–26
classification, 489–517
coding, 15–16
conflicts of interest in, 7
controversies, 7–8
depressive disorders, **104**
development of, 1–4
diagnostic classes of, **10**
diagnostic purpose of, 11–12
diagnostic reliability and field trials, 5–6
dimensional assessment of, 4–5
disruptive, impulse-control, and conduct disorders, **296**
dissociative disorders, **192**
versus DSM-V, xii, 4
elimination disorders, **233**
feeding and eating disorders, **218**
final approval of, 6
gender dysphoria, **283**
indicating diagnostic certainty, 16
mental disorder definition, 12
multiaxial system discontinued, 17
neurodevelopmental disorders, **32**
obsessive-compulsive and related disorders, **148**
"other specified" category, 16, 25
overview, 9–11
paraphilic disorders, **287**
pattern of chapter placement, 9
peer review process, 6
proposed disorders for further study, 469–481, **470**
recording a diagnosis, 12–14
principal diagnosis, 13
reason for visit, 13
useful information for, **14**
schizophrenia spectrum, **62**
self-rated level 1 cross-cutting symptom measure—Adult, **435–436**
sexual dysfunctions, **275**
sleep-wake disorders, **241**
somatic symptom and related disorders, **202**
Task Force, 2–4
trauma- and stressor-related disorders, **170**

"unspecified" category, 16
use of, 11
editions 1952 to 2013, **xxiii**
history of, xviii–xix
overview, xvii–xviii
Disinhibited social engagement disorder, 21, 174–176
description of, 174
diagnostic criteria for, 174–176
DSM-5 classification, 496
specifiers, 176
Disinhibition, description of, 451, 467
Disorders of sex development, 284, 285, 286
Disruptive, impulse-control, and conduct disorders, 295–310
antisocial personality disorder, 306
changes to diagnostic category, 24, 295–297
conduct disorder, 302–306
DSM-5 classification, **296,** 500–501
intermittent explosive disorder, 299–302
kleptomania, 307–309
oppositional defiant disorder, 297–299
other specified disruptive, impulse-control, and conduct disorder, 309
pyromania, 306–307
unspecified disruptive, impulse-control, and conduct disorder, 309–310
Disruptive mood dysregulation disorder, 19–20, 104, 105–108
description of, 105
diagnostic criteria for, 106–108
DSM-5 classification, 493
Dissociative amnesia, 21, 194–196
description of, 194–195
diagnostic criteria for, 195–196
DSM-5 classification, 496
specifier, 196
Dissociative disorders, 191–199
changes to diagnostic category, 21, 191–192
depersonalization/derealization disorder, 196–198
dissociative amnesia, 194–196
dissociative identity disorder, 192–194
DSM-5 classification, **192,** 496
other specified dissociative disorder, 198–199
unspecified dissociative disorder, 198, 199

Dissociative fugue, 21, 192, 195. *See also* Dissociative amnesia
Dissociative identity disorder, 21, 192–194
    description of, 192–193
    diagnostic criteria for, 193–194
    DSM-5 classification, 496
Down syndrome, 33
DSM. *See Diagnostic and Statistical Manual of Mental Disorders*
Dyscalculia, 49, 51
Dyslexia, 49, 50–51
Dysmorphophobia. *See* Body dysmorphic disorder
Dysthymia. *See* Persistent depressive disorder

Eating disorders. *See* Feeding and eating disorders
Educational and occupational problems
    description of, 427
    DSM-5 classification, 515
EEG. *See* Encephalogram
"Effort syndrome," 123
Electroencephalogram (EEG), 240
Elimination disorders, 18, 233–238
    changes to diagnostic category, 22, 233–234
    DSM-5 classification, **233**, 498
    encopresis, 235–237
    enuresis, 234–235
    other specified elimination disorder, 237
    unspecified elimination disorder, 237, 238
Emotional lability, description of, 461
Empathy, description of, 457, 459, 460, 462, 463
Encopresis, 18, 22, 235–237
    description of, 235
    diagnostic criteria for, 236
    DSM-5 classification, 498
    subtypes, 236–237
Enuresis, 18, 22, 234–235
    description of, 234
    diagnostic criteria for, 234–235
    DSM-5 classification, 498
    subtypes, 235
Erectile disorder
    description of, 278
    DSM-5 classification, 500
Erotomanic type, 65

Étienne-Dominique Esquirol, Jean, xviii
Excoriation (skin-picking) disorder, 20, 161–162
    description of, 161
    diagnostic criteria for, 161–162
    DSM-5 classification, 495
Exhibitionistic disorder, 288–289
    description of, 288
    diagnostic criteria for, 288–289
    DSM-5 classification, 509

Factitious disorder, 22, 212–214
    description of, 212–213
    diagnostic criteria for, 213–214
    DSM-5 classification, 497
FDA. *See* U.S. Food and Drug Administration
Feeding and eating disorders, 18, 217–232
    anorexia nervosa, 223–226
    avoidant/restrictive food intake disorder, 221–223
    binge-eating disorder, 228–230
    bulimia nervosa, 226–228
    changes to diagnostic category, 22, 217–218
    DSM-5 classification, **218**, 497
    other specified feeding or eating disorder, 230–231
    pica, 218–219
    rumination disorder, 219–221
    unspecified feeding or eating disorder, 230, 231
Feighner, John, xx
Feighner criteria, xx, 149
Female orgasmic disorder
    description of, 278–279
    DSM-5 classification, 500
Female sexual interest/arousal disorder, 23
    description of, 279
    DSM-5 classification, 500
Fetishistic disorder, 291–292
    description of, 291
    diagnostic criteria for, 292
    DSM-5 classification, 510
Fragile X syndrome, 33
Freud, Sigmund, 135, 149, 208
Frontotemporal lobar degeneration, coding with etiological medical condition, **368**

Frotteuristic disorder, 289
    description of, 289
    diagnostic criteria for, 289
    DSM-5 classification, 509
Functional neurological symptom disorder.
        See Conversion disorder

GAF. *See* Global Assessment of Functioning
        Scale
Gambling disorder, 24, 356–358
    changes to diagnostic category, 313
    description of, 356
    diagnostic criteria for, 356–358
    specifiers, 356–358
Gélineau, Jean-Baptiste-Édouard, 249
Gender dysphoria, 283–286
    changes to diagnostic category, 23–24,
        274, 283
    in children, 23–24
    DSM-5 classification, **283,** 500
    gender dysphoria in children, 283–284
    other specified gender dysphoria, 286
    unspecified gender dysphoria, 286
Gender dysphoria in adolescents and adults,
        285–286
    description of, 285
    diagnostic criteria for, 285–286
    DSM-5 classification, 500
    specifiers, 285–286
Gender dysphoria in children, 283–284
    description of, 283
    diagnostic criteria for, 283–284
    DSM-5 classification, 500
    specifiers, 284
Generalized anxiety disorder, 139–141
    description of, 139
    diagnostic criteria for, 139–141
    DSM-5 classification, 495
General personality disorder, 391–393
    description of, 391
    diagnostic criteria for, 391–393
Genito-pelvic pain/penetration disorder, 23
    description of, 279–280
    DSM-5 classification, 500
Global Assessment of Functioning (GAF)
        Scale, 17
Global developmental delay, 35–36
    description of, 35
    DSM-5 classification, 490

Grandiose type, 65
Grandiosity, description of, 462
Grief, versus major depressive episode, 109*n*1
Gull, Sir William, 217
Guze, Samuel, xx

Hair-pulling disorder. *See* Trichotillomania
Hallucinations, xviii, 65, 86
Hallucinogen persisting perception
        disorder, 335
    description of, 335
    diagnostic criteria for, 335
    DSM-5 classification, 503
Hallucinogen-related disorders, 330–335
    DSM-5 classification, 502–503
    hallucinogen persisting perception
        disorder, 335
    other phencyclidine- and other
        hallucinogen-induced disorders,
        330–333, 335
    phencyclidine and other hallucinogen
        use disorders, 330–333
    phencyclidine intoxication and other
        hallucinogen intoxication, 333–335
    unspecified phencyclidine- and
        unspecified hallucinogen-related
        disorders, 335
Hallucinogens, **81, 100, 117, 143,** 194, **362**
    diagnoses associated with substance
        class, **314**
Hippocrates, xviii
Histrionic personality disorder, 399–400
    description of, 399
    diagnostic criteria for, 399–400
HIV (human immunodeficiency virus)
    coding with etiological medical
        condition, **368**
    major or mild neurocognitive disorder
        due to, 381–382, 508
Hoarding disorder, 20, 21, 156–159
    description of, 156
    diagnostic criteria for, 156–158
    DSM-5 classification, 495
    specifiers, 158–159
Hostility, description of, 457, 461
Housing and economic problems, 428
    coding, 428
    description of, 428
    DSM-5 classification, 515

Human immunodeficiency virus. *See* HIV
"Humors," xviii
Huntington's disease, 384
   coding with etiological medical
      condition, **369**
   diagnosis of, 384
   major or mild neurocognitive disorder
      due to, 384
Hyman, Steven E., 1
Hypersomnia. *See* Hypersomnolence
   disorder
Hypersomnolence disorder, 23, 245–249
   description of, 245–246
   diagnostic criteria for, 246–249
   DSM-5 classification, 498
   specifiers, 249
Hypnic jerks, 240. *See also* Non–rapid eye
   movement sleep arousal disorders
Hypochondriasis, 21, 202. *See also* Somatic
   symptom and related disorders
Hypocretin, 249
Hypomanic episode, 94–95
   coding, **96**
   diagnostic criteria for, 94–95
Hypopnea episode, 252–253. *See also*
   Obstructive sleep apnea hypopnea
Hysteria, 208
ICD. *See Manual of International Statistical
   Classification of Diseases, Injuries, and
   Causes of Death*
Identity, description of, 457, 459, 460, 462,
   463
Idiopathic central sleep apnea, 255
Idiopathic hypoventilation, 256
Illness anxiety disorder, 22, 205–207
   description of, 205–206
   diagnostic criteria for, 206–207
   DSM-5 classification, 497
   subtypes, 207
Impulse. *See also* Obsessive-compulsive
   disorder
   description of, 150
Impulse-control disorders, 147. *See also*
   Disruptive, impulse-control, and
   conduct disorders; Trichotillomania
   (hair-pulling disorder)
   changes to diagnostic category, 24
Impulsivity, description of, 458, 461
Inattention, 47

"Infantile autism," 40. *See also* Autism
   spectrum disorder
Inhalant intoxication, 337–338
   description of, 337
   diagnostic criteria for, 337–338
   DSM-5 classification, 503
Inhalant-related disorders, 336–338
   DSM-5 classification, 503
   inhalant intoxication, 337–338
   inhalant use disorder, 336–337
   other inhalant-induced disorders, 338
   unspecified inhalant-related disorder,
      338
Inhalants, **81, 117, 143, 362, 380**
   diagnoses associated with substance
      class, **314**
Inhalant use disorder, 336–337
   description of, 336
   diagnostic criteria for, 336–337
   DSM-5 classification, 503
Insomnia disorder, 23, 242–245
   description of, 242–243
   diagnostic criteria for, 243–245
   DSM-5 classification, 498
   specifiers, 245
Intellectual developmental disorder. *See*
   Intellectual disability; Unspecified
   intellectual disability
Intellectual disability (intellectual
   developmental disorder), 18, 32–36
   description of, 31, 32–34
   diagnostic criteria for, 34–35
   differentiated from autism spectrum
      disorder, 43
   DSM-5 classification, 489–490
   global developmental delay, 35–36
   unspecified intellectual disability, 36
Intellectual functioning, definition of, 34
Intelligence, definition of, 33
Intermittent explosive disorder, 24, 299–302
   description of, 299–300
   diagnostic criteria for, 300–302
   DSM-5 classification, 500
Internet gaming disorder, 25, 313, 476–477
   proposed disorder for further study,
      476–477
      proposed description of, 476
      proposed diagnostic criteria for,
         476–477

Intimacy, description of, 457, 459, 461, 462, 463
Intimacy avoidance, description of, 459, 464
Intoxication, description of, 315–316
IQ, 18, 31, 33, 35. *See also* Adaptive
　　functioning
Irregular sleep-wake type disorder, 23
　　description of, 259
Irresponsibility, description of, 458
"Irritable heart syndrome," 123

Jealous type, 65
Jet lag type sleep disorder, 23, 260
Jikoshu-kyofu, 166

Kanner, Leo, 40
Kasanin, Jacob, 75
Kleptomania, 24, 307–309
　　description of, 307–308
　　diagnostic criteria for, 308–309
　　DSM-5 classification, 501
Klismaphilia, 293
Koro, 166
Kraepelin, Emil, xviii, xix, 64, 71–72, 90
Kupfer, David J., 1, 2

Langfeldt, Gabriel, 70
Language disorder, 36–37
　　description of, 36–37
　　diagnostic criteria for, 37
　　DSM-5 classification, 490
Learning disorder, 31
Lehrbuch der Psychiatrie (Emil Kraepelin), xix
Level of personality functioning scale, **453–456**
Lewes, George Henry, xvii
Lewy body disease
　　coding with etiological medical
　　　　condition, **368**
　　major or mild neurocognitive disorder
　　　　with, 376–377
Linnaeus, Carolus, xviii

Major and mild neurocognitive disorders,
　　366–386
　　DSM-5 classification, 506–509
　　major neurocognitive disorder, 366–370
　　major or mild frontotemporal
　　　　neurocognitive disorder, 374–376
　　major or mild neurocognitive disorder
　　　　due to Alzheimer's disease, 373–374

major or mild neurocognitive disorder
　　due to another medical condition,
　　384–385
major or mild neurocognitive disorder
　　due to HIV infection, 381–382
major or mild neurocognitive disorder
　　due to Huntington's disease, 384
major or mild neurocognitive disorder
　　due to multiple etiologies, 385–386
major or mild neurocognitive disorder
　　due to Parkinson's disease, 383
major or mild neurocognitive disorder
　　due to prion disease, 382
major or mild neurocognitive disorder
　　due to traumatic brain injury,
　　378–379
major or mild neurocognitive disorder
　　with Lewy bodies, 376–377
major or mild vascular neurocognitive
　　disorder, 377–378
mild neurocognitive disorder, 371–373
substance/medication-induced major or
　　mild neurocognitive disorder,
　　379–381
unspecified neurocognitive disorder, 386
Major depressive disorder, 19, 95
　　DSM-5 classification, 493–494
　　recurrent episode, 112
　　single episode, 112
　　specifiers, 112
Major depressive episode (MDE), 108–112
　　coding and recording procedures, 110,
　　　　110
　　description of, 108
　　diagnostic criteria for, 108–112
　　versus grief, 109n1
Major neurocognitive disorder, 24, 366–370
　　coding, 367–369
　　description of, 366
　　diagnostic criteria for, 367–370
　　specifiers, 370, 372–373
Major or mild frontotemporal
　　neurocognitive disorder, 374–376
　　description of, 374–375
　　diagnostic criteria for, 375–376
　　DSM-5 classification, 507
Major or mild neurocognitive disorder due
　　to Alzheimer's disease, 373–374
　　description of, 373

Major or mild neurocognitive disorder due
  to Alzheimer's disease *(continued)*
  diagnostic criteria for, 373374
  DSM-5 classification, 506–507
Major or mild neurocognitive disorder due
  to another medical condition, 384–385
  description of, 384
  diagnostic criteria for, 384–385
  DSM-5 classification, 508
Major or mild neurocognitive disorder due
  to HIV infection, 381–382, 508
  description of, 381
  diagnostic criteria for, 381–382
Major or mild neurocognitive disorder due
  to Huntington's disease, 384
  description of, 384
  diagnostic criteria for, 384
  DSM-5 classification, 508
Major or mild neurocognitive disorder due
  to multiple etiologies, 385–386
  description of, 385
  diagnostic criteria for, 385–386
  DSM-5 classification, 508–509
Major or mild neurocognitive disorder due
  to Parkinson's disease, 383
  description of, 383
  diagnostic criteria for, 383
  DSM-5 classification, 508
Major or mild neurocognitive disorder due
  to prion disease, 382
  description of, 382
  diagnostic criteria for, 382
  DSM-5 classification, 508
Major or mild neurocognitive disorder due
  to traumatic brain injury, 378–379
  description of, 378
  diagnostic criteria for, 378–379
  DSM-5 classification, 507
Major or mild neurocognitive disorder with
  Lewy bodies, 376–377
  description of, 376
  diagnostic criteria for, 376–377
  DSM-5 classification, 507
Major or mild vascular neurocognitive
  disorder, 377–378
  coding with etiological medical
    condition, **368**
  diagnostic criteria for, 377–378
  DSM-5 classification, 507

Male hypoactive sexual desire disorder
  description of, 280
  DSM-5 classification, 500
Manic depressive illness, xx
Manic episode, 92–94
  diagnostic criteria for, 92–93
  specifiers, 94
Manipulativeness, description of, 457
*Manual of International Statistical
  Classification of Diseases, Injuries, and
  Causes of Death,* xix, xx
  coding, 15–16
    for anxiety disorder due to substance/
      medication-induced anxiety
      disorder, **143**
    for delirium, **362**
    for hypomanic episode, **96**
    for major neurocognitive disorder,
      367–369
    for medication-induced movement
      disorders and other adverse
      effects of medication, **409**
    for other conditions that may be a
      focus of clinical attention, **421**
    for substance/medication-induced
      bipolar and related disorder,
      100
    for substance/medication-induced
      depressive disorder, **117**
    for substance/medication-induced
      major or mild neurocognitive
      disorder, **380–381**
    for substance/medication-induced
      obsessive-compulsive and related
      disorder, **164**
    for substance/medication-induced
      psychotic disorder, 80, **81**
    for substance/medication-induced
      sexual dysfunction, **282**
    for substance/medication-induced
      sleep disorder, **268**
  ICD-9, 13
  ICD-10, 13–14
MDE. *See* Major depressive episode
Medication-induced acute akathisia, 411
  DSM-5 classification, 510
Medication-induced acute dystonia
  description of, 410
  DSM-5 classification, 510

Medication-induced movement disorders, 25, 407–413
  antidepressant discontinuation syndrome, 412
  changes to diagnostic category, 408–409, **409**
  DSM-5 classification, 510–511
  medication-induced acute akathisia, 411
  medication-induced acute dystonia, 410
  medication-induced postural tremor, 411
  neuroleptic-induced parkinsonism, 409
  neuroleptic malignant syndrome, 410
  other adverse effect of medication, 413
  other medication-induced movement disorder, 411
  other medication-induced Parkinsonism, 409
  tardive akathisia, 411
  tardive dyskinesia, 411
  tardive dystonia, 411
Medication-induced postural tremor, 411
  description of, 411
  DSM-5 classification, 510
Mental deficiency, 30
Mental disorders. *See also* Other mental disorders
  classification of, xviii
  coding for unspecified, 16
  definition of, 12
  humoral theories of, xviii
Mental retardation, 18, 30, 31, 33. *See also* Intellectual disability (intellectual developmental disorder)
Mild neurocognitive disorder, 24, 371–373
  description of, 371
  diagnostic criteria for, 371–372
  specifiers, 372–373
Mirin, Steven M., 1
Mixed type, 65
Monomania, 148. *See also* Obsessive-compulsive disorder
Mood disorders, 89–121
  bipolar and related disorders, 90–103
  changes to diagnostic category, 89–90
  depressive disorders, 103–120
Morton, Richard, 217
Motor disorders, 51–57
  developmental coordination disorder, 51–52

DSM-5 classification, 491
  stereotypic movement disorder, 52–53
  tic disorders, 54–57
Multiaxial system, discontinuation of, 17
"Multiple personality disorder." *See* Dissociative identity disorder
Munchausen syndrome, 213. *See also* Factitious disorder

Narcissistic personality disorder, 400, 462–463
  description of, 400
  diagnostic criteria for, 400
  proposed description of, 462
  proposed diagnostic criteria for, 462–463
Narcolepsy, 23, 249–252
  autosomal dominant cerebellar ataxia, deafness, and narcolepsy, 250
  with cataplexy but without hypocretin deficiency, 250
  description of, 249
  diagnostic criteria for, 250–252
  DSM-5 classification, 498
  secondary to another medical condition, 250
  specifiers, 252
  subtypes, 252
  without cataplexy but with hypocretin deficiency, 250
National Institutes of Health (NIH), 2
Necrophilia, 293
Negative affectivity, description of, 451, 466–467
Neurasthenia, 123–124
Neurobehavioral disorder associated with prenatal alcohol exposure, 477–478
  proposed disorder for further study, 477–478
    proposed description of, 477
    proposed diagnostic criteria for, 477–478
"Neurocirculatory asthenia," 123
Neurocognitive disorders, 359–387, **361**
  changes to diagnostic category, 24, 359–360
  delirium, 360–366
  DSM-5 classification, 506–509
  major and mild neurocognitive disorders, 366–386

Neurodevelopmental disorders, 29–59
  attention-deficit/hyperactivity disorder, 44–49
  autism spectrum disorder, 40–44
  changes to diagnostic category, 18–19, 31
  communication disorders, 36–40
  description of changes to, 30–31
  DSM-5 classification, 489–491
  intellectual disabilities, 32–36
  motor disorders, 51–57
  other neurodevelopmental disorders, 57–58
  specific learning disorder, 49–51
Neuroleptic-induced parkinsonism, 409
  DSM-5 classification, 510
Neuroleptic malignant syndrome
  description of, 410
  DSM-5 classification, 510
Neuroses, 124
New York Academy of Medicine, xix
Nicotine. *See* Tobacco-related disorders
Night eating syndrome, 231
Nightmare disorder, 261–263
  description of, 261
  diagnostic criteria for, 261–263
  DSM-5 classification, 499
NIH. *See* National Institutes of Health
Non-24-hour sleep-wake type disorder
  description of, 259–260
Nonadherence to medical treatment, 430–431
  coding, 430–431
  description of, 430–431
Non–rapid eye movement sleep arousal disorders, 260–261
  description of, 260
  diagnostic criteria for, 260–261
  DSM-5 classification, 499
Non-substance-related disorders, 356–358
  DSM-5 classification, 506
  gambling disorder, 356–358
Nonsuicidal self-injury, 479–481
  proposed disorder for further study, 479–481
    proposed description of, 479–480
    proposed diagnostic criteria for, 480–481
NREM. *See* Non–rapid eye movement sleep arousal disorders

Obsessional jealousy, 166
Obsessive-compulsive and related disorder due to another medical condition, 164–165
  description of, 164
  diagnostic criteria for, 164–165
  DSM-5 classification, 495
Obsessive-compulsive and related disorders, 124
  body dysmorphic disorder, 153–156
  changes to diagnostic category, 20–21, 147–148, **148**
  DSM-5 classification, 495
  due to another medical condition, 20
  excoriation (skin-picking) disorder, 161–162
  hoarding disorder, 156–159
  insight specifier for, 20–21
  medication-induced, 20
  obsessive-compulsive and related disorder due to another medical condition, 164–165
  obsessive-compulsive disorder, 148–153
  other specified obsessive-compulsive and related disorder, 165–166
  substance/medication-induced obsessive-compulsive and related disorder, 162–164
  tic-related specifier, 21
  trichotillomania (hair-pulling disorder), 159–160
  unspecified obsessive-compulsive and related disorder, 165, 166
Obsessive-compulsive disorder (OCD), 148–153
  description of, 148–149
  diagnostic criteria for, 149–150
    compulsions, 148, 151–153
    obsessions, 148, 150–151
  DSM-5 classification, 495
  specifiers, 153
Obsessive-compulsive personality disorder, 402–403, 463–464
  description of, 402–403
  diagnostic criteria for, 403
  proposed description of, 463
  proposed diagnostic criteria for, 463–464

Obstructive sleep apnea hypopnea, 23, 252–254
description of, 252–253
diagnostic criteria for, 253–254
DSM-5 classification, 498
specifiers, 254
OCD. *See* Obsessive-compulsive disorder
Opioid intoxication, 341–342
description of, 341
diagnostic criteria for, 341–342
DSM-5 classification, 503
Opioid-related disorders, 339–343
description of, 338
DSM-5 classification, 503
opioid intoxication, 341–342
opioid withdrawal, 342
other opioid-induced disorders, 343
unspecified opioid-related disorder, 343
Opioids **117, 143** 255, **268, 282, 362**
diagnoses associated with substance
class, **314**
Opioid use disorder, 339–341
description of, 339
diagnostic criteria for, 339–341
DSM-5 classification, 503
Opioid withdrawal, 342
description of, 342
diagnostic criteria for, 342
DSM-5 classification, 503
Oppositional defiant disorder, 24, 297–299
description of, 297
diagnostic criteria for, 297–299
DSM-5 classification, 500
Orgasm, 275. *See also* Sexual dysfunctions
Other adverse effects of medication, 413
description of, 413
DSM-5 classification, 510–511
Other alcohol-induced disorders, 322–323
description of, 322
Other caffeine-induced disorders, 325
description of, 325
Other cannabis-induced disorders, 329
description of, 329
Other circumstances of personal history,
429–431
DSM-5 classification, 516–517
nonadherence to medical treatment,
430–431
problems related to access to medical and
other health care, 430

Other conditions that may be a focus of
clinical attention, 413–431
abuse and neglect, 421–427
coding, **415–421**
description of, 413–414
DSM-5 classification, 511–517
educational and occupational problems,
427
housing and economic problems, 428
other circumstances of personal history,
429–431
other health service encounters for
counseling and medical advice, 429
other problems related to the social
environment, 428
problems related to crime or interaction
with the legal system, 428–429
problems related to other psychosocial,
personal, and environmental
circumstances, 429
relational problems, 414
Other hallucinogen intoxication
description of, 333
diagnostic criteria for, 334–335
DSM-5 classification, 502–503
Other hallucinogen use disorders, 330,
331–333
description of, 330
diagnostic criteria for, 331–333
DSM-5 classification, 502
Other health service encounters for
counseling and medical advice, 429
coding, 429
description of, 429
DSM-5 classification, 516
Other inhalant-induced disorders, 338
description of, 338
DSM-5 classification, 503
Other medication-induced movement
disorder, 411
description of, 411
DSM-5 classification, 510
Other medication-induced Parkinsonism,
409
Other mental disorders, DSM-5
classification, 510
Other neurodevelopmental disorders, 57–58
diagnostic criteria for, 58
DSM-5 classification, 491

Other neurodevelopmental disorders
  (continued)
  other specified neurodevelopmental
    disorder, 57–58
  unspecified neurodevelopmental
    disorder, 57–58
Other opioid-induced disorders, 343
  DSM-5 classification, 503
Other personality disorders, 403–405
  DSM-5 classification, 509
  other specified personality disorder,
    404–405
  personality change due to another
    medical condition, 403–404
  unspecified personality disorder, 405, 406
Other phencyclidine- and other
  hallucinogen-induced disorders, 335
Other problems related to the social
  environment, 428
  coding, 428
  description of, 428
  DSM-5 classification, 515
Other sedative-, hypnotic-, or anxiolytic-
  induced disorders, 347
  description of, 347
  DSM-5 classification, 504
Other specified anxiety disorder, 144
  description of, 144
  diagnostic criteria for, 144
  DSM-5 classification, 491, 495
Other specified attention-deficit/
  hyperactivity disorder
  description of, 48
  diagnostic criteria for, 58
Other specified bipolar and related disorder,
  101–103
  description of, 101–102
  diagnostic criteria for, 102–103
  DSM-5 classification, 493
"Other specified" category, 16, 25
Other specified delirium, 365–366
  description of, 365
  diagnostic criteria for, 365–366
  DSM-5 classification, 506
Other specified depressive disorder,
  119–120
  description of, 119
  diagnostic criteria for, 119–120
  DSM-5 classification, 494

Other specified disruptive, impulse-control,
  and conduct disorder, 309
  description of, 309
  diagnostic criteria for, 309
  DSM-5 classification, 501
Other specified dissociative disorder,
  198–199
  acute dissociative reactions to stressful
    events, 199
  chronic and recurrent syndromes of
    mixed dissociative symptoms, 198
  description of, 198
  diagnostic criteria for, 198–199
  dissociative trance, 199
  DSM-5 classification, 496
  identity disturbance due to prolonged
    and intense coercive persuasion,
    198
Other specified elimination disorder, 237
  description of, 237
  diagnostic criteria for, 237
  DSM-5 classification, 498
Other specified feeding or eating disorder,
  230–231
  description of, 230
  diagnostic criteria for, 230–231
  DSM-5 classification, 497
Other specified gender dysphoria
  description of, 286
  DSM-5 classification, 500
Other specified hypersomnolence disorder,
  270–271
  description of, 270
  diagnostic criteria for, 270–271
  DSM-5 classification, 499
Other specified insomnia disorder, 269–270
  description of, 269
  diagnostic criteria for, 269–270
  DSM-5 classification, 499
Other specified neurodevelopmental
  disorder, 57–58
  description of, 57
  diagnostic criteria for, 58
  DSM-5 classification, 491
Other specified obsessive-compulsive and
  related disorder, 165–166
  description of, 165
  diagnostic criteria for, 165–166
  DSM-5 classification, 495

Other specified paraphilic disorder, 293
　　description of, 293
　　diagnostic criteria for, 293
　　DSM-5 classification, 510
Other specified personality disorder, 404–405
　　diagnostic criteria for, 405
Other specified schizophrenia spectrum and
　　　other psychotic disorder, 86–87
　　description of, 86
　　diagnostic criteria for, 86–87
　　DSM-5 classification, 492
Other specified sexual dysfunction
　　description of, 282–283
　　DSM-5 classification, 500
Other specified sleep-wake disorder,
　　271–272
　　description of, 271
　　diagnostic criteria for, 271–272
　　DSM-5 classification, 499
Other specified somatic symptom and
　　　related disorder, 214–215
　　description of, 214
　　diagnostic criteria for, 214–215
　　DSM-5 classification, 497
Other specified tic disorders, 56–57
　　description of, 56–57
　　diagnostic criteria for, 57
Other specified trauma- and stressor-related
　　　disorder, 188–189
　　description of, 188
　　diagnostic criteria for, 188–189
　　DSM-5 classification, 496
Other stimulant-induced disorders, 353
　　description of, 353
　　DSM-5 classification, 505
Other (or unknown) substance–related
　　　disorders, 356
　　description of, 356
　　DSM-5 classification, 505–506
Other tobacco-induced disorders, 355
　　description of, 355
　　DSM-5 classification, 505

Pain disorder, 21
Panic attacks, 20
Panic attack specifier, 135–137
　　description of, 135–136
　　diagnostic criteria for, 136–137
　　DSM-5 classification, 495

Panic disorder, 20, 133–135
　　description of, 133–134
　　diagnostic criteria for, 134–135
　　DSM-5 classification, 495
Paracelsus, xviii
Paranoid personality disorder, 394
　　description of, 394
　　diagnostic criteria for, 394
Paraphilic disorders, 286–294
　　changes to diagnostic category, 25, 274,
　　　286–287
　　DSM-5 classification, **287,** 509–510
　　exhibitionistic disorder, 288–289
　　fetishistic disorder, 291–292
　　frotteuristic disorder, 289
　　other specified paraphilic disorder, 293
　　pedophilic disorder, 291
　　sexual masochism disorder, 290
　　sexual sadism disorder, 290
　　transvestic disorder, 292–293
　　unspecified paraphilic disorder, 293, 294
　　voyeuristic disorder, 287–288
Parasomnias, 260–272
　　description of, 260
　　nightmare disorder, 261–263
　　non–rapid eye movement sleep arousal
　　　disorders, 260–261
　　other specified hypersomnolence
　　　disorder, 270–271
　　other specified insomnia disorder,
　　　269–270
　　rapid eye movement sleep behavior
　　　disorder, 263–265
　　restless legs syndrome, 265–266
　　substance/medication-induced sleep
　　　disorder, 266–269
　　unspecified hypersomnolence disorder,
　　　270, 271
　　unspecified insomnia disorder, 269, 270
Parkinson's disease, 152
　　coding with etiological medical
　　　condition, **369**
　　major or mild neurocognitive disorder
　　　due to, 383
PCP. *See* Phencyclidine
Pedophilic disorder, 291
　　description of, 291
　　diagnostic criteria for, 291
　　DSM-5 classification, 510

Persecutory type, 65
Perseveration, description of, 464
Persistent complex bereavement disorder, 25, 473–474
    proposed description of, 473
    proposed diagnostic criteria for, 473–474
Persistent depressive disorder (dysthymia), 20, 105, 112–115
    description of, 112–113
    diagnostic criteria for, 113–115
    DSM-5 classification, 494
Persistent (chronic) motor or vocal tic disorder, 55–56
    description of, 55
    diagnostic criteria for, 55–56
    DSM-5 classification, 491
Personality change due to another medical condition, 25, 403–404
    description of, 403–404
    diagnostic criteria for, 404
Personality disorders, 389–406
    alternative DSM-5 model for, 449–467
    changes to diagnostic category, 25, 389–391
    Cluster A personality disorders, 394–397
    Cluster B personality disorders, 397–400
    Cluster C personality disorders, 400–403
    description of, 452
    DSM-5 classification, 509
    general criteria for, 452
    general personality disorder, 391–393
    Level of Personality Functioning Scale, **453–456**
    other personality disorders, 403–405
    proposed description of, 449–452
    specific personality disorders, 457–467
Personality disorder—trait specified, 466–467
    proposed description for, 466
    proposed diagnostic criteria for, 466–467
Pervasive developmental disorder, 30, 40
    not otherwise specified, 18
Phencyclidine (PCP), **81, 100, 117, 143,** 194, **362**
    diagnoses associated with substance class, **314**
Phencyclidine and other hallucinogen use disorders, 330–333

Phencyclidine intoxication and other hallucinogen intoxication, 333–335
    description of, 333
    diagnostic criteria for, 333
    DSM-5 classification, 502
Phencyclidine use disorder
    description of, 330
    diagnostic criteria for, 330–331
    DSM-5 classification, 502
Phobia. *See also* Specific phobia disorder
    description of, 128
Pica, 18, 218–219
    description of, 218
    diagnostic criteria for, 218–219
    DSM-5 classification, 497
Pinel, Philippe, xviii
Posttraumatic stress disorder (PTSD), 20, 21, 124, 176–183
    for children 6 years and younger, 180–181
    description of, 176–178
    diagnostic criteria for, 178–183
    DSM-5 classification, 496
Postural tremor, medication-induced, 411
Pramipexole, 152
Premature (early) ejaculation
    description of, 280
    DSM-5 classification, 500
Premenstrual dysphoric disorder, 19–20, 104–105, 115–116
    description of, 115
    diagnostic criteria for, 115–116
    DSM-5 classification, 494
Prion disease
    coding with etiological medical condition, **368**
    major or mild neurocognitive disorder due to, 382
Problems related to access to medical and other health care, 430
    coding, 430
    description of, 430
Problems related to crime or interaction with the legal system, 428–429
    coding, 428
    description of, 428
    DSM-5 classification, 516
Problems related to other psychosocial, personal, and environmental circumstance, DSM-5 classification, 516

Problems related to other psychosocial, personal, and environmental circumstances, 429
coding, 429
description of, 429
Provisional tic disorder, 56
description of, 56
diagnostic criteria for, 56
DSM-5 classification, 491
Pseudocyesis, 215
Psychological factors affecting other medical conditions, 22, 210–212
description of, 210–211
diagnostic criteria for, 211–212
DSM-5 classification, 497
specifiers, 212
Psychoneurotic disorders, 124
Psychosis, definition of, 61
Psychotic disorder due to another medical condition, 82
description of, 82
diagnostic criteria for, 82
DSM-5 classification, 492
Psychoticism, description of, 451, 467
PTSD. *See* Posttraumatic stress disorder
Public Law 111-256 (Rosa's Law), 35
"Punding" behaviors, 152
Purging disorder, 231
Pyromania, 24, 306–307
description of, 306
diagnostic criteria for, 306–307
DSM-5 classification, 501

Rapid eye movement (REM) sleep behavior disorder, 23, 263–265
description of, 263–264
diagnostic criteria for, 264–265
DSM-5 classification, 499
RDC. *See* Research Diagnostic Criteria
Reactive attachment disorder, 18–19, 21, 171–174
description of, 171
diagnostic criteria for, 171–174
DSM-5 classification, 496
specifiers, 174
Reading disorders, 49
Regier, Darrel A., 1, 2
Relational problems, 414
DSM-5 classification, 511

other problems related to primary support group, 414
problems related to family upbringing, 414
REM. *See* Rapid eye movement sleep behavior disorder
A Research Agenda for DSM-V (Kupfer et al. 2002), 2
Research Diagnostic Criteria (RDC), xx–xxi
Resolution, 276. *See also* Sexual dysfunctions
Restless legs syndrome, 23, 265–266
description of, 265
diagnostic criteria for, 265–266
DSM-5 classification, 499
Restricted affectivity, description of, 464
Rett's disorder, 18, 40
Rigid perfectionism, description of, 463–464
Risk taking, description of, 457–458, 461
Robinowitz, Carolyn, 2
Robins, Eli, xx
Rome Diagnostic Criteria, 236, 237
Rosa's Law (Public Law 111-256), 35
Ruiz, Pedro, 2
Rumination disorder, 18, 22, 219–221
description of, 219–220
diagnostic criteria for, 220–221
DSM-5 classification, 497

Schizoaffective disorder, 19, 75–78
description of, 75–76
diagnostic criteria for, 76–78
DSM-5 classification, 492
specifiers, 78
Schizoid personality disorder, 394–395
description of, 394–395
diagnostic criteria for, 395
Schizophrenia, 71–75
description of, 71–72
diagnostic criteria for, 72–75
DSM-5 classification, 492
specifiers, 75
Schizophrenia spectrum and other psychotic disorders, xviii–xix, 19, 61–88
brief psychotic disorder, 68–70
catatonia associated with another mental disorder (catatonia specifier), 83
catatonic disorder due to another medical condition, 84–85
changes to diagnostic category, 19, 62–63

Schizophrenia spectrum and other psychotic
    disorders *(continued)*
  clinician-rated dimensions of psychosis
      symptom severity, 87
  coding for unspecified, 16
  delusional disorder, 64–67
  description of changes to, 61–63
  DSM-5 classification, **62**, 491–492
  other specified schizophrenia spectrum
      and other psychotic disorder, 86–87
  psychotic disorder due to another
      medical condition, 82
  schizoaffective disorder, 75–78
  schizophrenia, 71–75
  schizophreniform disorder, 70–71
  schizotypal (personality) disorder, 63
  substance/medication-induced psychotic
      disorder, 79–81
  unspecified catatonia, 85–86
  unspecified schizophrenia spectrum and
      other psychotic disorder, 86–87
Schizophreniform disorder, 70–71
  description of, 70
  diagnostic criteria for, 70–71
  DSM-5 classification, 492
Schizotypal personality disorder, 19, 63,
    395–397, 464–466
  description of, 395–396
  diagnostic criteria for, 396–397
  DSM-5 classification, 491
  proposed description of, 464–465
  proposed diagnostic criteria for, 465–466
Schneider, Kurt, 72
Scully, James E., Jr., 2
Sedative, hypnotic, or anxiolytic agents, **81,
    100, 117, 143, 268, 282, 362, 381**
  diagnoses associated with substance
      class, **314**
Sedative, hypnotic, or anxiolytic
    intoxication, 345–346
  description of, 345
  diagnostic criteria for, 345–346
Sedative-, hypnotic-, or anxiolytic-related
    disorders, 343–347
  DSM-5 classification, 504
  other sedative-, hypnotic-, or anxiolytic-
      induced disorders, 347
  sedative, hypnotic, or anxiolytic
      intoxication, 345–346

sedative, hypnotic, or anxiolytic use
    disorder, 343–345
sedative, hypnotic, or anxiolytic
    withdrawal, 346–347
unspecified sedative-, hypnotic-, or
    anxiolytic-related disorder, 347
Sedative, hypnotic, or anxiolytic use
    disorder, 343–345
  description of, 343
  diagnostic criteria for, 343–345
  DSM-5 classification, 504
Sedative, hypnotic, or anxiolytic
    withdrawal, 346–347
  description of, 346
  diagnostic criteria for, 346–347
  DSM-5 classification, 504
Selective mutism, 18–19, 20, 127–128
  description of, 127
  diagnostic criteria for, 127–128
  DSM-5 classification, 494
Self-direction, description of, 457, 459, 460,
    462, 463
Separation anxiety disorder, 18–19, 20,
    124–126
  description of, 125
  diagnostic criteria for, 125–126
  DSM-5 classification, 494
Separation insecurity, description of, 461
Sexual dysfunctions, 275–283
  acquired, 23
  changes to diagnostic category, 23, 274
  delayed ejaculation, 276–278
  description of, 275–276
  DSM-5 classification, **275,** 500
  erectile disorder, 278
  female orgasmic disorder, 278–279
  female sexual interest/arousal disorder,
      279
  generalized, 23
  genito-pelvic pain/penetration disorder,
      279–280
  lifelong, 23
  male hypoactive sexual desire disorder,
      280
  other specified, 23
  other specified sexual dysfunction,
      282–283
  premature (early) ejaculation, 280
  situational, 23

specifiers, 278
substance/medication-induced sexual
    dysfunction, 280–282
subtypes, 278
unspecified, 23, 282–283
Sexual excitement, 275. *See also* Sexual
    dysfunctions
Sexual masochism disorder, 290
    description of, 290
    diagnostic criteria for, 290
    DSM-5 classification, 510
Sexual sadism disorder, 290
    description of, 290
    diagnostic criteria for, 290
    DSM-5 classification, 510
Shared psychotic disorder, 19
Sharfstein, Steven S., 2
Shift work type sleep-wake disorder, 258,
    259–260
Shubo-kyofu, 166
Skin-picking. *See* Excoriation (skin-picking)
    disorder
Sleep disorder related to a general medical
    condition, 22–23
Sleep disorder related to another medical
    disorder, 22–23
Sleep-related hypoventilation, 23, 256–257
    description of, 256
    diagnostic criteria for, 256–257
    DSM-5 classification, 499
    specifiers, 257
    subtypes, 257
Sleep terrors, 260, 261. *See also* Non–rapid
    eye movement sleep arousal disorders
Sleep-wake disorders, 239–272
    breathing-related sleep disorders,
        252–257
        central sleep apnea, 254–255
        changes to diagnostic category, 252
        obstructive sleep apnea hypopnea,
            252–254
        sleep-related hypoventilation,
            256–257
    changes to diagnostic category, 22–23,
        240–242
    circadian rhythm sleep-wake disorders,
        257–260
    DSM-5 classification, **241,** 498–499
    hypersomnolence disorder, 245–249

pa
uns
Sleepw
    eye
Slow-wa
    eye n
Snoring, 2
    apnea
Social anxiet   ... phobia), 20,
    131–133
    description of, 131
    diagnostic criteria for, 131–133
    DSM-5 classification, 495
    specifiers, 133
Social (pragmatic) communication disorder,
    39
    description of, 39
    diagnostic criteria for, 39
    DSM-5 classification, 490
Social phobia. *See* Social anxiety disorder
"Soldier's heart," 123
Somatic symptom and related disorders,
    201–215
    changes to diagnostic category,
        201–203
    conversion disorder (functional
        neurological symptom disorder),
        207–210
    DSM-5 classification, **202,** 496–497
    factitious disorder, 212–214
    illness anxiety disorder, 205–207
    other specified somatic symptom and
        related disorder, 214–215
    psychological factors affecting other
        medical conditions, 210–212
    somatic symptom disorder, 203–205
    unspecified somatic symptom and
        related disorder, 214, 215
Somatic symptom disorder, 203–205
    changes to diagnostic category, 21–22
    description of, 203–204
    diagnostic criteria for, 204–205
    DSM-5 classification, 496
    specifiers, 204–205
Somatic type, 65

147. *See also* Body
...sorder; Somatic
...nd related disorders
...rning disorder, 18, 31, 49–51
...ription of, 49
...iagnostic criteria for, 49–51
DSM-5 classification, 490–491
essential features of, 49
Specific phobia disorder, 20, 128–131
description of, 128–129
diagnostic criteria for, 129–131
DSM-5 classification, 494–495
specifiers, 131
Speech sound disorder, 37–38
description of, 37
diagnostic criteria for, 37–38
DSM-5 classification, 490
Spitzer, Robert, xx
Spouse or partner abuse, psychological, 426
coding, 426
description of, 426
DSM-5 classification, 514
Spouse or partner neglect, 425–426
coding, 426
description of, 425
DSM-5 classification, 514
Spouse or partner violence, physical, 424–425
coding, 424–425
description of, 424
Spouse or partner violence, sexual, 425
coding, 425
description of, 425
DSM-5 classification, 513
A Standard Classified Nomenclature of Disease (American Medical Association 1933), xix
Statistical Manual for the Use of Institutions for the Insane (American Medico-Psychological Association 1918), xix
Stereotypic movement disorder, 52–53
description of, 52–53
diagnostic criteria for, 53
DSM-5 classification, 491
Stimulant intoxication, 350–351
description of, 350
diagnostic criteria for, 350–351
DSM-5 classification, 504–505

Stimulant-related disorders, 348–353
description of, 348
diagnoses associated with substance class, **314**
DSM-5 classification, 504–505
other stimulant-induced disorders, 353
stimulant intoxication, 350–351
stimulant use disorder, 348–350
stimulant withdrawal, 352
unspecified stimulant-related disorder, 353
Stimulant use disorder, 348–350
description of, 348
diagnostic criteria for, 348–350
DSM-5 classification, 504
Stimulant withdrawal, 352
description of, 352
diagnostic criteria for, 352
DSM-5 classification, 505
Stressor-related disorders. *See also* Brief psychotic disorder
changes to diagnostic category, 21
Stuttering. *See* Childhood-onset fluency disorder
Substance intoxication delirium, 362
Substance/medication-induced anxiety disorder, 141–142
description of, 141
diagnostic criteria for, 141–142
DSM-5 classification, 495
Substance/medication-induced bipolar and related disorder, 99–100
coding, 99–100, **100**
diagnostic criteria, 99–100
DSM-5 classification, 493
Substance/medication-induced depressive disorder, 116–118
coding, 117, **117**
description of, 116
diagnostic criteria for, 116–118
DSM-5 classification, 494
Substance/medication-induced major or mild neurocognitive disorder, 379–381
coding, **380–381**
description of, 379
diagnostic criteria for, 379–380
DSM-5 classification, 507

Substance/medication-induced
   neurocognitive disorder, coding with
   etiological medical condition, **368**
Substance/medication-induced obsessive-
   compulsive disorder, 20, 162–164
   coding, **164**
   description of, 162
   diagnostic criteria for, 162–163
   DSM-5 classification, 495
Substance/medication-induced psychotic
   disorder, 79–81
   coding, **81**
   description of, 79
   diagnostic criteria for, 79–81, **81**
Substance/medication-induced sexual
   dysfunction, 23, 280–282
   coding, 281, **282**
   description of, 280
   diagnostic criteria for, 281–282
   DSM-5 classification, 500
Substance/medication-induced sleep
   disorder, 266–269
   coding, **268**
   description of, 266–267
   diagnostic criteria for, 267–269
   DSM-5 classification, 499
Substance-related and addictive disorders,
   311–358, **317–318**
   alcohol-related disorders, 316–323
   caffeine-related disorders, 323–325
   cannabis-related disorders, 325–329
   changes to diagnostic category, 24, 312–316
   diagnoses associated with substance
      class, **314**
   DSM-5 classification, 501–506
   hallucinogen-related disorders, 330–335
   inhalant-related disorders, 336–338
   non-substance-related disorders, 356–358
   opioid-related disorders, 339–343
   other (or unknown) substance-related
      disorders, 356
   sedative-, hypnotic-, or anxiolytic-related
      disorders, 343–347
   stimulant-related disorders, 348–353
   tobacco-related disorders, 353–356
Substance use disorder, 24
Suicidal behavior disorder, 478–479
   proposed description of, 478–479
   proposed diagnostic criteria for, 479

Suicide, 111, 203. *See also* Suicidal behavior
   disorder
Sydenham, Thomas, xviii

Taijin kyofusho, 166
Tardive akathisia, 411
   description of, 411
   DSM-5 classification, 510
Tardive dyskinesia, 25, 411
   description of, 411
   DSM-5 classification, 510
Tardive dystonia, 411
   description of, 411
   DSM-5 classification, 510
Tay-Sachs disease, 33
Telephone scatologia, 293
Tic disorders, 54–57
   description of, 54
   other specified tic disorder, 56–57
   persistent (chronic) motor or vocal tic
      disorder, 55–56
   provisional tic disorder, 56
   Tourette's disorder, 54–55
   unspecified tic disorder, 56–57
Tobacco-related disorders, **268,** 353–356
   DSM-5 classification, 505
   other tobacco-induced disorders,
      355
   tobacco use disorder, 353–355
   tobacco withdrawal, 355
   unspecified tobacco-related disorder,
      356
Tobacco use disorder, 353–355
   description of, 353
   diagnostic criteria for, 353–355
   DSM-5 classification, 505
Tobacco withdrawal, 355
   description of, 355
   diagnostic criteria for, 355
   DSM-5 classification, 505
Tourette's disorder, 54–55
   description of, 54
   diagnostic criteria for, 54–55
   DSM-5 classification, 491
Transient situational disturbances, 30
Transvestic disorder, 292–293
   description of, 292
   diagnostic criteria for, 292–293
   DSM-5 classification, 510

Trauma- and stressor-related disorders,
    169–190
  acute stress disorder, 183–186
  adjustment disorders, 186–188
  changes to diagnostic category, 21,
    169–171
  disinhibited social engagement disorder,
    174–176
  DSM-5 classification, **170,** 496
  other specified trauma- and stressor-
    related disorder, 188–189
  posttraumatic stress disorder, 176–183
  reactive attachment disorder, 171–174
  unspecified trauma- and stressor-related
    disorder, 188–189
Traumatic brain injury, 378–379
  coding with etiological medical
    condition, **368**
  major or mild neurocognitive disorder
    due to, 378–379
Trichotillomania (hair-pulling disorder), 20,
    159–160
  description of, 159
  diagnostic criteria for, 159–160
  DSM-5 classification, 495

Undifferentiated somatoform disorder, 21
Unspecified alcohol-related disorder,
    322–323
  description of, 323
  DSM-5 classification, 501
Unspecified anxiety disorder, 144, 145
  description of, 144
  diagnostic criteria for, 145
  DSM-5 classification, 495
Unspecified attention-deficit/hyperactivity
    disorder, 48–49
  description of, 48–49
Unspecified bipolar and related disorder,
    101–102, 103
  description of, 101–102
  diagnostic criteria for, 103
  DSM-5 classification, 493
Unspecified caffeine-related disorder, 325
  description of, 325
  DSM-5 classification, 502
Unspecified cannabis-related disorders, 329
  description of, 329
  DSM-5 classification, 502

Unspecified catatonia, 85–86
  description of, 85, 86
  diagnostic criteria for, 85
"Unspecified" category, 16
Unspecified communication disorder, 40
  diagnostic criteria for, 40
  DSM-5 classification, 490
Unspecified delirium, 365, 366
  description of, 365
  diagnostic criteria for, 366
  DSM-5 classification, 506
Unspecified depressive disorder, 119–120
  description of, 119
  diagnostic criteria for, 120
  DSM-5 classification, 494
Unspecified disruptive, impulse-control,
    and conduct disorder, 309–310
  description of, 309
  DSM-5 classification, 501
Unspecified dissociative disorder, 198, 199
  description of, 198
  diagnostic criteria for, 199
  DSM-5 classification, 496
Unspecified elimination disorder, 237, 238
  description of, 237
  diagnostic criteria for, 238
  DSM-5 classification, 498
Unspecified feeding or eating disorder, 230, 231
  description of, 230
  diagnostic criteria for, 231
  DSM-5 classification, 497
Unspecified gender dysphoria
  description of, 286
  DSM-5 classification, 500
Unspecified hallucinogen-related disorders,
    335
  DSM-5 classification, 503
Unspecified hypersomnolence disorder, 270,
    271
  description of, 270
  diagnostic criteria for, 271
  DSM-5 classification, 499
Unspecified inhalant-related disorder, 338
  description of, 338
  DSM-5 classification, 503
Unspecified insomnia disorder, 269, 270
  description of, 269
  diagnostic criteria for, 270
  DSM-5 classification, 499

Unspecified intellectual disability
(intellectual developmental disorder),
36
description of, 36
diagnostic criteria for, 36
DSM-5 classification, 490
Unspecified neurocognitive disorder, 386
description of, 386
diagnostic criteria for, 386
DSM-5 classification, 509
Unspecified neurodevelopmental disorder,
57–58
description of, 57
diagnostic criteria for, 58
DSM-5 classification, 491
Unspecified obsessive-compulsive and
related disorder, 165, 166
description of, 165
diagnostic criteria for, 166
DSM-5 classification, 495
Unspecified opioid-related disorder, 343
DSM-5 classification, 503
Unspecified paraphilic disorder, 293, 294
description of, 293
diagnostic criteria for, 294
DSM-5 classification, 510
Unspecified personality disorder, 404–405
description of, 404–405
diagnostic criteria for, 405
Unspecified phencyclidine-related disorder,
335
DSM-5 classification, 503
Unspecified schizophrenia spectrum and
other psychotic disorder, 86–87
description of, 86
diagnostic criteria for, 87
DSM-5 classification, 492
Unspecified sedative-, hypnotic-, or
anxiolytic-related disorder, 347
description of, 347
DSM-5 classification, 504
Unspecified sexual dysfunction, 282–283
DSM-5 classification, 500
Unspecified sleep-wake disorder, 271, 272
description of, 271
diagnostic criteria for, 272
DSM-5 classification, 499

Unspecified somatic symptom and related
disorder, 214, 215
description of, 214
diagnostic criteria for, 215
DSM-5 classification, 497
Unspecified stimulant-related disorder, 353
description of, 353
DSM-5 classification, 505
Unspecified tic disorder, 56–57
description of, 56–57
diagnostic criteria for, 57
DSM-5 classification, 491
Unspecified tobacco-related disorder, 356
description of, 355
DSM-5 classification, 505
Unspecified trauma- and stressor-related
disorder, 188–189
description of, 188
diagnostic criteria for, 189
DSM-5 classification, 496
Unspecified type, 65
Urophilia, 293
U.S. Food and Drug Administration (FDA), 12

Vascular disease. *See* Major or mild vascular
neurocognitive disorder
Vascular neurocognitive disorder, 377–378
Vitamin B_{12} deficiency, 143
Voyeuristic disorder, 287–288
description of, 287–288
diagnostic criteria for, 288
DSM-5 classification, 509
V/Z codes, 16, 25

WHO. *See* World Health Organization
WHODAS 2.0. *See* World Health
Organization, Disability Assessment
Schedule 2.0
Winokur, George, xx
Withdrawal, description of, 315–316, 459
World Health Organization (WHO), xix, 2, 235
Disability Assessment Schedule 2.0, 440,
441–442
World Psychiatric Association, 2

Zoophilia, 293